Ophthalmology Review Manual

Ophthalmology Review Manual

Second Edition

Kenneth C. Chern, MD

Assistant Clinical Professor
Francis I. Proctor Foundation
University of California, San Francisco
Partner
Peninsula Ophthalmology Group
Burlingame, California

Michael A. Saidel, MD

Assistant Professor
Director, Cornea Service
Section of Ophthalmology
University of Chicago
Chicago, Illinois

Wolters Kluwer | Lippincott Williams & Wilkins
Health

Philadelphia • Baltimore • New York • London
Buenos Aires • Hong Kong • Sydney • Tokyo

Senior Executive Editor: Jonathan Pine
Product Manager: Ryan Shaw
Vendor Manager: Alicia Jackson
Senior Manufacturing Manager: Benjamin Rivera
Senior Marketing Manager: Angela Panetta
Design Coordinator: Teresa Mallon
Production Service: SPi Global

Two Commerce Square
2001 Market Street
Philadelphia, PA 19103 USA
LWW.com

Printed in China

Library of Congress Cataloging-in-Publication Data
Ophthalmology review manual / [edited by] Kenneth C. Chern, Michael Saidel. — 2nd ed.
p. ; cm.
Includes bibliographical references and index.
ISBN 978-1-60831-007-4
1. Eye—Diseases—Outlines, syllabi, etc. 2. Ophthalmology—Outlines, syllabi, etc. I. Chern, Kenneth C. II. Saidel, Michael.
[DNLM: 1. Eye Diseases—Outlines. WW 18.2]

RE50.O63 2012
617.7—dc22

2010052082

To purchase additional copies of this book, call our customer service department at (800) 638-3030 or fax orders to (301) 223-2320. International customers should call (301) 223-2300.

Visit Lippincott Williams & Wilkins on the Internet: at LWW.com. Lippincott Williams & Wilkins customer service representatives are available from 8:30 am to 6 pm, EST.

10 9 8 7 6 5 4 3 2 1

Preface to the Second Edition

With this second edition, we provide a newly revamped reference. New contributors have brought the latest in ophthalmology with updated images, new sections on clinical trials, and the state of the art in medical treatments. As with the first edition, the outline format provides a quick reference to the management and differential diagnosis of clinical problems. We hope that this edition will provide with as much success as its predecessor an updated reference and board review platform for residents and practicing ophthalmologists alike.

Kenneth C. Chern
Michael A. Saidel

Acknowledgments

We are thankful to previous contributors to the *Review Manual*. In this second edition, new contributors have brought new insights and strengths to each section. We are sincerely thankful for their efforts. Dr. Greenwald would like to thank Nikki Batra, CO, for her help in preparation of the pediatrics section. We are grateful to our families for their support in this second edition of the *Review Manual*.

Contributors

Irma Ahmed, MD, FRCS
Retina Macula Specialists, PC
Chicago, Illinois

Sophie J. Bakri, MD
Consultant
Associate Professor of Ophthalmology
Director, Vitreoretinal Surgery Fellowship Mayo Clinic
SW Rochester, Minnesota

Paul W. Brazis, MD
Professor of Neurology
Consultant in Neurology and Neuro-Ophthalmology
Departments of Neurology and Ophthalmology
Mayo Clinic–Jacksonville
Jacksonville, Florida

Susan Carter, MD
Clinical Associate Professor
Institute of Ophthalmology and Visual Science
New Jersey Medical School
Newark, New Jersey
Ophthalmic Plastic and Reconstructive Surgeon
The Eye Center
Warren, New Jersey

Kenneth C. Chern, MD
Assistant Clinical Professor
Francis I. Proctor Foundation
University of California
San Francisco, California
Partner
Peninsula Ophthalmology Group
Burlingame, California

Cynthia S. Chiu, MD, FACS
Associate Professor
Director, Comprehensive Ophthalmology & Optometry
University of California
San Francisco California

Mandi D. Conway, MD, FACS
Professor, Basic Sciences
University Arizona College of Medicine, Phoenix Campus
Professor, Clinical Ophthalmology
Tulane University School of Medicine
New Orleans, Louisiana

Mark J. Greenwald, MD
Professor and Chief
Ophthalmology and Visual Science
University of Chicago Medical Center
Chicago, Illinois

Seenu M. Hariprasad, MD
Associate Professor and Director
Clinical Research
Chief, Vitreoretinal Service
Program Director
Fellowship in the Diseases and Surgery of the Retina, Vitreous, and Macula
Department of Ophthalmology and Visual Science
The University of Chicago
Chicago, Illinois

David Hinkle, MD
Massachusetts Research and Surgery Institution
Cambridge, Massachusetts

H. Jane Kim, MD
Oculoplastic Fellow
Clinical Instructor
Department of Ophthalmology
University of California, San Francisco
San Francisco, California

Edward Y. Koo, MD
Associate Clinical Professor of Ophthalmology
UCSF School of Medicine
Diplomate, American Board of Ophthalmology
Chairman
Department of Ophthalmology
Mills-Peninsula Health Services
Peninsula Ophthalmology Group
Burlingame, California

Rohit Krishna, MD
Associate Professor
Director of Glaucoma
Department of Ophthalmology
Vision Research Center of Kansas City
University of Missouri-Kansas City School of Medicine
Sabates Eye Centers, PC
Kansas, Kansas

Andrew G. Lee, MD
Professor of Ophthalmology
Professor of Ophthalmology in Neurology and Neurological Surgery
Weill Cornell Medical College
New York, New York
Clinical Professor
Department of Ophthalmology and Visual Sciences
University of Texas Medical Branch at Galveston
Galveston, Texas
Adjunct Professor
Department of Ophthalmology
Baylor College of Medicine
Houston, Texas
Adjunct Professor
Department of Ophthalmology and Visual Sciences
University of Iowa
Iowa City, Iowa
Chair
Department of Ophthalmology
The Methodist Hospital
Houston, Texas

Tamer H. Mahmoud, MD, PhD
Associate Professor, Vitreoretinal Surgery
Program Director, Vitreoretinal Fellowship
Kresge Eye Institute
Wayne State University
Detroit, Michigan

Andrew A. Moshfeghi, MD, MBA
Medical Director
Assistant Professor of Ophthalmology
Vitreoretinal Diseases and Surgery
Bascom Palmer Eye Institute
University of Miami Miller School of Medicine
Palm Beach Gardens, Florida

Prithvi Mruthyunjaya, MD
Assistant professor of ophthalmology
Duke Eye Center
Durham, North Carolina

Michael D. Ober, MD, FACS
Partner, Retina Consultants of Michigan
Southfield, Michigan
Adjunct Teaching Faculty
Henry Ford Hospital
Detroit, Michigan

Michael A. Saidel, MD
Assistant Professor
Director, Cornea Service
Section of Ophthalmology
University of Chicago
Chicago, Illinois

Andrew Sorenson, MD
Department of Ophthalmology
Corneal, Refractive, and Cataract Surgery
California Pacific Medical Center
San Francisco, California

Sunil K. Srivastava, MD
Cole Eye Institute
Cleveland Clinic Foundation
Cleveland, Ohio

David G. Telander, MD, PhD
UC Davis, Department of Ophthalmology
Sacramento, California

Ryan D. Vincent, MD
Clinical Assistant Professor
Glaucoma Service
Department of Ophthalmology
Vision Research Center of Kansas City
University of Missouri-Kansas City
Sabates Eye Centers
Kansas, Kansas

Cuong D. Vu, MD
Retina Associates, PC
Annapolis, Maryland

Contents

CHAPTER

1

Cornea: External Disease

Kenneth C. Chern • Michael A. Saidel

ANATOMY AND PHYSIOLOGY

Tear Film

The tear film is composed of three major layers, each produced by specialized cells. The adequacy and stability of the tear film are important in the maintenance of a healthy corneal surface. The normal pH of the tear film is 6.5 to 7.6. Tear film osmolarity is 296 to 308 mOsm (Figure 1.1; Table 1.1).

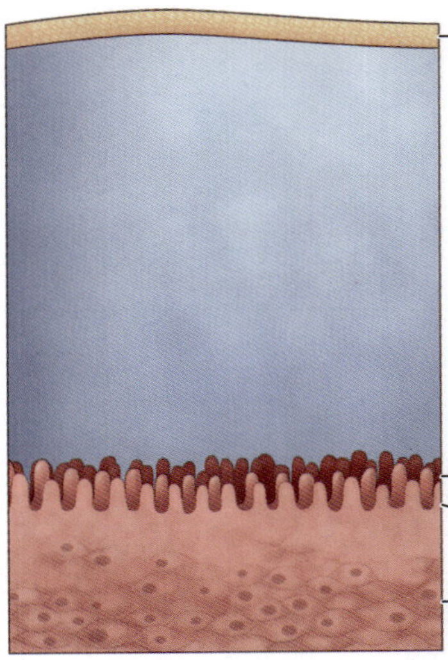

FIGURE 1.1. Structure of the tear film.

Conjunctiva

The conjunctiva is a nonkeratinizing stratified squamous epithelium with goblet cells. The conjunctiva extends from the limbus into the superior and inferior fornices to the gray line of the eyelid margin. The majority of goblet cells are concentrated in the fornices and at the caruncle. The conjunctiva is closely adherent to the superior and inferior tarsus by fine septa.

Cornea

The cornea has five distinct layers (Figure 1.2; Table 1.2). Maintenance of the orderly arrangement of the collagen fibers and the relative deturgescence of the corneal layers is important in permitting the cornea to remain optically clear.

The refractive index of the cornea is 1.376. To account for the combined optical power of the anterior and

Table 1.1

Composition and function of the tear film

Layer	Source	Components	Function
Mucin	Conjunctival goblet cells	Mucin	Interface between the hydrophobic epithelium and aqueous layer of tears
Aqueous	Main and accessory lacrimal glands	Electrolytes, glucose, antibacterial substances (lysozyme, immunoglobulins [predominantly IgA], lactoferrin)	Provide nutrition and health of epithelium
Lipid	Meibomian glands	Lipid	Decrease tear evaporation and stabilize tear film

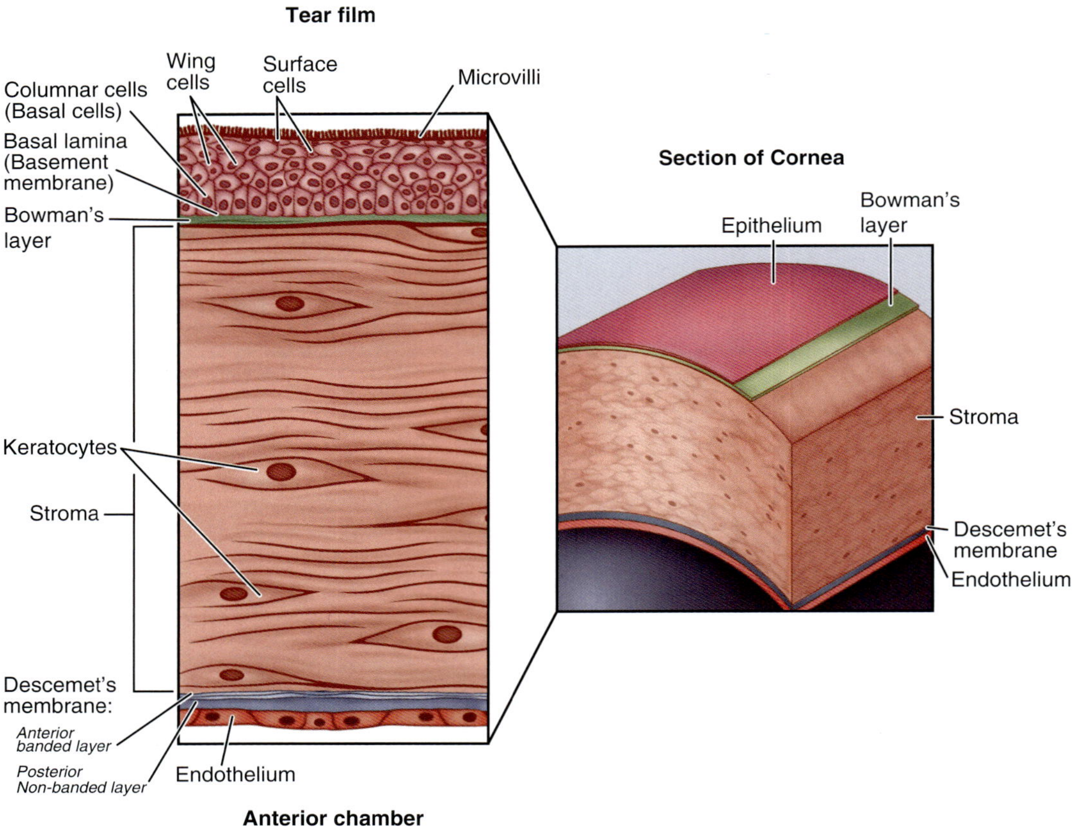

FIGURE 1.2. The five major layers of the cornea from anterior to posterior are the epithelium, Bowman layer, stroma, Descemet membrane, and endothelium.

posterior curvatures of the cornea, a refractive index of 1.3375 is used to calibrate the keratometer.

The cornea is innervated by the long posterior ciliary nerves that branch from the ophthalmic divisions of cranial nerve V1.

Epithelium

The corneal epithelium is a stratified squamous epithelium that originates from limbal stem cells found in the palisades of Vogt and the interpalisade rete ridges. The epithelium has three predominant layers (Table 1.3).

Table 1.2

Layers of the cornea

Layer	Thickness (µm)	Composition	Function
Epithelium	50	Nonkeratinizing stratified squamous epithelium	Barrier to microbial invasion
Bowman layer	10	Compact layer of unorganized collagen fibers	Structural support, barrier to infection and damage
Stroma	500	Orderly arrangement of collagen lamellae	Main substance of cornea
Descemet membrane	10–12	Basement membrane material	Very strong membrane, structural integrity of cornea
Endothelium	5	Monolayer of endothelial cells	Pump to remove fluid from the stroma

Table 1.3

Layers of the corneal epithelium

Layer	Description
Basal cell	Single layer of columnar cells found adjacent to the Bowman layer
Wing cells	Two to three layers of cells with elongated processes
Surface cells	Three layers of flattened epithelial cells with microvilli in contact with the tear film

Bowman Layer

Bowman layer or membrane is an acellular layer of compact collagen fibers. If damaged, Bowman's does not regenerate, and scarring results.

Stroma

The thickest layer is the corneal stroma composed of type I collagen and glycosaminoglycans (mostly keratin sulfate) with scattered keratocytes. The lamellae are in orderly sheets that permit the dissection of a lamellar plane with a blunt instrument.

The imbibition pressure of the stroma = IOP – Swelling pressure.

Descemet Membrane

Descemet membrane is the basement membrane deposited by the endothelium.

- The anterior banded zone is formed before birth and is 3 to 4 mm thick.
- The posterior nonbanded zone is continually added throughout life.
- Guttae and Hassall-Henle bodies are focal excrescences (outgrowths) of Descemet membrane.
- In Fuchs dystrophy, central guttae precede stromal and epithelial edema and corneal decompensation.

Endothelium

The corneal endothelium is a monolayer of hexagonal cells that are not thought to divide or regenerate if damaged. At birth, the endothelium has 3,500 to 4,000 cells/mm^2. With age, the cell count declines with 1,500 to 2,000 cells/mm^2 present at adulthood. Corneal edema will occur when cells fall below 500 cells/mm^2.

Sclera

- Made of type I collagen, proteoglycans and fibroblasts.
- Axenfeld loop is a branch of the posterior ciliary nerve that forms a visible intrascleral loop.
- Senile scleral plaques are $CaPO_4$ anterior to insertion of medial and lateral recti that become dehydrated leading to bluish color.
- Grayish scleral appearance can be due to scleral thinning allowing the underlying choroid to become visible.

LABORATORY DIAGNOSIS

Diagnostic Tests

The majority of corneal disease can be diagnosed using the slit lamp and careful examination; however, a number of diagnostic tests are available to help confirm the diagnosis or provide additional information. Below are listed some of the common tests and their applications (Table 1.4).

LID DISORDERS

Anterior Blepharitis

Summary

A chronic inflammatory process of the eyelids, which may result secondarily in corneal changes.

Etiology

- Staphylococcal blepharitis is due to chronic colonization of the lid margins with staphylococcal species, marked by the presence of fibrin collarettes on the lashes.
- Seborrheic blepharitis is due to oily changes of the skin and is marked by greasy scales crusted on the lashes. These changes incite inflammatory processes in the eyelids. Inflammatory substances fall onto the ocular surface, where further inflammatory changes may occur. Seborrheic blepharitis is not characterized by corneal ulceration.

Signs and Symptoms

Patients complain of itching, irritation, tearing, or foreign body sensation, or a combination of these, with crusting on the lid margins and lashes.

Demographics

All races and ages may be affected.

Table 1.4

Diagnostic testing for corneal disease

Test	Specimen	Methodology	Diagnostic utility
Microbacterial cultures	Conjunctiva, cornea swab Biopsy of cornea or conjunctiva	Blood, chocolate, or other specialized nutrient agar	Bacteria
		Sabouraud agar	Fungi
		Lowenstein-Jensen media	Mycobacteria
		Nonnutrient agar	*Acanthamoeba*
		Herpes culture medium	HSV, VZV
		Chlamydia culture medium	*Chlamydia*
Microscopy	Conjunctival or corneal scraping	Giemsa stain	Cell morphology, bacteria, fungi, *Acanthamoeba*
		Gram stain	Bacteria
		Calcofluor white	Fungi, *Acanthamoeba*
		KOH	Fungi
		Gomori methenamine-silver stain	Fungi
	Tissue specimens	H&E	Structure
		Congo red	Birefringence with amyloid
		PAS	Highlights basement membranes, goblet cells
	Confocal	Scanning confocal microscopy	Amoeba, fungi, infectious crystalline keratopathy. Also to follow refractive patients
Impression cytology	Conjunctiva	PAS, etc.	Goblet cells
DFA	Conjunctival scraping	Adenovirus DFA	Adenoviral antigen
		Herpes DFA	Herpes antigen
DNA amplification	Conjunctival scraping	PCR	*Chlamydia*, viruses, bacteria
Tear sampling	Tear film	Schirmer's	Tear production
Pachymetry	Cornea	Pachymeter	Corneal thickness
Specular microscopy	Endothelium		Observe endothelial cell morphology and number
Corneal topography	Anterior surface of cornea	Placido disk, corneoscope photo, or computerized topographic unit	Surface irregularity and astigmatism

DFA, direct fluorescent antibody; H&E, hematoxylin and eosin; HSV, herpes simplex virus; KOH, potassium hydroxide; PCR, polymerase chain reaction; PAS, periodic acid–Schiff; VZV, varicella-zoster virus.

Ophthalmic Findings

- Eyelids may be red and thickened and may show telangiectasias.
- There may be ulceration and notching (ptilosis) of the lid margin (Figure 1.3).
- Hordeolum and chalazion formation is seen more frequently.
- Lashes may be lost (madarosis) or misdirected.
- Secondary corneal changes may be seen including pannus, punctate epithelial keratitis, and marginal infiltrates, because of a type IV hypersensitivity.

Systemic Findings

- Seborrheic blepharitis is associated with rosacea.
- Patients with seborrheic blepharitis may also have oily skin and dandruff.

Special Tests

Lid cultures should be taken periodically to guide antibiotic therapy.

Pathology

Chronic inflammation is present.

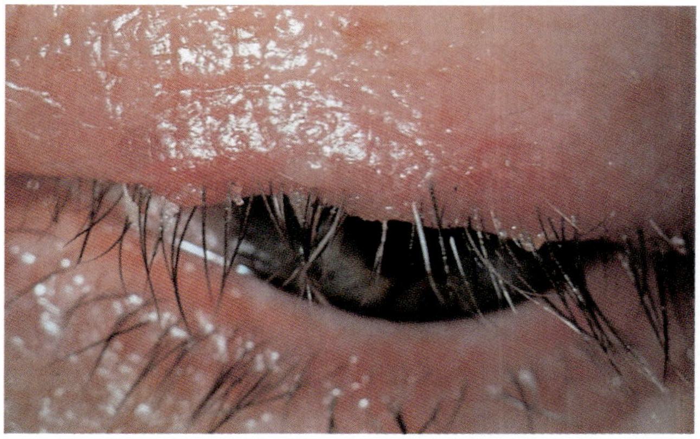

FIGURE 1.3. Crusting, lash loss, and ulceration of the lid margin caused by staphylococcal lid disease.

Disease Course

Chronic with exacerbations and remissions

Treatment and Management

Lid hygiene, consisting of warm-water soaks to loosen debris, followed by lid margin scrubs (with plain water, diluted baby shampoo, or an antibiotic drop) should be performed daily.

Medications

Antibiotics may be useful, guided by culture results. If chronic use is required, antibiotics should be rotated to minimize resistance.

Follow-Up

Patients often return frequently, since the problem is chronic. Often, no change in therapy is needed—just explanation, support, and empathy.

Differential Diagnosis

Unilateral disease is unusual, and a masquerade syndrome should be considered. Sebaceous gland carcinoma presents with unilateral eyelid ulceration, lid distortion, and lash loss. This requires a full-thickness biopsy and pathologic examination.

Posterior Blepharitis

Other names: meibomian gland dysfunction, meibomitis.

Summary

Meibomian gland dysfunction and inflammation of the meibomian glands change the composition of the lipid layer, resulting in instability of the tear film. Release of inflammatory mediators irritates the lid margin and ocular surface.

Etiology

Genetic predisposition in some patients, since seen more commonly in patients with rosacea

Signs and Symptoms

Burning and stinging.
Symptoms worse upon waking in the morning.
Redness and ocular irritation.
Sore eyelids.

Demographics

Very common, may be more frequent in patients with rosacea.

Ophthalmic Findings

- Foamy tears and oily tear film (Figure 1.4).
- Thickened and inspissated meibomian gland secretions.

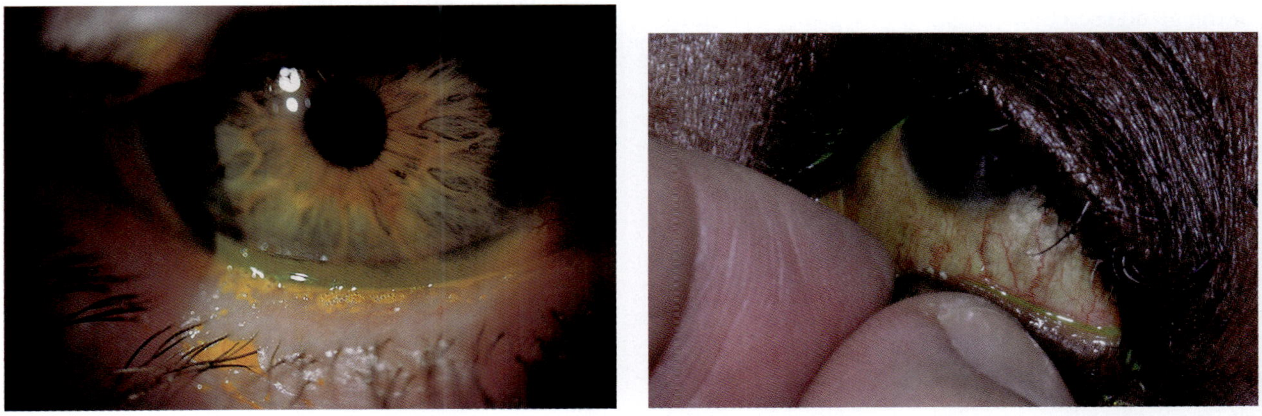

A B

FIGURE 1.4. A: Foamy tears along the lower lid from saponification of the lipid layer in meibomian gland dysfunction. B: Inspissation of meibomian glands in posterior blepharitis.

- Stenotic or occluded meibomian gland orifices.
- Meibomian gland cysts and chalazia.
- Telangiectasia of the lid margins.
- Inferior interpalpebral staining with rose bengal or lissamine green.

Systemic Findings

Telangiectasia on the cheeks and nose.
Rosacea.

Disease Course

- Chronic disease with episodes of exacerbation.
- If severe, can lead to corneal neovascularization.

Treatment and Management

- Hot compresses.
- Oral doxycycline or tetracyclines.
- Topical steroids and antibiotic.
- Artificial tears.

Differential Diagnosis

- Staphylococcal blepharitis.
- Keratoconjunctivitis sicca (KCS).

Hordeolum

Summary

An acute focal swelling of the eyelid secondary to obstruction of a sebaceous gland orifice (usually a meibomian gland, but may be a gland of Zeis or lash follicles). Internal hordeola occur at the posterior eyelid from meibomian gland inspissation. External hordeola, or styes, occur on the anterior eyelid in the glands of Zeis or lash follicles.

Etiology

Underlying meibomitis is usually present, with thickening of the gland secretions, stasis of oily gland secretions, and inspissation of the orifice. Staphylococcal infection is often present secondarily.

Signs and Symptoms

Patients present with an eyelid lump or swelling and erythema, which is often tender. There may be blurring of vision secondary to induced astigmatism and an oily tear film.

Demographics

All individuals may be affected.

Ophthalmic Findings

Lid tenderness, erythema, swelling, and focal mass. The blocked meibomian gland orifice is usually visible.

Systemic Findings

None.

Special Tests

None.

Pathology

Inflammation is caused as the oily material extends from the blocked gland into the surrounding tissue. A chalazion is present when lipogranulomatous inflammation occurs in response to lipids from meibomian or Zeis glands.

Disease Course

Generally self-limited as the lesion spontaneously drains. Granuloma formation may develop if the hordeolum does not drain, and a chalazion results, which is a nontender and uninflamed nodule.

Treatment and Management

- Frequent warm compresses at onset encourage spontaneous drainage.
- Incision and drainage may be required (usually for cosmetic purposes).
- Intralesional steroid injection.

Medications

A local superinfection may require topical (or rarely, oral) antibiotics.

Follow-Up

None required.

Differential Diagnosis

Preseptal cellulitis may present as a diffuse infectious lid inflammation with absence of a focal mass. There is usually a history of trauma as the inciting event for infection. Insect bites and contact dermatitis are usually discerned by history. Recurrent chalazia in the same location, particularly in an older individual, should raise the suspicion for sebaceous cell carcinoma and may require biopsy.

Contact Dermatitis

Summary

Rapid onset of periorbital erythema, with thickening and swelling of the eyelid skin.

Etiology

- Type IV hypersensitivity reaction to a topically applied substance, usually a medication.

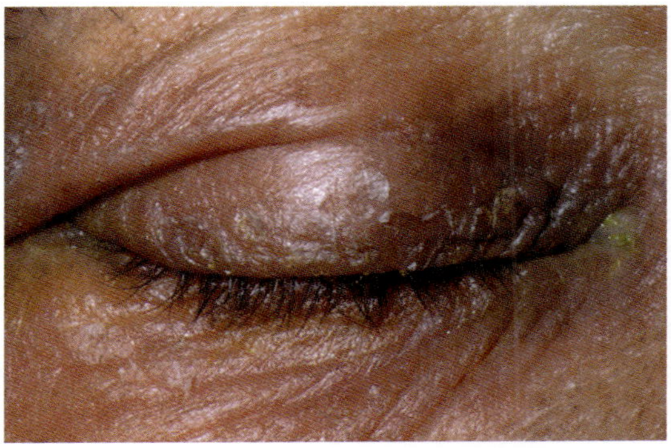

FIGURE 1.5. Severe red, scaly, and itchy periocular skin secondary to the topical use of medications such as neomycin ointment.

- Chief offenders include atropine, pilocarpine, epinephrine, apraclonidine, brimonidine, prostaglandins, antivirals, and antibiotics, particularly neomycin and other aminoglycosides.

Signs and Symptoms

Periorbital redness, crusting, and itching. There may be a mild watery discharge.

Ophthalmic Findings

- Periorbital edema, erythema, and thickening.
- The skin may have a shiny, scaly, leathery appearance and texture (Figure 1.5).

Systemic Findings

None.

Special Tests

None.

Pathology

Type IV allergic reaction, involving delayed type hypersensitivity mediated by T cells.

Disease Course

Chronic until the offending agent removed.

Treatment and Management

- Identification of the offending agent, which must be discontinued.
- Cold compresses.

Medications

Oral antihistamines may help, as may application of a mild steroid preparation.

Follow-Up

Resolution should be apparent in approximately 2 weeks. Conservative measures should be used first, with addition of steroids at that time if necessary.

Differential Diagnosis

There is usually little confusion with this clinical appearance and supporting history of a recent addition of an offending agent.

Atopic Dermatitis

Summary

Chronic superficial inflammation of the skin, frequently associated with underlying manifestations of allergic eye disease (atopic keratoconjunctivitis).

Etiology

A form of type I hypersensitivity reaction involving immunoglobulin E (IgE) overproduction, eosinophils, and mast cells, with release of histamine and other inflammatory mediators.

Signs and Symptoms

Itching, burning, watering, and photophobia are prominent. Skin thickening and mucous discharge may be evident.

Demographics

Onset generally in the teens and early years of adulthood, extending until approximately age 60 years, at which time the disease process seems to burn itself out.

Ophthalmic Findings

- "Allergic shiners" or increased pigmentation of the periorbital skin (Figure 1.6).
- Scaling and woody, thickened (often described as leathery or lichenified) eyelid skin, which may lead to ectropion, ptosis, and/or lagophthalmos with secondary ocular surface changes.

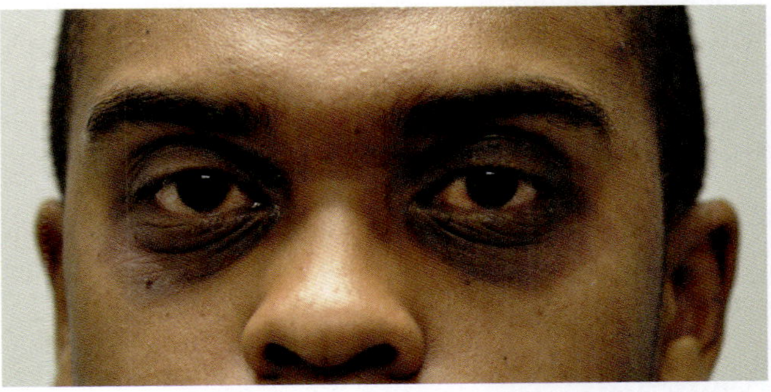

FIGURE 1.6. Periorbital skin pigmentation known as Allergic Shiners.

- Inferior fornix subepithelial fibrosis.
- Punctate epithelial keratitis and corneal epithelial defects, which may scar or develop microbial ulceration.
- Associations with subcapsular cataracts, keratoconus, increased incidence of herpes simplex virus (HSV) eye disease (bilateral in some cases), and retinal detachment.

Systemic Findings

Asthma, atopic dermatitis or eczema, and allergic rhinitis or hay fever often coexist in the same individual and are frequently found in other family members.

Special Tests

Generally none. Rarely, a skin biopsy may be considered to assist with diagnosis. A conjunctival scraping may show eosinophils and mast cells.

Pathology

A prominence of mast cells and eosinophils is seen in the mucosal tissues.

Disease Course

Chronic, with exacerbations and remissions.

Treatment and Management

Any identifiable triggers should be avoided. Disease control is optimized by both local and systemic medications. Lid and tear abnormalities must also be addressed. Cold compresses.

Medications

- Artificial tears.
- Topical nonsteroidal anti-inflammatory drugs (NSAIDs), antihistamines, mast cell stabilizers (cromolyn, lodoxamide, olopatadine, bepotastine): may be continued indefinitely.
- Steroids: should be the first drug to be discontinued.
- Oral nonsedating antihistamines are a useful addition to therapy and may help to limit the number of topically applied agents (and preservative toxicity to a fragile ocular surface).
- Cyclosporin has been used topically and systemically in severe cases.
- Epithelial defects should be treated with prophylaxis against microbial infection with topical broad-spectrum antibiotics.

Follow-Up

Regular intervals should be scheduled based on disease severity.

Differential Diagnosis

Vernal keratoconjunctivitis may present similar ocular findings, but the dermatitis is absent and generally affects young male patients.

Reference

Foster CS, Calonge M. Atopic keratoconjunctivitis. *Ophthalmology* 1990;97:992–1000.

Ichthyosis

Summary

Widespread abnormality of keratinization of the skin.

Etiology

Inherited. All inheritance patterns are seen, with autosomal dominant being most common and X-linked recessive the most severe.

Signs and Symptoms

Dry, scaly skin giving the appearance of a dirty neck, often referred to as the "dirty neck syndrome."

Demographics

Becomes apparent in the first year of life.

Ophthalmic Findings

- Secondary lid abnormalities are seen, including ectropion, lagophthalmos, and resulting corneal exposure.
- Pre-Descemet stromal deposits are seen, which are gray, punctate, and linear opacities without affecting vision.
- Congenital cataracts may be present.
- Prominent corneal nerves.

Systemic Findings

Skin changes as described above.

Special Tests

None.

Pathology

Abnormal keratinization of the skin.

Disease Course

Chronic.

Treatment and Management

Supportive measures for secondary ocular abnormalities. Not responsive to steroids.

Medications

None specific.

Follow-Up

As required depending on degree of ocular involvement.

Reference

Jay B, Blach RK, Wells RS. Ocular manifestations of ichthyosis. *Br J Ophthalmol* 1968;52:217–226.

Ectodermal Dysplasia

Summary

A group of congenital, nonprogressive abnormalities of epidermis and at least one of the following: hair, nails, teeth, sweat glands.

Etiology

Various inheritance patterns are seen.

Signs and Symptoms

Demographics

Congenital.

Ophthalmic Findings

- Blepharitis.
- Ankyloblepharon.
- Hypoplastic lacrimal ducts.
- Dry eye.
- Corneal scarring and neovascularization.
- Cataract.
- Glaucoma.

Systemic Findings

Skin changes as described above.

Special Tests

None.

Pathology

Reduction in number of sweat glands, sebaceous glands and hair follicles, depending on the type.

Disease Course

Children with anhidrotic ectodermal dysplasia cannot sweat properly, making hyperpyrexia a problem.

Treatment and Management

Supportive measures for secondary ocular abnormalities.

Medications

None specific.

Follow-Up

As required, depending on degree of ocular involvement.

Rosacea

Summary

Chronic disorder affecting the facial skin and eyes.

Etiology

Unknown. Multiple mechanisms have been implicated, including vascular changes of the skin, sunlight-induced damage, and type IV hypersensitivity reactions. Antigens including the human follicle mite Demodex have been implicated as inciting inflammatory agents.

Signs and Symptoms

Patients complain of ocular irritation, redness, foreign body sensation, and burning. Facial flushing, eyelid margin telangiectasias, erythema, pustules, papules, and rhinophyma may be noted.

Demographics

All ages, but generally aged 30 to 60 years. Rosacea is more common in whites and more frequently diagnosed in women, but the disease is more severe in affected male patients.

Ophthalmic Findings

- Lid telangiectasias.
- Blepharitis.
- Meibomitis.
- Chalazia.
- Conjunctival injection.
- Tear deficiency and instability.
- Corneal punctate epithelial keratitis.
- Corneal vascularization.
- Inferior spade-shaped corneal infiltrates.

Systemic Findings

The skin of the face and upper body is affected. Facial flushing, telangiectasias (Figure 1.7), erythema, pustules, papules, and rhinophyma may be noted.

Special Tests

None.

Pathology

No unique features.

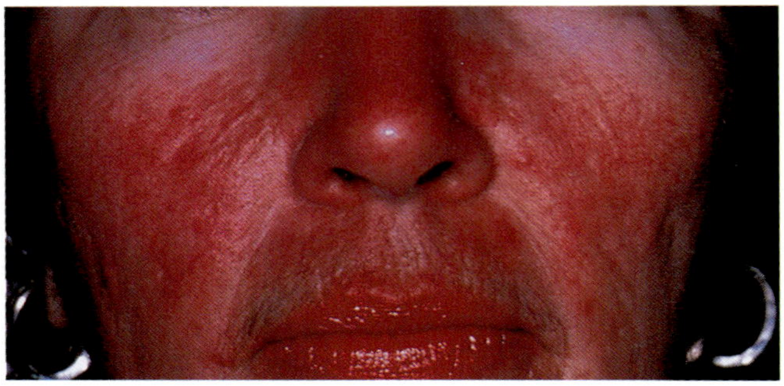

FIGURE 1.7. The typical rosacea facies with dilated, telangiectatic vessels on the cheeks and nose.

Disease Course

Chronic with exacerbations and remissions.

Treatment and Management

Local measures for lid hygiene, bacterial superinfection, and tear disturbances should be applied as required.

Medications

- Chronic use of oral tetracycline (doxycycline or minocycline) is advocated and may dramatically improve both skin and ocular disease.
- Topical metronidazole gel or cream has also been helpful.
- Topical antibiotic use should be guided by culture results and rotated if used long term.
- Topical steroid can be used to decrease sterile inflammation.

Follow-Up

Regular follow-up intervals are warranted for secondary ocular changes and monitoring during therapy.

Differential Diagnosis

- Contact dermatitis.
- Systemic lupus erythematosus (SLE).
- Seborrheic dermatitis.
- Acne vulgaris may give similar skin changes but usually is distinguished by history and clinical features.
- Rhinophyma may rarely be confused with basal cell carcinoma, and biopsy undertaken if necessary.

Reference

Knox CM, Smolin G. Rosacea. *Int Ophthalmol Clin* 1997;37:29–40.

CONJUNCTIVAL DISORDERS

Anatomy

Follicles

Follicles are focal collections of lymphocytes in the substantia propria of the conjunctiva. Follicles are most prominent in the inferior fornix as gelatinous elevations 1 to 5 mm in size with blood vessels coursing around the base of the follicles.

Common Causes

- Viral infections (adenovirus, herpes, molluscum contagiosum).
- Chlamydia (adult inclusion, trachoma).
- Drugs (atropine, epinephrine, glaucoma medications, trifluridine).

Papillae

Papillae represent a nonspecific response to conjunctival irritation. Because of inflammation, pinpoint blood vessels in the tarsal conjunctiva become dilated, leaking fluid and inflammatory cells. A papillary response can best be seen on the superior tarsal conjunctiva as multiple small bumps, each with a central core of vessels.

Common Causes

- Bacterial infection.
- Allergy/Atopy.
- Floppy eyelid syndrome.

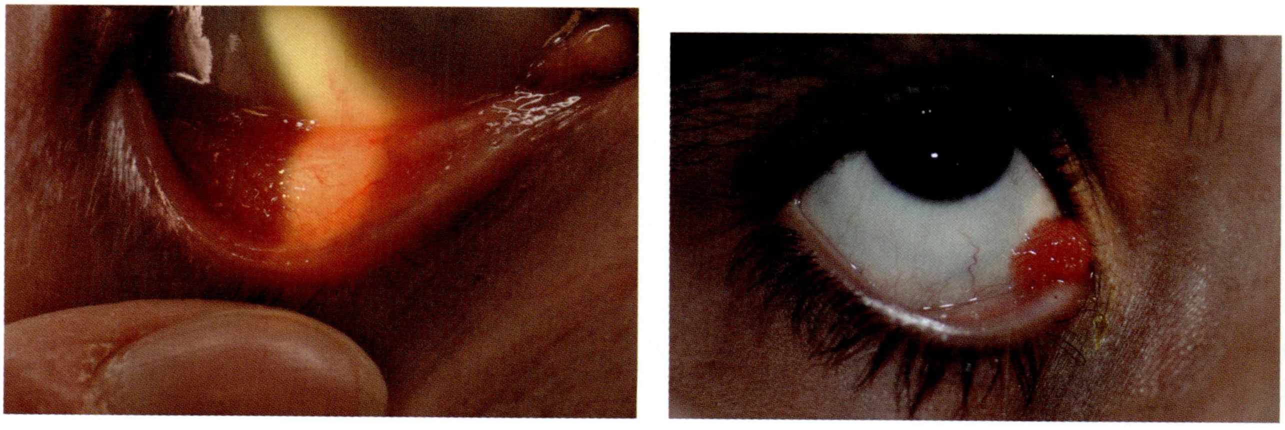

A B

FIGURE 1.8. **A:** Follicles in the lower fornix with typical gelatinous, dome-shaped appearance. **B:** Papillae on the upper tarsal conjunctiva.

Inflammation of any cause (eye rubbing, surface keratinization, etc.).

Giant Papillae and Cobblestone Papillae

The size of papillae is usually restricted by the fibrous septa attaching the conjunctiva to the underlying tarsus. With severe and chronic inflammation, these septa rupture, and the giant papillae coalesce to form the giant papillae. Stellate scarring can occur on the top of the papillae.

Common Causes

- Contact lens–associated giant papillary conjunctivitis (soft contact lenses more frequently).
- Vernal keratoconjunctivitis.

Membranes and Pseudomembranes

Damage to the conjunctival vessels and the epithelial surface by severe inflammation can cause exudation of fibrin, inflammatory cells, necrotic cells, and serous fluid. Coalescence of this material on the surface forms the membrane. Removal of a membrane causes bleeding from the raw epithelial surface; however, a pseudomembrane does not cause bleeding of the underlying surface. The differentiation of membranes from pseudomembranes is mostly of academic interest.

Common Causes

Severe epidemic keratoconjunctivitis (EKC).
Ligneous conjunctivitis.
Alkali or acid burns.
Stevens-Johnson syndrome (SJS).
Ocular cicatricial pemphigoid (OCP).
Gonococcal conjunctivitis.
Corynebacterium diphtheriae conjunctivitis.
Beta-hemolytic streptococcus conjunctivitis.

Allergic/Hypersensitive Conjunctivitis

Phlyctenule

Summary

A phlyctenule is a focal lymphocytic nodule usually at the limbus or on the bulbar conjunctiva that leads to localized fibrosis and vascularization. Phlyctenules are thought to be a type IV hypersensitivity reaction and can be a feature of staphylococcal blepharoconjunctivitis.

Etiology

The actual pathogenesis is unclear; however, phlyctenules are presumably a type IV hypersensitivity reaction to *Staphylococcus* organisms or tuberculosis (TB).

Signs and Symptoms

Foreign body sensation.
Redness.

Demographics

Any age group may be affected without sex predilection.

Ophthalmic Findings

- Unilateral.
- Conjunctival injection.
- Pearly nodule at limbus or on bulbar conjunctiva.
- Staphylococcal lid disease.
- Inflammatory mound with ulcerated apex (Figure 1.9).
- Leash of vessels from conjunctiva.

Special Tests

- Lid cultures.
- Purified protein derivative (PPD) skin test, chest x-ray, if TB suspected.

Pathology

Focal lymphocytic nodules at limbus.

Disease Course

Fibrosis and vascularization of the nodule may occur, and a pannus may form at the peripheral cornea.

Treatment and Management

Direct treatment of the underlying cause (e.g., staphylococcal blepharitis).

Medications

Antibiotic ointment.
Low-dose steroid drops.

Differential Diagnosis

Pterygium.
Fuchs marginal keratitis.
Conjunctival intraepithelial neoplasia (CIN).
Conjunctival granuloma.

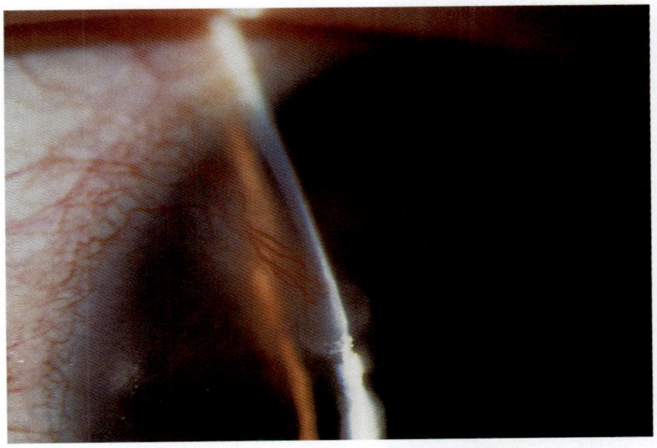

FIGURE 1.9. Elevated, ulcerated fibrovascular growth on the cornea in a 25-year-old patient with a phlyctenule.

References

Abu el-Asrar AM, Tabbara KF. Tetracycline treatment of phlyctenulosis. *Ophthalmology* 1994;101:1161–1162.

Ballintine EJ, Rotbart DC, Takimura Y. Phlyctenulosis. *Am J Ophthalmol* 1972;73:459–460.

Hay Fever (Allergic) Conjunctivitis

Summary

An immediate type I, IgE-mediated hypersensitivity reaction induced by airborne allergens. This occurs more frequently in patients with atopy or asthma.

Etiology

Type I hypersensitivity reaction to airborne allergens.

Signs and Symptoms

Severe itching.
Eyelid swelling.
Tearing.
Discharge.
Rapid development after exposure.

Ophthalmic Findings

Mucosal discharge.
Conjunctival hyperemia.
Papillary conjunctival reaction.
Conjunctival chemosis.
Eyelid swelling.
Caruncular hyperemia.

Systemic Findings

Rhinorrhea and sneezing.
Possibly asthma.

Special Tests

Conjunctival cytologic study with Wright stain shows eosinophils or granules.

Pathology

Seasonal allergic conjunctivitis is accompanied by increased mast cell numbers.

Disease Course

Seasonal exacerbation when exposed to allergen.

Treatment and Management

Cold compresses.
Vasoconstrictors.
Antihistamines.
NSAID.
Mast cell stabilizers.
Topical steroids.

Medications

See above.

Differential Diagnosis

Vernal conjunctivitis.
Medicamentosa.
Atopic keratoconjunctivitis.

Reference

Bonini S, Magrini L, Rotiroti G, et al. The eosinophil and the eye. *Allergy* 1997;52(Suppl):44–47.

Atopic Keratoconjunctivitis

Summary

Atopic keratoconjunctivitis is a chronic conjunctival inflammatory condition that occurs in patients with atopy, that is, three or more of the following features:

1. Typical, eczematoid skin lesions.
2. Pruritus.
3. Relapsing eczematoid dermatitis.
4. Personal or family history of asthma or allergic rhinitis.

Etiology

Hypersensitive immune system reacting to many antigens.

Signs and Symptoms

Itching.
Foreign body sensation.
Mucoid discharge.
Red eyes.

Ophthalmic Findings

- Periocular scaly skin and thickening of the eyelids: allergic shiners.
- Medium-sized papillae that can appear milky when confluent (Figure 1.10A).
- Conjunctival edema.
- Elevated limbal nodules: Horner-Trantas dots.
- Extensive corneal neovascularization may occur.
- Pseudogerontoxon (arc-shaped peripheral corneal opacity similar in appearance to a senile gerontoxon [Figure 1.10B]).
- Conjunctival scarring (forniceal foreshortening and symblephera) may occur.
- Posterior subcapsular or shield-shaped anterior lens opacities.

Systemic Findings

- Skin lesions.
- Flexural lichenification in adults (eczema).
- Facial and extensor involvement in infants or children.

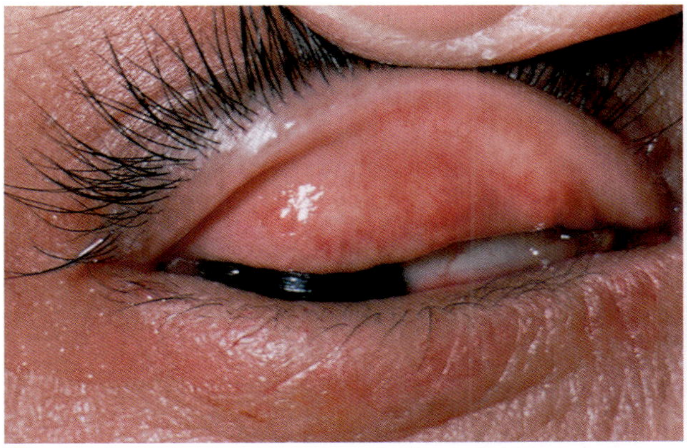

A

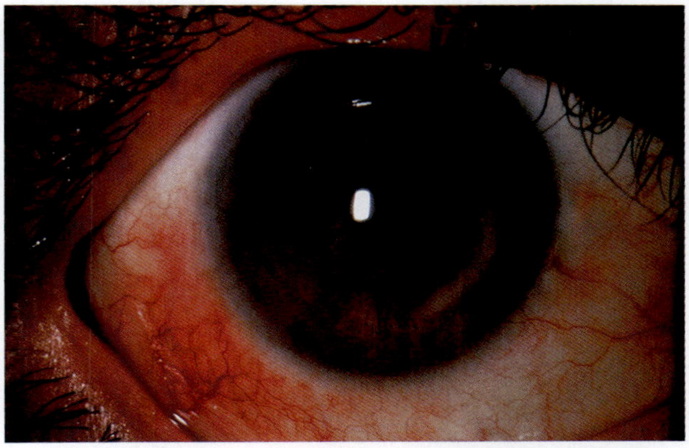

B

FIGURE 1.10. A: Confluent papillae and milky edema on the superior tarsus in an atopic patient. B: An arc-shaped deposition known as a pseudogerontoxon.

- Chronic relapsing dermatitis.
- Asthma.
- Allergic rhinitis.
- Family history of asthma or allergic rhinitis.

Special Tests

Conjunctival cytologic studies with eosinophils (less degranulated and less numerous than vernal).

Disease Course

- Chronic, progressive corneal pannus formation.
- Conjunctival scarring with long-standing disease.
- Bilateral ocular HSV infection may be seen.
- Patients typically older than those with vernal keratoconjunctivitis.

Treatment and Management

- Removal of environmental triggers.
- Treatment is based on the severity of the condition and consists of topical vasoconstrictors, topical cromolyn sodium and other mast cell stabilizers, antihistamines, and NSAID drops.
- Short-term steroids or cyclosporin A for severe cases.

Medications

Disodium cromolyn.
Lodoxamide.
Levocabastine.
Epinastine
Bepotastine.
Ketotifen.
Olopatadine.
Oral antihistamines.
Topical or oral steroids.
Cyclosporin A: for refractory cases.

Differential Diagnosis

Vernal conjunctivitis.
Giant papillary conjunctivitis.
Hay fever.

Reference

Casey R, Abelson MB. Atopic keratoconjunctivitis. *Int Ophthalmol Clin* 1997;37:111–117.

Vernal Keratoconjunctivitis

Summary

Vernal keratoconjunctivitis is a seasonally recurring, bilateral inflammation of the conjunctiva that occurs predominantly in male children and young adults who often have a history of atopy. There are two forms, palpebral and limbal.

Etiology

Hypersensitivity to airborne allergens superimposed on an atopic predisposition.

Signs and Symptoms

Itching.
Photophobia.
Blurred vision.
Copious mucous discharge.

Demographics

Male children and young adults.
Hot, dry climates.

Ophthalmic Findings

- Blepharospasm and ptosis.
- Predominantly palpebral inflammation.
- Diffuse papillary hypertrophy more prominent on upper palpebral conjunctiva.
- Breakdown of conjunctival septae forming cobblestones (Figure 1.11A).
- Bulbar conjunctival hyperemia.

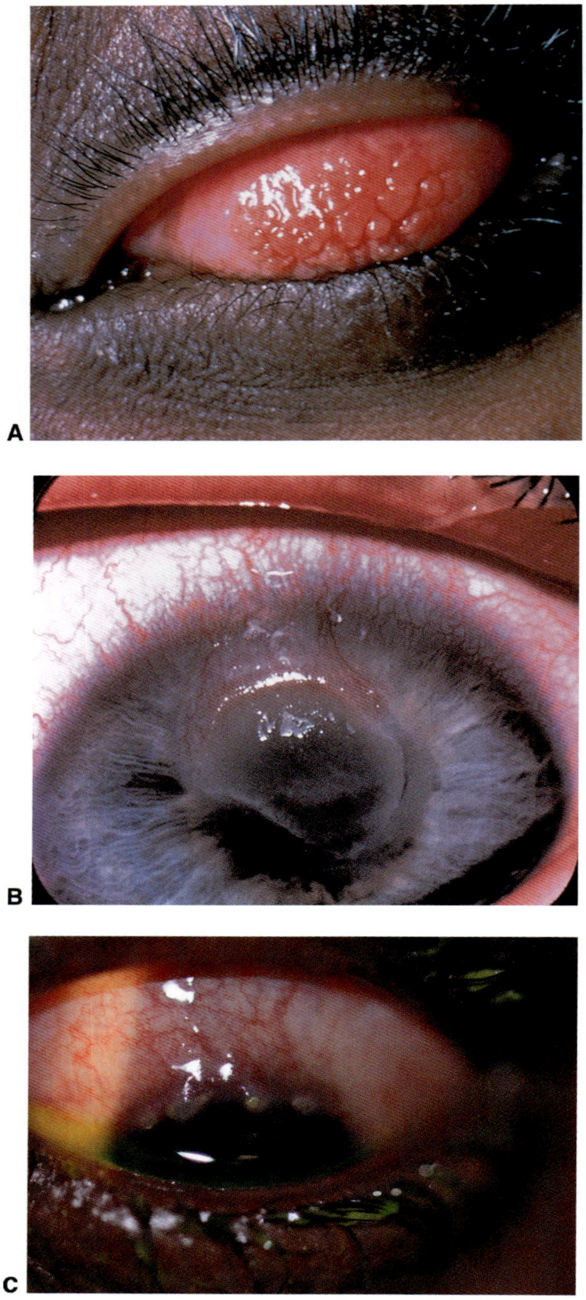

FIGURE 1.11. **A:** "Cobblestone" giant papillae in vernal conjunctivitis. **B:** Shield ulcer on the cornea in another patient with vernal conjunctivitis. **C:** Horner-Trantas dots in limbal vernal keratoconjunctivitis.

- Thickened gelatinous limbus with scattered opalescent mounds called Horner-Trantas dots (Figure 1-11C).
- Fine punctate epithelial erosions: "flour dusting."
- Superior corneal pannus, may progress to 360 degrees.
- Shield ulcer (Figure 1.11B).
- Pseudogerontoxon: whitish partial stromal arcus.

Systemic Findings

Atopic dermatitis (eczema).
Asthma.

Pathology

- Horner-Trantas dots: degenerated eosinophils in hypertrophied limbal tissue.
- Infiltration of the conjunctival epithelium with eosinophils, plasma cells, lymphocytes, and monocytes.

Disease Course

- Seasonal springtime exacerbations.
- Often resolves by puberty.

Treatment and Management

Antihistamines.
Mast cell stabilizers.
Oral topical and supratarsal steroids.
Topical cyclosporin A.
Climatotherapy: home air-conditioning or relocate to cooler climate.

Differential Diagnosis

Atopic keratoconjunctivitis.
Giant papillary conjunctivitis secondary to contact lenses.

Reference

Smolin G. Ocular allergy: The Third Annual Thygeson Lecture. *Cornea* 1998;17:253–256.

Infectious Conjunctivitis

Neonatal Conjunctivitis

Other name: ophthalmia neonatorum.

Summary

Neonatal conjunctivitis occurs within the first month of life. The most common causes include chemical irritation and infections with microorganisms including *Neisseria gonorrhoeae* (Figure 1.12), HSV, *Chlamydia*, and other organisms (Table 1.5).

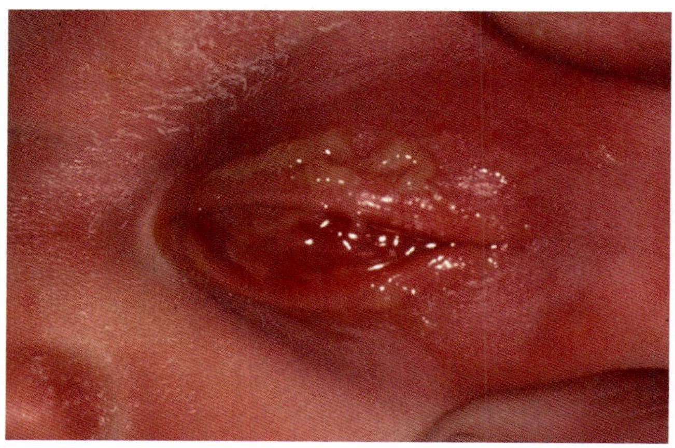

FIGURE 1.12. Gonococcal conjunctivitis in a neonate. (Courtesy of Mark Greenwald.)

Table 1.5

Neonatal conjunctivitis

	Chemical conjunctivitis	Gonococcus	*Chlamydia* (inclusion blennorrhea)	Other bacteria (*Staphylococcus, Haemophilus*, etc.)	Herpes simplex virus (HSV-2 most common)
Signs and Symptoms	Red eye, photophobia; swollen lids (for all five conditions) Neonates are unable to form follicles				
Onset after birth	1 d	3–5 d	5–10 d	5–10 d	5–30 d
Ophthalmic findings	Clear discharge Lid edema Conjunctival chemosis	Hyperacute purulent discharge (Figure 1.10) Lid edema Conjunctival chemosis Marked papillary conjunctivitis Keratitis and in some cases corneal perforation	Clear or mucopurulent discharge Papillary reaction Pseudomembrane formation (rare) Epithelial keratitis Preauricular node	Clear or mucopurulent discharge Papillary reaction Pseudomembrane formation (rare) Epithelial keratitis Preauricular node	Clear, serous discharge Unilateral or bilateral involvement Dendritic keratitis
Systemic findings	None	Meningitis, septicemia	Pneumonitis		Viremia Meningoencephalitis
Special tests		Cultures on chocolate agar Smears show intracellular Gram-negative diplococci	Conjunctival scrapings for inclusion bodies *Chlamydia* cultures Immunofluorescent tests for *Chlamydia*	Cultures Smears for bacteria	Conjunctival scrapings for giant cells *Herpes* culture
Disease course	Resolves spontaneously, with conjunctival scarring in some cases	Corneal ulceration and perforation	Can become chronic producing a follicular reaction		Treatment to prevent systemic spread and later complications
Treatment/ management	None usually May only need irrigation with saline to remove discharge	Systemic ceftriaxone Topical antibiotic drops	Systemic treatment to prevent pneumonitis: erythromycin, azithromycin, and topical tetracycline ointment can be added	Topical broad-spectrum antibiotics	Topical trifluridine drops Systemic acyclovir

Table 1.6

Bacterial conjunctivitis

	Gonococcal	Nongonococcal
Etiology	Spread from genital area via infected secretions	Trauma Foreign bodies, contact lenses wear Topical or systemic immunosuppression Ocular surface disease (dry eye, trichiasis, etc.) If chronic or recurrent, consider nasolacrimal duct obstruction
Signs and symptoms	Pain, red eyes, discharge, photophobia	
Demographics	Any age, but more common in sexually active adults	Any age, more common in elderly persons
Ophthalmic findings	Copious hyperacute purulent discharge Lid swelling and chemosis Intense papillary reaction Preauricular node Corneal ulceration and perforation	Mucopurulent discharge Papillary reaction Eyelid swelling Preauricular node
Systemic findings	Other sexually transmitted diseases	None
Special tests	Gram stain for intracellular Gram-negative diplococci Cultures on chocolate agar	Cultures Gram stain
Disease course	Can penetrate intact corneal epithelium leading to perforation	Can be self-limited and may resolve without treatment
Treatment/management	Systemic ceftriaxone Topical antibiotics	Broad-spectrum topical antibiotic Oral antibiotics if preseptal cellulitis is also present

Etiology

- Chemical: postpartum instillation of drops or ointment (usually from the use of silver nitrate) used for prophylaxis against infection.
- Infectious: ocular contact with infected vaginal secretions.
- Be suspicious in mothers with premature rupture of membranes.

Demographics

Newborns.

Bacterial Conjunctivitis

Summary

Conjunctivitis caused by bacteria is very common and in most cases is benign and self-limited. There is considerable overlap in the presenting findings from different bacteria. It is important to rule out possible infection by *N. gonorrhoeae* or *N. meningitidis* (Table 1.6). The most common etiologic organisms of bacterial conjunctivitis are *Streptococcus pneumoniae, Staphylococcus aureus*, and *Haemophilus influenzae*.

Viral Conjunctivitis

Summary

The most common cause of viral conjunctivitis is adenovirus (EKC); however, other viruses, including HSV, coxsackievirus, Enterovirus, and Newcastle disease viruses can affect the conjunctiva. Conjunctivitis from other viruses with conditions such as measles, influenza, and mumps is much less common (Table 1.7).

Chlamydia Conjunctivitis

Adult Inclusion Conjunctivitis

Summary

Adult inclusion conjunctivitis is a sexually transmitted conjunctivitis caused by *Chlamydia*. It should be considered in any case of chronic follicular conjunctivitis.

Etiology

- Spread by contact with infected genital secretions.
- *Chlamydia trachomatis* serotypes D to K.

Table 1.7

Viral conjunctivitis

	Adenovirus (see also section on EKC)	Herpes simplex	Acute hemorrhagic conjunctivitis	Newcastle disease conjunctivitis	Other viral conjunctivitis
Other names	EKC PCF		Apollo 11 conjunctivitis		
Etiology	Adenovirus	Herpes simplex virus	Coxsackievirus A24 or enterovirus 70	Newcastle disease virus	Various other viruses
Signs and symptoms	Red eye Clear, watery discharge Photophobia	Red eye Clear or mucoid discharge Photophobia Usually unilateral	Sudden onset of subconjunctival hemorrhage Red eye Clear, watery discharge Photophobia	Red eye Clear, watery discharge Photophobia	Red eye Clear, watery discharge Photophobia
Demographics	Any age		Affects groups of people who are in close proximity Hand-to-eye transmission	Poultry workers, veterinarians (virus most commonly affects turkeys and chickens)	
Ophthalmic findings	Follicular conjunctivitis Punctate epithelial keratitis Eyelid swelling Tender preauricular node	Follicular conjunctivitis Conjunctival chemosis Subconjunctival hemorrhages Pseudomembranous conjunctivitis (rare) Conjunctival dendritic ulcers	Large subconjunctival hemorrhage Follicular conjunctivitis Preauricular node Lid edema	Lid edema Small preauricular node Epithelial keratitis	
Systemic findings	Usually none	History of herpetiform rash	Malaise, flulike syndrome Can result in lumbosacral radiculomyelitis	Headaches, malaise, arthralgias	Dependent on particular virus
Special tests	Adenoviral DFA	Herpes culture			
Disease course	Sudden onset in one eye with the fellow eye affected 3–5 d later Self-limited, resolving in 7–14 d following onset	Self-limited, resolving within 1–2 wk	Patients are contagious before clinical symptoms manifest Highly contagious by infectious secretions Fellow eye affected soon after first eye	Self-limited disease	Usually self-limited
Treatment/ management	Supportive treatment with cool compresses and artificial lubricants Measures to prevent transmission to fellow eye and other people (e.g., hand washing)	Topical trifluridine Oral acyclovir	Supportive measures, usually resolves spontaneously within a week Hand washing and measures to prevent spread of secretions	Supportive therapy	Supportive therapy

EKC, epidemic keratoconjunctivitis; PCF, pharyngoconjunctival fever; DFA, direct fluorescent antibody.

Signs and Symptoms

Acute onset of conjunctivitis.
Irritation.

Demographics

Young, sexually active teenagers and adults.

Ophthalmic Findings

Unilateral or bilateral conjunctivitis.
Tarsal follicles, often more prominent inferiorly.
Small, nontender preauricular node.
Punctate epithelial keratopathy (PEK).
Superficial pannus.
Chronic mucopurulent discharge.

Systemic Findings

- Chlamydial genital infection, may be asymptomatic.
- Other sexually transmitted diseases.

Special Tests

- Giemsa stain for intracytoplasmic inclusions.
- *Chlamydia* organisms on direct fluorescent antibody (DFA) assay.
- Cultures for *Chlamydia* organisms.

Disease Course

Chronic irritation and mild mucopurulent discharge.

Treatment and Management

Treatment of choice is systemic antibiotics:

1. Oral azithromycin.
2. Tetracycline.
3. Erythromycin.
4. Doxycycline.

Also treat sexual partners who may also be harboring chlamydial infection.

Differential Diagnosis

EKC.
Toxicity.
Molluscum contagiosum.
Psittacosis.

Trachoma

Summary

Trachoma, caused by *C. trachomatis*, is a major cause of blindness worldwide. Infection leads to conjunctival and corneal scarring, trichiasis, and dry eye.

Etiology

- Spread by contact with infected ocular secretions; can be spread by flies and other fomites.
- *C. trachomatis* serotypes A to C.

Demographics

- Found in hot, dry climates, often in underdeveloped countries.
- Can occur in epidemics when many people live in close proximity.

Ophthalmic Findings

Early:

- Follicular conjunctivitis (Figure 1.13).
- Mucopurulent discharge.
- Tender preauricular node.
- Punctate epithelial keratitis.

Late:

- Conjunctival scarring including Arlt line.
- Entropion, trichiasis.
- Scarring of limbal follicles (Herbert pits).
- Superior superficial corneal neovascularization.

Systemic Findings

None.

Special Tests

Helpful only in acute infection: cultures, DFA.

Disease Course

Resolution of early infection with scarring occurring years to decades later.

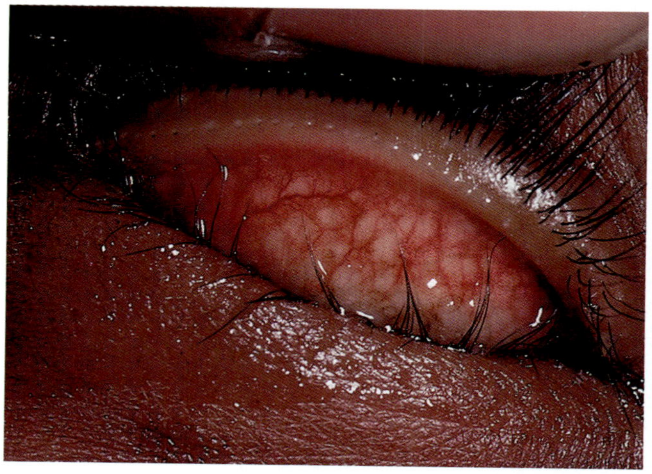

FIGURE 1.13. Follicular conjunctivitis in a 5-year-old child in a trachoma endemic area.

Treatment and Management

Early treatment:

- Oral azithromycin.
- Topical tetracycline, azithromycin, or erythromycin.

Late treatment:

- Management of complications such as dry eye and bacterial superinfection.
- Surgery for trichiasis or entropion.

Cicatricial Conjunctivitis

Differential Diagnosis

- Any severe infection producing a membrane or pseudomembrane:
  - Bacterial (*Neisseria*, beta-hemolytic *Streptococcus*, *Corynebacterium*, *Haemophilus* organisms).
  - Viral (EKC, HSV).
  - Chlamydial.
- Systemic medications:
  - Practolol.
  - D-penicillinamine.
- Topical medications: particularly glaucoma medications such as epinephrine and pilocarpine.
- Dermatobullous diseases:
  - Toxic epidermal necrolysis.
  - Dermatitis herpetifomis.
  - Pemphigus vulgaris.
  - Porphyria cutanea tarda.
- Autoimmune:
  - Stevens-Johnson syndrome.
  - Ocular cicatricial pemphigoid.
  - Systemic lupus erythematosus.
  - Sarcoidosis.
  - Atopic blepharoconjunctivitis.
  - Progressive systemic sclerosis.
  - Sjögren syndrome.
- Trauma:
  - Chemical and thermal burns.
  - Conjunctival surgery.
  - Conjunctival injury.
  - Radiation exposure.

Reference

Holsclaw DS. Ocular cicatricial pemphigoid. *Int Ophthalmol Clin* 1998;38:95.

Ocular Cicatricial Pemphigoid

Summary

OCP is an autoimmune disease of unknown etiology affecting the skin and mucosa. The mainstay of treatment is immunosuppression, as well as prompt diagnosis and treatment of the many ocular complications of the disease (Figure 1.14).

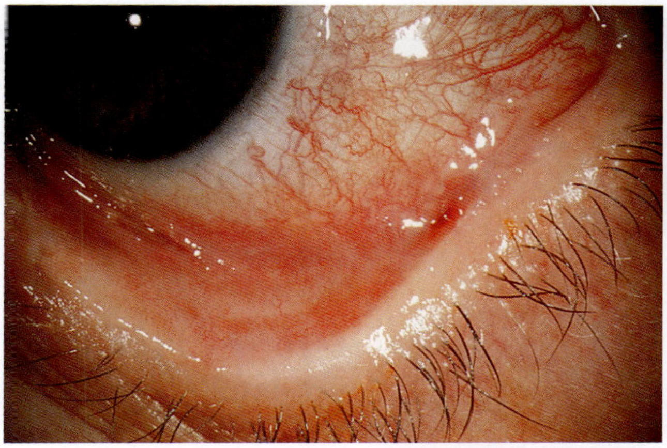

FIGURE 1.14. Ocular pemphigoid. Severe conjunctival foreshortening and symblepharon in a patient with moderately advanced ocular cicatricial pemphigoid. (From Tasman W, Jaeger E. *The Wills Eye Hospital atlas of clinical ophthalmology*, 2nd ed. Philadelphia, PA: Lippincott Williams & Wilkins, 2001.)

Etiology

- Autoimmune.
- Circulating antibodies and complement bind to the basement membrane of mucosal tissue at sites throughout the body. The initial stimulus for the formation of these autoreactive antibodies is not understood.

Signs and Symptoms

- Dry eye symptoms such as foreign body sensation.
- Chronic red eye.

Demographics

- Mean age of presentation is in the seventh decade of life.
- The disease may rarely present in the pediatric population.
- Women are affected twice as frequently as men.

Ophthalmic Findings

Chronic bilateral, papillary, cicatricial conjunctivitis with symblepharon formation (Figure 1.15A).
Forniceal foreshortening.
Diminished tear production.
Trichiasis.
Conjunctival keratinization.
Corneal ulcers, neovascularization, and scarring.

Systemic Findings

- Any mucosal surface may be affected in cicatrical pemphigoid.
- Oral mucosa is involved in 65% of patients with OCP, such as desquamative gingivitis (Figure 1.15B).
- Involvement of the larynx and esophagus may lead to life-threatening complications; it is important to elicit a

A 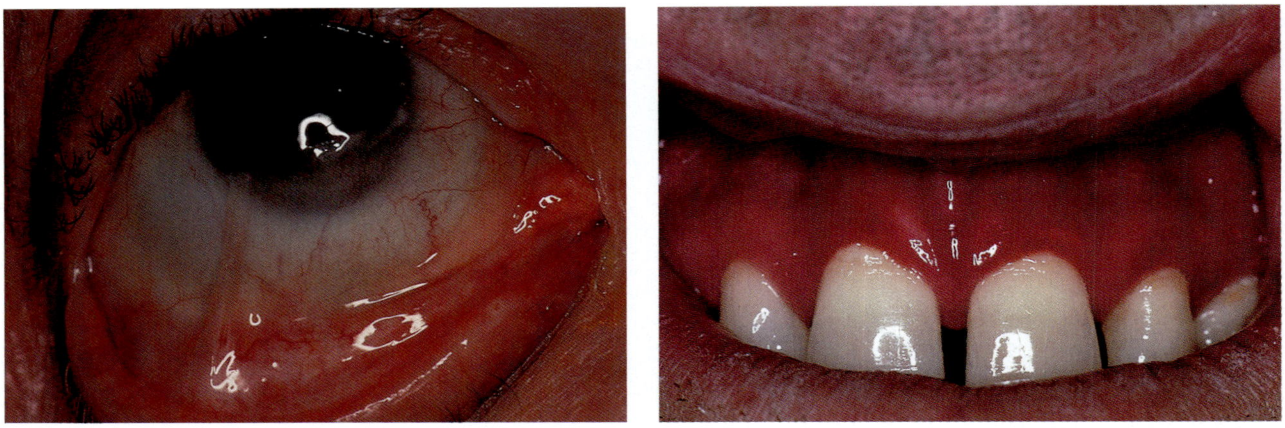 B

FIGURE 1.15. **A:** Symblephera in a patient with severe ocular cicatricial pemphigoid. **B:** Oral manifestations of pemphigoid include oral ulceration and gingivitis.

history of changes in speech or swallowing in patients with OCP.

- Vesiculobullous skin lesions that resolve without scarring, or erythematous plaques, which do scar.

Special Tests

Biopsy of the oral or conjunctival mucosa with direct immunofluorescence to detect the presence of linear deposition of immunoglobulin and complement on the basement membrane. This test is not available in all pathology departments. Specimens must be processed when fresh and must not be placed in formalin. Therefore, before undertaking a biopsy, arrangements should be made for the proper handling and interpretation of the specimen.

Pathology

Linear deposition of immunoglobin, complement, and fibrinogen on the basement membrane of the conjunctival mucosa.

Disease Course

- Wide range in severity from mild to vision threatening.
- In severe cases, the combination of diminished tear production and trichiasis leads to recurrent corneal ulcers and corneal scarring that may be blinding.

Treatment and Medications

- After a diagnosis of active OCP has been confirmed by tissue biopsy, systemic immunosuppressive therapy should be initiated in most cases.
- Immunosuppressive therapy with cyclophosphamide is the mainstay, but this is an evolving field of study.
- Methotrexate, azathioprine, mycophenolate, and other immunosupressive agents have been used for patients who cannot tolerate cyclophosphamide.
- Emerging therapies such as rituximab and intravenous immunoglobulin have been advocated by some.
- Often, patients are treated with prednisone while cyclophosphamide therapy is being initiated.
- The prednisone is withdrawn once the cyclophosphamide has reached a therapeutic level.
- Immunosuppressive treatment is usually continued for 9 to 12 months.
- Consultation with an internist for assistance in the management of these immunosuppressive medications and the development of extraocular manifestations of the disease is important.
- Formal OCP staging systems and serial photographs are useful to monitor progression of disease.
- Definitive surgical treatment of any trichiasis or other procedures should be undertaken when the eye is in remission during immunosuppressive therapy.
- Specific ocular complications of OCP such as dry eye, keratinization, and corneal ulcers should be treated as they arise.

Differential Diagnosis

Conjunctival scarring and trichiasis may be seen in association with many conditions:

- Bacterial and viral conjunctivitis.
- Chlamydial infection.
- Long-term use of glaucoma medications.
- Atopic keratoconjunctivitis.
- Chemical or thermal burns.
- Radiation exposure.
- Trauma.
- Sarcoidosis.
- SJS.
- Other dermatobullous disorders.

References

Bernauer W, Elder MJ, Leonard JN, et al. The value of biopsies in the evaluation of chronic progressive conjunctival cicatrisation. *Graefes Arch Clin Exp Ophthalmol* 1994;32:533–537.

Elder MJ, Lightman S, Dart JKG. Role of cyclophosphamide and high dose steroid in ocular cicatricial pemphigoid. *Br J Ophthalmol* 1995;79:264–266.

Foster CS. Cicatricial pemphigoid. *Trans Am Ophthalmol Soc* 1986;84:527–663.

Foster CS, Chang PY, Ahmed AR. Combination of Rituximab and intravenous immunoglobulin for recalcitrant ocular cicatricial pemphigoid: a preliminary report. *Ophthalmology* 2010;117(5):861–869.

Holsclaw DS. Ocular cicatricial pemphigoid. *Int Ophthalmol Clin* 1998;38:89–106.

Saw VP, Dart JK, Rauz S, et al. Immunosuppressive therapy for ocular mucous membrane pemphigoid strategies and outcomes. *Ophthalmology* 2008;115(2):253–261.e1.

Tauber J, Sainz de la Maza M, Foster CS. Systemic chemotherapy for ocular cicatricial pemphigoid. *Cornea* 1991;10:185–195.

Stevens-Johnson Syndrome

Other name: erythema multiforme major.

Summary

Acute mucocutaneous eruption usually associated with medication or infection, with a prodrome of malaise and fever, followed by erythematous skin lesions involving 10% to 20% of body surface area and two mucosal sites.

Etiology

Unknown, but most of the cases are drug related or postinfectious (Table 1.8).

Signs and Symptoms

- Malaise and fever.
- Cutaneous and mucosal eruptions.
- Red eyes.
- Photophobia.

Demographics

- Male-to-female predominance of 3 to 1.
- Usually occurring in people between 10 and 30 years of age.
- SJS may be more common among people with AIDS.

Table 1.8

Triggers for Stevens-Johnson syndrome

Medications	Antibiotics (penicillin, sulfonamides) Anticonvulsants (phenytoin) Nonsteroidal anti-inflammatory agents
Infections	Herpes simplex virus Measles *Mycoplasma pneumoniae*
Autoimmune	HLA subtypes (including Aw33, B12, DRw53, and others)

Ophthalmic Findings

Acute stage of the disease:

- Desquamative bullous rash of the skin of the eyelids.
- Mucopurulent conjunctivitis.
- Episcleritis.
- Severe papillary conjunctivitis.
- Ulcerative conjunctivitis with pseudomembranes.

Chronic ocular complications:

- Cicatricial conjunctivitis.
- Trichiasis.
- Entropion.
- Symblepharon.
- Dry eye.
- Keratinization.
- Corneal infections and scarring.

Progressive conjunctival scarring may occur even after the acute systemic disease has resolved.

Systemic Findings

- Skin lesions: erythematous macules or papules smaller than 3 mm that classically develop a target appearance. As the disease progresses, these lesions may coalesce. Despite their dramatic appearance, the cutaneous manifestations of SJS often resolve without sequelae.
- Other mucosal surfaces in the body, particularly the oral mucosa, may become involved.
- SJS may become a life-threatening condition as a result of superinfection, electrolyte imbalance, or severe volume depletion.

Special Tests

Usually none. A biopsy can be performed in cases that are not clinically obvious.

Pathology

Dermal and epidermal lymphocytic and histocytic infiltrate. Eosinophils may be seen in patients with drug-induced SJS.

Treatment and Management

- The systemic manifestation of SJS often makes the patient's condition medically unstable, and admission to a medical ward or burn unit may be required.
- Patients with ulcerative conjunctivitis and/or epithelial corneal defects should receive prophylactic topical antibiotics and should be monitored for infection.
- Bandage contact lenses, plastic wrap, symblepharon rings, amniotic membrane, and daily lysis of symblepharon have all been advocated for the prevention of symblepharon.
- Topical and systemic steroids are often used during the acute phase of the disease, but their use is controversial.

- Corneal transplantation has a poor prognosis. Keratoprosthesis has been used with some success.
- Amniotic membrane transplantation and limbal stem cell transplantation have been used.
- The ocular chronic complications of SJS are often the most troublesome sequelae of the disease. Trichiasis, entropion, symblepharon, dry eye, keratinization, and corneal infection and opacification must all be managed as they arise.

References

Foster CS, Fong LP, Azar D, et al. Episodic conjunctival inflammation after Stevens-Johnson syndrome. *Ophthalmology* 1988;95:453–462.

Holland EG, Palmon FE, Webster GF. Erythema multiforme, Stevens-Johnson syndrome and toxic epidermal necrolysis. In: Mannis MJ, Macsai MS, Huntley AC, eds. *Eye and skin disease*. New York, NY: Lippincott-Raven Publishers, 1996:273–284.

Mondino BJ. Cicatricial pemphigoid and erythema multiforme. *Ophthalmology* 1990;97:939–952.

Sayegh RR, Ang LP, Foster CS, et al. The Boston keratoprosthesis in Stevens-Johnson syndrome. *Am J Ophthalmol* 2008; 145(3):438–444.

Graft Versus Host Disease

Summary

Graft versus host disease (GVHD) is a severe complication following bone marrow transplantation in which transplanted immunocompetent cells attack the host tissues. Ocular involvement during the acute phase can range from conjunctival erythema to frank epithelial sloughing. Late complications include scarring and dry eye.

Etiology

Transplanted immune cells from the donor reacting against the immunoincompetent host following bone marrow transplantation.

Signs and Symptoms

Acute:

Red eyes.
Photophobia.
Serous or bloody tears.
Membrane formation.

Chronic:

Dry eye.
Foreign body sensation.
Chronic red eye.
Superior limbic keratoconjunctivitis.

Demographics

- Patients after bone marrow transplantation.
- Acute phase (within 100 days), chronic phase (after 100 days).

Ophthalmic Findings

Acute:

- Conjunctival hyperemia and papillary reaction.
- Chemosis and serosanguineous exudation.
- Membrane or pseudomembrane formation.
- Epithelial sloughing.
- Heals with cicatrization, symblephera.

Chronic:

- Cicatricial conjunctival changes similar to OCP.
- Dry eye.
- Superior Limbic Keratoconjunctivitis.

Systemic Findings

Skin: maculopapular rash with bulla formation.
Liver: elevated liver enzyme and bilirubin values.
Gut: diarrhea.

Pathology

- Subepithelial lymphocytic infiltrate with bulla formation.
- Lymphocytic infiltration of the lacrimal gland.

Disease Course

- Progressive conjunctival and corneal scarring with symblephera formation, entropion, and trichiasis.
- Dry eye with lacrimal gland involvement and loss of goblet cells.

Treatment and Management

- High-dose systemic steroids.
- Local treatment for superinfection, dry eyes.

Differential Diagnosis

OCP.

Reference

Jabs DA, Wingard JR, Green WR, et al. The eye in bone marrow transplantation, III: conjunctival graft-versus-host disease. *Arch Ophthalmol* 1989;1007:1343–1348.

Chemical Burns

See p. 74.

Miscellaneous Causes of Conjunctivitis

Floppy Eyelid Syndrome

Summary

Floppy eyelid syndrome occurs primarily in overweight individuals and is characterized by softening of the upper tarsus and laxity allowing easy eversion, especially while sleeping, causing chronic irritation and inflammation.

Etiology

- Extreme laxity of the upper eyelid with spontaneous eversion.
- Direct contact of the everted lids with bedsheets leads to chronic irritation.

Signs and Symptoms

Redness.
Irritation.
Discharge.

Demographics

Overweight individuals.
No sex predilection.

Ophthalmic Findings

- Upper lid laxity and floppy tarsus (Figure 1.16).
- Confluent small to large papillae on the upper palpebral conjunctiva.
- Mucous discharge.
- Punctate corneal epitheliopathy.
- Superficial corneal vascularization.
- May be unilateral if patient sleeps on one side.

Systemic Findings

Obesity.
Sleep apnea syndrome.

Special Tests

None.

Disease Course

- Chronic and persistent before intervention.
- May be easily confused with other conditions such as medicamentosa and allergy.

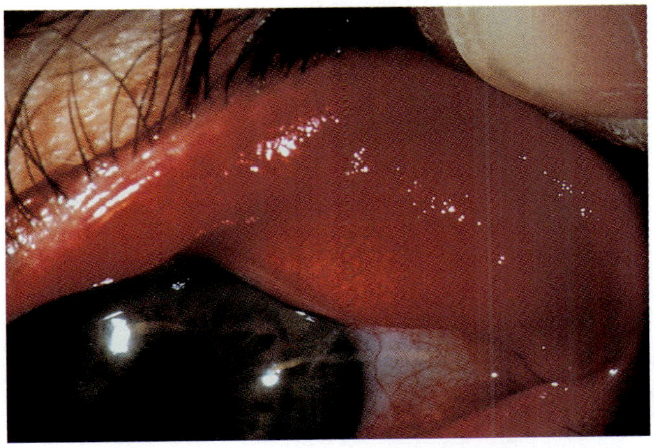

FIGURE 1.16. Spontaneous eyelid eversion with gentle elevation of the eyelid. Notice the tarsal kink with loss of its normal fibrous rigidity.

Treatment and Management

- Cover affected eye with shield at night.
- Patch eye at night.
- Surgical tightening procedure may be necessary.

Medications

Lubricants.

Differential Diagnosis

Vernal conjunctivitis.
Giant papillary conjunctivitis.
Atopic conjunctivitis.
Bacterial conjunctivitis.
Toxic conjunctivitis.

References

Culbertson W, Ostler W. Floppy eyelid syndrome. *Am J Ophthalmol* 1981;92:568–575.
McNab AA. Floppy eyelid syndrome and obstructive sleep apnea. *Ophthal Plast Reconstr Surg* 1997;13:98–114.

Giant Papillary Conjunctivitis

Summary

Giant papillary conjunctivitis is a descriptive term for a conjunctivitis caused by mechanical irritation, most frequently by contact lens use. The hallmark is the presence of giant papillae on the superior tarsal conjunctiva.

Etiology

Chronic mechanical trauma or irritation of the conjunctiva by contact lenses, exposed sutures, or prostheses.

Signs and Symptoms

- Itchy eyes.
- Mucoid discharge, worse when wearing lenses.
- Decreased comfort and wearing time of lenses.

Demographics

Contact lens wearers, more common in patients with poor lens hygiene or overnight wear.

Ophthalmic Findings

- Giant papillae on superior tarsal conjunctiva with apical scarring.
- Mucoid discharge.

Systemic Findings

None.

Disease Course

May resolve spontaneously with removal of irritant but may leave residual scars.

Treatment and Management

- Discontinuation of contact lens wear.
- Change of lenses to disposable soft contact lenses, low-water-content lenses, or gas-permeable hard contact lenses.
- Topical mast cell stabilizers.
- Increased enzyme tablet use.
- Topical steroids, if condition is severe.

Differential Diagnosis

Vernal conjunctivitis.

Dry Eyes

Keratoconjunctivitis Sicca

Other names: Sjögren syndrome (KCS with dry mouth).

Summary

Dry eyes is an extremely common ophthalmic condition caused by decreased tear production, increased tear evaporation, or instability of the tear film. Many associated conditions can result in dry eyes, making diagnosis and treatment more complicated.

Etiology

Three major causes:

1. Decreased tear production:
   - Sjögren syndrome.
   - Non-Sjögren syndrome.
   - Infiltration of the lacrimal gland such as with sarcoidosis.
   - Decreased corneal sensation.
   - Use of certain medications (anticholinergics, antihistamines).
2. Evaporative dry eye:
   - Meibomitis.
   - Goblet cell loss (SJS, cicatricial pemphigoid).
   - Exogenous irritants.
   - Abnormal lid anatomy.
   - Thyroid eye disease.
   - Cosmetic lid surgery.
   - Lagophthalmos.
   - Low-humidity environments (airplanes, air-conditioned rooms, desert climate).

Signs and Symptoms

Sandy, gritty sensation.
Constant foreign body sensation.
Redness.
Blurred vision.
Worse symptoms with wind and dry climates.

Demographics

- More common in elderly individuals and in women.
- Patients with thyroid eye disease or systemic autoimmune diseases may also be predisposed.

Ophthalmic Findings

- Increased interpalpebral fissure height.
- Lagophthalmos or incomplete blink.
- Decreased tear lake.
- Lissamine green or rose bengal staining of conjunctiva (Figure 1.17); fluorescein staining of cornea.
- Keratinization of the cornea or conjunctiva.
- Superficial corneal neovascularization.
- Blepharitis or meibomitis.
- Excessive mucus formation.
- Corneal filaments.
- Malposition of the puncta.

Systemic Findings

Sjögren syndrome: systemic sicca condition with dry mouth, dry skin, trouble swallowing, often associated with autoimmune diseases such as rheumatoid arthritis, SLE.

Special Tests

Schirmer testing: with or without topical anesthesia. Standardized strips of filter paper absorb tears. Consistent measurements of less than 5 mm of wetting at 5 minutes may be indicative of dry eyes.

Tear break-up time (TBUT): Instill fluorescein into the tear film. Observe the surface of the tear film for areas of disruption. Normal TBUT is generally greater than 10 seconds.

Treatment and Management

- Treat underlying cause (e.g., blepharitis, lid malposition, meibomitis).
- Aqueous tear replacements.

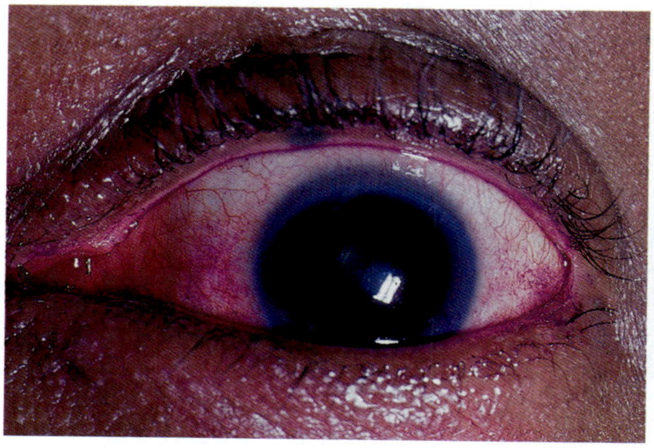

FIGURE 1.17. Interpalpebral rose bengal staining in a patient with KCS.

- Punctal occlusion or tarsorrhaphy in severe cases.
- Decrease evaporative loss with increased humidity, moist chambers, or ointments.
- Topical cyclosporine.
- Topical steroids.

Differential Diagnosis

- Meibomitis.
- Exposure keratopathy.
- Toxic keratopathy: Patients may be sensitive to preservatives in many over-the-counter eyedrops.

Vitamin A Deficiency

Summary

Without vitamin A, mucous membranes undergo squamous metaplasia with loss of goblet cells and subsequent xerosis. This condition is more common in developing countries where the diet may be nutritionally deficient.

Etiology

Deficiency of vitamin A leads to abnormal development of mucous membranes and metaplasia from columnar epithelium to stratified squamous epithelium.

Signs and Symptoms

Sandy, gritty irritation.
Foreign body sensation.

Demographics

- Nutritional deficiency:
  - Malnourished children in developing countries.
  - Fad diets and alcoholics.
- Fat malabsorption syndromes (e.g., cystic fibrosis): Vitamin A is a fat-soluble vitamin.

Ophthalmic Findings

- Conjunctival metaplasia to stratified squamous epithelium with loss of goblet cells.
- White keratinized conjunctival plaque (Bitot spot).
- Corneal drying and diffuse, confluent punctate keratopathy.
- Corneal ulceration and keratomalacia.
- Bacterial superinfection.
- Nyctalopia (night blindness) (vitamin A is necessary for the production of rhodopsin and phototransduction).

Systemic Findings

Metaplasia of mucous membranes of the lung and gut.
Systemic vitamin A deficiency has a 50% untreated mortality rate.

Disease Course

High incidence of bacterial superinfection and ulceration.

Treatment and Management

- Oral vitamin A supplementation.
- Topical vitamin A ointment (may be of limited benefit).

CONGENITAL CORNEAL ABNORMALITIES

Anterior Segment Dysgenesis

Summary

A group of congenital abnormalities of the anterior segment involving developmental arrest or incomplete migration of mesodermal or neural crest tissues (Table 1.9).

Signs and Symptoms

External examination in the newborn period may reveal abnormalities, prompting referral. For milder asymptomatic abnormalities, diagnosis may be made at the time of a routine examination. Visual deficits are variable.

Table 1.9

Anterior segment dysgenesis

Condition	Inheritance	Anterior segment findings	Other findings
Posterior embryotoxon	Autosomal dominant	Anteriorly displaced Schwalbe line	
Axenfeld-Rieger syndrome	Autosomal dominant(75%)	Posterior embryotoxon and prominent iris processes attaching to Schwalbe line, anterior iris stromal hypoplasia	Glaucoma, skeletal abnormalities, hypertelorism, hypoplastic shoulder, maxillary hypoplasia, microdontia, bony malformations
Peters anomaly	Sporadic	Absence of posterior corneal tissue and leukoma, ±iris adhesions to leukoma, ±lens-corneal adhesions	Glaucoma; microphthalmos; persistent hyperplastic primary vitreous; retinal dysplasia; mental retardation; urogenital, craniofacial, and skeletal abnormalities

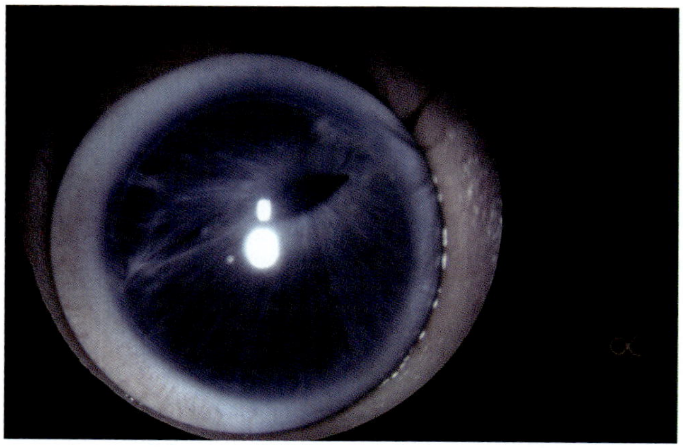

FIGURE 1.18. Anterior segment dysgenesis. (Courtesy of Mark Greenwald.)

Demographics

None specific.

Ophthalmic Findings and Systemic Findings

See Figure 1.18.

Posterior embryotoxon: prominent anteriorly displaced Schwalbe line (Figure 1.19A) visible on slit-lamp examination as a white arc that is central to the limbus. May be seen in up to 30% of normal individuals; causes no deficits. It is usually dominantly inherited.

Axenfeld-Rieger syndrome: Previous nomenclature has been compressed to include overlapping entities that are characterized by having posterior embryotoxon, iris strands (Figure 1.19B), iris and pupillary abnormalities (Figure 1.19C), and glaucoma in 50%. Often associated with dental, cranial, facial, or skeletal abnormalities. Axenfeld-Reiger syndrome is most often autosomal dominant, but it may be sporadic.

Peters anomaly: central corneal opacity, usually with strands of adherent iris. The lens may have an anterior polar cataract or keratolenticular adhesion (Figure 1.19D). Glaucoma is common. Associated ocular abnormalities include microphthalmos, persistent hyperplastic primary vitreous, and retinal dysplasia. In 60% of cases, systemic abnormalities may be found: mental retardation, urogenital, craniofacial, and skeletal abnormalities. Sixty percent of cases are bilateral.

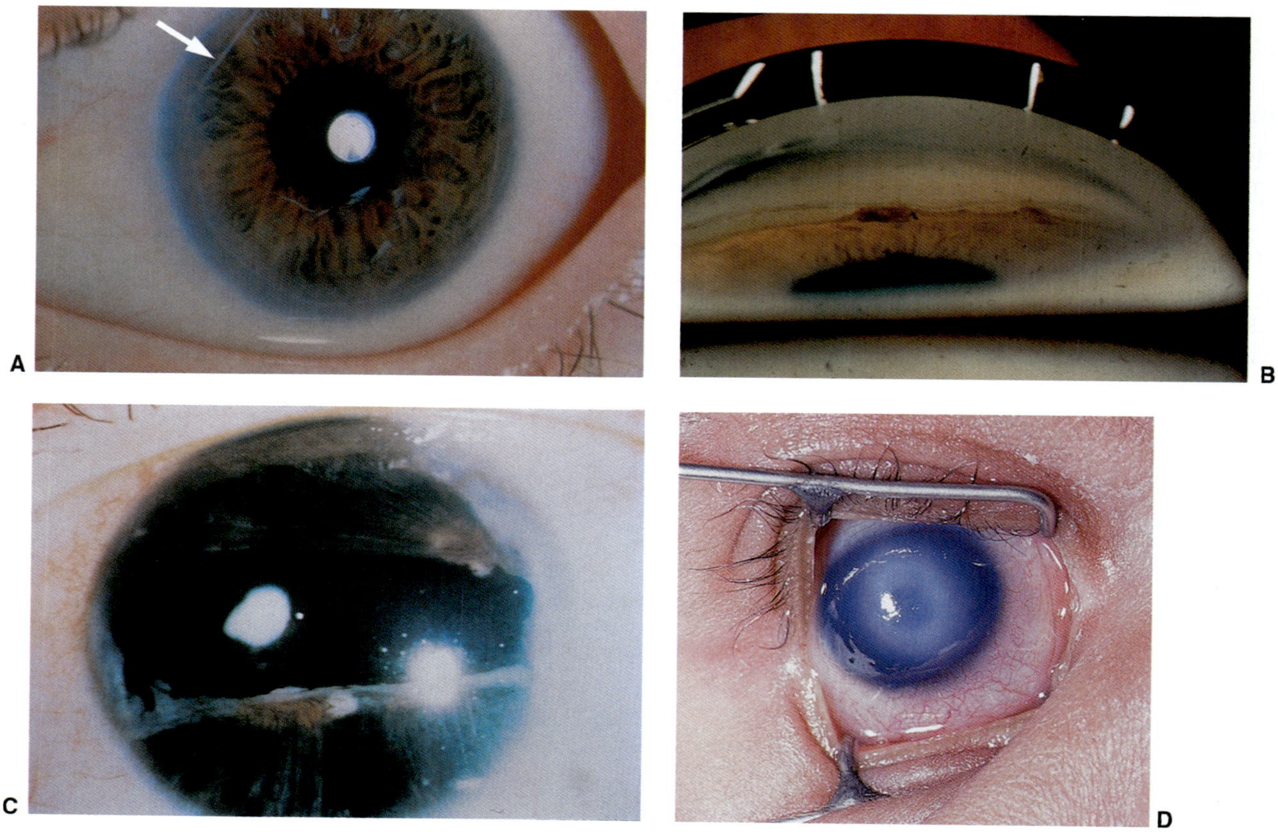

FIGURE 1.19. **A:** Posterior embryotoxon (*arrow*) is a congenital anterior displacement of Schwalbe line. **B:** Broad peripheral iridocorneal adhesions to Schwalbe line is found in Axenfeld anomaly. **C:** Further along the spectrum of anterior segment dysgenesis is Rieger anomaly with iris abnormalities. **D:** Central corneal opacity corresponding to an area of absent Descemet membrane. In many cases, the iris is adherent to the edge of this defect.

Special Tests

Gonioscopy should be included in the ocular examination if one of these abnormalities is suspected. Anterior segment ultrasound may be helpful to determine the lens position in Peters anomaly if surgery is considered.

Pathology

Peters anomaly is remarkable for a focal absence of Descemet membrane and endothelium in the area of central opacity.

Disease Course

Nonprogressive.

Treatment and Management

- Secondary complications such as glaucoma and amblyopia require ongoing care and follow-up.
- Peters anomaly may require penetrating keratoplasty (PKP).

Differential Diagnosis

Other causes of congenital corneal opacities should be considered in the differential diagnosis of Peters anomaly.

Reference

Waring GO III, Rodriques MM, Labison PR. Anterior chamber cleavage syndromes: a stepladder classification. *Surv Ophthalmol* 1975;20:3–27.

Aniridia

Summary

Aniridia is a bilateral developmental abnormality of the iris. A variably sized stump of iris is present in the periphery, which, if small, is obscured by overlying sclera, giving the appearance of no iris.

Etiology

- Familial, autosomal dominant in 85% of cases.
- Fifteen percent are sporadic cases, attributable to abnormality of the short arm of chromosome 11 (Miller syndrome).
- Two percent are familial, autosomal recessive: termed Gillespie syndrome.

Signs and Symptoms

Photophobia, pendular nystagmus, poor vision.

Demographics

None specific.

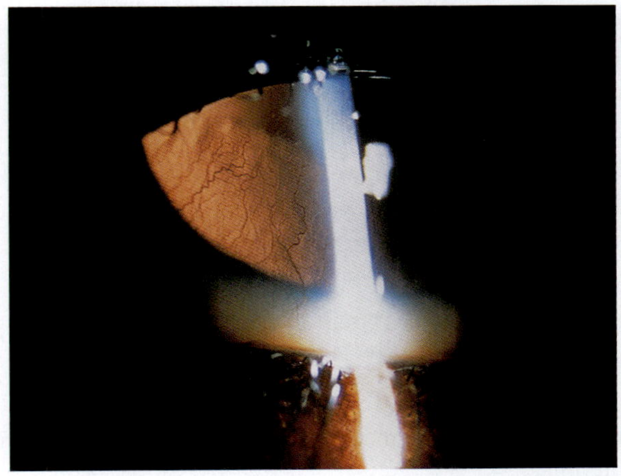

FIGURE 1.20. Retroillumination of the cornea of an aniridic patient with a rudimentary iris and superficial corneal vascularization.

Ophthalmic Findings

Variably hypoplastic iris.

Superficial corneal pannus due to limbal stem cell deficiency (Figure 1.20).

Foveal hypoplasia.

Amblyopia.

Strabismus.

High frequency of glaucoma, superficial corneal vascularization, and opacification.

Lens abnormalities and optic nerve hypoplasia also seen.

Systemic Findings

Miller syndrome: Wilms tumor of the kidney, Aniridia, Genitourinary abnormalities, mental Retardation. (WAGR syndrome)

Gillespie Syndrome: structural abnormalities of cerebellum; do not develop Wilms tumor.

Special Tests

Family history to determine sporadic cases, which then require workup for Wilms tumor (intravenous pyelogram [IVP] or ultrasound).

Pathology

Hypoplasia of iris.

Disease Course

Stable.

Treatment and Management

Strabismus, amblyopia, and glaucoma require usual care.

Medications

None specific.

Follow-Up

Require indefinite follow-up for corneal changes, lens abnormalities, and glaucoma.

Reference

Nelson LB, Spaeth GC, Nowinski TS, et al. Aniridia: a review. *Surv Ophthalmol* 1984;28:621–642.

Iridocorneal Endothelial Syndromes

Summary

A group of nonfamilial unilateral syndromes marked by corneal and iris abnormalities with a high association with glaucoma.

Etiology

Corneal endotheliopathy in which endothelial cells can proliferate and migrate, causing endothelization of the iris.

Signs and Symptoms

None in early disease; decreased vision in Chandler syndrome as corneal edema develops; iris abnormalities may be noted as a cosmetic abnormality.

Demographics

More common in women, findings present from early adulthood.

Ophthalmic Findings

Differentiated into three individual syndromes (Table 1.10).

Systemic Findings

None.

Special Tests

Specular microscopy provides useful information regarding the status of the endothelium.

Pathology

Abnormality of cells lining the cornea, trabecular meshwork, and anterior iris surface, which elaborate excessive basement membrane material and may contract, causing iris and pupil abnormalities.

Disease Course

Slowly progressive. Glaucoma control is problematic because of endothelialization and descemetization of the angle and filtering blebs.

Treatment and Management

Glaucoma management. Conservative management of corneal edema with sodium chloride drops and ointments is recommended. Can recur after penetrating or endothelial transplantation.

Medications

As required for glaucoma and corneal edema.

Follow-Up

Regular examination is indicated to monitor for glaucoma and corneal edema.

Differential Diagnosis

Findings similar to those of the iridocorneal endothelial (ICE) syndromes may be seen bilaterally in posterior polymorphous membranous dystrophy and Fuchs dystrophy, and in Axenfeld and Rieger syndromes. Iris melanoma should be considered in the differential of true unilateral findings but is notable for its lack of other iris abnormalities that are seen in the ICE syndromes.

Reference

Shields MB. Progressive essential iris atrophy, Chandler syndrome and the iris nevus syndrome: a spectrum of disease. *Surv Ophthalmol* 1979;24:3–20.

Birth Trauma

Summary

Unilateral congenital clouding of the cornea attributable to injury at birth.

Table 1.10

Iridocorneal endothelial syndrome

Syndrome	Findings
Iris nevus syndrome or Cogan-Reese syndrome	Diffuse endothelization of the iris with multiple flat pigmented iris nodules
Chandler syndrome	Corneal edema at relatively low or normal IOP with ipsilateral glaucoma, silver or dystrophic appearance to the corneal endothelial cells; iris abnormalities and pupillary distortion may or may not be present
Essential iris atrophy	Ectopic pupil due to peripheral anterior synechiae, which precede full-thickness stretch defects or holes in the iris, located opposite the displaced pupil

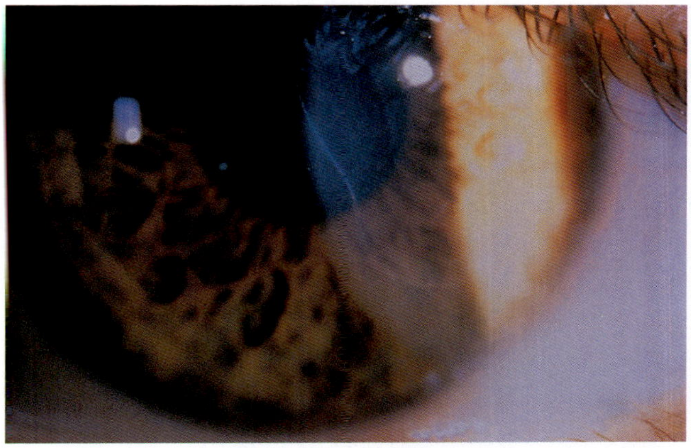

FIGURE 1.21. Vertically oriented Haab striae in a child with congenital glaucoma corresponding to ruptures of Descemet membrane secondary to the elevated pressures.

Etiology

Usually attributable to forceps delivery.

Signs and Symptoms

Cloudy cornea at birth, decreased vision as a result of high astigmatism later in life.

Demographics

None specific.

Ophthalmic Findings

- Acutely, corneal edema.
- Later, vertical or obliquely oriented breaks of Descemet membrane are seen, marked by scrolls or ridges of Descemet membrane (Figure 1.21).
- High degree of astigmatism and late endothelial decompensation are also seen.

Systemic Findings

None.

Special Tests

None.

Pathology

Breaks, scrolls, ridges, and duplication of Descemet membrane may be seen.

Disease Course

See findings above.

Treatment and Management

Correction of astigmatism and amblyopia management.

Medications

Generally not required. Sodium chloride drops and ointment may speed short-term resolution of corneal edema.

Follow-Up

As required for amblyopia if present. Yearly examinations, at minimum, during childhood to monitor vision and refraction.

Differential Diagnosis

Congenital glaucoma may also present with breaks in Descemet membrane and corneal edema; breaks are usually peripheral and arcuate or paracentral and horizontal.

Reference

Cotran PR, Bajant AM. Congenital corneal opacities. *Int Ophthalmol Clin* 1992;32:93–105.

CORNEAL DISORDERS

Developmental Disorders

Microcornea And Megalocornea

Summary

Small (horizontal diameter <10 mm, or 9 mm in a newborn) and large (horizontal diameter >13 mm) corneas, respectively.

Etiology

Undergrowth or overgrowth of the optic cup during development. Microcornea is generally autosomal dominant; megalocornea usually X-linked recessive.

Signs and Symptoms

Small-appearing (Figure 1.22A) or large-appearing (Figure 1.22B) eye.

Demographics

Megalocornea seen in male patients due to X-linked inheritance pattern.

Ophthalmic Findings

Refractive errors (hyperopia in microcornea, myopia in megalocornea), glaucoma, other ocular abnormalities.

Systemic Findings

- Microcornea is associated with myotonic dystrophy, fetal alcohol syndrome, Weill-Marchesani, Ehlers-Danlos, and Rieger syndromes, and Norrie disease.

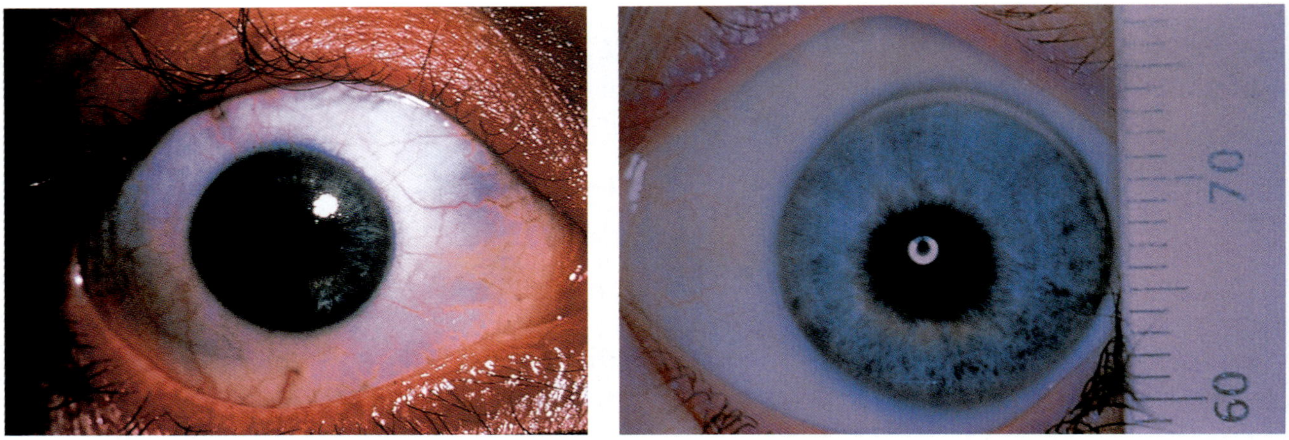

FIGURE 1.22. **A:** Microcornea. Microcornea is a descriptive term for a cornea with a diameter less than 11 mm. **B:** Megalocornea. Congenital enlargement of the cornea (and often the whole globe) with a diameter of almost 14 mm.

- Megalocornea is associated with Marfan syndrome, Down syndrome, mucolipidosis type II, craniosynostosis, facial abnormalities, dwarfism, mental retardation, and ichthyosis.

Special Tests

None.

Pathology

Cornea is normal, other than its size.

Disease Course

Nonprogressive.

Treatment and Management

Refractive correction.

Medications

None.

Follow-Up

Minimally, annual examination during childhood for refraction, and lifelong for glaucoma.

Differential Diagnosis

A variety of related conditions must be distinguished:

Nanophthalmos: small, anatomically normal globe.
Microphthalmos: small globe with multiple abnormalities.
Anterior megalophthalmos: large anterior segment with multiple abnormalities.
Buphthalmos: large globe attributable to infantile glaucoma.

Cornea Plana

Summary

Congenitally flat cornea, with a radius of curvature of less than 40 diopters (D), but commonly 30 to 33 D (similar to the scleral radius of curvature).

Etiology

Autosomal dominant or recessive. Occurs because of developmental arrest of the growth in utero that leads to the usual increase of corneal curvature relative to that of the sclera.

Signs and Symptoms

Poor vision because of high refractive error.

Demographics

More common in persons of Finnish descent.

Ophthalmic Findings

Congenital flat cornea (Figure 1.23).
High-level hyperopia.
May also have glaucoma, indistinct limbus, microcornea, sclerocornea, and other ocular abnormalities.

Systemic Findings

Associated with osteogenesis imperfecta, mucopolysaccharidosis, and trisomy 13.

Special Tests

Keratometry or topography quantitate the radius of curvature.

Pathology

Cornea is normal, other than its shape.

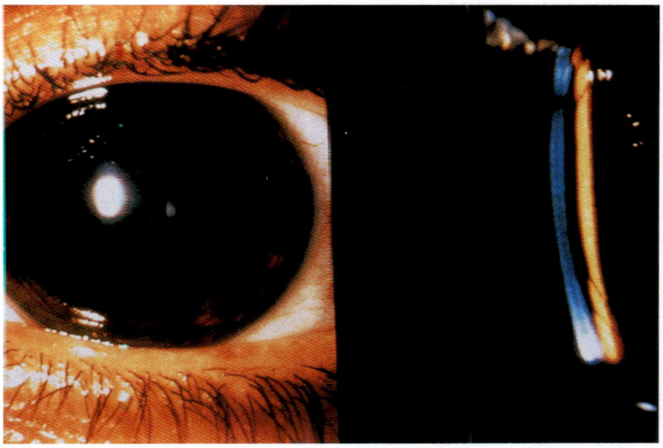

FIGURE 1.23. Patient with cornea plana, a congenital flat cornea, with keratometry readings of less than 40 D. The slit beam highlights the flat curvature of the cornea. The cornea is clear with no scarring or vascularization.

Disease Course

Nonprogressive.

Treatment and Management

Correction of refractive error.

Medications

None.

Follow-Up

Minimally, annual examination in childhood for vision and refraction, and lifelong for glaucoma.

Differential Diagnosis

None.

Sclerocornea

Summary

Congenital replacement of clear cornea with scleral tissue, usually bilateral.

Etiology

Developmental abnormality.

Signs and Symptoms

- Extra amount of sclera resulting in small or absent clear cornea (Figure 1.24).
- Poor vision.

Demographics

None specific.

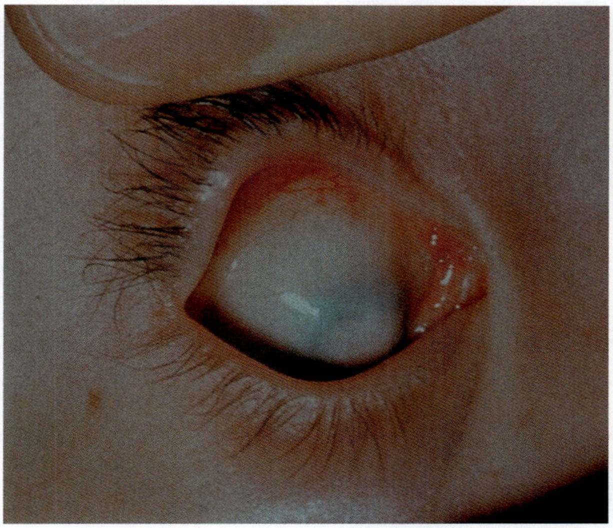

FIGURE 1.24. The cornea is opaque and replaced with disordered collagen lamellae similar to the sclera.

Ophthalmic Findings

Partial or complete replacement of clear cornea with white vascularized scleral tissue. Anterior chamber angle abnormalities and glaucoma are common, as are cornea plana and high-level refractive errors.

Systemic Findings

Associated with deafness, cerebellar and skeletal abnormalities, trisomy 13 and 18.

Special Tests

None.

Pathology

Collagen fibers of scleral thickness and orientation.

Disease Course

Nonprogressive.

Treatment and Management

PKP may be required if central cornea is opaque.

Medications

None.

Follow-Up

Required to monitor for glaucoma.

Differential Diagnosis

Must be distinguished from other conditions causing congenital corneal opacities:

Tears in Descemet membrane: birth trauma, congenital glaucoma.
Ulcers: HSV, congenial rubella, neurotrophic corneas.
Metabolic conditions: bilateral diffuse opacity, usually systemic abnormalities.
Peters anomaly: unilateral or bilateral central opacity.
Endothelial dystrophies: bilateral corneal edema.
Dermoids: unilateral or bilateral, white vascularized mass that may have hair and lipid.

References

Cotran PR, Bajart AM. Congenital corneal opacities. *Int Ophthalmol Clin* 1992;32:93–105.
Waring GO, Rodriques MM, Labison PR. Anterior chamber cleavage syndromes: a stepladder classification. *Surv Ophthalmol* 1975;20:3–27.

Thygeson's Superficial Punctate Keratopathy

Summary

Superficial punctate keratopathy (SPK) is an idiopathic bilateral keratopathy characterized by 10 to 20 discrete clusters of raised epithelial lesions in an otherwise quiet eye. Patients often have a foreign body sensation and photophobia out of proportion to apparent signs.

Etiology

Unknown. A viral origin has been proposed, but not definitively established.

Signs and Symptoms

Photophobia, blurred vision, foreign body sensation, tearing.

Demographics

Usually affects younger adults; occurs in male and female patients equally.

Ophthalmic Findings

- Quiet conjunctiva with no injection.
- Bilateral disease.
- Ten to twenty discrete clusters of whitish epithelial dots (Figure 1.25A) with pooling of fluorescein around the elevated areas (Figure 1.25B).

Systemic Findings

None.

Special Tests

None.

Pathology

None.

Disease Course

- Based on spontaneous resolution over several weeks to months.
- Episodes recur over many years but often "burn out."

Treatment and Management

- Artificial lubricants and tears for symptomatic relief.
- Bandage contact lens for symptomatic relief.
- Low-concentration topical corticosteroid such as prednisolone acetate 1/8%. Topical corticosteroids quickly alleviate the symptoms; however, they may prolong the disease course and make recurrences more frequent.
- In recalcitrant cases, topical cyclosporine 1% drops.

Differential Diagnosis

Punctate epithelial erosions.
EKC.
Exposure keratitis.
Recurrent erosion.

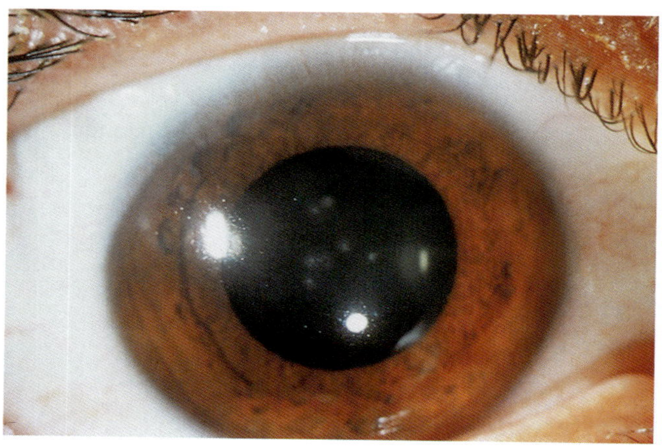

A

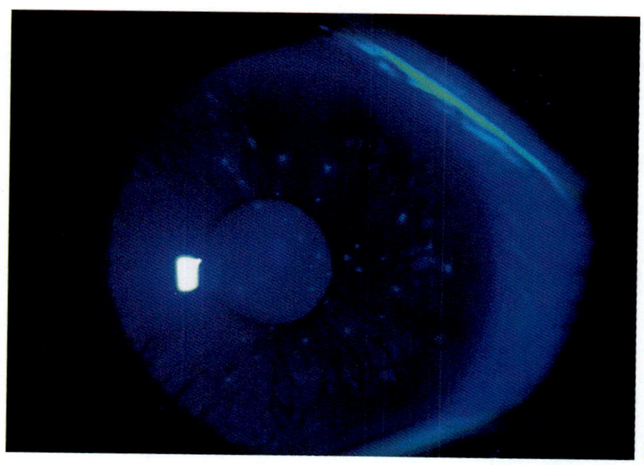

B

FIGURE 1.25. A: Multiple clusters of elevated epithelium in Thygeson's SPK. The conjunctiva is completely quiet and uninflamed. B: These elevated clusters have fluorescein pooling around them.

Superior Limbic Keratoconjuctivitis (of Theodore)

Summary

Superior limbic keratoconjunctivitis (SLK) is a bilateral condition predominately affecting middle-aged women with chronic irritative symptoms, foreign body sensation, and tearing. This condition may occur more frequently in patients with thyroid eye disease and after upper eyelid blepharoplasty.

Etiology

Loose, redundant conjunctiva with a tight upper lid causing folding and rubbing of the superior conjunctiva upon itself.

Signs and Symptoms

Foreign body sensation, tearing, redness, light sensitivity, blepharospasm, and constant eye blinking.

Demographics

Middle-aged women most frequently.

Ophthalmic Findings

- Loose redundant, inflamed superior conjunctiva (Figure 1.24).
- Papillary response of the superior tarsal conjunctiva.
- Superior corneal filaments.
- Bilateral, asymmetric disease.

Systemic Findings

Thyroid function test to rule out Graves disease, which occurs in a higher frequency in patients with SLK. Associated with graft versus host disease.

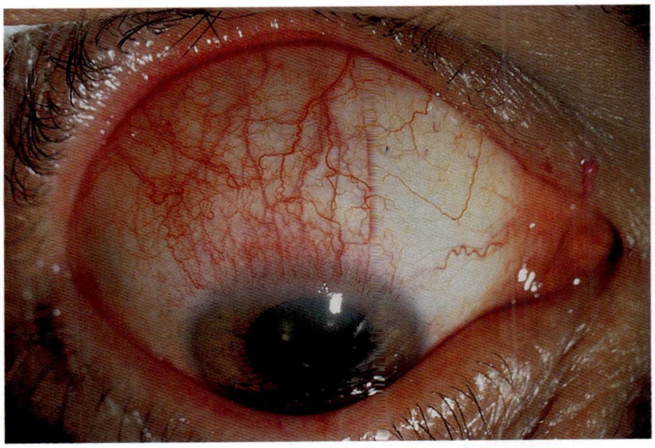

FIGURE 1.26. Superior conjunctival injection in a patient with superior limbic keratoconjunctivitis. Additional findings include a superficial superior corneal pannus and a conjunctival papillary response.

Special Tests

Rose bengal or lissamine green staining reveals a wedge-shaped area of conjunctival staining of the superior bulbar conjunctiva corresponding to an area of conjunctival keratinization.

Pathology

Keratinized epithelium on the superior bulbar conjunctiva. Conjunctival scraping may be helpful in diagnosing this disease.

Disease Course

- Chronic irritative symptoms.
- Patients are often very aware of their eyes and reluctant to have anything near their eyes.

Treatment and Management

- Topical artificial tearing and lubricants.
- Application of a bandage soft contact lens to alleviate irritative symptoms.
- Application of 1% silver nitrate to the superior bulbar conjunctiva.
- Conjunctival resection of the superior bulbar conjunctiva.

Medications

None.

Follow-Up

None.

Differential Diagnosis

Dry eye, essential blepharospasm, foreign body, floppy eyelid syndrome.

Peripheral Staphylococcal Marginal Keratitis

Summary

Staphylococcal marginal keratitis is an inflammatory condition characterized by circumferential corneal infiltrates that are located usually in the corneal stroma adjacent to the limbus with an intervening lucent area.

Signs and Symptoms

Symptoms include photophobia, foreign body sensation, redness, and tearing.

Ophthalmic Findings

- Arc-shaped anterior stromal infiltrate with a clear lucent interval between the infiltrate and the limbus.

- Occurs most commonly where the lid crosses the limbus.
- The infiltrate can have an overlying epithelial defect.
- The limbal vessels adjacent to the infiltrate can be more prominent with a superficial pannus growing toward the infiltrate.
- Often, evidence of previous staphylococcal marginal disease with superficial mild stromal scarring and thinning.
- May occur in conjunction with blepharitis and staphylococcal lid disease.

Systemic Findings

None.

Special Tests

None.

Etiology

Type III hypersensitivity to bacterial antigens or an immune reaction to a bacterial exotoxin.

Disease Course

- Chronic recurrent episodes.
- May correspond to severity of lid disease.

Treatment and Management

- Treatment of the blepharitis with lid hygiene and topical antibiotics.
- The lesions often respond rapidly to a low dose of topical corticosteroids such as prednisolone acetate 0.12%3. Often, an antibiotic/steroid combination is used.

Differential Diagnosis

- Other causes of corneal ulcers (including *H. influenzae*, *Staphylococcus*, *Moraxella* species).
- Bacterial corneal infection.
- Herpes simplex keratitis.

Recurrent Erosion

Summary

Recurrent erosion is a condition whereby the corneal epithelium is poorly adherent to the underlying basement membrane and patients experience frequent irritative symptoms corresponding to epithelial erosions.

Etiology

- Previous traumatic corneal abrasion.
- Basement membrane dystrophy such as map-dot-fingerprint dystrophy.
- Disorders involving the anterior stroma and basement membrane such as lattice corneal dystrophy and Reis-Bucklers dystrophy.
- Ruptured corneal bullae with bullous keratopathy.

Signs and Symptoms

Severe pain, photophobia, tearing, and redness, often wake patients in the middle of the night or are first apparent upon waking in the morning.

Demographics

None.

Ophthalmic Findings

- Unilateral or bilateral areas of loose or wrinkled epithelium and epithelial defects.
- Can sometime occur in the same location as a previous erosion or trauma.
- May have evidence of dry eye, exposure, or a corneal dystrophy.

Systemic Findings

None.

Special Tests

- Instillation of fluorescein dye highlights areas of missing epithelium.
- Adjacent areas of missing epithelium may have fluorescein diffusion underneath the epithelial layer.

Pathology

None.

Disease Course

The epithelium usually heals within several days; however, patients may experience frequent and severe episodes of recurrent erosions.

Treatment and Management

Topical lubricants and artificial tears: These measures are useful for all patients; however, they rarely prevent a recurrence.

Bandage soft contact lens: helps to protect the epithelial surface from further damage and greatly reduces pain.

Stromal micropuncture: most appropriate if the erosions are located outside the visual axis. A bent, 27-gauge needle is used to make a small puncture through the basement membrane, perhaps allowing the epithelium to adhere more firmly. Recurrences after micropuncture may still occur.

Epithelial debridement: The new epithelium may adhere more firmly to the underlying basement membrane.

Excimer laser phototherapeutic keratotomy: may be helpful in removing debris and superficial scarring that may interfere with adhesion of epithelium to the underlying surface.

Medications

- Hypertonic saline solutions.
- Artificial tears and lubricants.

Differential Diagnosis

The main differential is identifying the cause of the recurrent erosion and addressing the underlying disease.

Toxic Medicamentosa

Summary

A toxic keratopathy can be induced by many medications, preservatives, and other ocular irritants. With removal of the toxic substances, the epithelium often slowly returns to normal.

Etiology

Exposure to epithelial toxic and irritative substances, including the persistent use of any topical medication, preservatives in ocular preparations, and environmental irritants.

Common Causes

- Aminoglycoside topical antibiotics such as tobramycin and gentamicin.
- Trifluridine.
- Proparacaine and other topical anesthetics.
- Preserved artificial tears.
- Chlorine and other material included in pools.

Signs and Symptoms

Redness, pain, light sensitivity, foreign body sensation.

Ophthalmic Findings

- Coarse PEK, often diffusely distributed, but may be concentrated in the inferior cornea.
- Trail of conjunctival staining leading to inferior punctum.

Systemic Findings

None.

Special Tests

None.

Disease Course

- The epithelial keratopathy persists as long as the irritant is present.
- With discontinuation of the irritant, the keratopathy may take weeks to months to resolve.

Treatment and Management

- Artificial lubricants and preservative-free artificial tears.
- Discontinuation of the irritant.

Differential Diagnosis

- Thygeson's SPK.
- EKC.
- Atopic keratoconjunctivitis.
- Dry eye.

Exposure Keratitis

Summary

Exposure keratopathy is a condition due to a poor tear surfacing over the cornea and subsequent drying of the surface.

Etiology

- Poor or incomplete lid closure with condition such as Bell palsy, lower lid ectropion, poor blink, or lagophthalmos.
- Adults should be queried about previous lid surgery which may interfere with complete closure of the eye.

Signs and Symptoms

Tearing, redness, foreign body sensation.

Ophthalmic Findings

- Coarse, discrete, or confluent PEK primarily in the interpalpebral fissure.
- Staining with lissamine green or rose bengal in the interpalpebral fissure on the cornea and conjunctiva.
- Incomplete blink or lagophthalmos.

Systemic Findings

- Proptosis preventing adequate lid closures such as with thyroid eye disease.
- Poor blink secondary to Bell palsy or slow blinking rate.
- Nocturnal lagophthalmos.
- Previous eyelid surgery with shortening of the upper or lower eyelids.
- Cicatricial ectropion or restriction of lid motion.

Special Tests

- Staining with rose bengal.
- Observation of the frequency and adequacy of the tear blink.
- Schirmer testing.

Disease Course

With chronic untreated exposure, the cornea is predisposed to infection or the cornea may thin or in some cases perforate.

Treatment and Management

- Frequent topical artificial tears and ointments.
- Increase ambient air humidity.

- Taping the eyelids closed at bedtime.
- Use of moist chamber goggles or plastic wrap over the eye to prevent moisture evaporation.
- Partial or complete tarsorrhaphy.
- Treatment of the underlying condition.
- Gold weights.

Differential Diagnosis

Thygeson's SPK.
EKC.
Toxic medicamentosa.
Dry eye.

Neurotrophic Keratitis

Summary

Neurotrophic keratitis is an epithelial healing disorder secondary to denervation of the corneal surface. Causes for this include previous infection with herpes simplex or zoster, damage to the trigeminal nerve, or the postsurgical period, such as with a corneal transplant.

Etiology

Secondary to loss of the trophic influence from the innervation of the cornea.

Signs and Symptoms

Painless blurred vision, occasionally tearing and light sensitivity.

Ophthalmic Findings

Epithelial defect with ragged epithelial edges, PEK, dull gray epithelium (Figure 1.27).

Systemic Findings

May have evidence of previous herpes simplex or zoster infection, injury to the fifth cranial nerve.

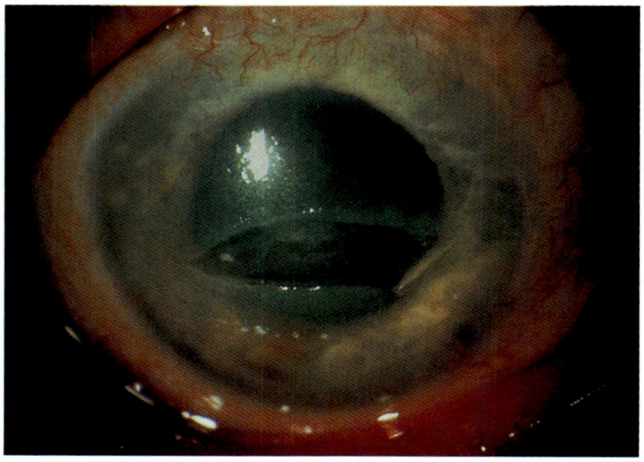

FIGURE 1.27. Following an episode of herpes zoster ophthalmicus, the neurotrophic cornea has a chronic epithelial defect in the exposed interpalpebral fissure.

Special Tests

Cornea sensation is invariably decreased in these cases.

Disease Course

- Chronic and indolent nonhealing epithelial ulcer.
- May become superinfected with bacteria or fungi.
- Thinning of the underlying cornea stroma.

Treatment and Management

- Artificial tears, ointments.
- Prolonged patching.
- Bandage soft contact lens.
- Tarsorrhaphy.
- Amniotic membrane.
- Gunderson flap.

Differential Diagnosis

Corneal abrasion.
Herpetic geographic ulcer.
Bacterial corneal ulcer.

TUMORS OF CONJUNCTIVA AND CORNEA

Conjunctival Squamous Papilloma

Summary

Fingerlike projections of conjunctiva composed of a fibrovascular core covered by acanthotic squamous epithelium.

Etiology

May be associated with human papillomavirus types 6 and 11.

Signs and Symptoms

Cosmetic change, occasionally foreign body sensation.

Demographics

Usually young individuals.

Ophthalmic Findings

- Sessile or pedunculated, with broad or narrow base.
- Surface has red dots corresponding to the central vasculature (Figure 1.28).
- May occur anywhere on the conjunctival surface and be unilateral or bilateral.

Systemic Findings

None.

Special Tests

None.

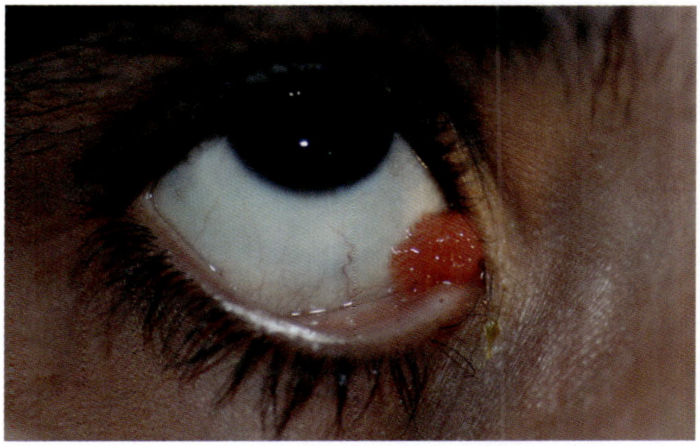

FIGURE 1.28. Conjunctival papilloma demonstrating the typical vascular fronds. These can be either pedunculated or sessile.

Pathology

Acanthotic nonkeratinized epithelium, characterized by irregular hyperchromatic nuclei, surrounded by clear cytoplasm.

Disease Course

Generally benign. May undergo dysplastic change, with increased keratinization, inflammation of adjacent conjunctiva with symblepharon formation, and spread to tarsal surface.

Treatment and Management

Excision with cryotherapy to base and surrounding epithelium. Recurrences frequent, particularly if incomplete excision.

Medications

Mitomycin C or interferon alpha-2b have been used with differing success.

Follow-Up

None required.

Differential Diagnosis

Pyogenic granuloma: usually a history of preceding inflammation or trauma, more fleshy in appearance, without the surface red dots seen on the surface of a papilloma.

Kaposi sarcoma: seen in patients with acquired immunodeficiency syndrome (AIDS).

Conjunctival Intraepithelial Neoplasm and Invasive Squamous Cell Carcinoma of The Conjunctiva

Summary

Squamous dysplasia and carcinoma of the ocular surface. Spectrum ranges from dysplasia without violation of Bowman membrane (CIN) to the rarer invasive squamous cell carcinoma.

Etiology

- Abnormal maturation of epithelial cells.
- Risk factors include ultraviolet (UV) radiation exposure, exposure to petroleum derivatives and human papillomavirus (types 6 and 8 are associated with benign disease, types 16 and 18 with malignancy).

Signs and Symptoms

- Foreign body sensation.
- Redness, irritation.
- Rapid and visible growth on the ocular surface.

Demographics

Generally fair-skinned men in older age groups with a history of high levels of sun exposure.

Ophthalmic Findings

- Unilateral translucent or gelatinous thickening of the conjunctiva with a variable degree of keratinization and leukoplakia.
- Dilated feeding vessels may be present (Figure 1.29).
- May be nodular or diffuse.
- Generally arises at the limbus in the interpalpebral zone.
- The adjacent cornea may be involved: An area of frosted gray corneal epithelium with fimbriated edge is characteristic.

Systemic Findings

Usually none.

Special Tests

- Surface cells may be examined with impression cytology or scraping.

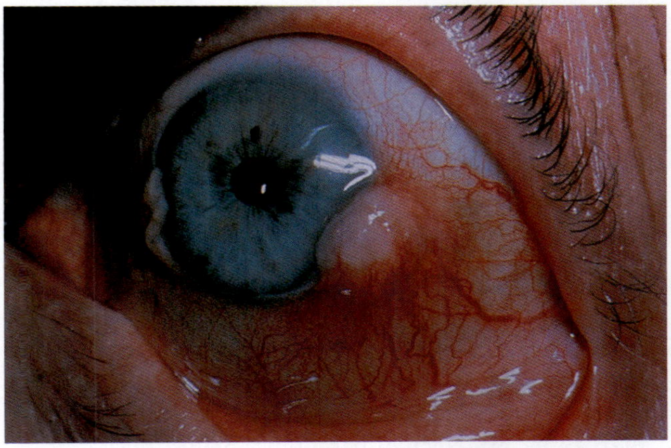

FIGURE 1.29. The elevated fleshy limbal masses with dilated feeding vessels in squamous cell carcinoma of the conjunctiva.

- Rose bengal or lissamine green dye may be helpful in outlining the affected area.
- Pathologic examination is necessary for accurate diagnosis and determination of completeness of excision.

Pathology

- Epithelial cells are seen in disarray, with abnormal maturation and alteration of nuclear to cytoplasmic ratio or frank anaplasia.
- CIN refers to partial-thickness neoplasia and is graded as mild, moderate, or severe on the basis of cellular abnormalities.
- Carcinoma *in situ* refers to full-thickness neoplasia.
- Both CIN and carcinoma *in situ* have an intact basement membrane underlying the abnormal epithelial cells. If invasion through the basement membrane into the substantia propria has occurred, the diagnosis on pathologic examination is that of invasive squamous carcinoma.

Disease Course

Slowly progressive. Most cases do not progress to invasive squamous carcinoma. Intraocular extension and metastasis are rare.

Treatment and Management

- Wide local excision with double freeze-thaw cryotherapy to the margins and base is indicated.
- Some authors recommend frozen sections at the time of excision.
- If corneal involvement is present, the cells should be scraped for removal, leaving Bowman membrane intact if possible, since this functions as a barrier to deeper involvement.
- Despite tumor-free surgical margins, there is a 5% recurrence rate.

Medications

Topical mitomycin C and interferon alpha-2b have been advocated. Use of topical dinitrochlorobenzene (DNCB), urea, and thiotepa has also been described in selected cases.

Follow-Up

Lifelong for recurrence.

Differential Diagnosis

- A variety of benign and malignant entities may be difficult to distinguish.
- A biopsy for cytology should be undertaken when the clinical diagnosis is not certain.
- Benign conditions in the differential diagnosis include pterygium, pinguecula, papilloma, nevus, dyskeratosis, pyogenic granuloma, and corneal pannus.
- Malignant melanoma usually is distinguished clinically by a regular, smooth surface that lacks gelatinous or leukoplakic surface features.

References

Lee GA, Hirst LW. Ocular surface squamous neoplasia. *Surv Ophthalmol* 1995;39:429–450.

Maskin SL. Regression of limbal epithelial dysplasia with topical interferon. *Arch Ophthalmol* 1994;112(9):1145–1146.

Wilson MW, Hungerford JL, George SM, et al. Topical mitomycin C for the treatment of conjunctival and corneal epithelial dysplasia and neoplasia. *Am J Ophthalmol* 1997;124(3):303–311.

Melanocytic Lesions

Nevi

Summary

A benign proliferation of melanocytes; this is the most common pigmented lesion of the conjunctiva.

Etiology

Congenital proliferation of melanocytes.

Signs and Symptoms

Pigmented lesion seen.

Demographics

Noticed first in young individuals.

Ophthalmic Findings

- Elevated, pigmented lesion of conjunctiva on the bulbar surface, plica, caruncle, or lid margin (Figure 1.30.).
- Cystic spaces, representing the nests of cells seen on pathologic examination, are diagnostic of nevi.
- The lesion is mobile.

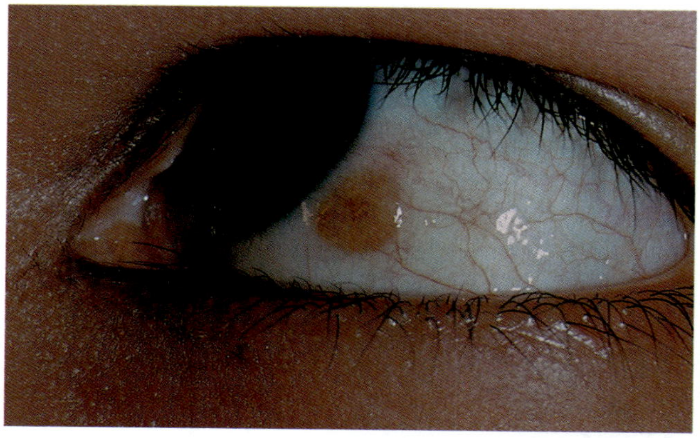

FIGURE 1.30. Conjunctival nevus. This lesion was noticed to grow in this teenage boy. The nevus was freely mobile and had clear cystic spaces within its substance.

- Involvement of the palpebral or forniceal conjunctiva is rare and raises suspicion of malignant melanoma.
- Twenty to thirty percent are nonpigmented.

Systemic Findings

None.

Special Tests

None.

Pathology

Melanocytes proliferate in the basal layer of the epithelium and form clusters or nests.

Disease Course

Generally stable. An increase in size at puberty may be noted. The nevus may seem to disappear later in life as the pigmented cells move into deeper tissue layers.

Treatment and Management

None required. Excision may be performed for cosmetic purposes, or if there is a question of diagnosis.

Medications

None.

Follow-Up

None required.

Differential Diagnosis

Other pigmented tumors and racial pigmentation should be considered. Secondary melanosis may occur with Addison disease, pregnancy, adrenochrome deposition from epinephrine drops, and postinflammatory pigmentation.

Reference

Jakobiec FA, Folberg R, Iwamoto T. Clinicopathological characteristics of premalignant and malignant lesions of the conjunctiva. *Ophthalmology* 1989;96:147–166.

Primary Acquired Melanosis

Summary

Premalignant pigmented lesion of the ocular surface.

Etiology

Dysplasia of melanocytes.

Signs and Symptoms

Appearance of a pigmented lesion.

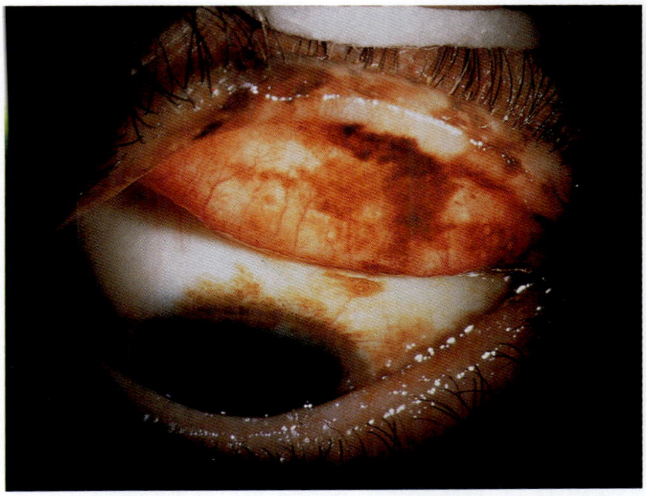

FIGURE 1.31. Primary acquired melanosis. Conjunctival pigmentation in a white patient. In some cases this represents a premalignant condition.

Demographics

Middle-aged, fair-skinned individuals.

Ophthalmic Findings

Diffuse, flat patchy pigmentation on bulbar conjunctiva (Figure 1.31).

Systemic Findings

None.

Special Tests

None.

Pathology

Abnormal melanocytes with varying amounts of atypia based on cellular features.

Disease Course

Pigment may be seen to appear and disappear. Up to 30% may give rise to malignant melanoma.

Treatment and Management

Biopsy, if increased thickness, vascularity, or spread. Cryotherapy to adjacent tissue at time of biopsy.

Medications

None.

Follow-Up

Lifelong because of malignant potential.

Differential Diagnosis

Malignant melanoma: usually fixed to the underlying tissues, prominent dilated vessels.

Reference

Jacobiec FA, Folberg R, Iwamoto T. Clinicopathological characteristics of premalignant and malignant melanocytic lesions of the conjunctiva. *Ophthalmology* 1989;96:147–166.

Ocular Melanocytosis

Summary

Congenital melanosis of the eye.

Etiology

Nonheritable congenital lesion.

Signs and Symptoms

Increased pigmentation of the eye.

Demographics

Increased frequency in whites.

Ophthalmic Findings

Increased slate-gray pigmentation of the episclera, sclera, and uveal tract, usually unilateral (Figure 1.32).

Systemic Findings

None.

Special Tests

None.

Pathology

Increased number of melanin-containing cells in affected tissues.

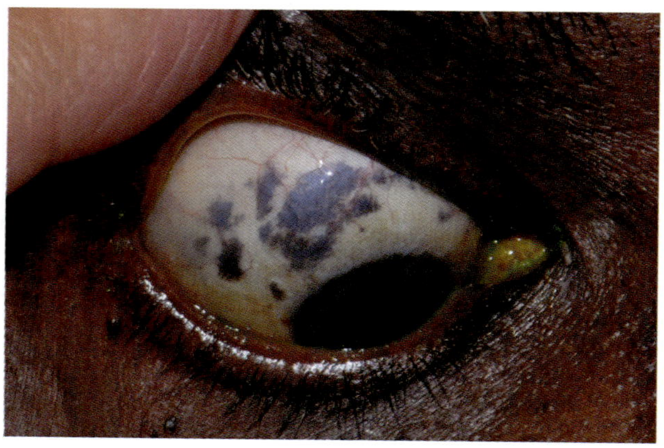

FIGURE 1.32. In ocular melanosis, the pigment is found deeper at the level of the episclera and sclera and appears gray or bluish.

Disease Course

Increased risk of uveal melanoma in affected white individuals.

Treatment and Management

None.

Medications

None.

Follow-Up

Yearly examination for individuals at risk for uveal melanoma.

Differential Diagnosis

Oculodermal melanocytosis (nevus of Ota) is differentiated by blue-gray pigmentation of the skin in the ipsilateral trigeminal nerve distribution, in addition to ocular melanocytosis. This is more common in Asians and blacks and is associated with ipsilateral glaucoma, Duane syndrome, retinitis pigmentosa, and congenital cataract.

Reference

Velazquez N, Jones IS. Ocular and oculodermal melanocytosis associated with uveal melanoma. *Ophthalmology* 1983;90:1472–1476.

Melanoma

Summary

Melanocytic malignancy of the ocular surface.

Etiology

Seventy-five percent of cases arise from primary acquired melanosis (PAM) and 20% from preexisting nevi; 5% arise *de novo*.

Signs and Symptoms

Development of a mass that is usually pigmented. Growth or thickening of an existing lesion may be noted, or an increase in vascularity.

Demographics

Usually affects white patients in the fifth and sixth decades of life.

Ophthalmic Findings

Pigmented mass with prominent vascularity that is fixed to the underlying tissues (Figure 1.33).

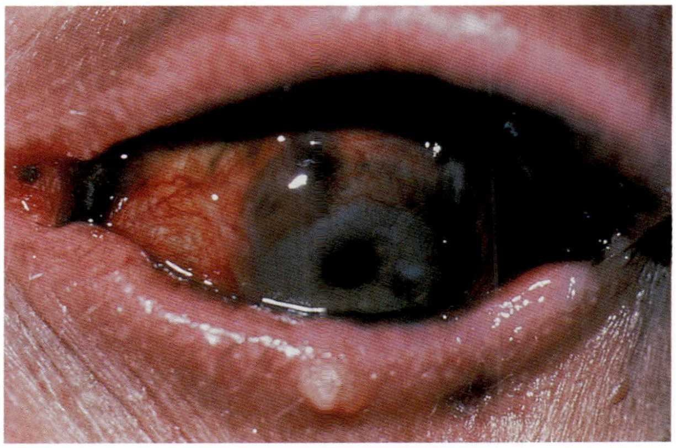

FIGURE 1.33. Malignant melanoma of the conjunctiva with multiple elevated pigmented nodules. Extensive disease such as this may require exenteration.

Systemic Findings

Metastasis to local lymph nodes.

Special Tests

Pathologic examination required at time of excision. Prognostic features include the extent of tissue involvement and degree of atypia of the cells.

Pathology

Proliferation of pleomorphic melanocytes, with mitotic figures and loss of normal cellular polarity, involving the entire epithelium and invasion into the underlying substantia propria.

Disease Course

Overall tumor-related mortality is 25%.

Treatment and Management

- Complete excision of tumor with wide (4 mm) margins, with cryotherapy to the base and adjacent conjunctiva of the lesion.
- Topical mitomycin C has been used to treat residual tumor.
- Workup for presence of systemic metastases with oncologist.

Medications

None.

Follow-Up

Lifelong for recurrence, including palpation of the regional lymph nodes.

Differential Diagnosis

- Ocular melanosis.
- Nevus.
- PAM.
- Foreign body.
- Pigmented deposits.

References

Jakobiec FA, Folberg R, Iwamoto T. Clinicopathological characteristics of premalignant and malignant melanocytic lesions of the conjunctiva. *Ophthalmology* 1989;96:147–166.

Shields CL, Shields JA, Gündüz K, et al. Conjunctival melanoma: risk factors for recurrence, exenteration, metastasis, and death in 150 consecutive patients. *Arch Ophthalmol* 2000;118(11):1497–1507.

Vascular Tumors

Pyogenic Granuloma

Summary

Benign vascular tumor.

Etiology

May occur following inflammation or trauma to the ocular surface. Seen as a postoperative change after strabismus surgery or chalazia incision and drainage.

Signs and Symptoms

Fleshy lump or mass on the conjunctiva.

Demographics

Usually, young individuals.

Ophthalmic Findings

- Bright red mass that is mobile (Figure 1.34).
- Any conjunctival surface may be affected; rarely, this lesion may be found on the cornea.

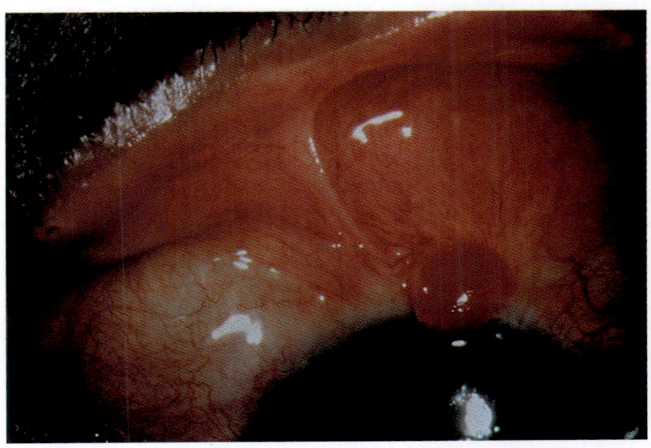

FIGURE 1.34. The red, fleshy, pedunculated mass is a pyogenic granuloma.

Systemic Findings

None.

Special Tests

None.

Pathology

Vascular tumor. Contrary to the name, there is no granuloma formation.

Disease Course

May slowly increase in size.

Treatment and Management

May decrease with topical or intralesional steroids or may be excised for cosmetic reasons.

Medications

Steroids may be used as an alternate to excision.

Follow-Up

None required.

Differential Diagnosis

Kaposi sarcoma occurs in the immunosuppressed population. This is a reddish-bluish vascular conjunctival lesion that may be diffuse or nodular.

Reference

Cameron JA, Mahmod MA. Pyogenic granulomas of the cornea. *Ophthalmology* 1995;102:1681–1687.

Kaposi Sarcoma

Summary

Ocular Kaposi sarcoma is almost exclusively seen in patients immunosuppressed with AIDS. It presents as multiple, discrete, red, painless, slow-growing patches on the conjunctiva.

Etiology

Associated with infection with Kaposi sarcoma–associated herpes virus/human herpes virus 8 (KSHV/HHV-8).

Signs and Symptoms

Painless.
Cosmetically deforming.

Demographics

AIDS patients predominantly, but can be found in other patients immunosuppressed for organ transplantation.

Ophthalmic Findings

Single or multiple discrete flat or elevated red, fleshy nodules.

Systemic Findings

Kaposi sarcoma can also be found on the skin and viscera.

Pathology

Dilated vascular channels within a stroma of spindle cells with mitotic figures.

Disease Course

Slow, gradual enlargement.

Treatment and Management

Observation.
Radiation.
Cryotherapy: discouraged, since it causes scarring.
Surgical excision: may be difficult to determine exact borders.
Systemic immune reconstitution: reports of regression of lesions on highly active antiretroviral therapy (HAART).
Liposomal doxorubicin, interferon α_{2a}: investigational treatments.

Differential Diagnosis

Lymphoma: pink, fleshy lesions, molded to globe.
Subconjunctival hemorrhage: resolves in 1 to 2 weeks.

References

Dugel PU, Gill PS, Frangieh GT, et al. Ocular adnexal Kaposi's sarcoma in acquired immunodeficiency syndrome. *Am J Ophthalmol* 1990;110:500–503.
Shuler JD, Holland GN, Miles SA, et al. Kaposi's sarcoma of the conjunctiva and eyelids associated with the acquired immunodeficiency syndrome. *Arch Ophthalmol* 1988;107:859–862.

Conjunctival Lymphoma and Benign Lymphoid Proliferation

Summary

Conjunctival lymphoid proliferations present as salmon-colored subconjunctival masses. Although often limited to the eye, a systemic workup is important, since 20% of patients develop systemic lymphoma.

Etiology

Proliferation of lymphoid tissue.

Signs and Symptoms

Painless, asymptomatic.

Demographics

Majority of patients are older than 50 years of age at presentation.

Ophthalmic Findings

- Unilateral or bilateral well-demarcated salmon-colored subconjunctival masses (Figure 1.35).
- Freely moveable over underlying sclera.
- No ulceration or scarring of adjacent conjunctiva.

Systemic Findings

Most patients do not have extraocular lymphoma.

Special Tests

Biopsy for special stains for clonality of lymphocytes.

Pathology

Spectrum from small, benign, monotonous lymphocytes to larger, anaplastic cells with mitoses.

Disease Course

- May be difficult to separate benign from malignant lesions without a biopsy.
- Twenty percent of patients subsequently develop systemic lymphoma.

Treatment and Management

- Radiotherapy to lesions.
- Chemotherapy.
- Consultation with oncologist.

Differential Diagnosis

Granuloma: cat scratch disease, Parinaud oculoglandular fever.

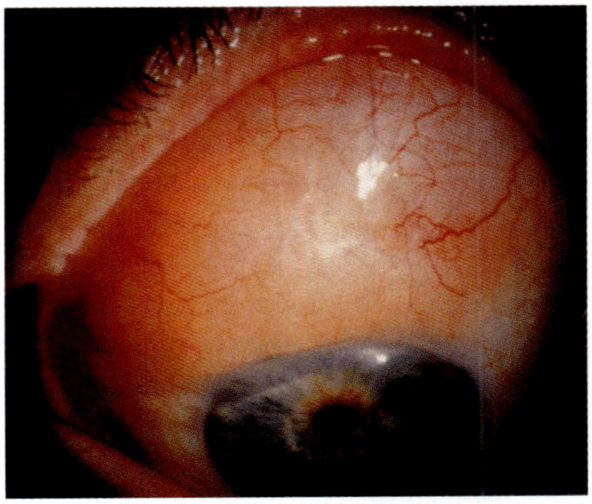

FIGURE 1.35. Lymphoma presenting as a painless salmon-colored mass in the superior fornix.

DEGENERATIONS

Pinguecula

Summary

Pinguecula is a degenerative process of the conjunctiva (usually nasal) caused by sun exposure.

Etiology

UV radiation exposure is presumed to cause excessive production of elastin by conjunctival fibroblasts.

Signs and Symptoms

Redness.
Foreign body sensation.

Demographics

Individuals exposed to UV radiation.

Ophthalmic Findings

- Raised, yellowish-brown nasal conjunctival mass.
- Gelatinous appearance of the affected conjunctiva.
- May progress to a pterygium.
- Freely moveable over underlying sclera.

Systemic Findings

None.

Special Tests

None.

Pathology

- Elastotic degeneration.
- Hyalinization of the subepithelial connective tissue of the substantia propria.
- Diffuse or lobular collections of eosinophilic granular material.
- Increased fibroblasts.

Disease Course

May progress to pterygium.

Treatment and Management

- Artificial tears.
- Nonsteroidal anti-inflammatory drops.
- Mild steroid drops.
- Excision if bothersome.

Medications

See above.

Differential Diagnosis

Episcleritis.
Granuloma.

Reference

Austin P, Jakobiec FA, Iwamoto T. Elastodysplasia and elastodystrophy as the pathologic bases of ocular pterygia and pinguecula. *Ophthalmology* 1983;90:96–109.

Pterygium

Summary

A pterygium describes a fibrovascular degenerative pannus extending from the conjunctiva onto the cornea.

Etiology

UV radiation exposure is presumed to cause excessive production of elastin by conjunctival fibroblasts.

Signs and Symptoms

Foreign body sensation.
Redness.
Decreased vision.

Demographics

- Occurs predominantly in individuals with significant sun exposure.
- Seen more frequently in equatorial populations.

Ophthalmic Findings

Conjunctival injection.
Astigmatism.
Decreased vision.
Localized fibrovascular growth, usually over the nasal cornea (Figure 1.36).
Corneal iron line (Stocker line).

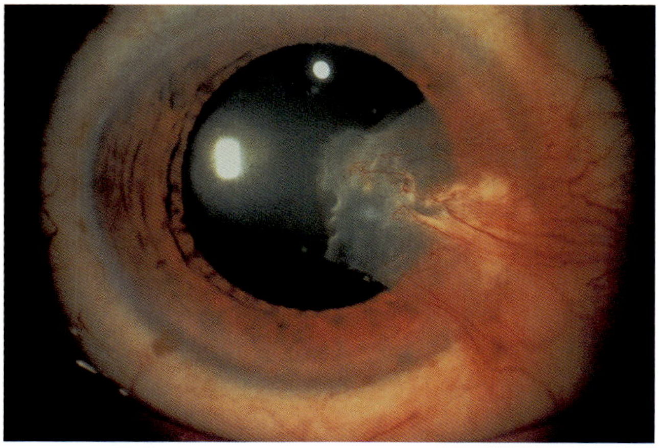

FIGURE 1.36. Typical pterygium encroaching on the central cornea.

Systemic Findings

Actinic changes of the skin.

Special Tests

None.

Pathology

- Elastotic degeneration.
- Hyalinization of the subepithelial connective tissue of the substantia propria.
- Diffuse or lobular collections of eosinophilic granular material.
- Increased fibroblasts.
- Lymphocytic infiltration.

Disease Course

Slowly progressive.

Treatment and Management

- Artificial tears.
- Nonsteroidal anti-inflammatory drops.
- Surgical excision with or without:
  Conjunctival autograft.
  Antimetabolite therapy (mitomycin C).
  Amniotic membrane graft.
  Bare sclera.

Differential Diagnosis

Pseudopterygium.
Squamous cell carcinoma.
CIN.
Fuchs marginal keratitis.

Reference

Hill JC, Maske R. Pathogenesis of pterygium. *Eye* 1989;3(Pt 2): 218–226.

Spheroidal Degeneration

Other names: Labrador keratopathy, climatic droplet keratopathy, Bietti nodular dystrophy, corneal elastosis.

Summary

This is a degeneration of the cornea consisting of yellowish-brownish proteinaceous deposits in the anterior stroma with extension onto the conjunctiva.

Etiology

Deposition of extracellular protein thought to be a result of actinic exposure, genetic predisposition, and age.

Signs and Symptoms

Irritation.
Blurred vision.

Demographics

- More common in male patients.
- More common in individuals with increased exposure to sun and wind.

Ophthalmic Findings

- Injection.
- Decreased acuity if severe.
- Often bilateral.
- Yellow-brown deposits in the superficial stroma, usually in interpalpebral fissure.
- May extend onto the conjunctiva.

Systemic Findings

None.

Special Tests

None.

Pathology

Extracellular proteinaceous deposits.

Treatment and Management

- Superficial keratectomy.
- PKP.

Medications

Lubricants.

Differential Diagnosis

- Salzmann nodular degeneration.
- Phlyctenulosis.

Reference

Gray RH, Johnson GT, Freedman A. Climatic droplet keratopathy. *Surv Ophthalmol* 1992;36:241–253.

Salzmann Nodular Degeneration

Summary

The condition of Salzmann nodular degeneration is seen in cases of long-standing keratitis or corneal irritation secondary to entities such as trachoma, interstitial keratitis, or phlyctenulosis. It is noninflammatory and consists of bluish or gray-white elevated subepithelial nodules located paracentrally.

Etiology

Unclear origin, but it is thought to be a response to long-standing irritation.

Signs and Symptoms

- Irritation.
- Pain if recurrent erosions occur.
- Decreased visual acuity.

Demographics

- More common in women.
- More common in middle-aged and older patients.

Ophthalmic Findings

- Gray or bluish subepithelial nodules (Figure 1.37).
- Recurrent erosion syndrome.
- No vascularization.
- Paracentral location often grouped circularly.

Systemic Findings

Possible systemic findings associated with trachoma or causes of interstitial keratitis.

Special Tests

None.

Pathology

Histologic study shows hyaline and fibrillar material replacement of Bowman membrane.

Disease Course

- Recurrent erosions can cause persistent irritation.
- Can encroach upon visual axis.

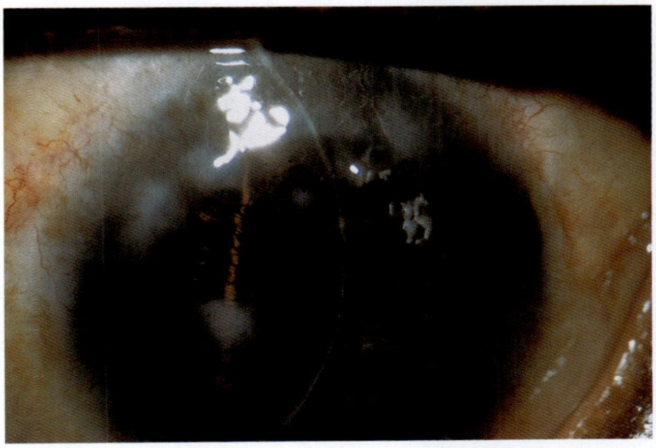

FIGURE 1.37. Multiple gray, elevated subepithelial nodules in Salzmann nodular degeneration.

Treatment and Management

Superficial keratectomy.
Lamellar keratoplasty.

Medications

Lubricating drops.

Reference

Wood TO. Salzmann's nodular degeneration. *Cornea* 1990;9:17–22.

Band Keratopathy

Summary

Band keratopathy, a degenerative change of the cornea, has many causes and is characterized by gray, plaquelike depositions of calcium hydroxyapatite in the superficial cornea, usually within the interpalpebral fissure. It begins peripherally and with progression coalesces to form a band of calcium across the cornea.

Etiology

Common: chronic ocular inflammation (juvenile idiopathic arthritis [JIA], HSV/varicella-zoster virus [VZV], pars planitis, Fuchs heterochromic iridocyclitis), silicone oil.
Rare: hypercalcemia, genetic predisposition, renal failure, chronic exposure to mercurial vapors.

Signs and Symptoms

Pain if erosions develop over calcified areas.
Blurred vision.

Demographics

No age predilection.

Ophthalmic Findings

- Injection.
- Decreased acuity.
- Band of calcific plaques in Bowman layer and anterior stroma in the interpalpebral fissure (Figure 1.38).
- Epithelial defects over calcium deposits.

Systemic Findings

Look for signs or causes of hypercalcemia.

Pathology

Early changes can be seen histologically as a fine basophilic deposition in Bowman membrane.

Disease Course

Progressive.

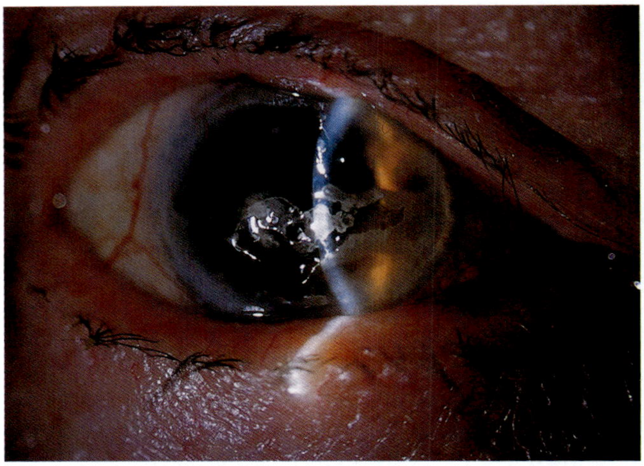

FIGURE 1.38. White calcific deposits and epithelial defect in the interpalpebral fissure in a patient with chronic uveitis.

Treatment and Management

Superficial keratectomy in conjunction with chelation with disodium ethylenediaminetetraacetate (EDTA).

Medications

Chelation with EDTA.

Reference

Braverman DE, Snyder WE. A case report and review of band keratopathy. *Metab Pediatr Syst Ophthalmol* 1987;10:39–41.

Dellen

Summary

Dellen are small elliptical excavations at the margin of the cornea that occur most often adjacent to the site of a paralimbal elevation, which causes an abnormality of the tear film and subsequent drying and thinning of the underlying cornea.

Etiology

Suspected to be caused by a localized disruption of the tear film adjacent to an area of elevation.

Signs and Symptoms

Redness.
Irritation.
Foreign body sensation.

Demographics

No age or race predilection.

Ophthalmic Findings

- No vascularization.
- Paralimbal elevation.

- Filtering bleb.
- Scleritis.
- Conjunctival mass.
- Elliptical or saucerlike depression of the peripheral cornea.
- May have overlying epithelial defect and cellular infiltrate.
- Pseudodescemetocele.

Systemic Findings

None.

Special Tests

None.

Pathology

Compacted epithelium and corneal stroma.

Disease Course

Improves with rehydration.

Treatment and Management

- Reduce paralimbal elevation if possible.
- Rehydrate cornea.

Medications

- Artificial tears and ointment.
- Antibiotics if epithelial defect is present.

Follow-Up

Routine based on degree of epithelial defect.

Differential Diagnosis

Corneal scar.
Old phlyctenule.

References

Baum J. Dellen or pseudodellen. *Cornea* 1990;9:182.
Baum JL, Mishima S, Boruchoff SA. On the nature of dellen. *Arch Ophthalmol* 1968;79:657–662.

Terrien Marginal Degeneration

Summary

Terrien marginal degeneration is a slowly progressive noninflammatory peripheral thinning of the cornea.

Etiology

Idiopathic.

Signs and Symptoms

Usually none.

Demographics

- No sex predilection.
- Occurs in the teens and twenties.

Ophthalmic Findings

- Against-the-rule astigmatism.
- Superficial vascularization.
- Leading edge of lipid deposition (Figure 1.39).
- Begins superiorly and spreads circumferentially.
- Steep medial edge of degeneration.
- Epithelium is intact.
- Perforation rare.

Systemic Findings

None.

Special Tests

None.

Pathology

Histiocytes possibly responsible for phagocytosis of collagen.

Disease Course

Slowly progressive, can progress to perforation.

Treatment and Management

Often no treatment is necessary. Tissue adhesive, full-thickness corneoscleral graft or lamellar patch graft for perforation or severe ectasia.

Medications

None.

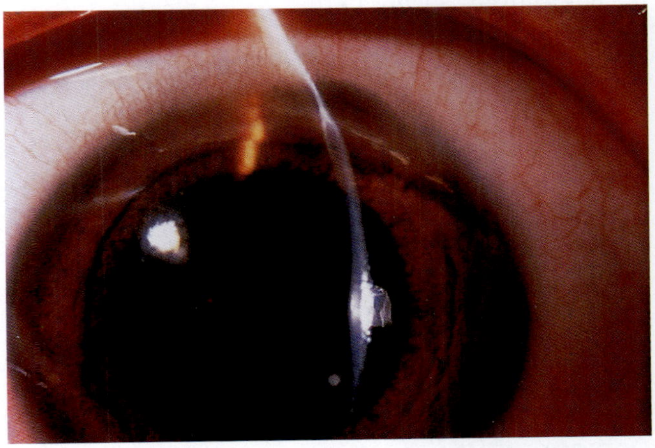

FIGURE 1.39. Superior thinning and superficial neovascularization of the cornea in Terrien marginal degeneration. Lipid is deposited along the leading border of the vessels.

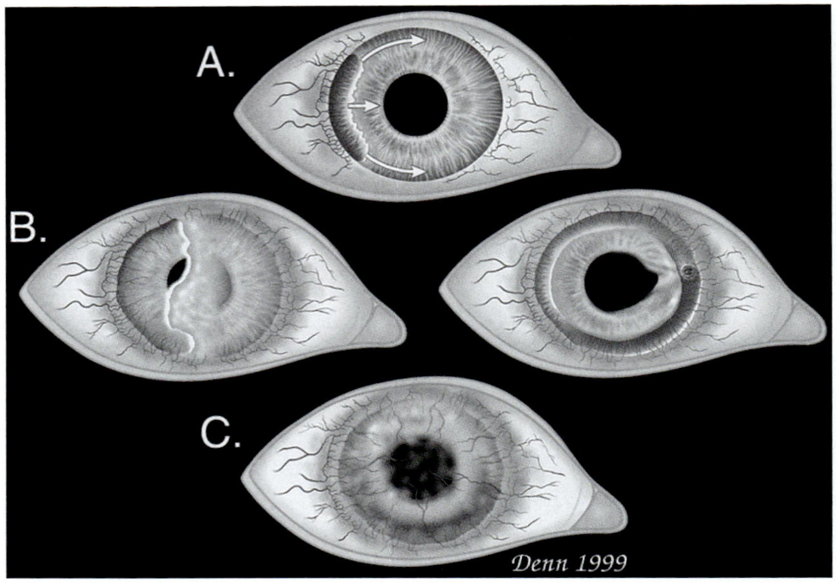

FIGURE 1.40. **A:** Mooren ulcer. Arrows indicate that progression may proceed in a circumferential or transverse manner. **B: Left,** transverse progression. **Right,** circumferential progression with a performation. **C:** End-stage Mooren ulcer with complete destruction of the corneal stroma. (From Zegans ME, Srinivasan M. Mooren's ulcer. *Int Ophthalmol Clin* 1998;38:81–88, with permission.).

Differential Diagnosis

- Furrow marginal degeneration.
- Pellucid marginal degeneration.

References

Binder PS, Zavala EY, Stainer GA. Noninfectious peripheral corneal ulceration: Mooren's ulcer or Terrien's marginal degeneration? *Ann Ophthalmol* 1982;14:425–426, 428–429, 432–435.

Krachmer JH, Feder RS, Belin MW. Keratoconus and related noninflammatory corneal thinning disorders. *Surv Ophthalmol* 1984;28:293–322.

Mooren Ulcer

Summary

A rare, idiopathic, painful ulceration of the peripheral cornea that may affect one or both eyes either simultaneously or consecutively (Figure 1.40).

Etiology

- Idiopathic.
- Several associations have been proposed, including prior ocular trauma, infection and surgery, helminth infection, and hepatitis C virus. There is limited and sometimes contradictory evidence regarding these associations.

Sign and Symptoms

Painful red eye.
Decreased vision.

Demographics

- Slight male preponderance.
- Any age, but most older than 35 years.

Ophthalmic Findings

- Unilateral disease most common.
- Peripheral ulceration of the cornea begins at the limbus with blood vessels extending into the area of ulceration.
- The central corneal edge of the ulcer is undermined, creating an overhanging edge (Figure 1.41).
- Opacities in the cornea central to the ulcer.
- The ulcer may progress in a circumferential or transverse manner.
- Eventually, complete destruction of the corneal stroma may occur.
- Perforation may occur at any stage of the disease.
- Necrotizing scleritis does not occur.

Systemic Findings

None.

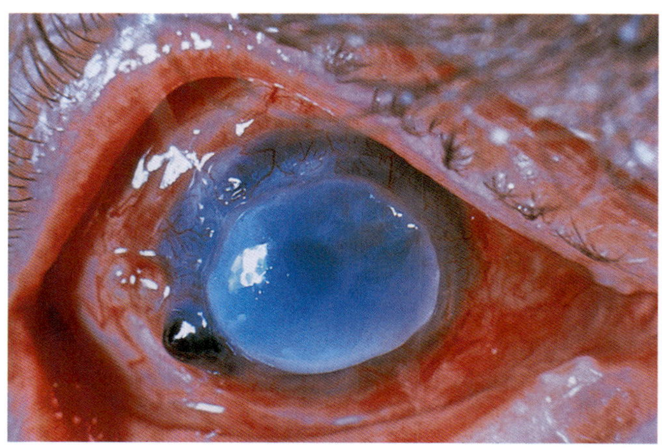

FIGURE 1.41. Mooren ulcer with circumferential corneal ulceration and an undermined leading edge centrally.

Special Tests

Since Mooren ulcer may be confused with peripheral ulcerative keratitis secondary to collagen-vascular diseases including rheumatoid arthritis, Wegener granulomatosis, polyarteritis nodosa (or microvascular polyangititis), and SLE, a complete history and examination focused on these entities should be performed. Antinuclear antibodies (ANA), antineutrophil cytoplasmic antibodies (ANCA), rheumatoid factor (RF), and anti-cyclic citrullinated peptide antibody (Anti-CCP) are helpful in excluding the presence of these rheumatic diseases.

Pathology

Mixed inflammatory cell infiltrate in the limbal conjunctiva and cornea with necrosis and disorganization of the stromal lamella.

Disease Course

Wide variation in the natural history of the disease ranging from limited peripheral thinning without any loss of vision to perforation of the cornea and complete loss of vision.

Treatment and Management

- Best treatment is controversial, but treatment generally begins with topical prednisolone acetate and conjunctival resection.
- In severe or bilateral cases, treatment with oral steroid and cytotoxic agents may be necessary.

Medications

Prednisolone acetate, prednisone, cyclophosphamide.

Differential Diagnosis

- Infectious keratitis (bacterial and herpetic infection).
- Autoimmune disorders (rheumatoid arthritis, Wegener granulomatosis, polyarteritis nodosa, SLE, relapsing polychondritis).
- Staphylococcal marginal disease, acne rosacea, radiation exposure, and mitomycin C exposure.

References

Brown SI, Mondino BJ. Therapy of Mooren's ulcer. *Am J Ophthalmol* 1984;98:1–6.

Lewallen S, Courtright P. Problems with current concepts of the epidemiology of Mooren's corneal ulcer. *Ann Ophthalmol* 1990;22:52–55.

Mooren A. *Ophthalmologische beobachturges 107*. Berlin, Germany: A Hirshwald, 1867.

Tauber J, Sainz de la Maza M, Hoang-Xuan T, et al. An analysis of therapeutic decision making regarding immunosuppressive chemotherapy for peripheral ulcerative keratitis. *Cornea* 1990;9:66–73.

Wang QS, Yuan J, Zhou SY, et al. Chronic hepatitis C virus infection is not associated with Mooren's ulcer. *Eye (Lond)* 2008;22(5):697–700. [Epub 2007 Jul 6.]

Wilson SE, Lee WM, Murakami C, et al. Mooren-type hepatitis C virus-associated corneal ulceration. *Ophthalmology* 1994;101:736–745.

Peripheral Ulcerative Keratitis Associated with Systemic Autoimmune Diseases

Summary

Ulceration of the peripheral cornea in association with an underlying autoimmune disease such as rheumatoid arthritis, Wegener granulomatosis, SLE, polyarterititis nodosa, and relapsing polychrondritis. Rheumatoid arthritis is the systemic condition most commonly associated with peripheral ulcerative keratitis.

Etiology

Autoimmune.

Signs and Symptoms

- Decreased vision often accompanied by a painful red eye.
- Occasionally symptoms may be minimal.

Demographics

- Patients with autoimmune disease.
- May be the first presentation of their autoimmune disease.

Ophthalmic Findings

- Peripheral ulceration of the cornea (Figure 1.42).
- Varying amounts of associated conjunctival and scleral inflammation.

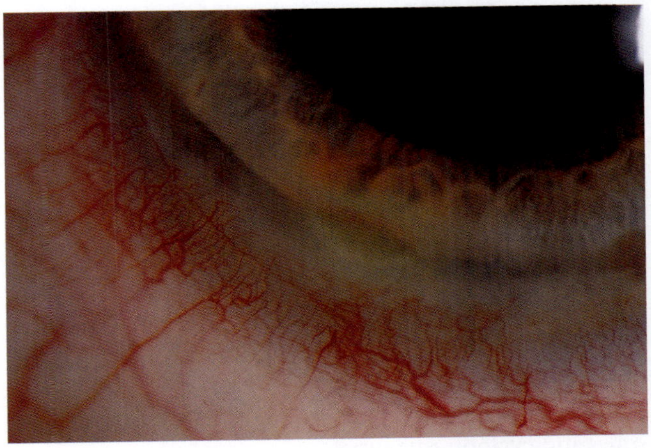

FIGURE 1.42. Inflammation of the peripheral cornea and adjacent sclera with loss of corneal substance in a patient with Wegener granulomatosis.

- There may be an uninvolved area of cornea between the limbus and the ulcer.
- Adjacent necrotizing scleritis.
- Anterior chamber reaction.
- Perforation of the cornea in severe cases.

Systemic Findings

Specific to the underlying condition (e.g., sinusitis [Wegener granulomatosis], inflammation of the ear cartilage [relapsing polychondritis]).

Special Tests

ANA: present in most patients with SLE.

ANCA: present in most patients with Wegener granulomatosis and many patients with polyarteritis nodosa.

RF: present in most patients with rheumatoid arthritis.

Anti-CCP: in the majority of patients with RA and a higher specificity than RF.

Urinalysis: Presence of red blood cells in the urine may suggest presence of vasculitis.

By themselves, none of these serologic markers confirms the diagnosis of an autoimmune disorder; however, if they are negative, it is unlikely that such a condition is present.

Pathology

Varies with the condition.

Disease Course

- Depends on the severity of the inflammation.
- Ranges from little effect on vision to perforation and complete loss of vision.
- Patients with peripheral ulcerative keratitis and an associated systemic autoimmune disease may be at increased risk for severe inflammation in other organ systems.

Treatment and Management

- Mild cases: topical steroids and conjunctival resection. Local measures alone are usually inadequate.
- Severe ocular cases or systemic autoimmune activity: systemic steroid, cytotoxic agents, and immunologic agents such as infliximab.
- Consultation with a rheumatologist should be obtained in all patients suspected of having peripheral ulcerative keratitis.
- Associated with a systemic autoimmune condition.

Medications

Topical prednisolone acetate, oral and intravenous prednisone, and cyclophosphamide.

Differential Diagnosis

Infectious keratitis (bacterial and herpetic infection), Mooren ulcer, staphylococcal marginal disease, acne rosacea, radiation exposure, and mitomycin C exposure.

References

Dana MR, Qian Y, Hamrah P. Twenty-five-year panorama of corneal immunology: emerging concepts in the immunopathogenesis of microbial keratitis, peripheral ulcerative keratitis, and corneal transplant rejection. *Cornea* 2000;19(5):625–643.

Forster CS, Forstot SL, Wilson LA. Mortality rate in rheumatoid arthritis patients developing necrotizing scleritis or peripheral ulcerative keratitis: effects of systemic immunosuppression. *Ophthalmology* 1984;91:1253–1263.

Gregory JK, Watson CS. Peripheral ulcerative keratitis in the collagen vascular diseases. *Int Clin Ophthalmol* 1996;36:21–30.

Murphy CC, Ayliffe WH, Booth A, et al.Tumor necrosis factor alpha blockade with infliximab for refractory uveitis and scleritis. *Ophthalmology* 2004;111(2):352–356.

Tauber J, Sainz de la Maza M, Hoang-Xuan T, et al. An analysis of therapeutic decision making regarding immunosuppressive chemotherapy for peripheral ulcerative keratitis. *Cornea* 1990;9:66–73.

CORNEAL DYSTROPHIES

The corneal dystrophies are a group of inherited disorders generally affecting the central cornea, with no signs of inflammation or vascularization. They are bilateral conditions that usually affect a single corneal layer, which provides for anatomic classification within the group. There is usually no systemic or other ocular abnormality, and the conditions are slowly progressive. These features are common to the group and serve to distinguish dystrophies from other corneal entities. The size and distribution of the opacities can often be helpful in classifying these conditions (Figure 1.43).

Anterior Cornea

Corneal Epithelial Basement Membrane Dystrophy

Summary

Epithelial basement membrane dystrophy (EBMD) is the most common dystrophy affecting the epithelium and anterior basement membrane. Patients are usually asymptomatic but can develop recurrent erosions over affected areas. Also known as map-dot-fingerprint dystrophy, anterior basement membrane dystrophy, and Cogan microcystic dystrophy.

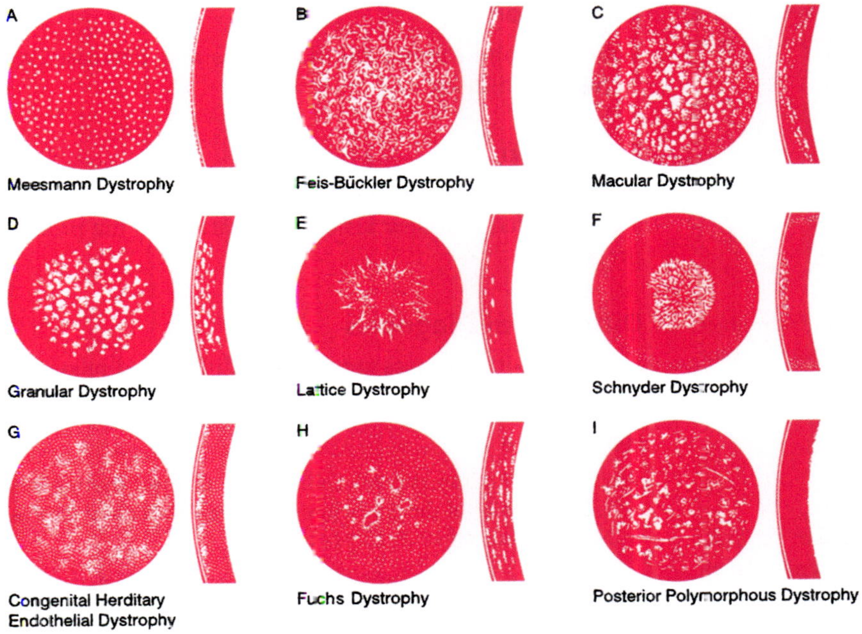

FIGURE 1.43. Patterns of the opacities in the corneal dystrophies. *En face* and corneal cross sections demonstrating the typical location of the opacities.

Etiology

Autosomal dominant or sporadic. There is an abnormality of basement membrane adhesion complex formation by dystrophic epithelial cells.

Signs and Symptoms

Recurrent erosions, marked by pain, tearing, and photophobia. Blurred vision may occur that is due to astigmatism of an irregular corneal surface.

Demographics

None specific. This is the most common corneal dystrophy.

Ophthalmic Findings

Maps (gray geographic opacities), dots (cysts), and fingerprints (fine linear subepithelial ridges) are present but may be subtle and may be best seen on retroillumination. Recurrent erosions are seen, as is epithelial breakdown with minor trauma.

Systemic Findings

None.

Special Tests

None.

Pathology

Thickened aberrant basement membrane material is present. Maps are fibrous plaques of accumulated subepithelial basement membrane and collagen. Dots are cysts of desquamated epithelial cells caught within the layers of the epithelium. Fingerprints are aberrant basement membrane material within the epithelium.

Disease Course

Chronic exacerbations and remissions.

Treatment and Management

- Artificial tears and hypertonic sodium chloride drops may be useful to help the epithelium adhere to the basement membrane.
- Erosions are managed with patching or bandage contact lenses in conjunction with topical antibiotics and cycloplegics until healed.
- Stromal micropuncture, creating small punctures and resultant scars through basement membrane into Bowman layer, helps epithelium adherence and should be considered for treatment of selected areas off the visual axis where erosions are occurring frequently.
- More recently, the excimer laser has been used, as there seems to be a firmer adhesion of epithelium to stroma after treatment. This is preferable to micropuncture for involved areas within the visual axis.

Medications

Lubricants and sodium chloride drops may decrease erosions in mild cases.

Follow-Up

Erosions must be closely followed until healed. Documentation of the location of the erosion is important to guide interventional therapy. Regular examinations are of limited utility, but patients should be encouraged to report erosions promptly.

Differential Diagnosis

Recurrent erosions may also occur with other corneal dystrophies, and in areas of previous trauma.

Reference

Waring GO, Rodriques MM, Laibson PR. Corneal dystrophies, I: dystrophies of the epithelium, Bowman's layer and stroma. *Surv Ophthalmol* 1978;23:71–122.

Reis-Bucklers Dystrophy

Summary

Reis-Bucklers corneal dystrophy is characterized by reticular opacities in the anterior cornea, specifically, Bowman layer.

Etiology

Autosomal dominant. Gene is *TGFBI*.

Signs and Symptoms

Recurrent erosions and decreased vision that is due to surface irregularity, and eventually, scarring.

Demographics

Appears in first or second decade of life.

Ophthalmic Findings

Subepithelial blue-gray reticular opacities form a honeycomb-like pattern that is most dense in the midperipheral cornea.

Systemic Findings

None.

Special Tests

None.

Pathology

Bowman layer is replaced with a fibrocellular material.

Disease Course

Slowly progressive. Erosions eventually diminish as scar tissue forms, with a resultant decrease in acuity.

Treatment and Management

Erosions are followed until healed. Superficial keratectomy, surgically or with the excimer laser, may be sufficient to remove superficial scarring.

Medications

Lubricants and sodium chloride drops may decrease erosions in mild cases.

Follow-Up

Erosions are followed until healed. Regular examinations are scheduled to follow vision and scarring as the process progresses.

Differential Diagnosis

Scars from other causes are rarely as diffuse and bilateral.

Reference

Waring GO, Rodriques MM, Laibson PR. Corneal dystrophies, I: Dystrophies of the epithelium, Bowman's layer and stroma. *Surv Ophthalmol* 1978;23:71–122.

Meesman Dystrophy

Summary

Meesman corneal dystrophy is an extremely rare epithelial dystrophy in which tiny, clear cysts can be found diffusely throughout the epithelium.

Etiology

Autosomal dominant defects in keratin genes.

Signs and Symptoms

- Can be asymptomatic.
- Erosions, blurred vision, and mildly decreased acuity resulting from irregular astigmatism and surface irregularity.

Demographics

Slit-lamp findings appear in the first decade of life; symptoms appear in the fourth or fifth decade.

Ophthalmic Findings

Clear epithelial cysts or vesicles are best seen in retroillumination.

Systemic Findings

None.

Special Tests

None.

Pathology

An extracellular material previously named "peculiar substance" is present. It is a periodic acid–Schiff (PAS)-positive material of unknown composition. Intracytoplasmic fibrogranular material is present, as are thickening of the basement membrane and epithelium and intraepithelial cysts.

Disease Course

Slowly progressive.

Treatment and Management

Erosions are managed with patching or bandage contact lenses in conjunction with topical antibiotics and cycloplegics until healed.

Medications

Lubricants and sodium chloride drops may decrease erosions.

Differential Diagnosis

Other corneal dystrophies.

Reference

Waring GO, Rodriques MM, Laibson PR. Corneal dystrophies, I: dystrophies of the epithelium, Bowman's layer and stroma. *Surv Ophthalmol* 1978;23:71–122.

Stromal Dystrophies

Granular Dystrophy, Type 1

Summary

Granular stromal dystrophy, type 1 is an autosomal dominantly inherited dystrophy in which multiple discrete white deposits develop throughout the stroma. Visual acuity is good in most cases. Type 2 granular corneal dystrophy (or Avellino corneal dystrophy) is characterized by having findings similar to both granular and lattice dystrophies.

Etiology

Autosomal dominant, with onset in early adolescence. Gene: *TGFBI*

Signs and Symptoms

Generally no erosions. Vision is stable until late in the course.

Demographics

Slit-lamp findings appear in the first decade of life; symptoms begin in midlife.

Ophthalmic Findings

Discrete white anterior stromal deposits that look like bread crumbs, snowflakes, or cigarette ash with intervening clear spaces. They begin in the superficial stroma and later extend more deeply (Figure 1.44).

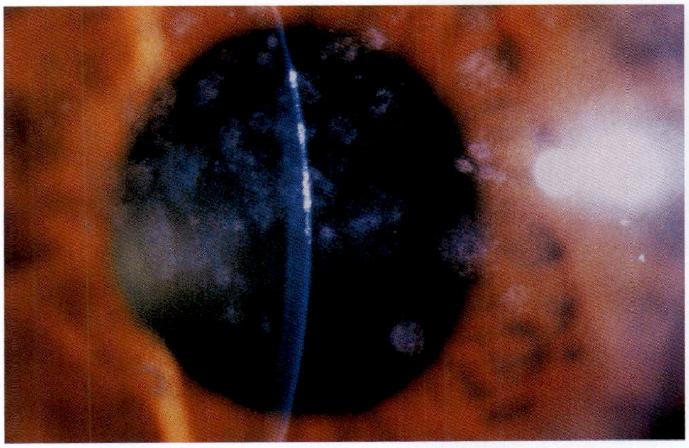

FIGURE 1.44. Granular corneal dystrophy. In this condition, the crystals are scattered throughout the corneal stroma and are most prominent centrally. The intervening stroma is clear.

Systemic Findings

None.

Special Tests

None.

Pathology

Deposition of a hyaline material, which stains red with Masson trichrome stain.

Disease Course

Slowly progressive in terms of the number, density, and depth of lesions. Vision gradually decreases but remains surprisingly good, despite numerous deposits.

Treatment and Management

Superficial keratectomy (surgical or excimer laser) is recommended to decrease the number and density of deposits as required based on visual acuity, but PKP may be required eventually.

Medications

None.

Follow-Up

Regular examinations to monitor vision are encouraged.

Differential Diagnosis

Other stromal dystrophies.

Reference

Waring GO, Rodriques MM, Laibson PR. Corneal dystrophies, I: dystrophies of the epithelium, Bowman's layer and stroma. *Surv Ophthalmol* 1978;23:71–122.

CORNEA

Lattice Dystrophy

Summary

Lattice stromal dystrophy is an autosomal dominant inherited dystrophy in which amyloid material is deposited in the stroma forming linear opacities.

Etiology

Autosomal dominant, with onset in early adolescence.
Gene: *TGFBI*.

Signs and Symptoms

Recurrent erosions. Vision usually begins to decrease by 20 to 40 years of age.

Demographics

Onset in early adolescence.

Ophthalmic Findings

Grayish, branching refractile lines are seen to be white with direct illumination and translucent on retroillumination. They are most prominent centrally and progress to the periphery, where small dots may also be seen (Figure 1.45).

Systemic Findings

Lattice corneal dystrophy, gelsolin type or type II lattice dystrophy, or Meretoja syndrome has systemic amyloidosis in association with corneal findings. Cranial and peripheral neuropathies are present, as are skin changes. A masklike face is characteristic. This is not a true corneal dystrophy.

Special Tests

None.

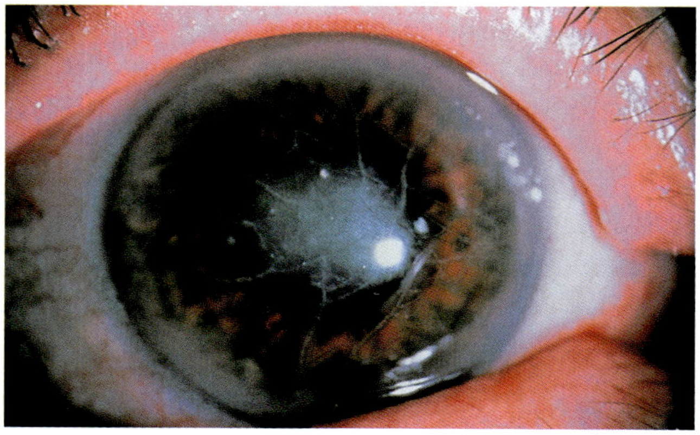

FIGURE 1.45. Lattice dystrophy. The lattice lines represent amyloid deposition within the stroma. The intervening stroma is clear.

Pathology

Deposition of amyloid, which stains with Congo red stain and demonstrates birefringence and dichromism.

Disease Course

Slowly progressive.

Treatment and Management

Erosions are managed with patching or bandage contact lenses in conjunction with topical antibiotics and cycloplegics until healed. Superficial keratectomy (surgical or excimer laser) or PKP may be required eventually for vision.

Medications

None.

Follow-Up

Erosions must be closely followed until healed. Regular examinations to monitor vision are encouraged.

Differential Diagnosis

Other stromal dystrophies.

Reference

Waring GO, Rodriques MM, Laibson PR. Corneal dystrophies, I: dystrophies of the epithelium, Bowman's layer and stroma. *Surv Ophthalmol* 1978;23:71–122.

Macular Dystrophy

Summary

Macular corneal dystrophy is the least common of the three major stromal dystrophies. Deposition of mucopolysaccharides in the stroma causes diffuse clouding of the cornea with scattered areas of denser opacities.

Etiology

Autosomal recessive, with onset in the first decade.
Gene: carbohydrate sulfotransferase 6 gene (*CHST6*)

Signs and Symptoms

Mild recurrent erosions. Vision usually begins to decrease between 10 and 30 years.

Demographics

Onset in early adulthood.

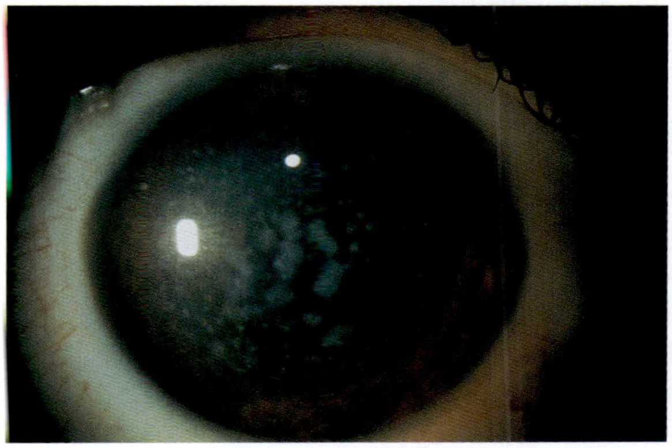

FIGURE 1.46. Macular corneal dystrophy. The cornea is diffusely cloudy, in contrast to granular and lattice dystrophies, with indistinct areas of denser opacification.

Ophthalmic Findings

Gray-white stromal opacities with superficial clouding between the opacities, which may involve full-thickness stroma and other corneal layers (Figure 1.46).

Systemic Findings

None.

Special Tests

None.

Pathology

Accumulation of glycosaminoglycans, leading to localized deposition of acid mucopolysaccharide and abnormal keratin sulfate. The mucopolysaccharide stains with Alcian blue and colloidal iron stains.

Disease Course

Slowly progressive.

Treatment and Management

Erosions are managed with patching or bandage contact lenses in conjunction with topical antibiotics and cycloplegics until healed. PKP may be required eventually for vision.

Medications

None.

Follow-Up

Erosions must be closely followed until healed. Regular examinations to monitor vision are encouraged.

Differential Diagnosis

Other stromal dystrophies.

Reference

Waring GO, Rodriques MM, Laibson PR. Corneal dystrophies, I: dystrophies of the epithelium, Bowman's layer and stroma. *Surv Ophthalmol* 1978;23:71–122.

Schnyder Corneal Dystrophy

Summary

Also known as central crystalline dystrophy of Schnyder; an avascular ring of lipid crystals accumulates in the central cornea. Patients may have systemic hyperlipidemia and a prominent arcus senilis.

Etiology

Autosomal dominant.

Gene: UbiA prenyltransferase domain containing 1 (*UBIAD1*)

Signs and Symptoms

Often, none. Vision is good until late in the course.

Demographics

None specific.

Ophthalmic Findings

- Diffuse, stromal haze, decreasing visual acuity worsening with age.
- In 50% fine yellow-white polychromatic stromal crystals are found in the central anterior stroma (Figure 1.47).
- Corneal arcus and limbal girdle of Vogt are seen in association with the crystals.

Systemic Findings

- Hyperlipidemia and cholesterolemia may be present.

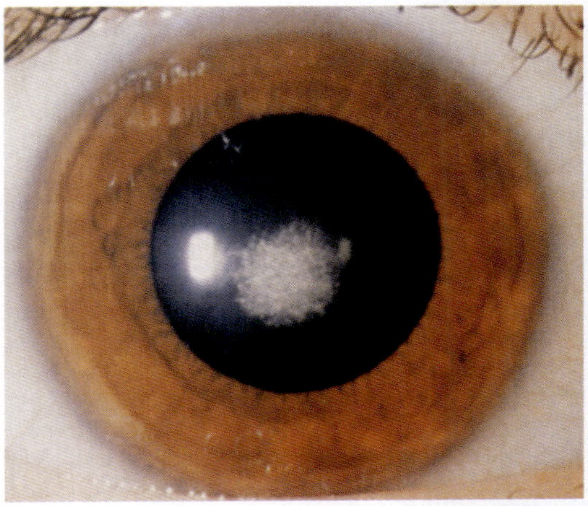

FIGURE 1.47. Characteristic central stromal crystals in Schnyder crystalline corneal dystrophy. The crystals are confined to the stroma. This patient's fellow eye had a similar appearance.

- Genu valgum may also be present, a deformity in which the knees are abnormally close together and the space between the ankles is increased ("knock-knee").

Special Tests

Blood lipid studies should be undertaken.

Pathology

Neutral fats and cholesterol are present in keratocytes and within the stroma among collagen fibrils.

Disease Course

Generally stable.

Treatment and Management

PKP is rarely required.

Medications

None.

Follow-Up

Periodic examinations for vision are recommended.

Differential Diagnosis

Crystalline deposits may be seen bilaterally with cystinosis, gout, multiple myeloma, Bietti tapetoretinal degeneration, and gold and thioridazine (Mellaril) toxicity. Systemic evaluation may be required if a family history of corneal dystrophy is absent. Unilateral focal crystals may be seen in infectious crystalline keratitis (ICK), frequently attributable to *Streptococcus viridans* infection.

Fleck Dystrophy

Summary

Fleck corneal dystrophy is a rare dystrophy in which diffuse comma-shaped opacities can be seen in the corneal stroma.

Etiology

Autosomal dominant.

Signs and Symptoms

None. Vision is unaffected.

Demographics

Rare.

Ophthalmic Findings

Subtle grayish specks that may extend into all layers. Under high magnification, specks are seen as rings with relatively less opacified centers.

Systemic Findings

None.

Special Tests

None.

Pathology

Keratocytes have intracytoplasmic vacuoles of glycosaminoglycans and lipids.

Disease Course

Stable.

Treatment and Management

None.

Medications

None.

Follow-Up

Periodic examination.

Differential Diagnosis

Other dystrophies.

Reference

Purcell JJ, Krachmer JH, Weineist TA. Fleck corneal dystrophy. *Arch Ophthalmol* 1977;95:440–444.

Posterior Cornea

Fuchs Corneal Dystrophy

Summary

Fuchs corneal dystrophy is a common disorder in which guttae develop along Descemet membrane, accompanied by loss of endothelial cells. As endothelial cells are lost, the cornea becomes edematous and cloudy.

Etiology

Autosomal dominant, with onset in later life.

Signs and Symptoms

Glare and blurred vision, often described as worse in the morning, attributable to corneal edema. Late in disease course, pain may be reported as a result of ruptured bullae.

Demographics

Most commonly noted in older women.

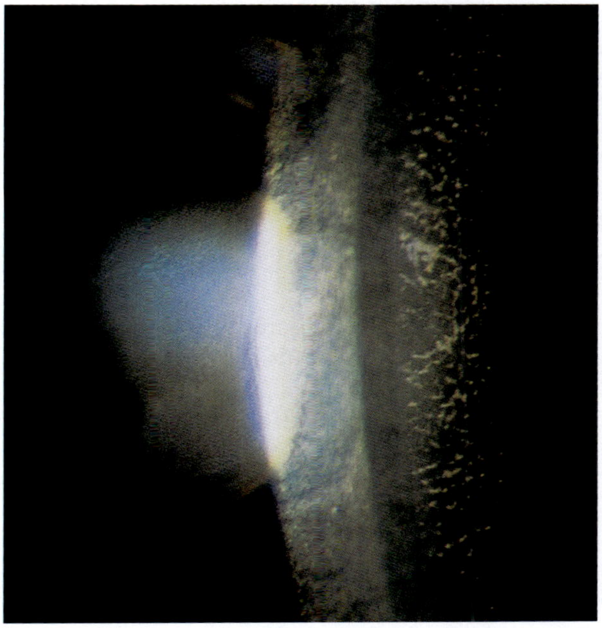

FIGURE 1.48. Slit-lamp photograph of a patient with Fuchs dystrophy. The endothelial reflex has a beaten-metal appearance centrally, and the stroma is diffusely edematous.

Ophthalmic Findings

- Diagnostic finding is that of confluent guttae on the endothelium, which may be pigmented (Figure 1.48).
- As disease progresses, corneal edema and epithelial bullae become present.
- Subepithelial scarring may develop as bullae rupture and heal.

Systemic Findings

None.

Special Tests

Specular microscopy to study the endothelial cells is helpful, and shows guttae as black spots. Serial pachymetry to assess degree of corneal edema and endothelial cell dysfunction.

Pathology

Endothelial cells become attenuated and diminished in number. Thickening of Descemet membrane and anvil-shaped focal excrescences (seen clinically as guttae) are diagnostic.

Disease Course

Slowly progressive to corneal edema. Progression may be accelerated by cataract surgery.

Treatment and Management

Initially, hypertonic sodium chloride drops and ointments and warm air from a hair dryer over the ocular surface may help corneal edema. Bullae should be managed as an abrasion or erosion, with antibiotic prophylaxis until healed. Eventually pain and decreased vision necessitate PKP or endothelial keratoplasty. Combined keratoplasty and cataract surgery should be undertaken together, if corneal edema is present when cataract surgery is contemplated.

Medications

Sodium chloride drops and ointments and medical reduction of intraocular pressure (IOP) often help mild corneal edema.

Follow-Up

Regular examinations for vision, edema, and IOP management.

Differential Diagnosis

Other causes of corneal edema must be considered but lack guttae.

Reference

Waring GO, Rodriques MM, Laibson PR. Corneal dystrophies, II: endothelial dystrophies. *Surv Ophthalmol* 1978;23:147–168.

Posterior Polymorphous Corneal Dystrophy

Summary

Bilateral corneal dystrophy affecting the posterior cornea in which the endothelium becomes multilayered and develops epithelial features.

Etiology

Autosomal dominant. May be related to abnormal development or differentiation of neural crest tissues.

Signs and Symptoms

Generally none.

Demographics

No particular group.

Ophthalmic Findings

Polymorphous opacities at the level of Descemet membrane are evident as vesicles or broad bands with irregular scalloped edges. There may be iris abnormalities, iridocorneal adhesion, ectopic pupil, glaucoma, and other anterior segment abnormalities.

Systemic Findings

None.

Special Tests

Specular microscopy to study endothelial cells may be helpful.

Pathology

Endothelial cells morphologically and immunopathologically resemble epithelial cells: they contain keratin, desmosomes, microvilli, and some fibroblast properties.

Disease Course

Stationary or slowly progressive, generally with normal vision. Rarely, endothelial decompensation may result in corneal edema.

Treatment and Management

Periodic observation and glaucoma management as necessary.

Medications

None specifically.

Follow-Up

Periodic examination for IOP and assessment of corneal edema.

Differential Diagnosis

ICE syndromes, which show similar anterior segment abnormalities but tend to be unilateral, occur in young women, and have no inheritance pattern.

References

Waring GO, Rodriques MM, Laibson PR. Corneal dystrophies, II: endothelial dystrophies. *Surv Ophthalmol* 1978;23:147–168.

Weiss JS, Møller HU, Lisch W, et al. The IC3D classification of the corneal dystrophies. *Cornea* 2008;27(Suppl 2):S1–S83.

Ectatic Disorders

Keratoconus

Summary

Bilateral noninflammatory ectasia of the cornea, marked by central or paracentral thinning with protrusion of the resulting cone.

Etiology

Unknown.

Signs and Symptoms

Decreased vision, contact lens intolerance, and difficulties fitting standard lenses; rarely, pain, photophobia, and tearing as a result of corneal hydrops (a spontaneous break in Descemet membrane with resulting corneal edema).

Demographics

Presents from adolescence to middle age.

Ophthalmic Findings

- Vogt striae (central vertical stress lines in the deep stroma) (Figure 1.49A).
- Fleischer ring (epithelial iron at the base of the cone, best seen with the cobalt blue filter).
- Paracentral thinning and bulging of the cone, which is thinnest at the apex; irregular astigmatism; and irregularity of the retinoscopic reflex.
- Munson sign (peaking of the lower lid in downward gaze) is a late finding (Figure 1.49B).
- Rupture of Descemet membrane and influx of fluid into the stroma results in hydrops (Figure 1.49C). Healing of hydrops can result in flattening of the cone and reduction in myopia.

Systemic Findings

Keratoconus has been associated with a large number of conditions, including atopy, vernal keratoconjunctivitis, Down syndrome, Marfan/syndrome, aniridia, floppy eyelid syndrome, obstructive sleep apnea syndrome, and retinitis pigmentosa.

Special Tests

Keratometry and corneal topographical mapping are helpful to document the high level of irregular astigmatism (Figure 1.49D).

Pachymetry of apex of cone to monitor extent of ectasia.

Pathology

Focal disruptions in Bowman and Descemet membranes are seen, as may be stromal thinning. These features are not particularly specific to keratoconus.

Disease Course

Progressive at variable rate. Bilaterality of disease almost always becomes evident if patients are followed over long periods.

Treatment and Management

Spectacle and then rigid gas-permeable contact lenses for astigmatism. Special fitting techniques become necessary.

For earlier stages of keratoconus without scarring, intrastromal ring segments can help improve the curvature of the surface, allowing a better contact lens fit.

PKP or deep anterior lamellar keratoplasty for scarring when satisfactory vision can no longer be achieved with contact lenses.

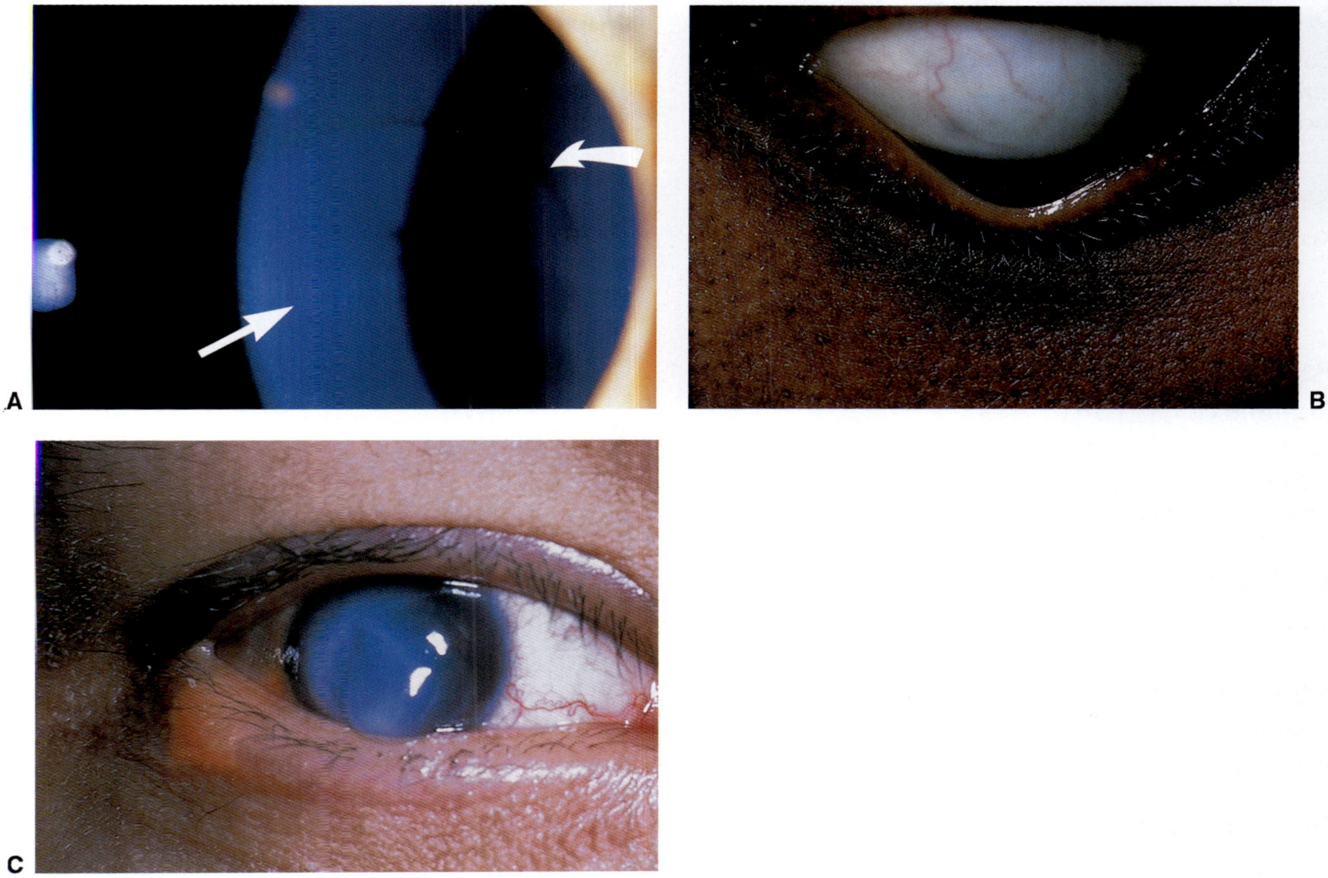

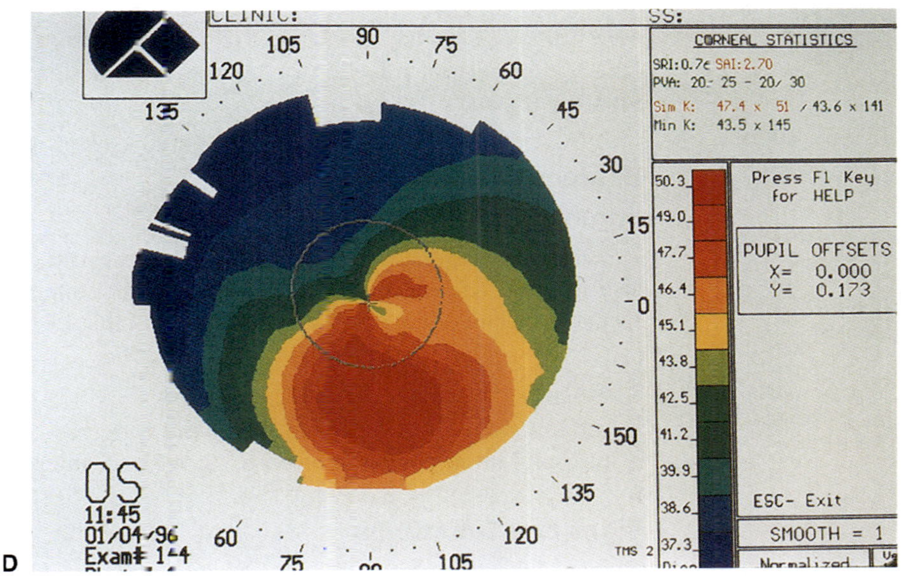

FIGURE 1.49. **A:** High-magnification view of the Vogt striae (*arrow*) and the Fleischer ring (*curved arrow*) seen in keratoconus. **B:** Munson sign is the distortion of the lid when looking downward. The apex of the cone can be more prominent in this position. **C:** Rupture of Descemet membrane allows stromal swelling and hydrops. **D:** Computerized topographic mapping in keratoconus showing inferior steepening (*red area*) corresponding to the cone.

Medications

Episodes of hydrops should be treated as a corneal abrasion, with the addition of hypertonic sodium chloride drops and ocular hypotensive agents to speed resolution of corneal edema. Cycloplegia and topical steroids help to reduce the accompanying inflammation.

Follow-Up

Episodes of hydrops must be followed closely until resolved. Periodic examination is warranted, with contact lens changes as required depending on the rate of progression.

Differential Diagnosis

Contact lens warpage may give a similar topographic picture. Other ectatic conditions may be distinguished by the location of thinning and corneal shape.

Reference

Krachmer JH, Felder RS, Belin MW. Keratoconus and related noninflammatory corneal thinning disorders. *Surv Ophthalmol* 1984;28:293–322.

Pellucid Marginal Degeneration

Summary

Painless bilateral noninflammatory ectasia of the cornea, marked by inferior peripheral thinning with adjacent protrusion of the central cornea, giving a "beer-belly cornea."

Etiology

Unknown.

Signs and Symptoms

Decreased vision secondary to irregular, against-the-rule astigmatism.

Demographics

None specific.

Ophthalmic Findings

Inferior thinning with intact epithelium.

Systemic Findings

None.

Special Tests

Keratometry and corneal topographical mapping are helpful to document the high irregular astigmatism.

Pathology

None specific. Corneal thinning may be seen.

Disease Course

Progressive at variable rate.

Treatment and Management

Spectacle and then rigid gas-permeable contact lenses for astigmatism. Special fitting techniques become necessary. Surgical correction requires large PKP or lamellar tectonic graft for peripheral thinning followed by central PKP.

Medications

None.

Follow-Up

Periodic examination as required depending on the rate of progression.

Differential Diagnosis

Other peripheral thinning disorders should be considered. Keratoglobus is distinguished by uniform thinning in the midperipheral cornea. Rheumatoid arthritis, polyarteritis nodosa, Wegener granulomatosis, and Mooren ulceration usually have inflammatory features, and Terrien marginal degeneration is marked by a lipid line.

Reference

Krachmer JH, Feder RS, Belin MW. Keratoconus and related noninflammatory corneal thinning disorders. *Surv Ophthalmol* 1984;28:293–322.

CORNEAL INFECTIONS

Viral Keratitis

Summary

Many viral infections can affect the cornea, most causing stromal infiltrates or a nummular keratitis. The accompanying systemic symptoms and findings can help to determine the specific infecting virus.

Etiology

Direct viral corneal infection or immune recognition of related antigens.

Epidemic Keratoconjunctivitis

Summary

In addition to conjunctival infection in EKC, adenovirus can also affect the corneal epithelium and stroma. The conjunctival manifestations are covered elsewhere (see Table 1.7).

Etiology

- Immune reaction to deposited adenoviral antigens.
- Infection with adenovirus serotypes 8, 19, or 37, subgroup D.

Signs and Symptoms

Glare and photophobia.

Ophthalmic Findings

- Subconjunctival hemorrhage.
- Bulbar conjunctival follicles.
- In severe cases, cicatrizing conjunctivitis with membrane formation (Figure 1.50A).
- PEK.
- Subepithelial infiltrates (Figure 1.50B) may persist for months to years.

Table 1.11

Ocular manifestations of herpetic disease

	Dendritic keratitis	Disciform keratitis	Interstitial keratitis	Iridocyclitis
Signs and symptoms	Red eye Foreign body sensation or ocular irritation Photophobia	Red eye Photophobia Foreign body sensation or ocular irritation	Red eye Photophobia Blurred vision	Red eye Photophobia Blurred vision
Ophthalmic findings	Classic ulcerated epithelial dendrite with terminal bulbs Elevated IOP Staining of the edges with rose bengal and the ulcer base with fluorescein (Figure 1.49) Decreased cirneal	Stromal edema over an area of endothelial involvement Keratic precipitates Elevated IOP Decreased corneal sensation Stromal immune ring	Stromal infiltration, necrosis, and scarring Ingrowth of stromal vessels	Stellate-appearing or nongranulomatous keratic precipitates Iridocyclitis Hypopyon or hyphema Iris atrophy Elevated IOP
Special tests	Corneal scraping for PCR, Tzanck preparation, DFA, or cultures			
Pathology	Multinucleated giant cells on Tzanck test	Stromal edema	Stromal necrosis with PMNs	
Treatment[a]	Epithelial debridement and patching Topical trifluridine or ganciclovir Oral acyclovir or valacyclovir Vidarabine ointment (second-line treatment) Idoxuridine drops or ointment (second-line treatment)	Topical corticosteroids ± acyclovir or valacyclovir	Topical corticosteroids ± acyclovir or valacyclovir	Topical corticosteroids ± acyclovir or valacyclovir Cycloplegia
Natural course	Up to 25% of patients have recurrent disease within 1 y of initial infection Patients with recurrent disease tend to have more recurrences	Stromal scarring	Stromal scarring with loss of stromal substance Ingrowth of stromal vessels and deposition of lipid	Resolution with pigmented keratic precipitates Iris atrophy
Systemic findings	Periocular vesicular dermatitis Cold sores or aphthous ulcers			

[a]See the Herpetic Eye Disease Study, p. 82.
IOP, intraocular pressure; PMNs, polymorphonuclear neutrophils.

CORNEA

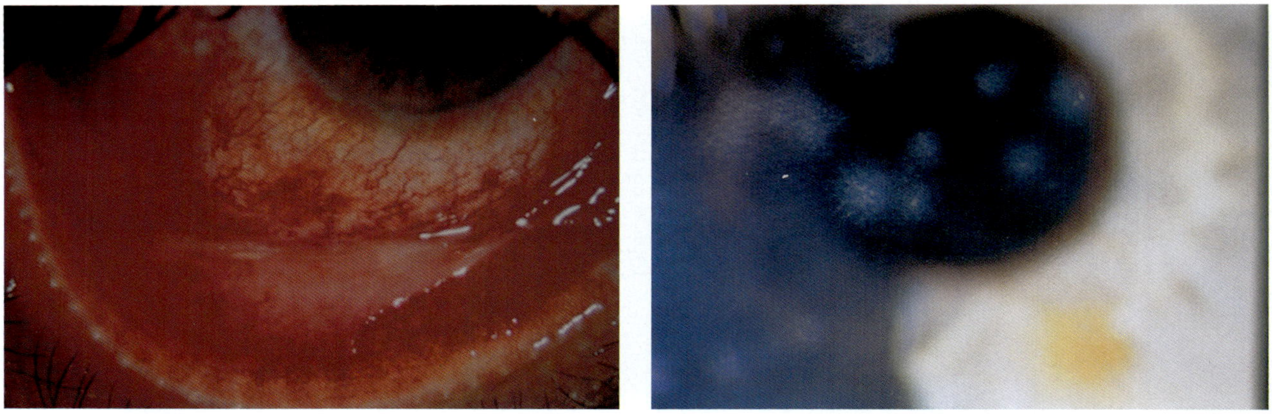

FIGURE 1.50. A: Membrane formation in a severe case of EKC. B: Persistent subepithelial infiltrates following a case of EKC.

Systemic Findings

None.

Special Tests

RPS Adeno Detector and Adenoclone of limited use with high clinical suspicion.

Disease Course

Days 2 to 30: diffuse epithelial keratitis.
Days 6 to 30: focal epithelial keratitis.
Day 14: subepithelial infiltrates.
Days 14 to 17: gray epithelial infiltrates.

Treatment and Management

- No treatment usually necessary.
- Artificial tears and topical NSAIDs for comfort.
- Low-dose topical corticosteroids to decrease density of infiltrates, but the infiltrates may recur when the steroid is stopped.
- Patient may have difficulty weaning off steroid.

Differential Diagnosis

Bacterial corneal infection: purulent discharge, deeper stromal infiltration.
Interstitial keratitis: stromal vessels, no epithelial defect.

Reference

Dawson CR, Hanna L, Wood TR, et al. Adenovirus 8 keratoconjunctivitis in the United States. *Am J Ophthalmol* 1970;69:473–480.

Herpes Simplex Keratitis

Summary

HSV affects a variety of ocular tissues, causing a periocular dermatitis, epithelial and stromal keratitis, and iridocyclitis.

Etiology

Infection by the HSV or immune reaction to viral antigens (Table 1.11; Figure 1.51).

Differential Diagnosis

VZV keratitis.

Varicella-Zoster Virus Keratitis

Summary

Reactivation of VZV in the trigeminal ganglion can cause a vesicular dermatomal eruption, as well as epithelial keratitis and iridocyclitis. Other manifestations such as stromal keratitis and scleritis are most likely immune action against the viral antigen, rather than from active viral replication.

Etiology

Reactivation of latent VZV from the trigeminal ganglion, presumably attributable to decreased immune containment of latent infection.

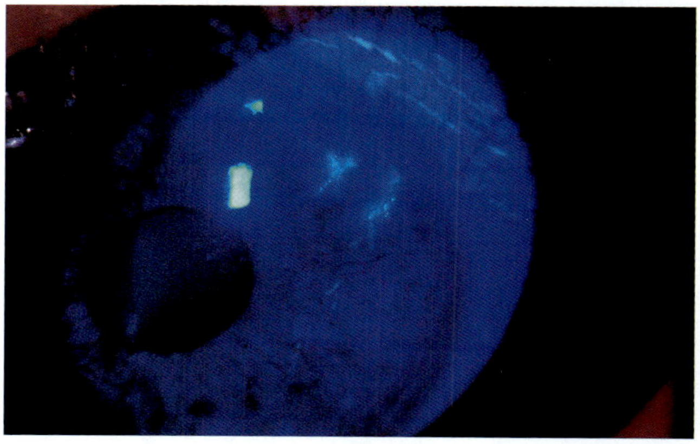

FIGURE 1.51. Classic ulcerated epithelial dendrite caused by HSV stained with fluorescein and viewed with the cobalt blue light.

Signs and Symptoms

- Red eye.
- Skin rash in dermatomal distribution, but can occur without a rash (*sine herpete*).
- Pain, photophobia.

Demographics

Trimodal demographics: young (children with chickenpox), middle-aged (immunosuppressed, AIDS patients), elderly (declining cell-mediated immunity).

Ophthalmic Findings

Hutchinson sign (dermatitis in the distribution of the nasociliary nerve).
Anesthetic cornea and conjunctiva.
Stellate, granulomatous, or nongranulomatous keratic precipitates.
Increased IOP.
Thin, multiple medusa shaped elevated dendrite (early dendrites).
Elevated, thick, ropy epithelial lesions (late mucous plaques).
Iridocyclitis.
Iris atrophy.
Horner syndrome.
Extraocular muscle palsy.
Scleritis.
Optic neuritis.
Interstitial keratitis.
Acute retinal necrosis.

Systemic Findings

Zoster dermatitis in the V_1 dermatome.

Special Tests

- Polymerase chain reaction (PCR) of epithelial lesions.
- Corneal scraping for Tzanck preparation (looking for multinucleated giant cells).

Disease Course

- Skin disease resolves in 2 to 3 weeks, leaving scars.
- Neurotrophic keratitis and nonhealing epithelial defects: can be difficult to manage (see p. 36).
- May have residual, persistent postherpetic neuralgia.
- Chronic uveitis may develop.

Treatment and Management

During acute phase: acyclovir.

Neurotrophic phase: lubrication, punctal occlusion, tarsorrhaphy, Gunderson flap, uveitis, amniotic membrane topical steroids.

Differential Diagnosis

HSV keratitis.

Bacterial Keratitis

Summary

Bacterial infection of the cornea usually associated with contact lens wear, trauma, or underlying ocular disease, such as dry eye or trichiasis.

Etiology

- Corneal infection by bacteria.
- In most cases, the corneal epithelium must be compromised to allow adherence and penetration of bacteria into the stroma; however, several bacteria are known to penetrate intact epithelium:
  H. influenzae.
  N. gonorrhoeae and *N. meningitidis*.
  Corynebacterium diphtheriae.
  Shigella species.
  Listeria monocytogenes.
- Contact lens wear, trauma, ocular surface disease (e.g., exposure, trichiasis, conjunctival scarring), and use of immunosuppressive medications (e.g., steroids) can damage the cornea, allowing bacterial invasion of the stroma.

Signs and Symptoms

Yellowish mucoid discharge.
Foreign body sensation.
Redness, photophobia.

Demographics

Patients who wear contact lenses overnight are at a 10 to 20 times higher risk for bacterial keratitis than with daily wear.

Ophthalmic Findings

Purulent discharge.
Epithelial defect.
Stromal infiltrate and ulceration (Figure 1.52).
Anterior chamber inflammation and/or hypopyon.

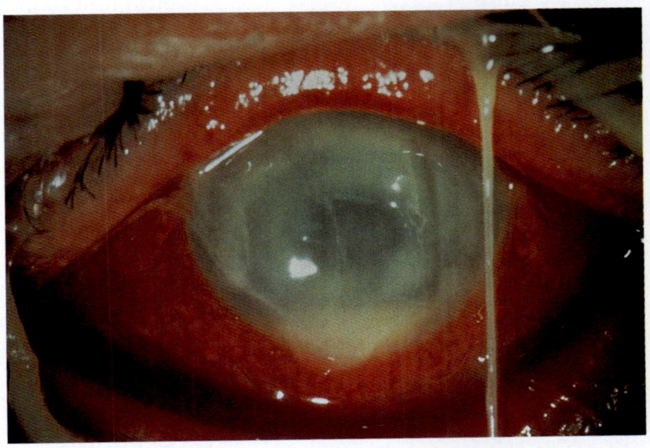

FIGURE 1.52. Severe corneal infection caused by *H. influenzae*. Copious purulent discharge, extensive stromal infiltration, hypopyon, and inflamed bulbar conjunctiva are evident.

Systemic Findings

Usually none.

Special Tests

- Corneal scraping for Gram stain.
- Cultures on blood agar, chocolate agar, and thioglycolate or cooked meat broth.

Disease Course

Untreated, bacterial keratitis can lead to stromal loss, perforation, panophthalmitis, and loss of the eye.

Treatment and Management

- Topical broad-spectrum antibiotics.
- Use culture results and antibiotic sensitivities to refine treatment regimen.
- In poorly compliant patients or severe disease:
    - Consider admission to hospital.
    - IV or subconjunctival antibiotics.
    - Debridement of necrotic tissue.
    - Therapeutic keratoplasty.
- Systemic antibiotics for *N. gonorrhoeae* and *N. meningitidis* infections.

Differential Diagnosis

Fungal keratitis.
Acanthamoeba keratitis.
Anesthetic abuse.
Medicamentosa.

Medications

See Table 1.12.

Fungal Keratitis

Keratomycosis

Summary

Fungal keratitis is caused by the invasion of cornea by filamentous fungi or yeast. The keratitis frequently appears as a dirty white, dry infiltrate with filamentous or feathery edges.

Table 1.12

Medications in the treatment of infectious keratitis

Organism	Antibiotics	Concentration
Topical drugs		
Gram-positive or Gram-negative organisms (severe infection)	Fortified vancomycin	25–50 mg/mL
	Fortified tobramycin	14 mg/mL
	Fortified cefazolin	50 mg/mL
Candida	Amphotericin B	0.15%
	Voriconazole	
Fusarium	Natamycin	5%
	Amphotericin B	0.15%
	Voriconazole	
Aspergillus	Amphotericin B	0.15%
	Voriconazole	
Acanthamoeba	PHMB or Chlorhexidine	0.01% or 0.02%
	Propamidine	
	Neomycin	
Capnocytophaga	Ciprofloxacin	0.3 mg/mL
Nocardia	Sulfacetamide	30%
Atypical mycobacterium	Amikacin	20–50 mg/mL
	Ciprofloxacin	0.3 mg/mL
Subconjunctival drugs		
Gram-positive or Gram-negative organisms (severe infection)	Cefazolin	50–100 mg/0.5 mL
	Ceftriaxone	50–100 mg/0.5 mL
	Tobramycin	20–40 mg/0.5 mL
	Clindamycin	34 mg/0.5 mL
	Vancomycin	25–50 mg/0.5 mL
Fungus	Amphotericin B	0.5 mg/0.5 mL

PHMB, polyhexamethylene biguanide.

Etiology

- Sixty genera of fungi reported.
  Yeast: *Candida*.
  Filamentous fungi: *Aspergillus*, *Fusarium*, *Curvularia*.
  Dimorphic fungi: *Blastomyces*.
- Risk factors:
  - Trauma: vegetable material or wood.
  - Topical corticosteroids.
  - Ocular surface disease.
  - Contact lens wear.

Signs and Symptoms

Eye redness, discharge, blurring of vision.

Demographics

- United States: 1,500 cases seen per year (5% to 10% of corneal infections).
- Increased risk of *Fusarium* keratitis in patients using Bausch & Lomb ReNu with MoistureLoc multipurpose contact lens solution (now off the market).

Ophthalmic Findings

Usually central keratitis.
Dry, dirty white lesion with filamentous or feathery edges (Figure 1.53).
Endothelial plaque under stromal lesion.
Hypopyon.
Immune ring.
Satellite lesions.

Systemic Findings

None.

Special Tests

Corneal scraping for Giemsa stain, potassium hydroxide (KOH), or silver stains.
Culture medium: Sabouraud dextrose agar (some fungi grow well on blood agar plates).
Confocal microscopy.

Pathology

Fungal hyphae or yeast forms within the corneal stroma.

Disease Course

- Usually slow, indolent growth.
- Unresponsive to antibiotics.
- Superficial lesions may respond with just mechanical debridement and heal in few days.
- Deep lesions may last for weeks, may be unresponsive to medications, and may cause corneal perforation.

Treatment and Management

Medical: Figure 1.54.
Surgical: keratectomy, therapeutic PKP.

Differential Diagnosis

- *Acanthamoeba* keratitis: severe pain, history of contact lens wear or exposure to contaminated water.
- Pneumococcal keratitis: advancing border, sharply demarcated lesion.
- *Pseudomonas* keratitis: melting appearance, stromal necrosis, rapid course.

References

Bernal MD, Acharya NR, Lietman TM, et al. Outbreak of Fusarium keratitis in soft contact lens wearers in San Francisco. *Arch Ophthalmol* 2006;124(7):1051–1053.

Johns KJ, O'Day DM. Pharmacologic management of keratomycoses. *Surv Ophthalmol* 1988;33:178–187.

Rosa RH, Miller MA, Alfonso EC. The changing spectrum of fungal keratitis in South Florida. *Ophthalmology* 1994;101:1005–1013.

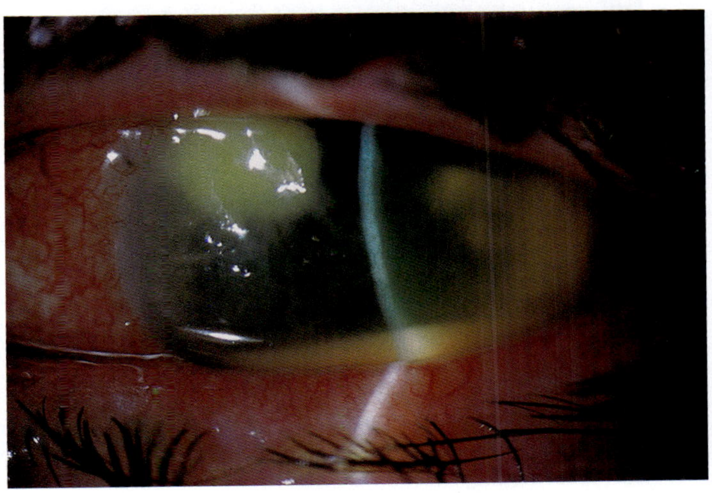

FIGURE 1.53. The dense stromal infiltrate has feathery, wispy edges suggestive of a fungal infection. Satellite lesions and a hypopyon are also present. A waxing and waning course, slow progression, and a history of topical steroid use also frequently occur with fungal keratitis.

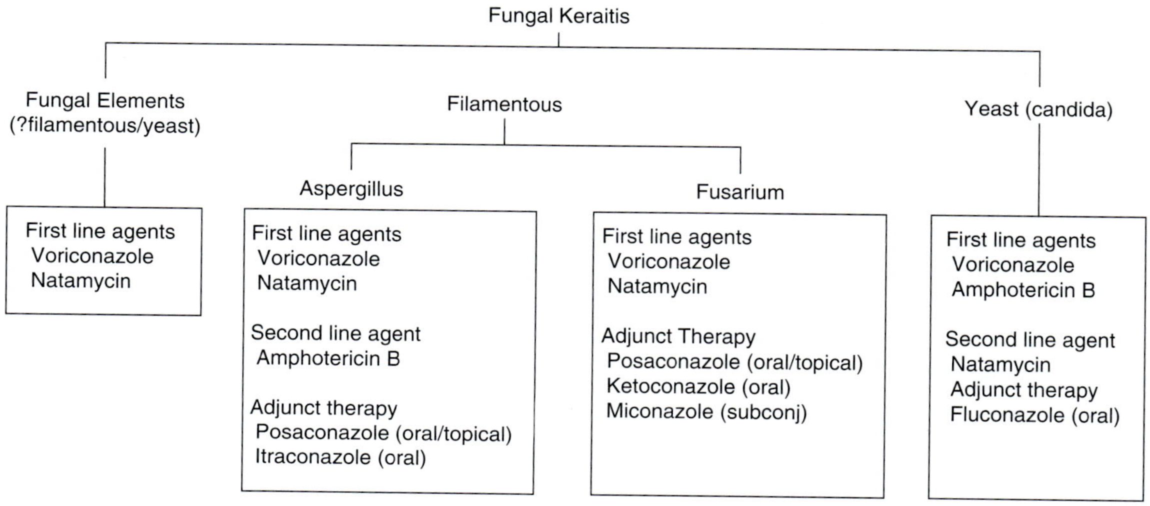

FIGURE 1.54. Algorithm for the medical therapy of fungal keratitis.

Parasitic Infections

Parasitic infections of the cornea are rare and unusual. *Acanthamoeba* and microsporidia are the most important parasites in corneal disease.

Acanthamoeba

Summary

Corneal infection by the protozoan, *Acanthamoeba*, causes an epithelial or stromal keratitis characterized by severe pain and photophobia.

Etiology

- Infection by the protozoan *Acanthamoeba*. *Acanthamoeba* exists either as an active trophozoite or, in harsh environmental conditions, as a protected cyst.
- Many patients have a history of contact lens wear, the use of homemade saline, or exposure to brackish water (streams, creeks, hot tubs).
- The use of AMO Complete MoisturePlus Multi-Purpose Solution (now off the market) was an independent risk factor for Acanthamoeba keratitis.

Signs and Symptoms

- Severe pain and photophobia, can be out of proportion to clinical findings.
- Foreign body sensation.

Demographics

Contact lens wearers.

Ophthalmic Findings

- Early:
  - Epithelial cysts.
- Late:
  - Epithelial defect.
  - Stromal infiltrate, may be ring shaped (Figure 1.55).
  - Scleritis.
  - Hypopyon.
  - Radial keratoneuritis (inflammation and enlargement of corneal nerves).

Systemic Findings

None.

Special Tests

- Corneal scraping for Giemsa, PAS, calcofluor white, or acridine orange stains to identify cysts.
- Confocal microscopy.
- Corneal biopsy for pathologic study.
- Culture on nonnutrient agar with *Escherichia coli* or *Enterobacter aerogenes* overlay.

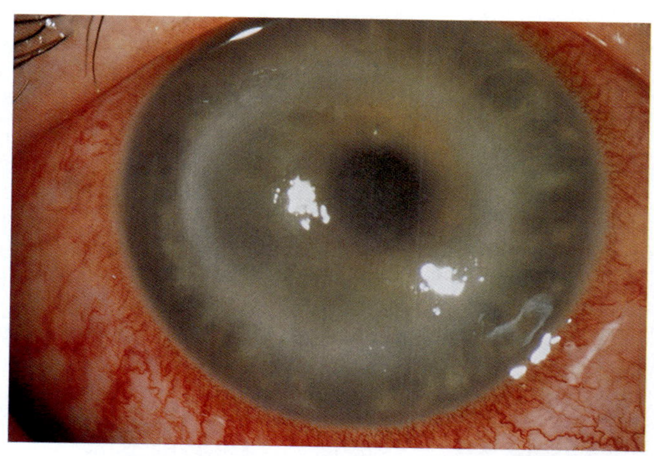

FIGURE 1.55. Ring-shaped stromal infiltrate is a late sign of Acanthamoeba keratitis in a former contact-lens wearer.

Pathology

Double-walled cysts can be seen in the corneal stroma using a Giemsa, PAS, or calcofluor white stain.

Disease Course

Untreated, disease progresses to involve full thickness of cornea and sclera.

Treatment and Management

- Epithelial debridement in early cases.
- Long-term medical therapy, sometimes requiring multiple medications for months, to eliminate cysts.
- PKP in progressive, recalcitrant cases.

Medications

Polyhexamethylene biguanide (PHMB) 0.01% or 0.02%.
Propamidine.
Neomycin.
Chlorhexidine.
Miconazole, itraconazole, fluconazole, clotrimazole.

Differential Diagnosis

Bacterial ulcer: copious purulent discharge.
Fungal ulcer: stromal infiltrate with feathery edges, satellite lesions.
Anesthetic abuse: can also have ring infiltrate, epithelial defect, and hypopyon.
HSV: history of dermatitis, epithelial dendrite, recurrent episodes.

References

Elder MJ, Kilvington S, Dart JK. A clinicopathologic study of in vitro sensitivity testing and Acanthamoeba keratitis. *Invest Ophthalmol Vis Sci* 1994;35:1059–1064.

Joslin CE, Tu EY, Shoff ME, et al. The association of contact lens solution use and Acanthamoeba keratitis. *Am J Ophthalmol* 2007;144(2):292–293.

Illingworth CD, Cook SD, Karabatsas CH, et al. Acanthamoeba keratitis: risk factors and outcome. *Br J Ophthalmol* 1995;12:1078–1082.

Larkin DF, Kilvington S, Dart JK. Treatment of *Acanthamoeba keratitis* with polyhexamethylene biguanide. *Ophthalmology* 1992;99:185–191.

Microsporidia

Summary

Microsporidia ocular infection causes a bilateral coarse PEK. Most reported patients are immunosuppressed with AIDS.

Etiology

Epithelial infection with microsporidia.

Signs and Symptoms

Foreign body sensation.
Pain, photophobia.

Demographics

AIDS patients most frequently, but has been reported in immunocompetent individuals.

Ophthalmic Findings

- Bilateral diffuse coarse PEK.
- Conjunctival injection.

Systemic Findings

Microsporidia can also colonize the nose and sinuses asymptomatically or the gastrointestinal tract, causing diarrhea.

Special Tests

Conjunctival scraping to look for intraepithelial organisms.

Pathology

Intraepithelial parasites.

Treatment and Management

- Albendazole: systemic treatment useful for patients with microsporidia in other sites (e.g., sinuses, gut).
- Topical fumagillin drops.

Differential Diagnosis

Dry eyes: PEK mostly in interpalpebral fissure.
Atopic keratoconjunctivitis: itching more prominent, fine PEK.

References

Cali A, Meisler DM, Lowder CY, et al. Corneal microsporidioses: characterization and identification. *J Protozoology* 1991;38:215S–217S.

Didier ES, Rogers LB, Brush AD, et al. Diagnosis of disseminated microsporidian Encephalitozoon hellem infection by PCR-Southern analysis and successful treatment with albendazole and fumagillin. *J Clin Microbiol* 1996;34:947–952.

Interstitial Keratitis

Summary

Interstitial keratitis is a descriptive term for a nonsuppurative stromal keratitis without epithelial disease. As the inflammation resolves, stromal neovascularization is often prominent.

Etiology

Various infectious and immune conditions. Causes of interstitial keratitis include:

- Bacterial:
  - Syphilis (congenital, acquired).
  - Lyme disease.
  - Mycobacterium (TB, leprosy).
- Viral:
  - Mumps.
  - HSV.
  - VZV.
  - Epstein-Barr virus.
- Parasitic:
  - Onchocerciasis.
  - Trypanosomiasis.
- Unknown: Cogan syndrome.

Signs and Symptoms

- Pain.
- Photophobia.

Ophthalmic Findings

Stromal infiltration and edema.
Mild anterior uveitis.
Intact epithelium.
Active or ghost stromal vessels (Figure 1.56).
Stromal thinning and scarring.
Deposition of lipid.

Systemic Findings

Cogan syndrome (etiology unknown): interstitial keratitis, vertigo, tinnitus, hearing loss.

Special Tests

Laboratory tests to determine underlying causes or origins.

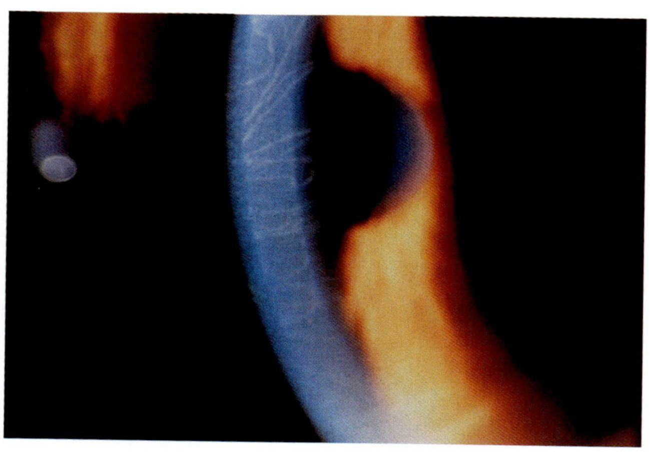

FIGURE 1.56. Bilateral midstromal ghost vessels are the residua of the interstitial keratitis in a patient with congenital syphilis.

Disease Course

- With time, active vessels become smaller in caliber and may become ghost vessels.
- Lipid deposition from exudation of fluid.

Treatment and Management

- Treatment of underlying disease.
- Topical steroids.
- Corneal transplantation for scarring.

DEPOSITS

Amiodarone Keratopathy

Summary

Patients taking amiodarone, a cardiac antianginal antiarrhythmic drug, may devolop a verticillate keratopathy (cornea verticillata), indistinguishable from chloroquine keratopathy and Fabry disease.

Etiology

Amiodarone deposition in epithelium.

Signs and Symptoms

- Usually asymptomatic.
- Evident as early as 2 weeks after initiation of drug therapy.

Demographics

Seen in 76% to 100% of patients with doses of amiodarone 200 to 800 mg/day.

Ophthalmic Findings

- Early stage: subtle intraepithelial vortex.
- Advanced stage: verticillate pattern with white or gray-brown deposits swirling outward from a point just below the pupil, sparing the limbus (Figure 1.57).
- Bilateral.
- Optic neuropathy (rare).

Pathology

Cytoplasmic lamellated inclusions in the basal epithelial cells of conjunctiva and cornea.

Disease Course

- Deposits slowly disappear with discontinuation of the drug.
- May be associated with irreversible loss of vision from optic neuropathy.

Treatment and Management

None; the keratopathy is not an indication for the cessation of the medication.

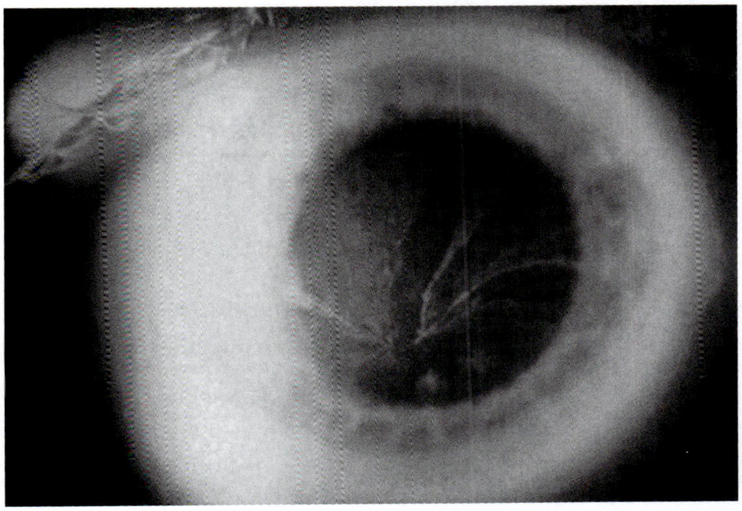

FIGURE 1.57. Whorling whitish amiodarone deposits follow the centripetal migration patterns of the corneal epithelium.

Differential Diagnosis

- Fabry disease.
- Other drugs that produce cornea verticillata: chloroquine, indomethacin, chlorpromazine.

Reference

D'Amico DS, Kenyon KR, Ruskin J. Amiodarone keratopathy: a drug-induced lipid storage disorder. *Arch Ophthalmol* 1981;99:257–261.

Acquired Amyloid Corneal Deposits

Summary

Acquired corneal amyloidosis is a degeneration in which a noncollagenous material, amyloid protein, is deposited in the corneal tissue (Table 1.13). This is seen in several chronic corneal conditions.

Etiology

Associated with chronic ocular conditions: trichiasis, bullous keratopathy, interstitial keratitis, trachoma, Hansen disease, trauma, and climatic droplet keratopathy.

Signs and Symptoms

Blurring of vision.

Demographics

May be seen in 3.5% of pathologic corneal specimens.

Ophthalmic Findings

Raised, yellow-pink nodular masses in the cornea.

Systemic Findings

None.

Pathology

Homogenous eosinophilic material. Green birefringence in polarized light of Congo-red–stained tissue.

Disease Course

Chronic.

Treatment and Management

No known way of preventing or limiting the condition. If vision is compromised, lamellar or PKP is an option.

Reference

Sandgren O. Ocular amyloidosis, with special reference to the hereditary forms with vitreous involvement. *Surv Ophthalmol* 1995;40:173.

Tyrosinemia Type Ii

Summary

Tyrosinemia type II leads to elevated tyrosine in the blood and urine.

Etiology

Autosomal recessive defect of hepatic cytosolic tyrosine aminotransferase.

Signs and Symptoms

Photophobia.
Injection.
Epiphora.
Blepharospasm.

Ophthalmic Findings

- Pseudodendrites.

Table 1.13

Chemical immunologic classification of amyloidosis of ophthalmic interest

Type of protein	Examples/symptoms	Remarks
1. AL and AH amyloid	Primary amyloidosis Myeloma-associated amyloidosis Systemic AL amyloidosis	Proteins derived from immunoglobulin light and heavy chain Ophthalmoplegia Lacrimal involvement
	Localized ocular AL and AH amyloid	Conjunctival amyloidosis Rare condition but the most common nonfamilial ophthalmologic manifestation of amyloidosis
2. AA Amyloid	Nephrotic syndrome Ophthalmic signs not seen	Reactive secondary amyloidosis with serum amyloid A protein
3. Transthyretin (TTR)-related amyloidosis	Vitreous involvement associated with the neuropathic type (CNS symptoms) Lacrimal dysfunction presenting as dry eye	
4. Gelsolin-related amyloidosis	Lattice dystrophy type II (Meretoja)	
5. Corneal amyloidosis	Lattice corneal dystrophy Granular Corneal Dystrophy, Type 2 (also known as Granular-lattice dysrophy and Avellino corneal dystrophy) Familial subepithelial amyloidosis (gelatinous drop–like dystrophy) Polymorphic amyloid degeneration Chronic ocular condition–related	Most common corneal manifestation of amyloidosis

CNS, central nervous system.
Adapted from Sandgren O. Ocular amyloidosis, with special reference to the hereditary forms with vitreous involvement. *Surv Ophthalmol* 1995;40:173; and the Sixth International Symposium on Amyloidosis, Oslo, Norway, 1990.

- Tarsal papillary hypertrophy.
- Nystagmus.
- Corneal neovascularization and scarring.

Systemic Findings

Hyperkeratotic lesions on palms, soles, elbows.
Mental retardation.
Ataxia.
Convulsions.

Special Tests

- Plasma/urine tyrosine levels.
- Liver biopsy.

Treatment and Management

- Dietary modification may modulate development of symptoms.

Differential Diagnosis

HSV keratitis.

Reference

Macsai MS, Schwartz TL, Hinkle D, et al. Tyrosinemia type II: nine cases of ocular signs and symptoms. *Am J Ophthalmol* 2001;132(4):522–527.

Cystinosis

Summary

Cystinosis is a rare form of inborn error of metabolism characterized by an abnormally high intracellular content of free cystine resulting in cystine crystal deposits in the kidney, bone marrow, lymph node, and eyes.

Etiology

Genetically determined defect in the cell resulting in cystine accumulation in the lysosomes (Table 1.14).

Signs and Symptoms

Photophobia: may be incapacitating and associated with blepharospasm.

Table 1.14

Phenotypes of cystinosis

Forms	Systemic findings	Ocular findings
Infantile form (Fanconi syndrome)	Growth retardation Progressive renal failure Autosomal recessive	Cystine deposition in the cornea and conjunctiva Peripheral retinopathy
Adult form	Benign	Asymptomatic; may see crystals in the cornea during routine examination
Adolescent form	Nephropathy, less severe Autosomal recessive	± Cornea and conjunctival deposits No retinopathy

Demographics

In infantile form, crystals are not present at birth but may be detected as early as 6 months of age.

Ophthalmic Findings

- Refractile, polychromatic crystals found in conjunctiva and all layers of the corneal stroma, most dense in the peripheral cornea.
- Crystals are fusiform or needle shaped.
- Ground-glass appearance of the conjunctiva.
- Iris stroma may be thickened with glistening dots on surface.
- Crystals are also seen in the uvea/choroid and retina.

Systemic Findings

Nephropathy.
Growth retardation.

Special Tests

- Contrast sensitivity: decreased in the infantile form.
- Conjunctival biopsy, with assay for cystine.
- Electron microscopy to detect crystals.

Treatment and Management

- Cystamine to prevent kidney damage; corneal deposits not reversed.
- Topical cysteamine.
- PKP in advanced cases.

Differential Diagnosis

Other causes of polychromatic corneal crystals:
Multiple myeloma.
Schnyder crystalline dystrophy.
Bietti crystalline dystrophy.
Gout.

References

Kaiser-Kupfer MI, Gazzo MA, Datiles MB, et al. A randomized placebo-controlled trial of cysteamine eye drops in nephropathic cystinosis. *Arch Ophthalmol* 1990;108:689–693.

Sanderson PO, Kuwabara T, Stark WJ, et al. Cystinosis: a clinical, histopathologic, and ultrastructureal study. *Arch Ophthalmol* 1974;91:270.

Iron Lines

Summary

Iron lines are faint yellow to dark brown discoloration in the corneal epithelium that is seen in different corneal conditions.

Etiology

Precise origin is unclear. The source of iron has been thought to be from tears or cellular breakdown. Iron is deposited at the site of contour change or the location of the pooling of tears.

Signs and Symptoms

None.

Ophthalmic Findings

Iron lines are seen with direct illumination and may be made more apparent using the cobalt blue light. Types (Figure 1.58A):

- Hudson-Stahli line: horizontal line at the junction of the middle and lower third of the cornea. It is bilateral and symmetric.
- Ferry line: line on the cornea anterior to a filtering bleb.
- Stocker line: line running parallel with the head of the pterygium.
- Fleischer ring: associated with keratoconus, the ring outlines the base of the cone (Figure 1.58B).
- Pigment adjacent to Coat white ring from a previous metallic foreign body.
- Iron lines seen following radial keratotomy and PKP.

Treatment and Management

Of no visual consequence.

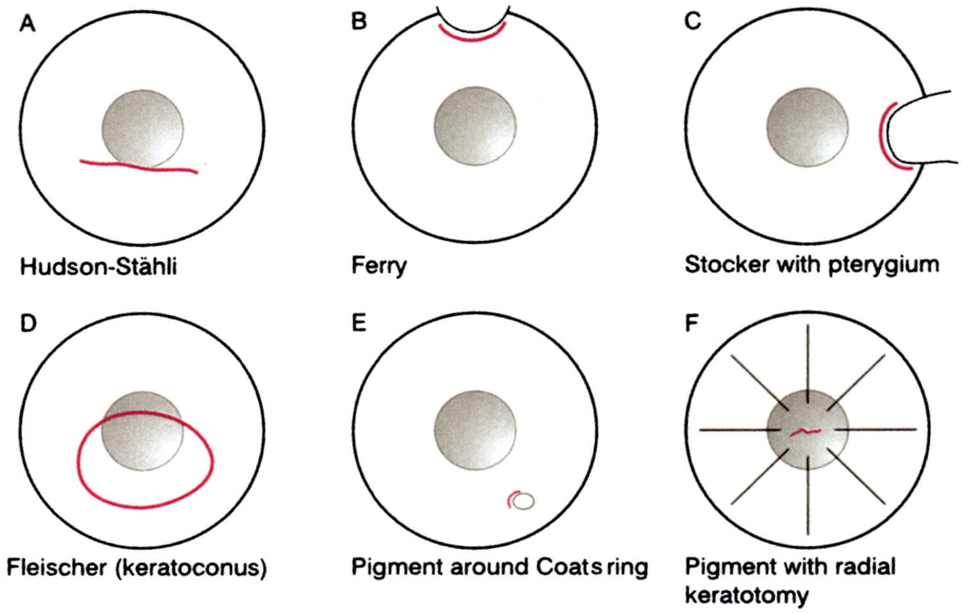

FIGURE 1.58. Circular iron line at the base of the cone in keratoconus. A–F: Pictures indicating common locations of corneal iron lines.

Reference

Barraquer-Somers E, Chan CC, Green WR. Corneal epithelial iron deposition. *Ophthalmology* 1983;90:729–734.

Fabry Disease

Summary

Fabry disease, an X-linked recessive metabolic disorder causing several systemic symptoms, is evident in the eye as a verticillate keratopathy, retinal aneurysm, and spoke-like posterior capsular cataract.

Etiology

X-linked recessive disorder caused by a deficiency of ceramide trihexosidase.

Demographics

Corneal changes seen within the first decade in 90% of affected male patients.

Ophthalmic Findings

- Cornea verticillata: fine subepithelial whorl-like lines emanating from a paracentral nodal point.
- Aneurysmal dilation and tortuosity of conjunctival and retinal vessels.
- Spokelike posterior capsular cataract.

Systemic Findings

Cutaneous angiokeratomas.
Subungal splinter hemorrhages.
Febrile crisis with peripheral extremity pain.
Renal failure.
Cardiovascular disease.
Neurologic changes: hemiplegia, cerebellar disorders, stroke.

Special Tests

- Alpha-galactosidase level in serum, leukocytes, cultured fibroblasts, tears.
- High-performance liquid chromatography for glycolipids in urine.

Pathology

- Accumulation of ceramide trihexoside throughout the cardiovascular and renal system and many ocular tissues including corneal epithelium.
- Birefringent lipid material located in the peripheral smooth muscle, endothelial cells of the blood vessel of conjunctiva, iris, ciliary body, retina, choroid, and orbit.

Treatment and Management

- Enzyme replacement with alpha-galactosidase (very expensive).
- Kidney transplantation if renal failure develops.
- Genetic counseling for women who are asymptomatic heterozygous Fabry carriers.

Differential Diagnosis

Medications causing cornea verticillata: amiodarone, chloroquine, indomethacin, chlorpromazine, quinacrine.

Reference

Sher N, Letson R, Desnick R. The ocular manifestation in Fabry's disease. *Arch Ophthalmol* 1979;97:671–676.

Chloroquine-Induced Keratopathy

Summary

Chronic use of chloroquine may result in a reversible keratopathy. Vision may not be affected, and the keratopathy is not an indication for cessation of chloroquine therapy.

Etiology

- Systemic treatment with chloroquine.
- Dose range: 100 mg/day over several years to 1,000 mg over as short a period as 3 weeks.

Signs and Symptoms

- Halos.
- With or without blurring of vision.

Ophthalmic Findings

- Fine punctate gray deposits in the corneal epithelium concentrated centrally and less dense peripherally. Pattern is initially diffuse and later becomes curvilinear or whorl-like (cornea verticillata).
- Bilateral.
- With or without toxic retinopathy.

Systemic Findings

With or without reversible neuromyopathy.

Pathology

Intralysosomal lipid accumulation.

Disease Course

Subepithelial deposits gradually eliminated with discontinuation of the drug.

Treatment and Management

- None.
- The keratopathy is not an indication for the cessation of chloroquine therapy.

Differential Diagnosis

- Fabry disease.
- Other drugs that produce cornea verticillata: chlorpromazine, indomethacin, amiodarone, quinacrine.

TRAUMA

Thermal Burns

Summary

Injury to the ocular surface by heat predominantly affects the corneal epithelium with limited damage to the underlying structures.

Etiology

Two groups:

Flame burns: caused by radiant heat, flash burns.

Contact burns: contact with hot objects or liquid.

The rapid-reflex eyelid closure and Bell phenomenon limit extent of burn.

Demographics

- Twenty percent involvement of the eyes in patients with significant burns involving the face.
- Thirty-one percent of eye injuries are corneal burn or abrasion. Only 7% result in permanent scarring.
- Curling irons: an increasingly frequent cause of corneal contact burns in the United States.

Ophthalmic Findings

- Abrasion in mild cases as coagulated epithelium sloughs.
- Severe burn may involve the deeper layers of the cornea. The involved tissue becomes opaque, described as having porcelain or ground-glass appearance.

Systemic Findings

In children, if child abuse is suspected, look for additional burns elsewhere on the body and other injuries.

Disease Course

In mild cases, stromal shrinkage and coagulation. Remodeled tissue can cause change in corneal curvature.

In severe burns, eschar tissue eventually sloughs, leaving thinned tissue behind that may later become ectatic or staphylomatous.

Treatment and Management

- Cycloplegics to relieve discomfort from secondary iridocyclitis; corticosteroids may sometimes be indicated.
- Pressure patching for epithelial abrasions.
- Topical antibiotics to prevent infections.
- Limited debridement of devitalized tissue and granulation tissue, together with full-thickness skin grafts to minimize eyelid scarring and ectropion formation.

Chemical Injury

Summary

Chemical injuries of the eye, depending on the type of chemical and the duration of contact, may produce either mild damage without sequelae or extensive involvement of the cornea and anterior segment resulting in permanent unilateral or bilateral visual impairment.

Etiology

Alkali: ammonia, lye, KOH, magnesium hydroxide, and lime (most common).

Acid: sulfuric (most common), sulfurous, hydrofluoric, acetic, chromic, and hydrochloric acids.
Other: solvents (alcohol, benzene, etc.).

Demographics

- Most patients are young.
- Exposure occurs in industrial accidents or at home, or from criminal assault.
- Alkali exposure is more frequent than acid injuries because of more frequent presence of household cleaning agents.

Ophthalmic Findings

Extent of damage dependent on strength (pH) of acid or base and duration of exposure. Alkali tends to penetrate deeper, since it causes saponification of cell membranes. Acids cause tissue coagulation that limits penetration. Solvents are primarily irritative to the ocular surface.

Area of involvement: extent of fluorescein staining.
Depth of corneal penetration: estimated by evaluating the loss of stromal clarity.
Extent of conjunctival damage: assessed by direct observation of vascular ischemia and/or necrosis of limbal and bulbar conjunctiva (Table 1.15; Figure 1.59).
Anterior segment fluorescein angiography: Document severity of anterior segment vascular ischemia.

Pathology

Alkali: saponification of the fatty acid component of cell membrane resulting in cell disruption and penetration.
Acid: protein precipitation and denaturation of the corneal epithelium and stroma.

Disease Course

Four distinct pathophysiologic and clinical phases:
I. Immediate.
II. Acute (days 0 to 7).
III. Early repair (days 7 to 21).
IV. Late repair (after 21 days).
In severe injury, secondary glaucoma may develop.

Treatment and Management

1. Emergency treatment:
   - Aggressive decontamination of ocular surface with copious irrigation and monitoring of pH.
   - Do NOT try to neutralize acids by instilling an alkali solution and vice versa.
   - Inspection and removal of debris in fornices.
2. Promote ocular surface epithelial recovery with proper corneal phenotypic transdifferentiation:
   - Tear substitutes.
   - Bandage contact lens.
   - Sodium hyaluronate.
   - Tenoplasty.
   - Limbal stem cell transplantation.
   - Amniotic membrane tissue.
3. Augment corneal repair by supporting keratocyte collagen production, and minimize ulceration related to collagenase activity:
   - Ascorbate.
   - Tetracycline.
   - Collagenase inhibitors.
4. Control inflammation:
   - Corticosteroids.
   - NSAIDs.
   - Amniotic membrane transplantation (controversial).

Table 1.15

Modified Hughes classification

Grade	Corneal opacity	Limbal ischemia	Limbal stem-cell loss	Prognosis
I (Figure 1.57A)	None	None	None	Excellent
II	Hazy with visible iris details	Less than 1/3 of limbus	Subtotal	Good
III (Figure 1.57B)	Stromal haze obscure iris details	1/3–1/2 of the limbus	Total Retention of some proximal conjunctional epithelium and vascularity	Guarded
IV	Opaque, no view of the iris or pupil	More than 1/2 of the limbus Ischemic necrosis of the proximal conjunctiva and sclera	Total Loss of proximal conjunctival epithelium	Dismal

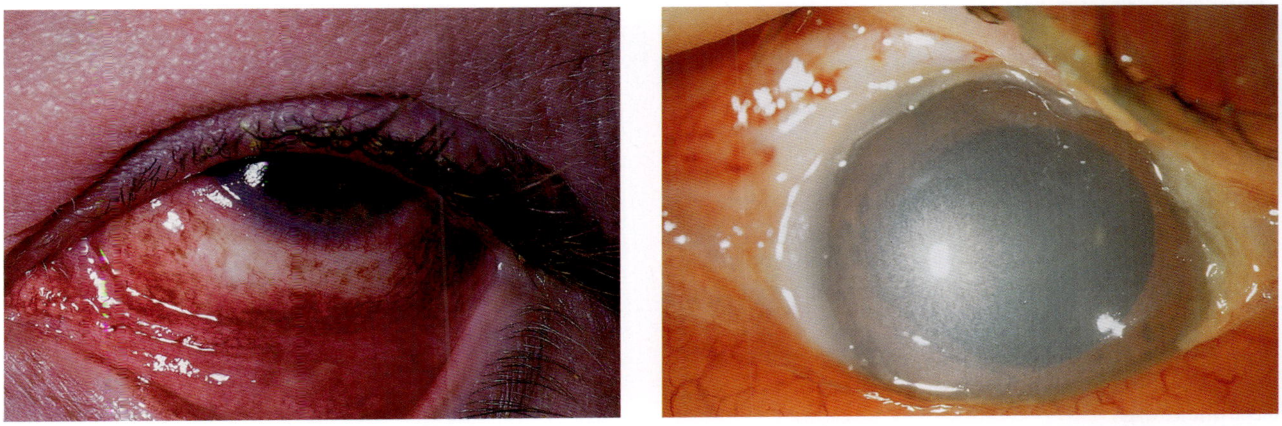

A B

FIGURE 1.59. **A:** Hughes grade I chemical burn in a patient who splashed cleaning fluid in his eye. The cornea is clear with an excellent view of the iris. The conjunctiva has an area of ischemia; the limbus is inflamed, but largely intact. **B:** Hughes grade III chemical burn. The cornea is hazy with complete loss of surface epithelium. The limbus and adjacent conjunctiva are white and ischemic. The prognosis is guarded in this eye.

5. Visual rehabilitation:
   - Lid repair.
   - Stem cell transplant.
   - Corneal graft.
   - Glaucoma surgery and management.

Reference

Wagoner MD. Chemical injuries of the eye: current concepts in pathophysiology and therapy. *Surv Ophthalmol* 1997;41:275–313.

Traumatic Hyphema

Summary

The presence of blood in the anterior chamber commonly caused by ocular trauma. In most cases, the blood clears from the anterior chamber without sequela; however, in certain circumstances, complications of increased IOP or corneal blood staining can occur.

Etiology

- Blunt or penetrating injury.
- Most hyphemas (71% to 94%) result from tears in the anterior face of the ciliary body, with disruption of the major arterial circle and its branches.

Demographics

- Common in young, active men and boys. Seventy percent of patients are younger than 20 years old.
- Male-to-female ratio is 3:1.
- Incidence: 20 per 100,000 per year.

Ophthalmic Findings

Types according to volume of blood in the anterior chamber:

Microscopic: no layered blood; circulating red blood cells only.
Grade I: less than one third of the anterior chamber.
Grade II: one third to half of the anterior chamber (Figure 1.60).
Grade III: greater than half of the anterior chamber.
Grade IV: total hyphema.

Evaluate for other signs of ocular and orbital trauma including iridodialysis, cyclodialysis, lens subluxation, corneal or scleral laceration, retinal detachment or commotio, and orbital fractures.

Special Tests

- Ultrasonography and radiologic imaging in extensive injury or if an intraocular foreign body is suspected.
- Sickle cell preparation may be indicated if sickle cell hemoglobinopathy is suspected.

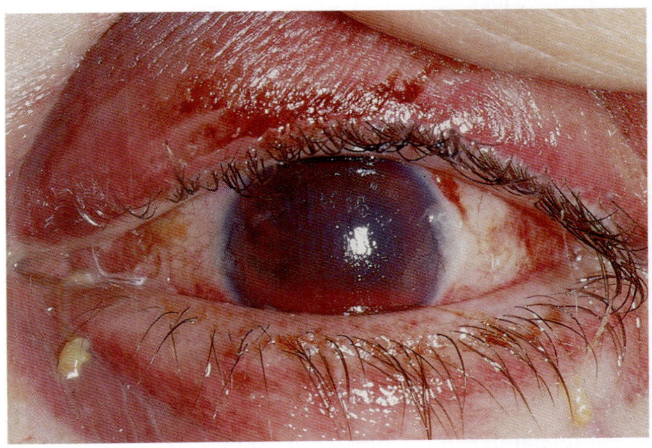

FIGURE 1.60. Traumatic hyphema occuring after a car accident with deployment of the air bag. The blood is layered along the inferior third of the anterior chamber. Epithelium irregularity and subconjunctival hemorrhage are also present.

Pathology

Red blood cell aggregate surrounded by a pseudocapsule of fibrin/platelet coagulum.

Disease Course

- Small hyphemas generally clear within 4 to 5 days.
- Hyphemas occupying half or more of the anterior chamber are more likely to be associated with delayed clearing, glaucoma, corneal blood staining, rebleeding, and poor visual outcome.
- Rebleeds in 2 to 5 days (before 7 days): incidence, 3.8% to 38%.
- Complications:

Glaucoma: may be acute or late. Danger of optic nerve damage if the IOP remains above 50 mm Hg for more than 5 days, above 45 mm Hg for more than 1 week, or above 35 mm Hg for more than 2 weeks.

Corneal blood staining: associated with larger hyphemas, rebleeding, and sustained increase in IOP.

Treatment and Management

- Supportive treatment: metal shield, head elevation.
- Medical treatment:

Cycloplegics.

Topical corticosteroids.

Aminocaproic acid or tranexamic acid may be used.

Intracameral tissue plasminogen activator (tPA) to lyse clot.

Glaucoma pressure control (avoid carbonic anhydrase inhibitors in sickle cell patients).

- Surgical management (anterior chamber wash-out) in severe cases.

Reference

Wilson FM. Traumatic hyphema. Pathogenesis and management. *Ophthalmology* 1980;87:910–919.

Traumatic Iritis

Etiology

Blunt trauma.

Signs and Symptoms

- Photophobia.
- Tearing.
- Ocular pain.

Ophthalmic Findings

- Minimal anterior chamber reaction.
- Perilimbal conjunctival injection.
- Decreased visual acuity.
- IOP is usually reduced but may be elevated, if associated with trabecular meshwork dysfunction.

Disease Course

May be a trigger for chronic uveitis.

Treatment and Management

- Topical cycloplegics.
- Topical corticosteroids, if with significant inflammation. If regimen is started, must be tapered slowly to prevent rebound iritis.

Differential Diagnosis

HLA-B27–associated iridocyclitis.

Ghost Cell Glaucoma

Summary

Ghost cell glaucoma is a secondary open-angle glaucoma that may develop a few weeks after onset of a posttraumatic vitreous hemorrhage.

Etiology

Transformed erythrocytes ("ghost cells") from vitreous hemorrhage block trabecular outflow.

Signs and Symptoms

History of trauma 2 or more weeks earlier.

Poor vision.

Pain with uninflamed eye.

Ophthalmic Findings

Vitreous hemorrhage.

Disruption of the anterior hyaloid.

Increased IOP.

Reduced visual acuity.

Mild to severe stromal edema.

Multiple small, tan cells in the aqueous.

Tan, white, or khaki layer of precipitate inferiorly.

Candy-stripe sign: double-layered hyphema of light khaki cells (older, degenerated red blood cells) on top of red layer (coexisting fresh blood cells).

Gonioscopy: wide open with discolored trabecular meshwork (fine khaki layer).

Fundus examination: khaki hue: degenerated hemoglobin.

Special Tests

Phase-contrast microscopic examination of unstained anterior chamber (AC) tap: spherical hollow cells with Heinz bodies (inclusions of denatured hemoglobin) at their periphery.

Pathology

- Ghost cells: transformed erythrocytes (spherical, more rigid, hollow structure).

- Ghost cells lower outflow facility three times more than same amount of fresh red blood cells.

Disease Course

- Transient or long-lasting, depending on the quantity of ghost cells present.
- No permanent damage to trabecular meshwork has been described.

Treatment and Management

- Medical therapy: beta-blockers, apraclonidine, carbonic anhydrase inhibitors.
- Irrigation of the anterior chamber with balanced salt solution (BSS).
- Vitrectomy may be necessary to remove the blood.

Differential Diagnosis

Neovascular glaucoma: shows typical rubeosis and synechial angle closure.

Hemosiderotic glaucoma: rare entity presenting years after initial hemorrhage.

Uveitic glaucoma: keratic precipitates and white cells in the anterior chamber.

Reference

Montenegro MH, Simmons RJ. Ghost cell glaucoma. *Int Ophthalmol Clin* 1995;35:111–115.

Lens Subluxation

Summary

Blunt trauma to the globe may result in the rupture of the zonules and subluxation of the lens.

Etiology

- Zonular rupture secondary to equatorial expansion from blunt trauma.
- Twenty-five percent or more of the zonule fibers must be disrupted to cause subluxation.
- Medical conditions that predispose the eye to lens subluxation with minimal trauma:
  - Syphilis.
  - Marfan syndrome.
  - Weill-Marchesani syndrome.
  - Homocystinuria.
  - Pseudoexfoliation syndrome.
  - Infantile glaucoma.

Signs and Symptoms

- Fluctuating vision.
- Decreased vision.

Ophthalmic Findings

- Iridodonesis.
- Phacodonesis.

Other Findings

Iris sphincter tears, iridodialysis, pigment disruption, and vitreous in the anterior chamber.

Disease Course

Concussive cataracts may develop.

Treatment and Management

- Subluxated lens is not necessarily an indication for surgical removal.
- If lens capsule is intact, surgery may be performed electively.
- Dilating or constricting drugs may minimize astigmatism from decentered lens.

Reference

Irvine JA, Smith RE. Lens injuries. In: Shingleton BJ, Hirsh PS, Kenyon KR, eds. *Eye trauma*. St. Louis, MO: Mosby, 1991.

DISORDERS OF THE LACRIMAL SYSTEM

Dacryocystitis

Summary

Dacryocystitis is an inflammation of the lacrimal sac associated with nasolacrimal duct obstruction.

Etiology

Stagnant fluid in nasolacrimal sac can become secondary superinfected due to poor drainage.

S pneumoniae: most common.

Staphylococcus aureus.

Pseudomonas aeruginosa.

Actinomyces.

Other Gram-negative bacilli.

H. influenzae: common in children.

Signs, Symptoms, and Ophthalmic Findings

- Acute dacryocystitis:
  - Severe pain.
  - Tearing.
  - Redness.
  - Purulent discharge.
  - Tender, swollen lacrimal sac.
- Silent or chronic dacryocystitis:
  - Tearing.
  - Minimal inflammation.
  - Chronic, recurrent conjunctivitis.

CORNEA

Special Tests

- Gram stain and cultures of discharge.
- Nasolacrimal duct irrigation.

Treatment and Management

Oral and topical antibiotics.
Dacryocystorhinostomy: most definitive treatment.
Dacryocystectomy: for elderly patients.

Differential Diagnosis

Lacrimal sac neoplasm.

Dacryoadenitis

Summary

Dacryoadenitis is an uncommon and usually unilateral inflammation of the lacrimal gland presenting as swelling of the temporal upper eyelid.

Etiology

- Acute dacryoadenitis:
  1. *S. aureus*.
  2. *S. pneumoniae*.
  3. *N. gonorrhoeae*.
  4. Epstein-Barr virus.
  5. Herpes zoster.
  6. Nonspecific orbital inflammation (pseudotumor).
- Chronic dacryoadenitis:
  1. Sjögren syndrome.
  2. Sarcoidosis.
  3. Syphilis.
  4. Tuberculosis.
  5. Cat scratch disease

Signs and Symptoms

Swelling of the lateral aspect of the upper eyelid.
Pain.
Discharge.
Fever.

Ophthalmic Findings

- Swelling and tenderness of the lacrimal gland (Figure 1.61).
- S-shaped curve of the upper eyelid.
- Ptosis.
- Globe may be shifted inferiorly and medially.
- Bulbar conjunctival injection, chemosis.
- Discharge.

Special Tests

- Computed tomography (CT) scan or MRI.
- Gram stain and culture of discharge.
- Biopsy may be indicated in some cases.

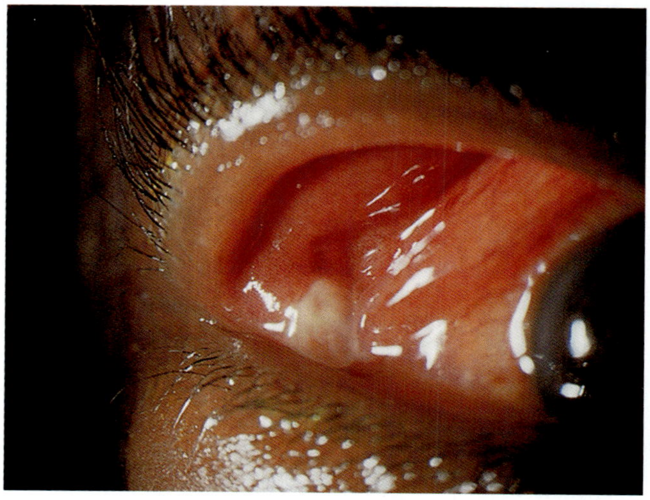

FIGURE 1.61. Acute dacryoadenitis caused by *Staphylococcus aureus*. The patient presented with redness, swelling, and tenderness over his lacrimal gland. There is purulent discharge when the lacrimal gland is massaged.

Treatment and Management

Oral dicloxacillin/cephalexin/clindamycin.
Topical sulfacetamide.
Oral steroids/NSAIDs for pseudotumor.

Differential Diagnosis

Hordeolum.
Benign lymphoid hyperplasia.
Malignant lymphoma.

Reference

Kennerdell JS, Dresner SC. The nonspecific orbital inflammatory syndromes. *Surv Ophthalmol* 1984;29:93–103.

EPISCLERITIS

Summary

A transient, relatively benign, self-limited inflammatory disease of the episclera.

Etiology

The majority are idiopathic. There are associated systemic disorders in 26% to 32% of cases:

- Collagen vascular disease or vasculitis (e.g., rheumatoid arthritis).
- Rosacea.
- Inflammatory bowel disease.
- Atopy.

- HSV.
- Chemical injury.
- Foreign material.
- Gout.
- Infectious (e.g., TB, syphilis, Lyme disease).

Signs and Symptoms

- Ocular redness without irritation (Figure 1.62).
- Acute in onset.
- Mild ocular discomfort, but no deep, aching pain.

Demographics

Fourth to fifth decade of life.

Male-to-female ratio: 1:0.8 to 1:2.8 (varies from study to study).

Bilaterality: 35% to 37% of cases.

Ophthalmic Findings

- Straight inflamed episcleral vessels radiating posteriorly from the limbus.
- Salmon-pink in natural sunlight.
- Moves with cotton-tipped applicator.
- Blanches with topical phenylephrine.
- Episcleral edema without scleral edema.
- Classification:

1. Simple episcleritis:
   Sectoral.
   Diffuse.
2. Nodular episcleritis: localized mobile nodule.

Special Tests

Topical phenylephrine 2.5%—will blanch episcleral vessels but not deeper scleral vessels (scleritis).

Directed laboratory tests indicated in multiple recurrences.

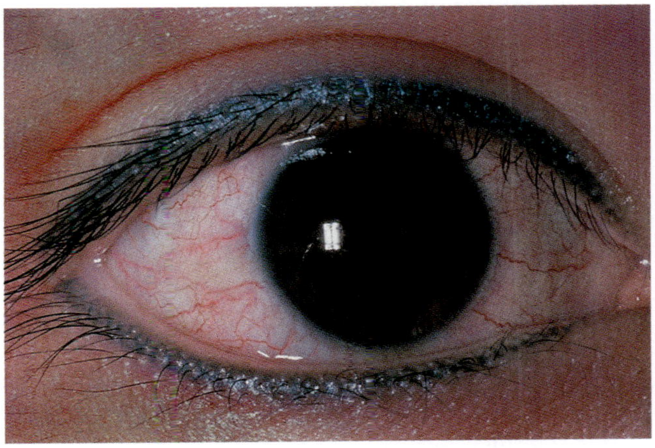

FIGURE 1.62. Diffuse superficial conjunctival injection in a case of episcleritis. These vessels blanch with the application of topical phenylephrine.

Pathology

Nongranulomatous inflammation with vascular dilation and perivascular infiltrates of lymphocytes and plasma cells.

Disease Course

- May resolve spontaneously.
- May recur in the same or different location (recurrence rate, 60%).

Treatment and Management

- Generally clears without treatment.
- Symptomatic relief with refrigerated artificial tears.
- Oral NSAIDs.
- Topical corticosteroid.

Differential Diagnosis

Conjunctivitis.

Scleritis.

References

Sainz de la Manza M, Jabbur NS, Foster CS. Severity of scleritis and episcleritis. *Ophthalmology* 1994;101:389–396.

Watson PG, Hayreh SS. Scleritis and episcleritis. *Br J Ophthalmol* 1976;60:163–191.

SCLERITIS

Summary

An inflammatory disease of the sclera associated with significant pain and, in some cases, underlying systemic immunologic disease or infection. It is important to diagnose and treat any underlying systemic disorder to prevent long-term ocular sequelae and visual loss.

Etiology

Inflammatory:

1. Rheumatoid arthritis.
2. Relapsing polychondritis.
3. Wegener granulomatosis.
4. Polyarteritis nodosa.
5. Inflammatory bowel disease.
6. Systemic lupus erythematosus.
7. Ankylosing spondylitis.
8. Reiter syndrome.
9. Psoriatic arthritis.
10. Giant cell arteritis.
11. Sarcoidosis.

Infectious:

1. Bacteria.
2. Fungi.

3. Parasites.
4. Virus.

Metabolic:
1. Gout.

Signs and Symptoms

- Gradual onset.
- Severe boring (aching) ocular pain, worse at night and can awaken patient from sleep.

Demographics

- Fourth to sixth decades of life.
- More common in women: female-to-male ratio, 1.6:1.
- Bilateral in more than half of the cases (52%).
- Patients with necrotizing scleritis: 40% have visual loss, 29% die within 5 years of systemic complications.
- Systemic involvement: 20% to 50% of patients (Table 1.16).

Table 1.16

Systemic involvement in scleritis

Systemic disease	Prevalence of scleritis (%)
Relapsing polychondritis	14
Wegener granulomatosis	10
Inflammatory bowel disease	10
Polyarteritis nodosa	6
Rheumatoid arthritis	6

Ophthalmic Findings

Globe: tender to touch.
Violaceous hue in natural sunlight.
Criss-cross pattern of scleral vessels.
Scleral and episcleral edema (Table 1.17; Figure 1.63).
Corneal involvement:
  Acute stromal keratitis.
  Sclerokeratitis.
  Marginal keratolysis (melting).

Special Tests

Complete blood cell count (CBC) with differential.
Erythrocyte sedimentation rate.
RF.
Anti-CCP.
ANAs.
Urinalysis.
Serum uric acid.
Chest x-ray.
Syphilis serologies.
PPD with controls.

Table 1.17

Classification of scleritis

Location	Types	Findings
Immune mediated		
Anterior sclera	Diffuse scleritis (Figure 1.61A)	
	Nodular scleritis	Deep red to purple scleral nodule, immobile and separated from episcleritis
	Necrotizing scleritis with inflammation	Severe pain out of proportion to inflammatory signs Edges of lesion more inflamed than center May have severe loss of tissue Blue-gray appearance of sclera from extreme thinning
	Necrotizing scleritis without inflammation (scleromalacia perforans)	Necrotizing scleritis without signs of inflammation
Posterior sclera	Posterior scleritis	Proptosis Visual loss May have restricted motility Choroidal folds, exudative retinal detachment, papilledema, angle closure glaucoma Retraction of lower lid on upgaze
Infectious		
Exogenous	Posttraumatic Postsurgical Extension from adjacent infection (Figure 1.61B)	Subconjunctival abscess Mucopurulent discharge
Endogenous		Similar to immune-mediated

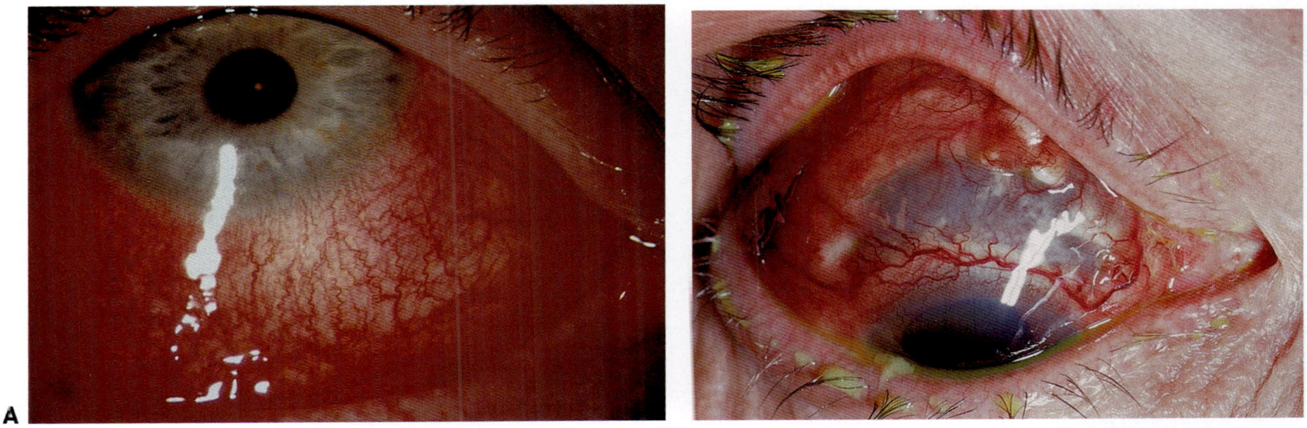

FIGURE 1.63. **A:** In natural lighting the diffuse anterior scleritis has a purplish hue indicative of dilation and inflammation of the deep episcleral and scleral vessels. **B:** Infectious scleritis caused by *Nocardia* species in a patient who had an infected scleral buckle removed. Under the area of scleral loss, the underlying uvea is visible.

Angiotensin-converting enzyme (ACE) and lysozyme.
ANCA.
HLA B-27.

Pathology

Immune complex deposition.

Disease Course

- Complications occur late in the disease course.
- Visual loss found in 27% to 37%.
- Uveitis develops in more than one third of the patients.

Treatment and Management

- Topical corticosteroids: inadequate in most cases.
- Oral nonsteroidal anti-inflammatory medications such as indomethacin.
- Oral corticosteroids.
- Systemic immunosuppressive therapy.

Differential Diagnosis

Episcleritis.

References

Benson WE. Posterior scleritis. *Surv Ophthalmol* 1988;32:297–316.
Sainz de la Maza M, Jabbur NS, Foster CS. Severity of scleritis and episcleritis. *Ophthalmology* 1994;101:389–396.
Watson PG, Hayreh SS. Scleritis and episcleritis. *Br J Ophthalmol* 1976;60:163–191.

MAJOR STUDY

The Herpetic Eye Disease Study

The Herpetic Eye Disease Study (HEDS) is a series of randomized, double-masked, placebo-controlled, multicenter clinical trials for potentially blinding HSV eye infections.

Topical Corticosteroids for HSV Stromal Keratitis

Patient Population

Patients with active HSV stromal keratitis receiving topical trifluridine.

Study Groups

Topical prednisolone phosphate versus placebo.

Outcome Measured

Treatment failure (worsening or no improvement of inflammation or an adverse event).

Results

- Corticosteroid therapy reduced the risk of persistent or progressive stromal keratouveitis by 68%.
- Time to resolution of stromal keratitis or uveitis was significantly shorter in the steroid-treated versus the placebo group.

Conclusions

- Compared with placebo, corticosteroid use significantly reduced the risk of persistent or progressive stromal keratouveitis.
- At 6 months, no clinically or statistically significant differences in visual outcome or recurrent herpetic eye disease were identified between the steroid-treated and placebo groups.

Reference

Wilhelmus KR, Gee L, Hauck WW, et al. Herpetic Eye Disease Study: a controlled trial of topical corticosteroids for herpes simplex stromal keratitis. *Ophthalmology* 1994;101:1883–1896.

Oral Acyclovir for HSV Stromal Keratitis

Patient Population

Patients with HSV stromal keratitis without epithelial involvement treated with topical trifluridine and prednisolone phosphate.

Study Groups

Ten weeks of oral acyclovir (400 mg five times per day) versus placebo.

Outcome Measured

Treatment failure (worsening or no improvement of inflammation or an adverse event).

Results

Median time to treatment failure was 84 days for the acyclovir-treated group versus 62 days for the placebo group.

Conclusions

- The difference in the median time to treatment failure between patients receiving oral acyclovir versus placebo was not statistically significant.
- Visual acuity improved over 6 months in more patients in the acyclovir group than in the placebo group.

Reference

Barron BA, Gee L, Hauck WW, et al. Herpetic Eye Disease Study: a controlled trial of oral acyclovir for herpes simplex stromal keratitis. *Ophthalmology* 1994;101:1871–1882.

Oral Acyclovir for HSV Iridocyclitis

Patient Population

Patients with iridocyclitis attributed to HSV treated with topical prednisolone phosphate and trifluridine.

Study Groups

Ten-week course of oral acyclovir (400 mg five times per day) versus placebo.

Outcome Measured

Persistence or worsening of ocular inflammation, toxicity from medication.

Results

Treatment failure occurred in 11 of 22 patients (50%) treated with acyclovir and 19 of 28 (68%) patients given placebo.

Conclusions

- The number of patients recruited for the trial was too small to achieve statistically conclusive results.
- The data showed a trend suggesting the benefit of oral acyclovir (400 mg five times per day) in the treatment of HSV iridocyclitis in patients receiving topical prednisolone phosphate and topical trifluridine.

Reference

The Herpetic Eye Disease Study Group. A controlled trial of oral acyclovir for iridocyclitis caused by herpes simplex virus. *Arch Ophthalmology* 1996;114:1065–1072.

Risk for HSV Epithelial Keratitis Recurrence in Patients with HSV Stromal Keratitis

Patient Population

Patients with active HSV stromal keratitis and/or iridocyclitis without epithelial disease. All patients received topical trifluridine for 10 weeks.

Study Groups

Ten-week course of either of the following:

1. Topical placebo.
2. Topical prednisolone phosphate.
3. Topical prednisolone phosphate and oral acyclovir.

Outcome Measured

Development of epithelial disease within 16 weeks.

Results

Epithelial keratitis occurred in:

1. One of forty-nine (2%) placebo-treated patients.
2. Nine of one hundred and thirty-eight (6.5%) patients treated with topical prednisolone alone.
3. Two of seventy-three (2.7%) patients treated with topical prednisolone and oral acyclovir.

Conclusions

- There was no significant difference in the occurrence of HSV epithelial keratitis in patients with stromal keratitis among the treatment groups: topical placebo, topical prednisolone phosphate, and topical prednisolone phosphate with oral acyclovir.
- Patients with a history of previous HSV epithelial keratitis were more likely to develop HSV epithelial keratitis during treatment of stromal keratitis/iridocyclitis.

Reference

Wilhelmus KR, Dawson CR, Barron BA, et al. Risk factors for herpes simplex virus epithelial keratitis recurring during treatment of stromal keratitis or iridocyclitis. *Br J Ophthalmol* 1996;80:969–972.

Oral Acyclovir for the Prevention of Stromal Keratitis

Patient Population

Patients with HSV epithelial keratitis treated with topical trifluridine.

Study Groups

Three-week course of oral acyclovir (400 mg b.i.d.) versus placebo.

Outcome Measured

Development of HSV stromal keratitis or iritis during the subsequent year.

Results

Seventeen of one hundred and fifty-three (11%) patients in the acyclovir group developed stromal keratitis versus 14 of 134 (10%) patients in the placebo group.

Conclusions

- No apparent benefit of acyclovir in the prevention of stromal keratitis.
- Development of stromal keratitis or iritis within 1 year was higher in patients with a previous history of stromal keratitis or iridocyclitis (23% vs. 9%).

Reference

The Herpetic Eye Disease Study Group. A controlled trial of oral acyclovir for the prevention of stromal keratitis or iritis in patients with herpes simplex virus epithelial keratitis. *Arch Ophthalmol* 1997;115:703–712.

Acyclovir for the Prevention of Recurrent HSV Eye Disease

Patient Population

Patients with HSV ocular disease in the preceding year.

Study Groups

Oral acyclovir (400 mg b.i.d.) versus placebo.

Outcome Measured

Development of ocular or nonocular HSV disease in the subsequent 12-month treatment period and 6-month subsequent follow-up.

Results

- Recurrent ocular HSV disease occurred in 19% of the acyclovir-treated patients versus 32% of the placebo group ($p < 0.001$).
- In patients with HSV stromal keratitis, recurrent disease occurred in 14% of acyclovir-treated patients versus 28% of the placebo group ($p < 0.005$).
- There was no rebound of HSV disease in the 6 months following discontinuation of oral acyclovir.

Conclusions

Oral acyclovir treatment decreased the rate of recurrent ocular HSV disease.

Reference

The Herpetic Eye Disease Study Group. Acyclovir for the prevention of recurrent herpes simplex virus eye disease. *N Engl J Med* 1998;339:300–306.

CHAPTER

2

Lens and Cataract

Edward Y. Koo

LENS ANATOMY AND PHYSIOLOGY

Normal Lens Anatomy

See Figure 2.1.

- Lens dimensions:
  - Biconvex shape, more convex posteriorly.
  - Infant: 6.4-mm wide and 3.5-mm long. Weighs approximately 90 mg.
  - Adult: 9.0-mm wide and 5.0-mm long. Weighs approximately 255 mg.
- Lens capsule:
  - Type IV collagen, which is the basement membrane for the lens epithelial cells.
  - Thickness: 2 to 23 μm. Thickest near periequator, thinnest central posteriorly.
- Lens epithelium:
  - Single row of nucleated lens epithelial cells beneath anterior capsule only.
  - Mitotically active lens epithelial cells found at equator of lens (lens bow).
  - Lens fibers at equator elongate and wrap around to join other epithelial cells forming anterior "Y" suture and posterior inverted "Y" suture.
- Zonules:
  - Fibers are 5 to 30 μm in diameter and provide support for the lens.
  - Originate from the nonpigmented epithelium of the pars plana and pars plicata of the ciliary body.
  - Insert on the lens capsule in the periequatorial region, 1.5 mm anteriorly and 1.25 mm posteriorly.

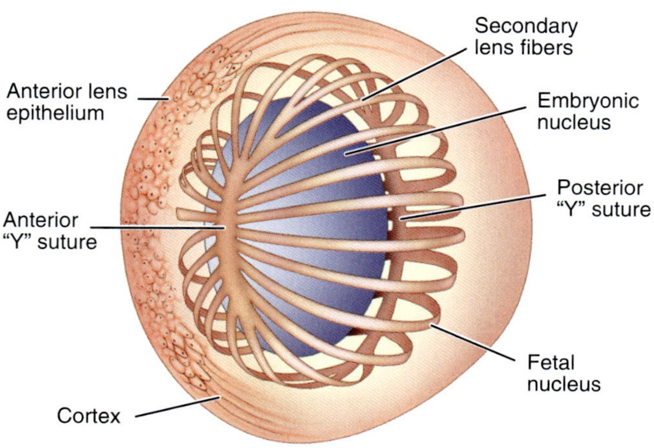

FIGURE 2.1. Anatomy of the fetal lens. Note the location of nucleated lens epithelial cells anteriorly and along the lens equator. The ends of the elongating lens fibers form the anterior and the posterior "Y" sutures.

Lens Embryology and Development

Time after gestation and lens development:

- Day 25: formation of optic vesicles from the forebrain (diencephalons).
- Day 27: elongation of surface ectodermal cells to form lens plate (placode).
- Day 29: invagination of surface ectoderm to form lens pit (fovea lentis).
- Day 33: formation of lens vesicle complete; optic vesicles form two-layered optic cup.
- Day 40: Primary lens fibers fill lens cavity forming embryonic nucleus.
- Week 7: Secondary lens fibers with nuclei at equator elongate and form Y sutures (upright Y suture anteriorly, inverted Y suture posteriorly) (Figure 2.2).

- Tunica vasculosa lentis:
  - Vasculature surrounding and nourishing the lens during development.
  - Usually regresses by birth (remnants include Mittendorf dot and persistent pupillary membranes).

Lens Biochemistry

Lens proteins (one third of lens mass):

- Water soluble (crystallins):
  - Alpha crystallin: 32% of lens proteins, largest of the crystallins.
  - Beta crystallin: 55% of lens proteins.
  - Gamma crystallin: 1.5% of lens proteins.

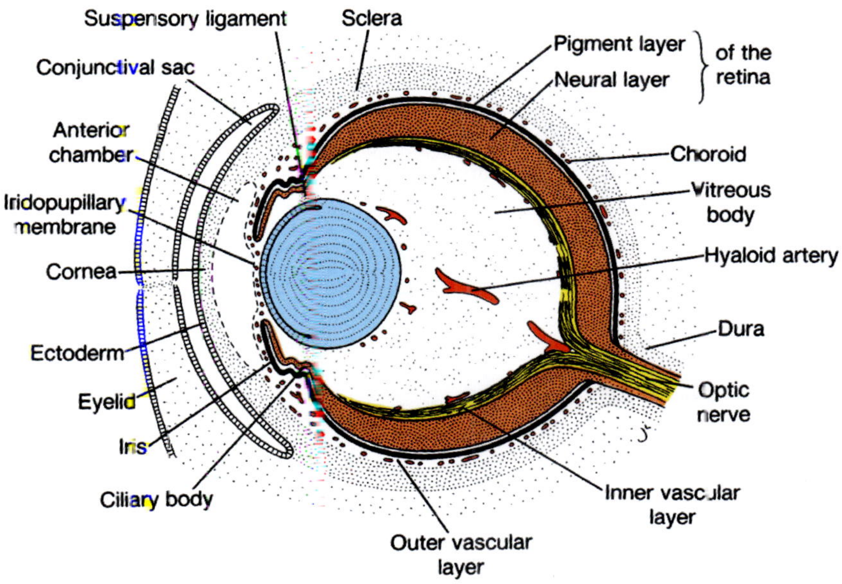

FIGURE 2.2. Invagination of surface ectoderm forms the lens. Elongation of the posterior lens epithelial cells forms the primary lens fibers obliterating the cavity. Nourishment is provided by the hyaloid artery that regresses before birth. (From Sadler T. *Langman's medical embryology,* 9th ed. Image Bank. Baltimore, MD: Lippincott Williams & Wilkins, 2003, with permission.)

- Water insoluble
  - Urea-insoluble fraction: mostly plasma membrane proteins.
  - Urea-soluble fraction.
- Proportion of water-insoluble proteins is increased in cataractous lenses.

Lens Physiology

- Ionic gradient:
  - Within the lens: Na^+ = 20 mmol, K^+ = 120 mmol.
  - Aqueous humor: Na^+ = 150 mmol, K^+ = 5 mmol.
- Lens epithelial cells supply metabolic demands for the lens.
- Anaerobic glycolysis responsible for bulk of adenosine triphosphate (ATP) production, since oxygen tension low.
- Hexose monophosphate shunt produces about 5% of ATP.
- Glutathione, vitamins C and E are antioxidants counteracting the damage of free radicals.

Accommodation

- Accommodation is a change in lens shape to allow focusing from distance to near (Figure 2.3).
- Theories of mechanism:

  Helmholtz: Most widely held theory
  - Circular muscle fibers of ciliary body contract decreasing equatorial circumlenticular space.
  - This reduces zonular tension, which allows the lens to become more spherical and increases optical power.
  - Amplitude of accommodation decreases with age as the lens substance becomes less flexible resulting in presbyopia (Table 2.1).

  Schachar
  - Circular muscle fibers of ciliary body contract increasing equatorial zonular tension while simultaneously decreasing zonular tension of anterior and posterior zonules.
  - This causes the central surface of the lens to steepen, the anterior-posterior diameter to increase, and the peripheral surface to flatten increasing optical power.

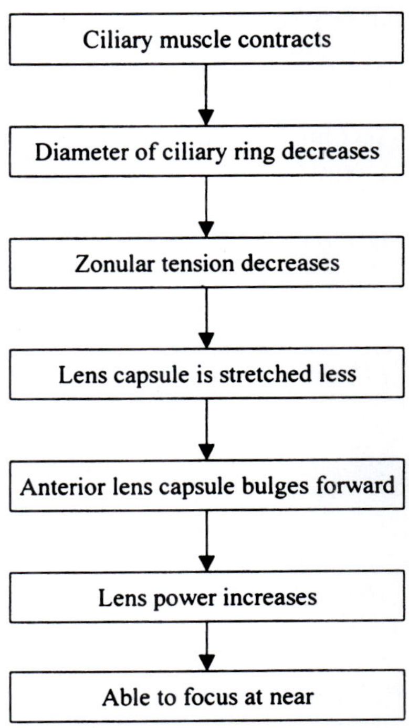

FIGURE 2.3. Cascade of accommodation.

Table 2.1

Amplitude of accommodation by age

Age (y)	Amplitude of accommodation (diopters)
10	14
20	10
30	7
40	4.5
50	2.5
60	1
70	0.25

Adapted from Katz M. The human eye as an optical system. In: Duane TD, ed. *Clinical ophthalmology*, vol 1. Philadelphia, PA: JB Lippincott Co., 1988:51.

- Amplitude of accommodation decreases with age as the equatorial diameter of the lens increases causing diminished baseline zonular tension due to decreasing distance between the lens and the ciliary body.

CONGENITAL ANOMALIES

Lens Coloboma

Summary

A notch in the peripheral lens caused by focal absence of the ciliary body and the zonules.

Signs and Symptoms

Irregular pupil. May be asymptomatic.

Ophthalmic Findings

- Usually located inferonasally.
- May be associated with other colobomata (iris, optic nerve, choroid) (Figure 2.4).
- Lens opacification may be noted in the region of the coloboma.

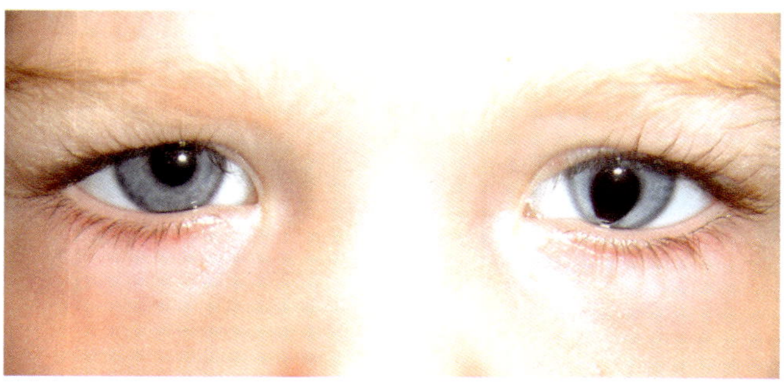

FIGURE 2.4. Photograph of a typical iris coloboma with a keyhole pupil located inferiorly and slightly nasally at approximately 7 o'clock position. The eye is slightly smaller than normal.

Systemic Findings

None.

Disease Course

Typically stationary.

Treatment and Management

Lens extraction if associated with visually significant cataract.

Mittendorf Dot

Etiology

Remnant of the posterior tunica vasculosa lentis.

Signs and Symptoms

Usually asymptomatic.

Ophthalmic Findings

- Whitish opacity generally connected inferonasal to the posterior capsule of the lens.
- May have remnant of hyaloid artery attached.

Systemic Findings

None.

Disease Course

Stationary.

Treatment and Management

None required.

ECTOPIA LENTIS

Ectopia lentis describes the condition of the natural lens being either partially or fully displaced from its normal anatomic position. There are many causes; the most common is trauma.

Signs and Symptoms

Monocular diplopia.
Change in refraction (marked astigmatism).

Ophthalmic Findings

Phacodonesis (tremulous lens on eye movement).
Iridodonesis (tremulous iris).
Cataract.
Pupil block with angle-closure glaucoma if lens displaced into anterior chamber.

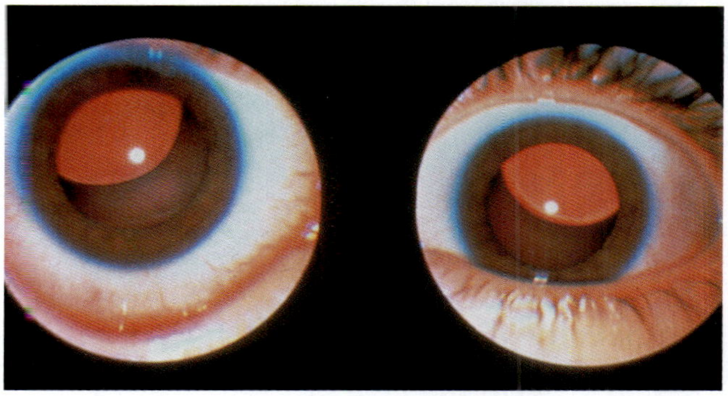

FIGURE 2.5. Bilateral superotemporal subluxation of the lens in Marfan syndrome. Because of weak zonules, bilateral intracapsular extractions were performed.

Marfan Syndrome

Summary

Marfan syndrome is an autosomal dominant disorder of collagen synthesis characterized by skeletal, cardiac, and ocular findings.

Etiology

An abnormality of fibrillin, a structural protein.

Demographics

Autosomal dominant inheritance.

Ophthalmic Findings

- Bilateral ectopia lentis (characteristically superotemporal) (Figure 2.5).
- Myopia.
- Increased incidence of retinal detachment.

Systemic Findings

Tall, thin stature.
Mitral valve prolapse.
Dilated aortic root and aortic dissection.
Arachnodactyly.
Hyperextensible joints.

Disease Course

Variable findings may present in adulthood.

Treatment and Management

- Most patients can be treated with spectacle correction.
- Pupillary dilation may be helpful.
- Lens extraction may be difficult.

Homocystinuria

Summary

Homocystinuria is an autosomal recessive systemic disorder of amino acid metabolism resulting in lenticular zonular fragility, seizures, and an increased risk for thromboembolic events.

Etiology

Abnormality of methionine metabolism.

Demographics

Autosomal recessive.

Ophthalmic Findings

Ectopia lentis (characteristically inferonasal subluxation).

Systemic Findings

Tall with light colored hair.
Seizures.
Osteoporosis.
Mental retardation.
Increased incidence of thromboembolism.

Disease Course

Eighty percent of patients have subluxed lenses by age 15 years.

Treatment and Management

A diet low in methionine, with supplemental cysteine and vitamin B_6 may reduce the incidence of ectopia lentis in these patients.

Miscellaneous Causes

Hyperlysinemia

Inborn error of metabolism associated with ectopia lentis, muscular hypotony, and mental retardation.

Sulfite Oxidase Deficiency

- A very rare autosomal recessive deficiency in sulfur metabolism.
- Associated with ectopia lentis, seizures, and mental retardation.

Microspherophakia

Summary

Microspherophakia is a congenital abnormality of lens development resulting in a small, spherical shaped lens that can dislocate anteriorly and cause pupillary block with resulting angle-closure glaucoma.

Etiology

Abnormal formation of secondary lens fibers during embryogenesis.

Ophthalmic Findings

- Myopia.
- Angle closure due to pupillary block.

- Lens may dislocate into anterior chamber.
- Abnormally small lens may be entirely visible through well-dilated pupil.

Systemic Findings

Usually associated with Weill-Marchesani syndrome.
May be an isolated abnormality or found in:
Lowe syndrome.
Alport syndrome.
Congenital rubella.

Disease Course

May develop angle-closure glaucoma.

Treatment and Management

- Iridotomy for pupillary block.
- Avoid miotics as they aggravate pupillary block.
- Cycloplegics may be helpful by moving the lens posteriorly and decreasing its anteroposterior diameter.

Weill-Marchesani Syndrome

Summary

Weill-Marchesani syndrome is an autosomal recessive condition characterized by short stature, small hands and feet, and microspherophakia.

Etiology

Autosomal recessive inheritance.

Signs and Symptoms

Myopia
Angle closure that is due to pupillary block.

Ophthalmic Findings

Microspherophakia.

Systemic Findings

Short stature.

Disease Course

May develop angle-closure glaucoma.

Treatment and Management

- Iridotomy for pupillary block.
- Avoid miotics as they aggravate pupillary block.
- Cycloplegics may be helpful by moving the lens posteriorly and decreasing its anteroposterior diameter.

Traumatic Cataract

Summary

Blunt, nonperforating injury to the eye may cause lens opacification either as an acute event or as a late sequela.

Etiology

Traumatic lens damage caused by blunt, nonperforating mechanical injury.

Signs and Symptoms

Blurry vision.
Fluctuating vision.

Ophthalmic Findings

Pigment from pupillary ruff imprinted on anterior lens capsule (Vossius ring).
Axially located stellate or rosette-shaped posterior lens capsule opacification that may progress to opacification of the entire lens.
Phacodonesis
Iridodonesis.
Retinal dialysis.
Rhegmatogenous retinal detachment.

Systemic Findings

Related to trauma.
Periorbital trauma (eyelid ecchymosis, bone fractures).

Disease Course

- Progression of cataract.
- May have progression to subluxation of lens.

Treatment and Management

- Surgical removal of cataract (intracapsular or pars plana approach if inadequate zonular support).
- Thorough examination of peripheral retina.

Traumatic Subluxation and Dislocation of Lens

Summary

Blunt ocular trauma can cause stretching of the zonular ring, stretching and rupture of the lens zonules, and lens subluxation.

Etiology

Concussive force transmitted to the lens with zonular disruption.

Signs and Symptoms

Fluctuating vision.
Impaired accommodation
High astigmatism
Monocular diplopia.

Ophthalmic Findings

Phacodonesis.
Iridodonesis.

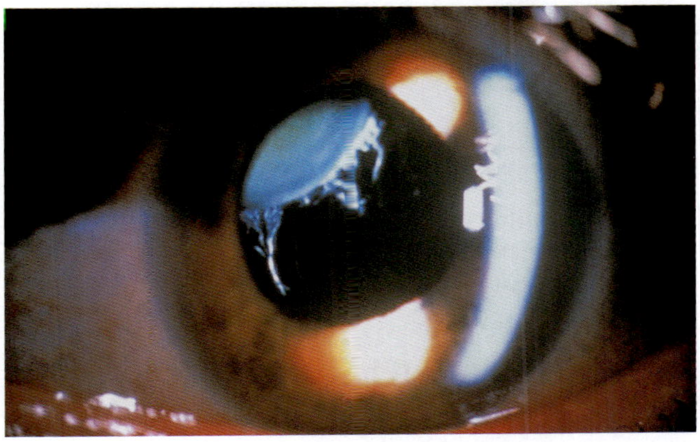

FIGURE 2.6. Traumatic subluxation of the lens. Note the torn zonules still attached to the lens and the slightly irregular pupil.

Torn zonules, subluxed lens (Figure 2.6).
Traumatic cataract.
Retinal dialysis.
Rhegmatogenous retinal detachment.

Systemic Findings

Related to trauma.
Periorbital trauma (eyelid ecchymosis, bone fractures).

Disease Course

- Progression of cataract.
- May have progressive subluxation of lens.

Treatment and Management

- Surgical removal of cataract (intracapsular or pars plana approach if inadequate zonular support).
- Thorough examination of peripheral retina.

EXFOLIATIVE DISORDERS

True Exfoliation (Glass-Blower Cataract)

Summary

Prolonged exposure to the infrared wavelengths can cause full-thickness delamination and peeling of the anterior lens capsule.

Etiology

Prolonged exposure to intense infrared wavelengths.

Signs and Symptoms

Decreased vision.

Ophthalmic Findings

Anterior capsular peeling.
Cortical cataract.

Systemic Findings

None.

Disease Course

Progression of cataract.

Treatment and Management

Surgical removal of cataract.

Pseudoexfoliation Syndrome

See also "Glaucoma/Exfoliation Syndrome," p. XX.

Summary

Abnormal fibrillar material is produced and deposited on the anterior lens capsule, iris, and other ocular structures. Open-angle glaucoma, poor pupil dilation, and weakened zonules are frequently found in these patients.

Etiology

Abnormal white fibrillogranular basement membrane-like material deposited on the anterior hyaloid face, ciliary processes, zonules, lens capsule, iris, cornea, and within the trabecular meshwork.

Signs and Symptoms

Usually none.

Ophthalmic Findings

Lens subluxation or dislocation.
Anterior capsular opacification or peeling, or both, often in a bull's-eye configuration (Figure 2.7).
Iris atrophy at pupillary margin.
Increased pigmentation of trabecular meshwork.
Open-angle glaucoma.

Systemic Findings

Pseudoexfoliative material has been found systemically in multiple organs of patients with this disease, usually of no consequence.

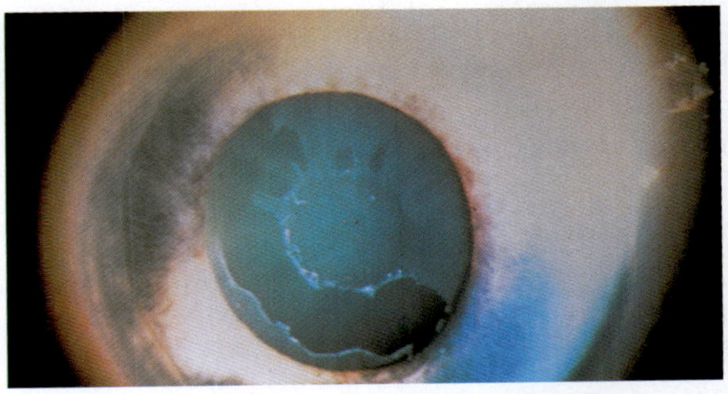

FIGURE 2.7. Pseudoexfoliative material deposited on the anterior lens capsule. The clear semicircular area is thought to be due to rubbing of the iris on the lens.

Disease Course

- Glaucoma may develop in 40% to 60% of patients.
- Spontaneous lens subluxation may develop in 5% of patients.

Treatment and Management

- Cataract extraction with careful attention to prevent zonular disruption.
- May need mechanical devices to achieve adequate pupil dilation.
- Vitreous loss is five times more frequent in this group of patients.
- Regular monitoring of intraocular pressure.

LENS-INDUCED UVEITIS AND GLAUCOMA

See also "Lens-Induced Glaucoma," p. XX.

Phacolytic Glaucoma

Summary

A condition in which denatured, liquefied lens proteins from a hypermature cataract leak into the anterior chamber through an intact lens capsule. This leads to glaucoma with macrophages ingesting the lens proteins resulting in blockage of the trabecular meshwork from both the engorged macrophages and the lens proteins.

Etiology

Leakage of lens proteins into the anterior chamber and occluding the trabecular meshwork.

Signs and Symptoms

Abrupt onset of pain, photophobia, and redness in cataractous eye that has had poor vision for a substantial length of time.

Ophthalmic Findings

Hypermature cataract.
Corneal edema.
Anterior chamber inflammation.
White flocculent material in anterior chamber and on lens capsule.
Markedly elevated intraocular pressure.

Special Studies

Microscopic examination of aqueous humor may reveal lipid-laden macrophages.

Systemic Findings

None.

Disease Course

Persistent inflammation and glaucoma until lens removed.

Treatment and Management

- Topical steroids and antiglaucoma medications to control inflammation and pressure.
- Definitive treatment is cataract extraction.

Phacoanaphylaxis (Phacoantigenic Uveitis)

Summary

Phacoanaphylaxis is characterized by immune recognition of lens material and a zonal granulomatous inflammatory reaction.

Etiology

An immune response to lens material elaborated after extracapsular cataract surgery or traumatic capsular rupture.

Signs and Symptoms

Pain.
Injection.
Photophobia.
Decreased vision.

Ophthalmic Findings

Large granulomatous keratic precipitates.
Anterior chamber inflammation.
Elevated intraocular pressure.

Special Tests

Microscopic examination of anterior chamber aspirate.

Pathology

Zonal granuloma with lens material and surrounding inflammatory cells.

Systemic Findings

None.

Disease Course

- After extracapsular cataract extraction or traumatic lens rupture.
- Onset typically occurs 1 to 14 days after exposure of the lens material to the host immune system, although latency of up to 1 year has been reported.
- The fellow eye may become involved at any time, particularly after extracapsular cataract surgery.

Treatment and Management

Topical steroids.
Surgical removal of lens or retained lens material.

Differential Diagnosis

Endophthalmitis.

Phacomorphic Glaucoma

Summary

Phacomorphic glaucoma is due to the enlargement of the lens in the anteroposterior dimension shallowing the anterior chamber and causing a secondary-angle closure glaucoma.

Etiology

Anteroposterior enlargement of the lens causing angle-closure glaucoma.

Signs and Symptoms

Attacks of angle closure.

Ophthalmic Findings

Hyperopia.
Small eye or shallow anterior chamber.
Large lens.

Systemic Findings

None.

Treatment and Management

Laser Iridotomy: temporizing treatment.
Lens extraction: definitive treatment.

Uveitis-Glaucoma-Hyphema Syndrome

Summary

Uveal irritation and resultant inflammation from a poorly fitting intraocular lens results in the uveitis-glaucoma-hyphema (UGH) syndrome. This most commonly results from older-generation iris-fixated and angle-supported anterior chamber lenses. May now occur more frequently with improper-sized (one-piece) lens in the sulcus.

Etiology

Uveal irritation from mobile intraocular lens in anterior chamber or sulcus.

Signs and Symptoms

Decreased, fluctuating vision.
Photosensitivity.

Ophthalmic Findings

Chronic low-grade anterior uveitis.
Glaucoma.
Recurrent hyphema.
Usually older design anterior chamber lens.
Can be improper-sized lens in sulcus as well.

Systemic Findings

None.

Treatment and Management

Removal and/or replacement of lens implant.

CATARACTS

Congenital Cataracts

Polar Cataracts

Demographics

Anterior polar: autosomal dominant transmission.
Posterior polar: sporadic or familial.

Etiology

Remnants of the tunica vasculosa lentis or abnormality of posterior capsule.

Signs and Symptoms

- Decreased vision (more so with posterior polar cataract, since it is closer to nodal point of eye).
- May be completely asymptomatic.

Ophthalmic Findings

- Opacity of the subcapsular cortex and lens capsule of either the anterior or posterior lens (Figure 2.8).
- Frequently bilateral, symmetric.

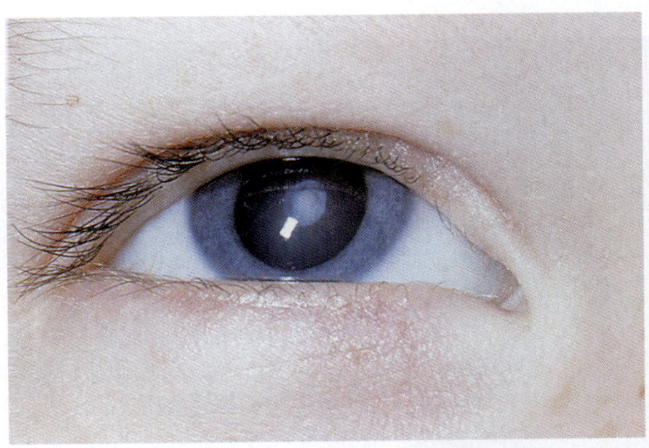

FIGURE 2.8. Anterior polar cataract and persistent pupillary membrane may be remnants of the hyaloid vasculature. (From Tasman W, Jaeger E. *The Wills Eye Hospital Atlas of Clinical Ophthalmology*, 2nd ed. Philadelphia, PA: Lippincott Williams & Wilkins, 2001, with permission.)

Systemic Findings

None.

Disease Course

- Anterior polar cataracts.
  Frequently bilateral.
  Nonprogressive; surgery is seldom required.
  May also be seen in patients with aniridia.
- Posterior polar cataracts.
  Nonprogressive, but in rare cases may worsen.
  Be cautious with lens extraction since lens capsule adjacent to cataract may be very thin.

Treatment and Management

Lens extraction if cataract is visually significant.

Sutural (Stellate) Cataract

Demographics

Autosomal dominant in most cases.

Etiology

Develops during fetal lens development (later, lens sutures are more branched).

Signs and Symptoms

Usually does not affect vision.

Ophthalmic Findings

Opacification of the Y sutures of the fetal nucleus (Figure 2.9).
Commonly bilateral, symmetric.

Systemic Findings

None.

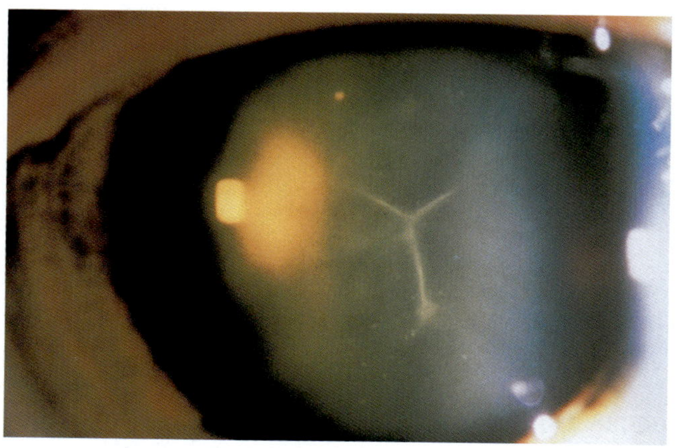

FIGURE 2.9. Sutural cataract with congenital opacification of the anterior "Y" suture. Usually does not affect vision and requires no treatment.

Disease Course

Nonprogressive.

Treatment and Management

None required, vision usually good.

Nuclear Cataract

Demographics

When inherited, autosomal dominant.

Etiology

Thought to be caused by abnormalities in development during early gestation affecting both the embryonic and fetal nucleuses.

Signs and Symptoms

Decreased vision.
Altered red reflex.
Sensory deprivation nystagmus.

Ophthalmic Findings

Opacities involving the embryonic and fetal lens nucleus, peripheral cortex unaffected.
Commonly bilateral, symmetric.
Microphthalmos.

Systemic Findings

None.

Disease Course

Nonprogressive.

Treatment and Management

Lens extraction early in life allows proper visual development.

Lamellar (Zonular) Cataract

Demographics

Autosomal dominant or related to toxic injury during gestation.
Most common type of congenital cataract.

Etiology

May occur in infants with hypocalcemia (or with maternal hypocalcemia).

Signs and Symptoms

Variable, depends on size of opacity.

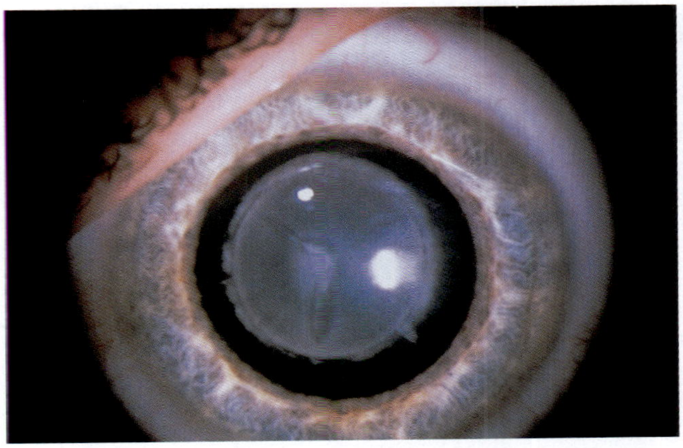

FIGURE 2.10. A lamellar cataract represents a focal insult during the development of the lens. The lens nucleus is clear (difficult to see, but surrounded by opacified lamellae), and the peripheral cortex is uninvolved.

Ophthalmic Findings

Opacification of discrete zones of lens fibers (Figure 2.10).
Clear nucleus centrally and clear peripheral cortex.
Commonly bilateral, symmetric.
Amblyopia.

Systemic Findings

Usually none, but hypocalcaemia may be noted.

Disease Course

Nonprogressive.

Treatment and Management

Lens extraction if visually significant.

Capsular Cataract

Etiology

Not known.

Signs and Symptoms

Usually does not affect vision.

Ophthalmic Findings

- Opacification of the lens epithelium and anterior capsule.
- Extends into anterior chamber (which differentiates this entity from anterior polar cataracts).

Systemic Findings

None.

Disease Course

Nonprogressive.

Treatment and Management

None required

Rubella Cataract

Etiology

- Maternal infection with the rubella virus during first trimester.
- Retention of lens nuclei causing opacification.

Signs and Symptoms

Decreased vision.
Sensory deprivation nystagmus.

Ophthalmic Findings

Cataract (may be nuclear or total).
Liquefied cortex is occasionally seen (morgagnian cataract).
Pigmentary retinopathy.
Microphthalmos.
Glaucoma.

Systemic Findings (Evidence of Systemic Rubella Infection)

Cardiac defects.
Mental retardation.
Deafness.

Pathology

Retained lens nuclei.

Disease Course

Nonprogressive.

Treatment and Management

- When visually significant, lens extraction may be considered.
- Surgery may be complicated by excessive postoperative inflammation, thought to be related to elaboration of live virus particles at the time of surgery. Live virus particles have been recovered from the lens up to 3 years of age.

Differential Diagnosis (Infectious Congenital Cataract)

Congenital toxoplasmosis.
Congenital varicella infection.

Metabolic Causes of Cataract

See Table 2.2; Figures 2.11 and 2.12.

LENS

Table 2.2

Metabolic causes of cataract

Disease	Inheritance	Enzymatic defect	Cataract type	Notes
Galactosemia	Autosomal recessive	Galactose-1-phosphate uridyl transferase (most commonly)	Oil droplet initially may progress to total opacification	75% of these patients develop cataracts soon after birth
Wilson disease (hepatolenticular degeneration)	Autosomal recessive	Low serum level of ceruloplasmin	Sunflower cataract (deposition of cuprous oxide in anterior lens capsule and subcapsular cortex) (Figure 2.11)	Kayser-Fleischer ring in Descemet membrane (Figure 2.12)
Diabetes mellitus	Multifactorial	May be related to sorbitol pathway (aldose reductase)	Rapid-onset "snowflake" cataract	Rapid cataract progression in young diabetic patient

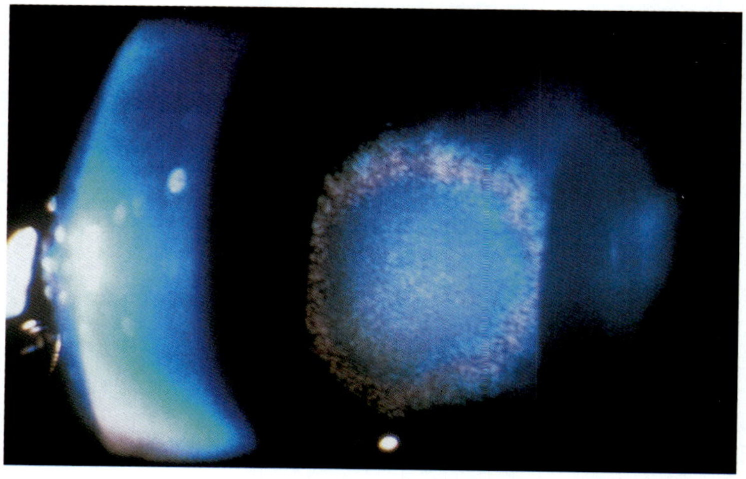

FIGURE 2.11. Copper deposits in the lens basement membrane (anterior lens capsule) producing the sunflower cataract in Wilson disease.

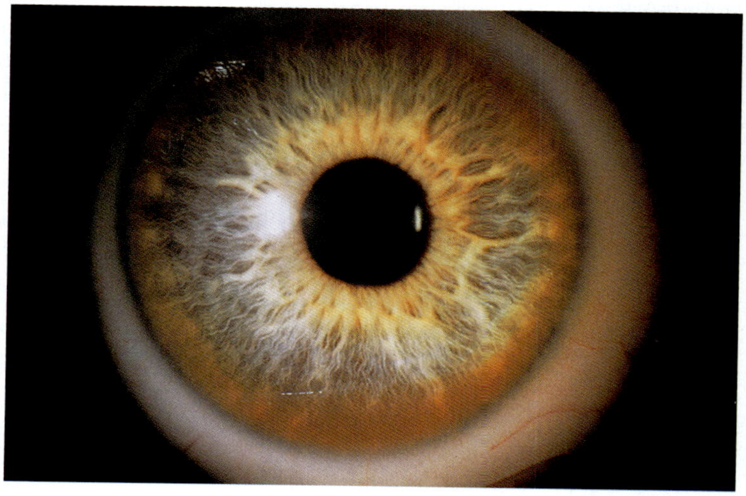

FIGURE 2.12. Copper deposits in Descemet membrane producing the brownish Kayser-Fleischer ring in Wilson disease.

Table 2.3

Genetic causes of cataract

Disease	Inheritance	Enzymatic defect	Cataract type	Ophthalmic findings
Fabry disease	X-linked recessive	Ceramide alphatribexosidase	Posterior spokelike opacities in males and carrier females	Cornea verticillata, renal failure
Down syndrome (trisomy 21)	N/A	N/A	Snowflake cataracts	Brushfield spots, myopia, strabismus keratoconus
Lowe oculocerebral syndrome	X-linked recessive	Decreased renal ammonia production	Thin, discoid lens Carriers have punctate cortical opacities	Glaucoma, mental retardation, aminoaciduria
Alport syndrome	X-linked dominant (most common)	Disorder of basement membranes, possibly collagen IV defect	Anterior lenticonus, anterior polar and cortical cataract	Deafness, nephropathy
Myotonic dystrophy	Autosomal dominant	Disorder of creatine kinase in skeletal muscles	Anterior and posterior subcapsular colored crystals ("Christmas tree" cataract) (Figure 2.13)	Ptosis, abnormal saccades, pigmentary retinopathy
Hallermann-Streiff syndrome	Unknown	Unknown	Mature cataract shortly after birth	Birdlike facies microphthalmia, glaucoma
Mannosidosis	Autosomal recessive	Alpha-mannosidase	Type I: posterior cortical spokelike Type II: punctate cortical opacities	Phenotype similar to Hurler disease
Niemann-Pick disease type A	Autosomal recessive	Sphingomyelinase	Anterior capsular brownish opacification and posterior cortical opacities	Cherry red spot, nystagmus, corneal clouding
Stickler syndrome (progressive arthro-ophthalmopathy)	Autosomal dominant	Disorder of type II collagen	Cortical wedges and flecks	High myopia, retinal detachment, short stature, arthropathy
Aniridia	$^{2}/_{3}$; Autosomal dominant, $^{1}/_{3}$ Sporadic	Unknown	Lamellar, cortical subcapsular opacities	Foveal hypoplasia, nystagmus, risk of Wilms tumor in sporadic patients

N/A, not applicable.

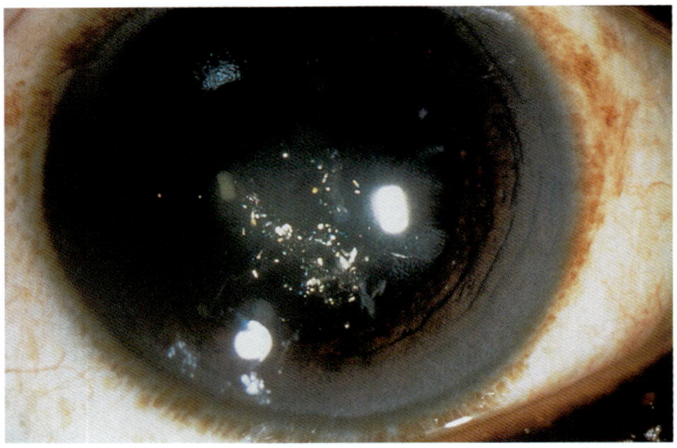

FIGURE 2.13. Colorful crystals in the "Christmas tree" cataract of a patient with myotonic dystrophy.

Genetic Causes of Cataract

See Table 2.3; Figure 2.13.

Drug-Induced Cataracts

See Table 2.4; Figure 2.14.

Age-Related Cataracts

Nuclear Sclerosis

Etiology

May be due to age-related increase in water-insoluble lens proteins.

Signs and Symptoms

- Decreased vision, especially at distance.
- Change in color perception (rarely noticed, since change is very gradual).
- Loss of contrast sensitivity.

Ophthalmic Findings

Bilateral, asymmetric yellowing or browning of lens.
Myopic shift in prescription.

Treatment and Management

Surgical removal.

Cortical Cataract

Etiology

Focal opacification of lens fibers.

Signs and Symptoms

Glare, haloes around lights.
Worse when pupil dilated.

Ophthalmic Findings

Multiple, wedge-shaped lens opacities.
Usually bilateral, but asymmetric.

Treatment and Management

Surgical removal.

Table 2.4

Drug-induced cataracts

Medication	Cataract type	Clinical significance
Phenothiazines	Anterior polar stellate pigmented opacities (Figure 2.14)	Usually visually insignificant
Corticosteroids	Posterior subcapsular cataracts	Significant reduction in acuity
Miotics (long-acting anticholinesterases, e.g., echothiophate iodide)	Nuclear or cortical with vacuoles	With long-term usage visually significant cataracts may develop
Amiodarone	Anterior lens pigment deposition	Usually visually insignificant

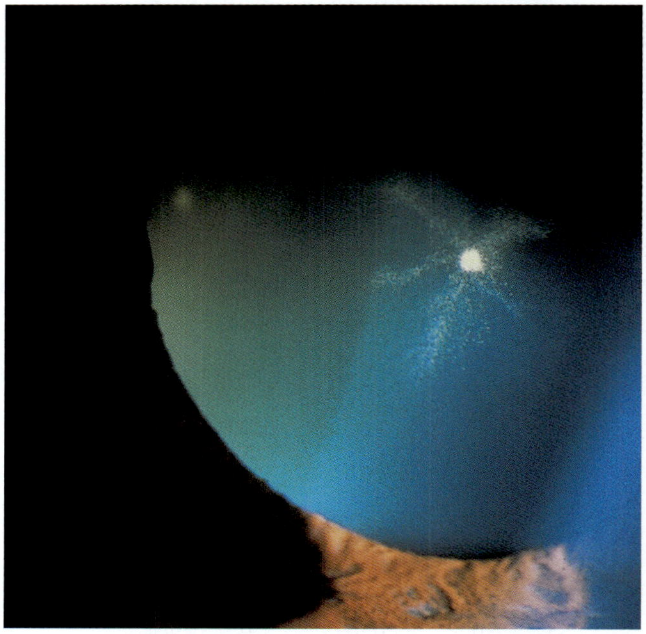

FIGURE 2.14. Stellate deposition of phenothiazine crystals in the anterior lens epithelium.

Posterior Subcapsular Cataract

Etiology

Age.
Trauma.
Inflammation or the use of steroids.
Ionizing radiation.
Diabetes Mellitus.
Smoking.

Signs and Symptoms

- Glare, monocular diplopia.
- Decreased vision, especially when pupil is small (with accommodation, at near, under bright conditions).

Ophthalmic Findings

- Plaque or granularity of posterior capsule.
- Usually axial in location, best seen with retroillumination (Figure 2.15).

Pathology

- Posterior migration and swelling of lens epithelial cells.
- When lens epithelial cells become swollen, they are known as *Wedl* or *bladder cells*.

Treatment and Management

Dilation of pupil (temporary solution).
Surgical removal.

Mature Cataract

Etiology

Generalized swelling and opacification of cortical lens fibers.

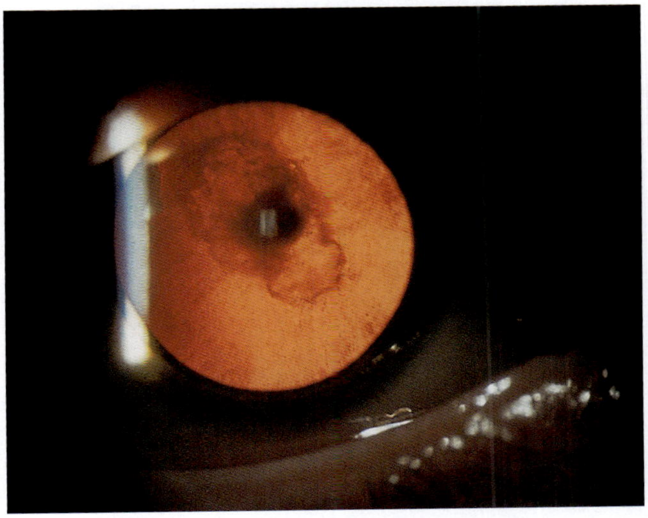

FIGURE 2.15. Posterior subcapsular cataract in retroillumination. Because these cataracts are axial and posterior, they frequently cause many symptoms.

Signs and Symptoms

Poor vision, usually at the level of hand motions.

Ophthalmic Findings

- White lens with water clefts (Figure 2.16).
- Lens may swell so large as to cause angle-closure glaucoma.

Treatment and Management

Surgical removal.

Hypermature Cataract

Etiology

Leakage of lens proteins through lens capsule.

Signs and Symptoms

Poor vision, usually at the level of hand motions.

Ophthalmic Findings

- White lens with water clefts.
- Wrinkled lens capsule from loss of lens substance.
- Ocular inflammation to lens proteins.
- Glaucoma from lens proteins occluding trabecular meshwork.

Treatment and Management

Surgical removal may be complicated by capsular tears, poor visibility from liquefied cortex.

Morgagnian Cataract

Etiology

Liquefaction of lens material allowing nucleus to move freely.

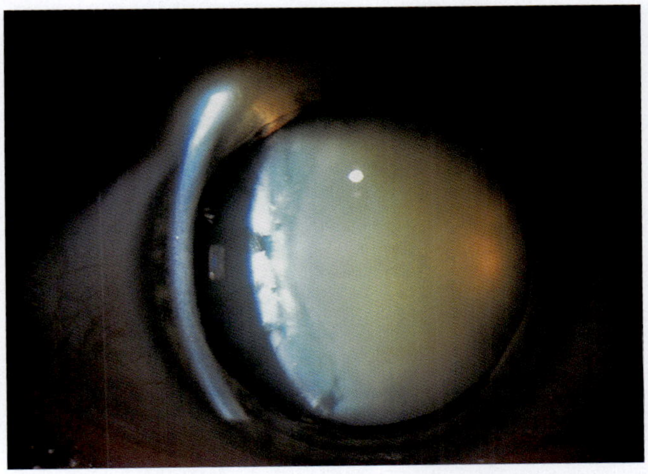

FIGURE 2.16. White, mature cataract with water clefts visible beneath the anterior capsule.

Ophthalmic Findings

Mature cataract with freely mobile nucleus.

Treatment and Management

Surgical removal.

Other Causes of Cataracts

Hypotony And Ocular Ischemic Syndrome

Etiology

Presumably attributable to lack of nutrition to the lens.

Alkali Burn

Etiology

Change in pH of anterior chamber, damage to ciliary body, anterior segment ischemia.

Cataract Masquerades

Differential Diagnosis of Leukocoria

- Children:
    - Retinoblastoma (Figure 2.17).
    - Persistent hyperplastic primary vitreous.
    - Retinopathy of prematurity.
    - Toxocariasis.
    - Coloboma of choroid.
    - Melanoma of ciliary body.
    - Coats disease.
    - Vitreous hemorrhage.
    - Retinal detachment.
    - Norrie disease.
    - Corneal opacity or Peters anomaly, or both.
    - Congenital cataract.
- Adults:
    - Mature cataract.
    - Intraocular inflammation:
        - Toxoplasmosis.
        - Endophthalmitis.
    - Intraocular tumors.
    - Retinal detachment.
    - Vitreous hemorrhage.
    - Corneal opacities.

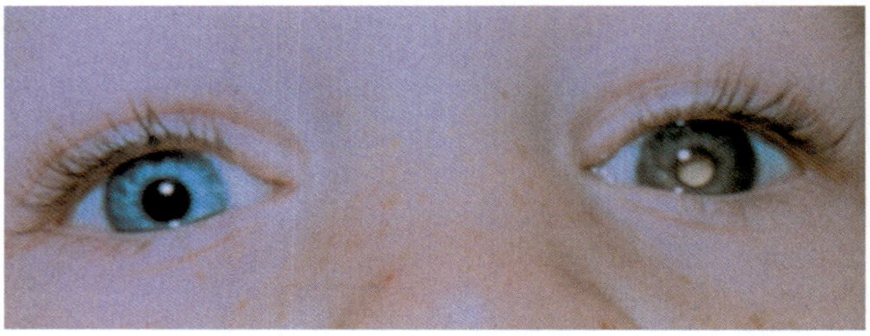

FIGURE 2.17. Retinoblastoma in the left eye, mimicking a cataract.

CHAPTER 3

Retina and Vitreous

Seenu M. Hariprasad • Irma Ahmed • Sophie J. Bakri • Mandi D. Conway • Tamer H. Mahmoud • Andrew A. Moshfeghi • Prithvi Mruthyunjaya • Michael D. Ober • Sunil K. Srivastava • David G. Telander • Cuong D. Vu

RETINAL ANATOMY

Macula and Fovea

The macula histologically contains more than two layers of ganglion cells (Figure 3.1).

Peripheral Retina

- Histological definition: any area with a single layer of ganglion cells.
- Terminates at the ora serrata located 6 mm posterior to the limbus nasally and 7 mm posterior to the limbus temporally.
- Continuous with the nonpigmented epithelium of the pars plana.

Retinal Layers

The layers of the retina are depicted in Figure 3.2.

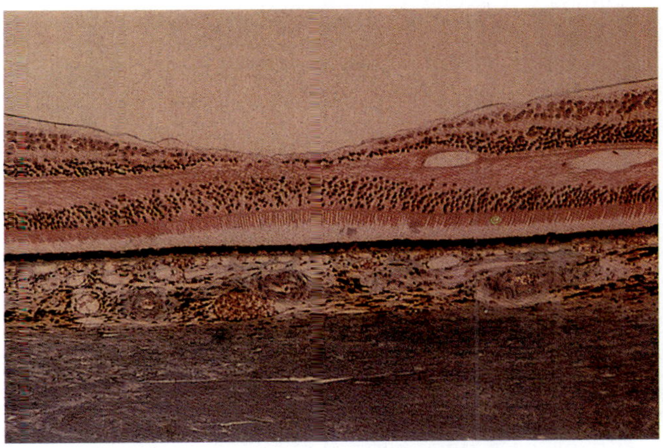

FIGURE 3.1. Histology of a normal macula. Note the multiple nuclei in the ganglion cell layer outside the fovea.

[1]A list of commonly used abbreviations may be found at the end of this chapter.

Retinal Circulation

Central retinal artery: supplies the inner two thirds of the retina.

Choriocapillaris: supplies the inner nuclear layer outward to the retinal pigment epithelium (RPE).[1]

Ophthalmic artery: gives off long and short posterior ciliary arteries.

Long posterior ciliary arteries: supply the choriocapillaris from the optic nerve to the equator.

Short posterior ciliary arteries: supply the optic nerve head and the peripapillary choroid.

Recurrent branches of the anterior ciliary arteries: supply the anterior choriocapillaris.

Vortex veins: one per quadrant; drain the choriocapillaris and form the superior ophthalmic vein that courses through the superior orbital fissure and drains into the cavernous sinus.

Choroid

Four layers:

1. Suprachoroidal space.
2. Stroma.
3. Choriocapillaris.
4. Bruch's membrane.

Nourishes the outer retina and acts as a heat sink for the retina.

Retinal Pigment Epithelium

- Single-layer hexagonal cuboidal cells of neuroectodermal origin.
- Cells in fovea are taller, thinner, and have more abundant, larger melanosomes.
- Functions of the RPE:
  1. Formation of the outer blood–ocular barrier between the choriocapillaris and the sensory retina via tight junctions. Pump functions to remove subretinal fluid.
  2. Phagocytosis of rod and cone outer segments.
  3. Vitamin A metabolism.

A

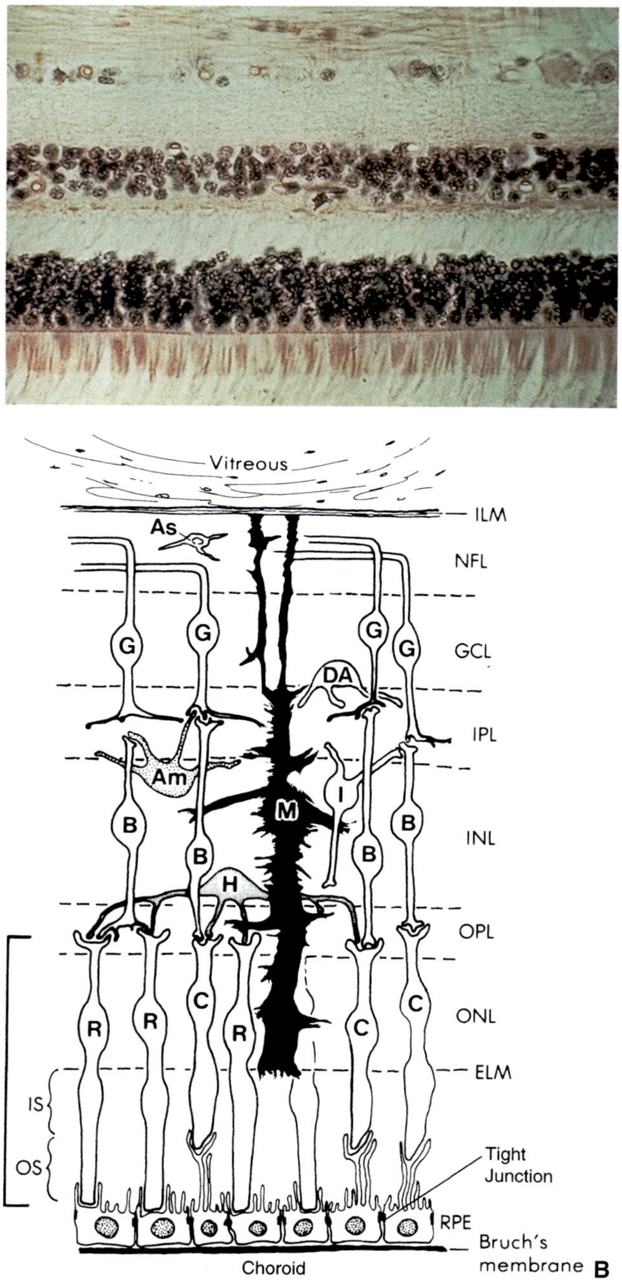

B

FIGURE 3.2. (**A**) Histopathology and (**B**) diagram of the nine retinal layers. The photoreceptors are located at the bottom.

4. Synthesis and degradation of extracellular matrix.
5. Atrophic, hypertrophic, and hyperplastic responses to disease.
6. Light absorption.
7. Heat exchange.
8. Formation of basal lamina.

Bruch Membrane

External to the RPE.
Five layers of Bruch membrane:

1. Basement membrane of the RPE.
2. Inner loose collagenous zone.
3. Middle layer of elastic fibers.
4. Outer loose collagenous zone.
5. Basement membrane of the choriocapillaris.

Photoreceptors

- Outer segments are involved in phototransduction.
- Inner segments transmit neuronal impulses along axons that synapse with the bipolar and horizontal cells.

Interneurons, Ganglion Cells, and Glial Cells

See Figure 3.2.

Retinal Layers

1. External limiting membrane: not a true membrane. It is the attachment site of adjacent photoreceptors and Müller cells.
2. Outer plexiform layer: interconnections of photoreceptor synaptic bodies, horizontal, and bipolar cells.
3. Inner nuclear layer: nuclei of bipolar, Müller, horizontal, and amacrine cells.
4. Middle limiting membrane: formed by the attachments of synaptic bodies of photoreceptor cells.
5. Inner plexiform layer: axons of bipolar, amacrine cells, and ganglion cell dendrites and synapses.
6. The nerve fiber layer: ganglion cell axons. The ganglion cell layer contains the ganglion cell bodies.
7. Inner limiting membrane (ILM): not a true membrane; made of footplates of Müller cells.

Ora Serrata

- Boundary between the retina and the pars plana.
- Retinal blood vessels terminate at the ora serrata, and the vascular supply is the watershed zone between the anterior and the posterior ciliary systems.

Vitreous

- Four cubic centimeters in volume.
- Constitutes four fifths of the entire eye.
- Composition is 99% water combined with mucopolysaccharide and hyaluronic acid, which imparts hyperviscosity.
- Peripheral vitreous attaches to the pars plana, retina, and optic nerve. The strongest attachments are at the vitreous base, optic nerve, and retinal vessels.

References

Apple DJ. Anatomy and histopathology of the macular region. *Int Ophthalmol Clin* 1981;21:1–9.

Blanks JC. Morphology of the retina. In: Ryan SJ, ed. *Retina*, 2nd ed., vol. 1. St. Louis, MO: Mosby, 1994:37–54.

RETINAL PHYSIOLOGY

Phototransduction

- Four classes of visual pigment:
  Rhodopsin in rods.
  Three pigments in cones.
- Rods and cones shed their outer segments.
- Retinal rod cells contain many stacked disklike membrane vesicles.
- Almost half of the protein in these membranes is a light-absorbing conjugated protein called *rhodopsin*.
- Rhodopsin consists of a protein opsin and tightly bound 11-cis retinal; the aldehyde form of vitamin A.
- Opsin is synthesized in the inner segments and transported to the base of the outer segment. Opsin is combined with 11-cis retinal to form rhodopsin (Figure 3.3).
- The tips of the rod outer segments are shed and phagocytized by the RPE. The rods shed at dawn and the cones shed at dusk. There is a net movement of vitamin A from the outer segments to the RPE during light adaptation, and the reversal of the flow in darkness.
- Depolarized state: In darkness, there are high levels of cyclic guanosine monophosphate (cGMP) in the outer segments that create open Na^+ channels.
- Hyperpolarized state: In the presence of light, there are decreased cGMP levels causing closure of the Na^+ channels, which leads to a decrease in neurotransmitter release. Cyclic GMP regulates protein phosphorylation. The bleaching of rhodopsin causes hydrolysis of cGMP through a series of biochemical reactions.
- Light triggers an electrical response in the retina. Presynaptic neurons are depolarized by an action potential (electrical transmission). This leads to an increase in intracellular calcium, which causes a release of neurotransmitters from the synaptic vesicles. Neurotransmitters stimulate postsynaptic receptors. There is then reuptake, catabolism, or diffusion of the neurotransmitter.
- There are three levels of neurotransmission:
  1. Light hyperpolarizes the photoreceptors causing a decrease in transmitter release.
  2. Bipolar and horizontal cells respond to the decreased neurotransmitter with graded potential.
  3. Ganglion cell generates an action potential.
- The neurotransmitters in the retina include the following:
  Acetylcholine.
  Dopamine.
  Gamma-aminobutyric acid: inhibits dopaminergic and cholinergic activity in the retina.
  Glutamate.
  Aspartate (causes excitation block of second order neurons).

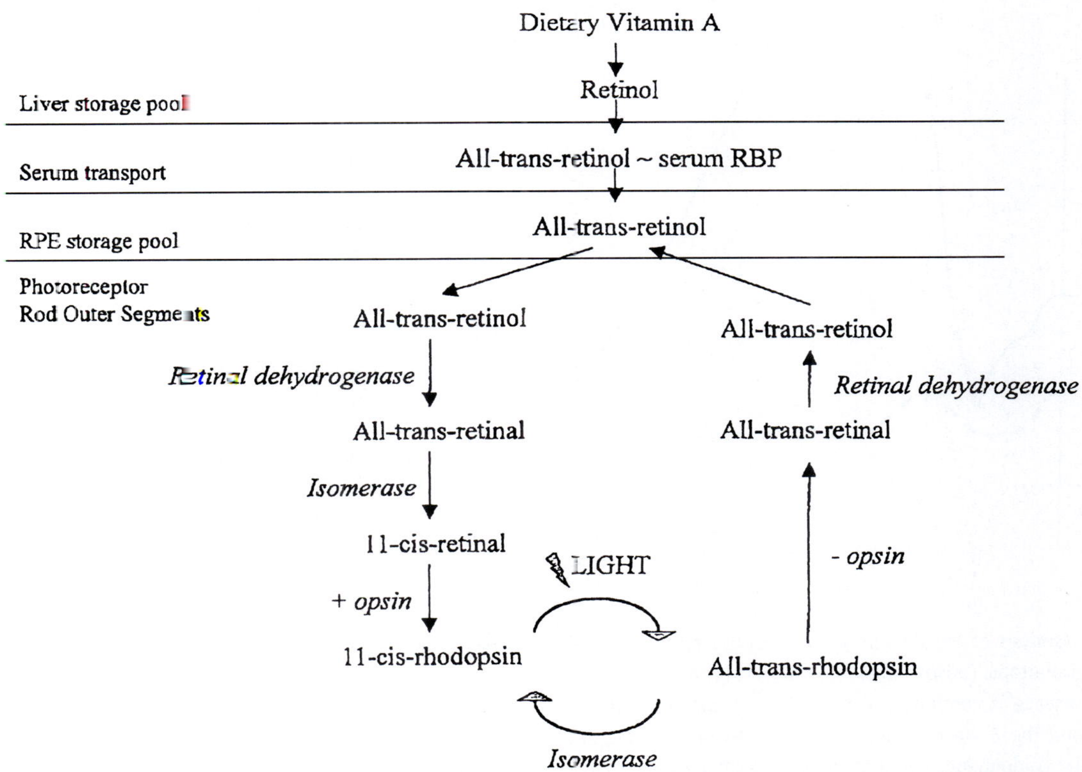

FIGURE 3.3. Biochemical cycle of vitamin A metabolism in the eye. (Adapted from *Retina and vitreous: basic and clinical science course,* Section 12. San Francisco, CA: American Academy of Ophthalmology, 1993:Figure 1–2.)

- Energy for visual excitation comes from adenosine triphosphate (ATP) generated from glucose metabolism. There are three pathways of glucose metabolism:
  1. Glycolysis.
  2. Tricarboxylic acid (TCA cycle): generates most of the ATP for the retina.
  3. Hexose monophosphate shunt.

Reference

Fundamentals and principles of ophthalmology: retina physiology. *Basic and clinical science course.* San Francisco, CA: American Academy of Ophthalmology, 1993:179–203.

RETINAL TESTING

Electrophysiological Testing

Electroretinogram

See Figure 3.4.

- Evoked by a brief flash of light.
- Negative a wave: photoreceptor depolarization.
- Positive b wave: Müller and bipolar cells.
- Scotopic electroretinogram (ERG): performed with a blue flash in the dark-adapted state; isolates rod response.

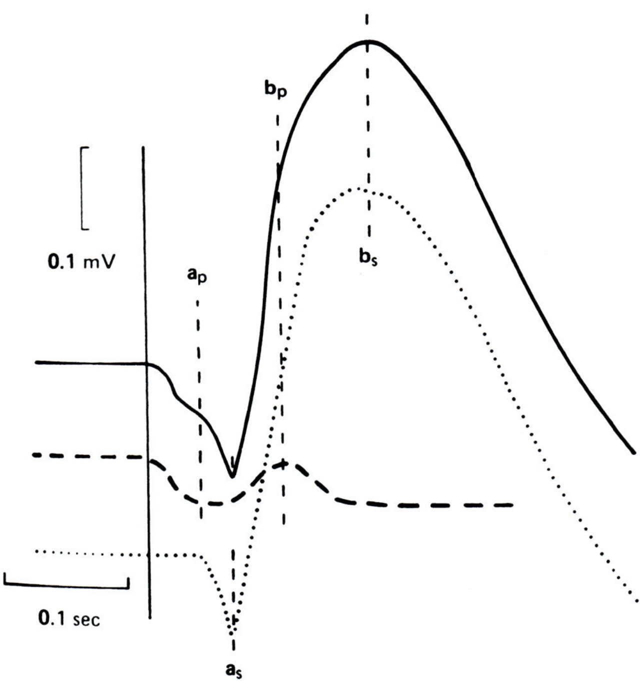

FIGURE 3.4. Analysis of the ERG in a dark-adapted eye (*solid line*) as the result of photopic (*dashed line*) and scotopic (*dotted line*) components. The *a* wave is composed of photopic (a_p) and scotopic (a_s) components, and the *b* wave is similarly composed of photopic (b_p) and scotopic (b_s) components. (From Miller NR. *Walsh and Hoyt's clinical neuro-ophthalmology,* 4th ed., vol. 1. Baltimore, MD: Williams & Wilkins, 1982:36, with permission.)

- Photopic ERG: performed with a bright white flash in the light-adapted state; isolates cone response.
- Clinical uses:
  - Help diagnose retinitis pigmentosa (RP), pattern dystrophies, and other retinal disorders.
  - Differentiates ischemic (decreased b:a wave amplitude) from nonischemic central retinal vein occlusion (CRVO).
  - Assesses retinal toxicity of intraocular foreign body (IOFB).

Multifocal ERG

- Mechanism is based on stimulating macular function while suppressing rod activity with a bright light.
- Clinical uses include objective assessment of macular function, for example, can be used to detect early hydroxychloroquine toxicity.

Electrooculogram

Electrooculogram (EOG) measures the RPE standing potential.

Arden ratio: maximum light adapted (light peak) to minimum dark adapted (dark trough). Normal value is greater than 1.75.

Clinical uses: dystrophies (i.e., Best disease, which has a normal ERG and an abnormal EOG).

Visual Evoked Potential

Visual evoked potential is the electrical signal generated by the occipital visual cortex.

- Tests macular function.
- Clinical uses:
  - Evaluates optic neuropathy, confirms projection of optic nerve fibers in albinism.
  - Verifies intact visual pathway in preverbal or uncooperative patients.

References

Grand MG, Bressler NM, Brown GC, et al. Retinal physiology and psychophysics. In: Denny M, Taylor F, eds. *Basic and clinical science course: retina and vitreous.* San Francisco, CA: American Academy of Ophthalmology, 1996:20–40.

Regillo C, Holekamp N, Johnson MW, et al. Retinal physiology and psychophysics. In: Skuta GL, Cantor LB, eds. *Basic and clinical science course: retina and vitreous.* San Francisco, CA: American Academy of Ophthalmology, 2008–2009:37–38.

Color Vision

Cones have three types of pigment: blue, green, and red.

- Red/green deficiency primarily represents X-linked inheritance.
- Blue/yellow deficiencies are usually seen in acquired diseases.

There are two types of color vision tests:

- Pseudoisochromatic plates (Ishihara, Hardy-Rand Littler) on which color numbers stand out from a background of dots. Useful in screening color-deficient individuals but does not classify the deficiency.
- Panel tests (Farnsworth panel D15, Farnsworth-Munsell 100-hue) discriminate between subtle shades of similar colors:
  - D15 test involves 15 color tiles that cover the visual spectrum. The subject arranges the tablets in perceived sequence; although the test is not very sensitive, it is fast and accurate.
  - D15 is useful in retinal diseases because it discriminates congenital from acquired defects.

Reference

Grand MG, Bressler NM, Brown GC, et al. Retinal physiology and psychophysics. In: Denny M, Taylor F, eds. *Basic and clinical science course: retina and vitreous.* San Francisco, CA: American Academy of Ophthalmology, 1996:20–40.

Retinal Imaging

Intravenous Fluorescein Angiography

- Sodium fluorescein absorbs blue light (465 to 490 nm) and emits green/yellow light (520 to 530 nm).
- Fluorescein is metabolized by the liver and excreted by the kidneys. One half of usual dose is usually administered in patients with renal failure.
- Pseudofluorescence occurs when nonfluorescent light passes through the entire filter system. The blue exciter filter overlaps into the yellow/green zone, and the yellow/green barrier filter overlaps into the blue zone. This causes nonfluorescent structures to appear fluorescent and can be detected by early photographs before dye injection.
- Side effects of fluorescein angiography (FA):
  - Nausea in 1% to 5% of patients. This usually occurs 30 seconds after injection and lasts approximately 2 to 3 minutes.
  - Extravasation and local tissue necrosis.
  - Intra-arterial injection.
  - Emesis.
  - Vasovagal reaction.
  - Allergic reaction.
  - Discoloration of the skin and urine.
  - Anaphylaxis.
  - Nerve palsy.
  - Neurologic problems.
  - Thrombophlebitis.
  - Pyrexia.
  - Death (extremely rare).
- Normal angiogram choroidal fluorescence (Table 3.1).
- Two categories of abnormalities (Figure 3.5):
  1. Hypofluorescence (Figure 3.6).
     - Blocked fluorescence.
     - Vascular filling defect.
  2. Hyperfluorescence
     - Pseudofluorescence (seen on red-free photographs before injection of fluorescein).
     - Optic nerve drusen.
     - Astrocytic hamartoma.
     - Sclera.
     - Exudate.
     - Scar.
     - Myelinated nerve fibers.
     - Foreign body.
     - Transmitted fluorescence: RPE window defect.
     - Abnormal vascular fluorescence: tortuosity, dilation, anastomoses, neovascularization (NV), aneurysms, telangiectasis, and tumors.
     - Leakage: may leak into the vitreous, the disk, the retina, or the choroid.

Table 3.1

Fluorescein angiography phases

Time after injection	Angiogram phase	Location of fluorescence
8–15 s	Choroidal phase	Patchy choroidal filling Cilioretinal artery (if present) will fill
10–30 s	Transit phase	Early filling of retinal arterioles
15–20 s	Laminar venous phase	Early venous return present as linear hyperfluorescence along walls of veins
20–25 s	Peak fluorescence	Filling of the perifoveal capillary net
30 s	Recirculation phase	Fluorescein recirculates through the liver and lower concentration of fluorescein flows through the retinal arteries
10 min	Late phase	Retinal vasculature devoid of fluorescein staining of choroid, Bruch membrane, and sclera

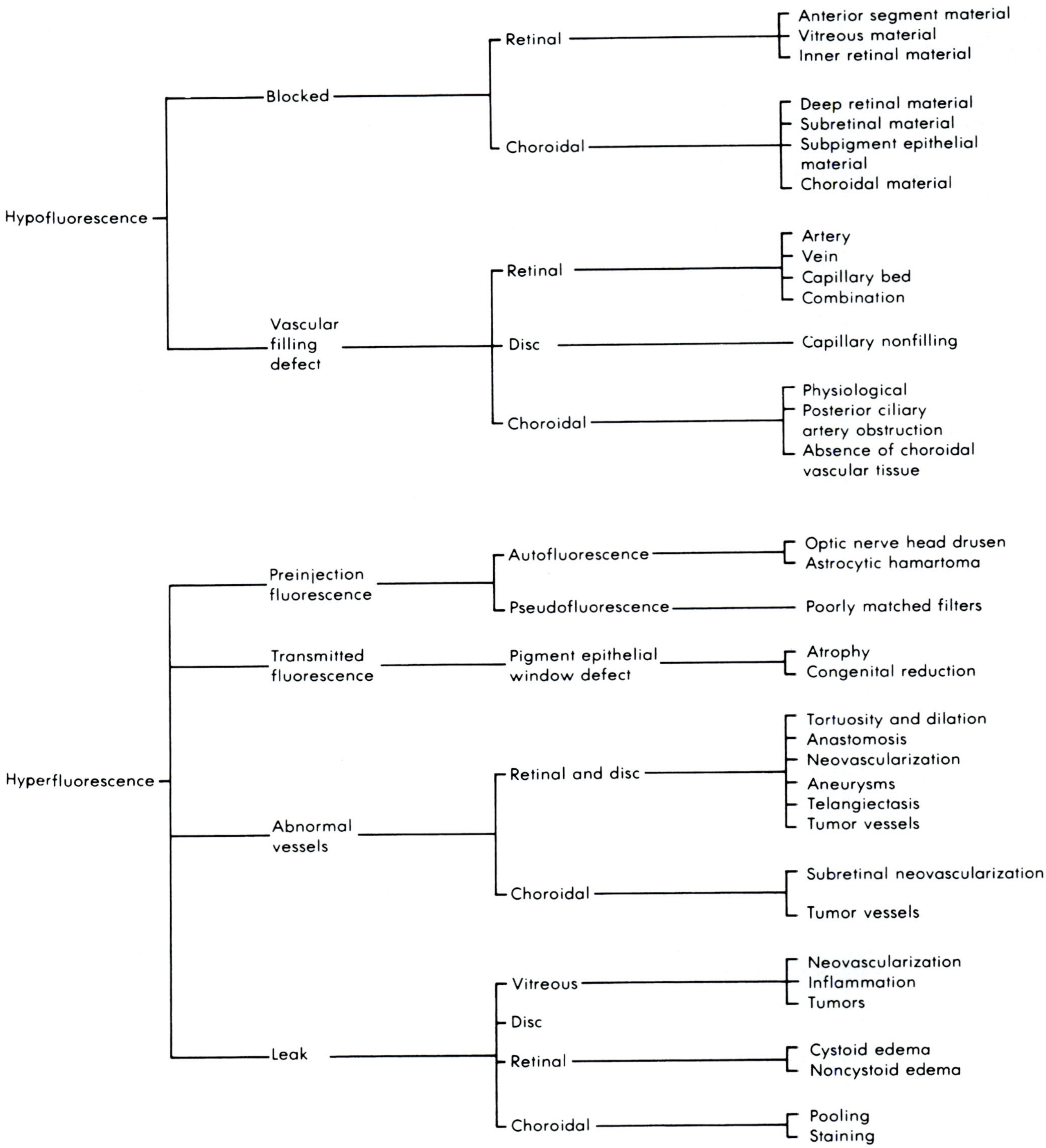

FIGURE 3.5. Flow sheet for abnormal FA.

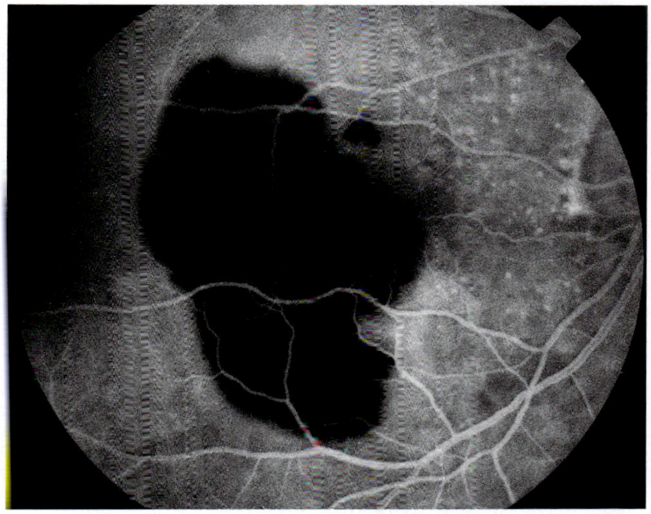

FIGURE 3.6. IVFA demonstrating hypofluorescence due to blockage by a large subretinal hemorrhage. The underlying choroidal fluorescence is obscured by the blood, but the retinal blood vessels are visible anterior to the blood.

Pooling: leakage of fluorescein dye into a distinct anatomic space (i.e., a sensory retinal detachment [RD] such as seen in central serous chorioretinopathy or an RPE detachment).

Staining: leakage of fluorescein diffusely into a tissue as in drusen, scar, or sclera.

Reference

Novotny HR, Alvis DL. A method of photographing fluorescence in circulating blood of the human eye. *Am J Ophthalmol* 1960;50:176.

Indocyanine Green Video Angiography

- Indocyanine green (ICG) video angiography is a water-soluble tricarbocyanine dye that absorbs and fluoresces in the near-infrared range.
- Less blockage of fluorescence by overlying pigment allowing enhanced imaging of the choroid.
- Because ICG dye is highly protein bound (98%), there is minimal escape from the choroidal vessels.
- ICG angiography allows visualization through retinal and subretinal hemorrhages, serous fluid, lipid, and pigment.
- Contraindications:
  Allergic reactions may occur in patients who have allergies to iodine.
  Avoid in liver failure patients, since the dye is metabolized by the liver.
  Avoid in pregnant women.
- Clinical uses of ICG angiography:
  Detection of choroidal neovascularization (CNV).
  Occult CNV with overlying hemorrhage.
  Recurrent CNV.
- Occult CNV with serous pigment epithelial detachment; detection of classic CNV with an area of occult choroidal neovascular membrane (CNVM) diagnosed by FA.
- Useful in evaluating intraocular tumors, choroiditis, choroidal vascular disorders, and choroidal infarctions.

Reference

Krupsky S, Friedman E, Foster CS, et al. Indocyanine green angiography in choroidal diseases. *Invest Ophthalmol Vis Sci* 1992;33:723.

Optical Coherence Tomography

- Noninvasive, noncontact and produces cross-sectional images of the retina described as "optical biopsy." It is based on low-coherence interferometry and uses light waves instead of ultrasound waves used in ultrasound. Reflected light waves from the retina form false-color images that represent the different retinal layers.
- Newer generations of spectral domain optical coherence tomography (OCT) are much faster with less motion artifact and show more details than the time-domain OCT scanners.
- Clinical uses include differentiating lamellar from full-thickness macular holes, highlighting vitreomacular traction, following treatment responses of cystoid macular edema (CME), neovascular macular degeneration. Spectral domain OCT also delineates external limiting membrane and outer segment-inner segment junctions, which if deficient may explain decreased visual acuity (VA) in many macular diseases (Figure 3.7).

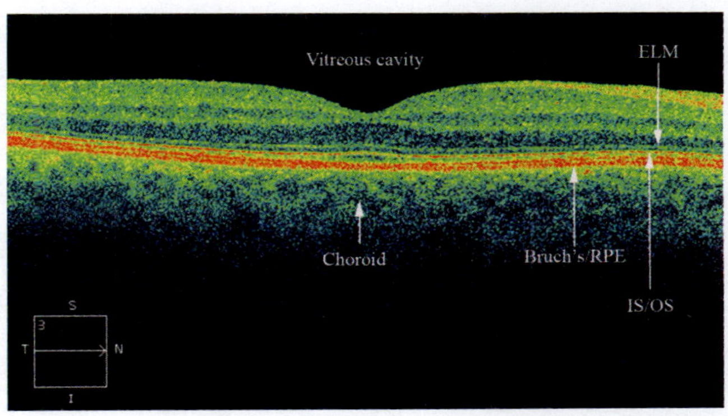

FIGURE 3.7. Normal Cirrus SD-OCT. ELM, external limiting membrane; I, inferior; IS/OS, inner segment outer segment junction; N, nasal; S, superior; T, temporal.

References

Kiernan DF, Mieler WF, Hariprasad SM. Spectral-domain optical coherence tomography: a comparison of modern high-resolution retinal imaging systems. *Am J Ophthalmol (Perspectives Invitation)* 2010;149(1):18–31.

Kiernan DF, Hariprasad SM, Chin EK, et al. Prospective comparison of high-definition-Cirrus™ and Stratus™ optical coherence tomography for quantifying retinal thickness. *Am J Ophthalmol* 2009;147(2):267–275.

Regillo C, Holekamp N, Johnson MW, et al. Retinal physiology and psychophysics. In: Skuta GL, Cantor LB, eds. *Basic and clinical science course: retina and vitreous.* San Francisco, CA: American Academy of Ophthalmology, 2008–2009: 37–38.

MACULAR DISEASE

Age-Related Macular Degeneration

Summary

Age-related macular degeneration (ARMD) is the leading cause of significant central visual impairment in the United States in patients over age 50 years. There are two main forms: nonexudative, in which there are no neovascular growths, and exudative, in which NV occurs.

Etiology

Pathogenesis unknown.

Genetic predisposition: allelic variants of genes encoding complement factor H, mutations at chromosome 1q31 at 10q26 and LOC387715 at 10q significantly increase risk of ARMD.

Associations with smoking, hypertension, high cholesterol level, and cardiovascular disease.

Possible nutritional deficiency.

Signs and Symptoms

Blurred vision.

Metamorphopsia.

Central/paracentral scotomas.

Demographics

Predominantly over age 55 years.

Associated with light irides, hyperopia, and female gender.

Nonexudative (nonneovascular) age-related macular degeneration.

Ophthalmic Findings of Nonexudative Age-Related Macular Degeneration

See Figure 3.8.

Drusen (large, soft drusen). By electron microscopy, this material at the level of Bruch membrane is formed of basal laminar and linear deposits. Drusen can be categorized according to size to the following:
- Small (<64 µm in diameter).
- Intermediate (64 to 124 µm in diameter).
- Large (≥125 µm in diameter).

Chorioretinal atrophy.

RPE hyperpigmentation.

Ophthalmic Findings of Exudative (Neovascular) Age-Related Macular Degeneration

See Figure 3.9.

Subretinal fluid.

Subretinal/vitreous hemorrhage (VH).

Subretinal/intraretinal exudates.

Pigment epithelial detachments.

RPE tears.

A 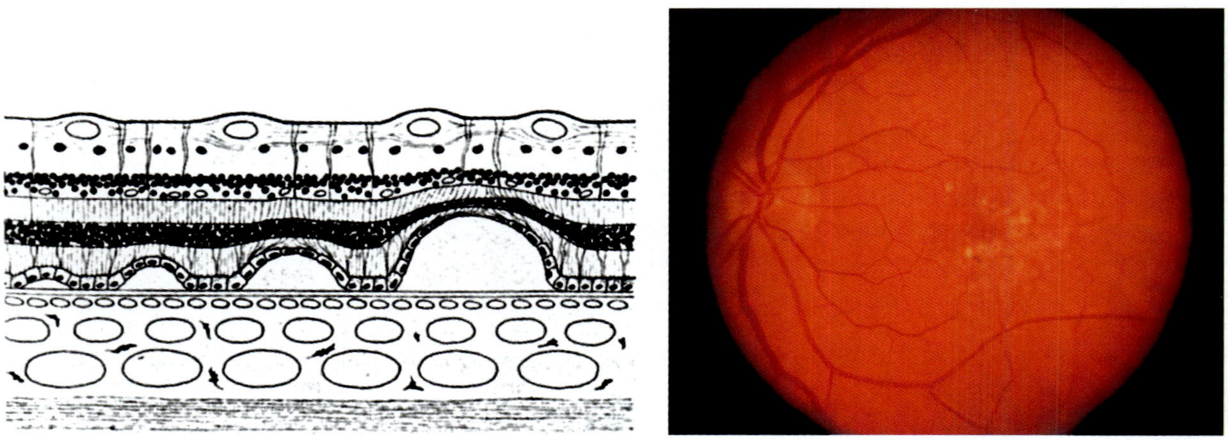 B

FIGURE 3.8. Age-related macular degeneration. **A:** Schematic section of retina shows progressively larger detachments of pigment epithelium. Drusen deposit between the pigment epithelium and Bruch membrane. **B:** Nonexudative age-related macular degeneration with drusen and retinal pigment epithelial changes.

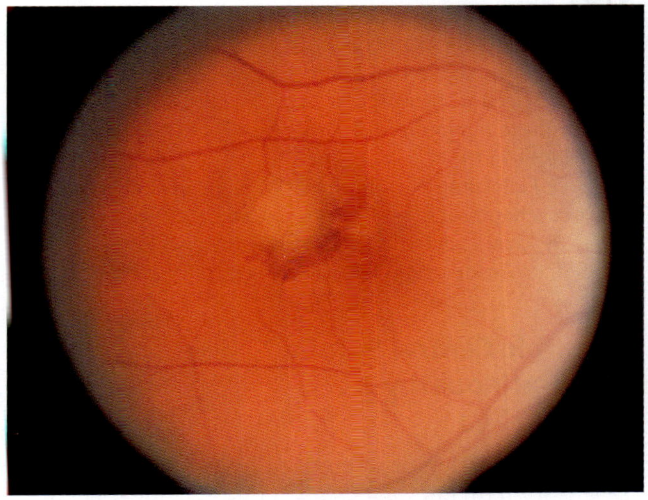

FIGURE 3.9. Exudative age-related macular degeneration with a CNVM surrounded by subretinal hemorrhage.

CNVMs.
Disciform scar.

Systemic Findings

None.

Special Tests

Intravenous fluorescein angiography (IVFA): to determine presence and localization of CNVM for treatment. Two main patterns of CNVM: classic (early bright hyperfluorescence with late leakage) and occult (early stippled hyperfluorescence with late leakage corresponding to fibrovascular pigment epithelium detachments [PEDs], or late leakage of undetermined source).

ICG angiography: may be helpful in evaluating PEDs, occult CNVM.

OCT is currently very useful for follow-up of patients with neovascular ARMD to determine the need of continued treatment and may replace IVFA in many instances (Figure 3.10).

Pathology

Irregular thickening of Bruch membrane leads to cracks through which abnormal neovascular growth from the choriocapillaris may occur.

Disease Course

- A grading scale was developed by the AREDS (Age-Related Eye Disease Study) depending on the presence in each eye of the following:
  One or more large drusen (1 point).
  Pigment abnormalities (1 point).
  Bilateral intermediate drusen (1 point).
  Neovascular ARMD (2 points).

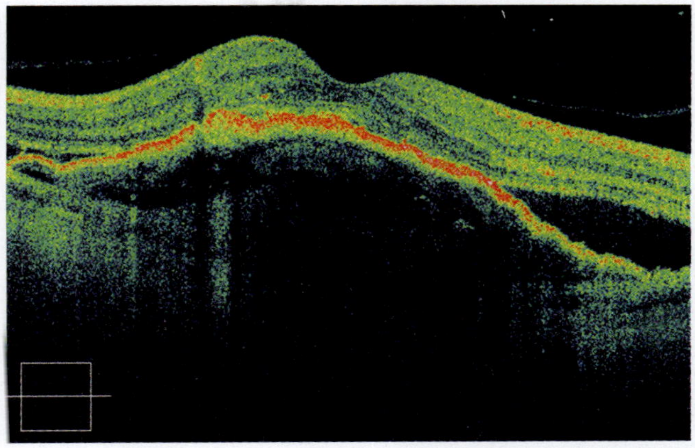

FIGURE 3.10. Cirrus SD-OCT of a patient with neovascular ARMD showing a large pigment epithelial detachment and subretinal fluid.

Points are summed in both eyes to determine the number-related risk of advanced ARMD as follows:

	5-year risk (%)	10-year risk (%)
0 factors	0.5	1
1 factor	3	7
2 factors	12	22
3 factors	25	50
4 factors	50	67

- Severe visual loss associated with advanced ARMD either CNV or geographic atrophy.

Treatment and Management

Education: Amsler grid testing.

Prophylactic laser photocoagulation was shown not to decrease the incidence of progression to neovascular late ARMD (see study section for the Complications of Age-Related Macular Degeneration Prevention Trial).

The current gold standard treatment are intravitreal anti-angiogenesis drugs. Ranibizumab (Lucentis) intravitreal injections have been proven efficacious in FDA registration trials to prevent vision loss and provide visual gain in patients with neovascular ARMD with classic as well as occult CNV (see study section for ANCHOR, MARINA, PIER, and PrONTO studies). Many treatment protocols have been adopted, ranging from monthly injections (MARINA and ANCHOR) to OCT-based guided treatment (PrONTO) to "Treat and Extend." Bevacizumab (Avastin) intravitreal injections are not FDA approved for use in the eye; however, this treatment modality has been shown in several pilot studies to be beneficial and is currently being tested head to head with ranibizumab in the Comparison of Age-related Macular Degeneration Treatment trial (see study section).

Photodynamic treatment with Verteporfin has also shown some value prior to the advent of antivascular endothelial growth factor (anti-VEGF) therapy in treating neovascular CNV (see study section for the TAP and VIP studies), and it is currently being evaluated for potential combination treatment with anti-VEGF treatment (see study section for the FOCUS and RADICAL studies).

Focal laser photocoagulation according to the MPS study is no longer used for subfoveal or juxtafoveal CNV but may still have a role in some extrafoveal CNV lesions (see study section for MPS study).

Submacular surgery and retinal translocation: may be performed to evacuate acute submacular hemorrhages or rotate the retina away from pathologic RPE/scar. Submacular surgery is not advocated for extracting CNVM associated with ARMD (see study section for the SST trial).

Low-vision aids.

Medications

According to the Age-Related Eye Disease Study I, taking a combination of vitamins (500 mg vitamin C, 400 IU vitamin E, 15 mg beta carotene, 80 mg zinc, and 2 mg cupric oxide to prevent zinc-induced anemia) may decrease the incidence of progression to advanced ARMD by 25% and moderate vision loss by 19% (refer to study section for the AREDS study).

Follow-Up

- If no CNVM, some authors advocate biannual examinations.
- Patients with active CNV are typically followed on a 4- to 6-week basis to determine the need for additional injections.

Differential Diagnosis

- Idiopathic central serous chorioretinopathy (ICSC) (may have RPE disturbances, serous RDs; seen in young, predominantly male patients).
- Myopic degeneration.
- Macular dystrophy (e.g., Best disease: has abnormal EOG).
- RPE pattern dystrophies.
- Bull's-eye maculopathies (central macular chorioretinal atrophy seen with various conditions such as chloroquine toxicity, cone dystrophy, fundus flavimaculatus).
- Trauma: choroidal rupture.

References

Age-Related Eye Diseases Study Research Group. A randomized, placebo-controlled, clinical trial of high-dose supplementation with vitamins C and E, beta carotene, and zinc for age-related macular degeneration and vision loss. AREDS report 8. *Arch Ophthalmol* 2001;119:1417–1436.

Ferris FL, Davis MD, Clemons TE, et al. Age-Related Eye Diseases Study (AREDS) Research Group. A simplified severity scale for age-related macular degeneration: AREDS report 18. *Arch Ophthalmol* 2005;123:1570–1574.

Macular Photocoagulation Study Group. Laser photocoagulation of subfoveal neovascular lesions in age-related macular degeneration: results of a randomized clinical trial. *Arch Ophthalmol* 1991;109:1219–1231.

Macular Photocoagulation Study Group. Argon laser photocoagulation for neovascular maculopathy after five years: results from randomized clinical trials. *Arch Ophthalmol* 1991;109:1109–1114.

Regillo C, Holekamp N, Johnson MW, et al. Retinal physiology and psychophysics. In: Skuta GL, Cantor LB, eds. *Basic and clinical science course: retina and vitreous*. San Francisco, CA: American Academy of Ophthalmology, 2008–2009:37–38.

Idiopathic Central Serous Chorioretinopathy

Summary

ICSC is a condition characterized by serous elevation of the sensory retina in the macula, typically affecting young male patients.

Etiology

- Pathogenesis unknown; thought to be due to a localized abnormality in the RPE fluid pump.
- May be exacerbated by corticosteroid use.

Signs and Symptoms

Blurred vision.

Metamorphopsia.

Micropsia.

Hyperopic shift in refraction (due to elevation of sensory retina).

Demographics

Young to middle-aged adults.

Male-to-female ratio is 8:1 to 10:1.

"Type A" personality.

Ophthalmic Findings

- Serous RD in macula.
- Subretinal yellowish precipitates.
- Atrophic RPE changes (evidence of previous episodes) in ipsilateral or contralateral eye.
- Extramacular RPE tracts.

Systemic Findings

None.

Special Tests

IVFA: classic "smokestack" with focal point of hyperfluorescence that rises and then diffuses laterally in 15% to 20% of cases. Majority have focal point of hyperfluorescence that increases slightly.

OCT shows subretinal fluid and can be used as guide of gradual spontaneous regression and resolution and follow response to treatment (Figure 3.11).

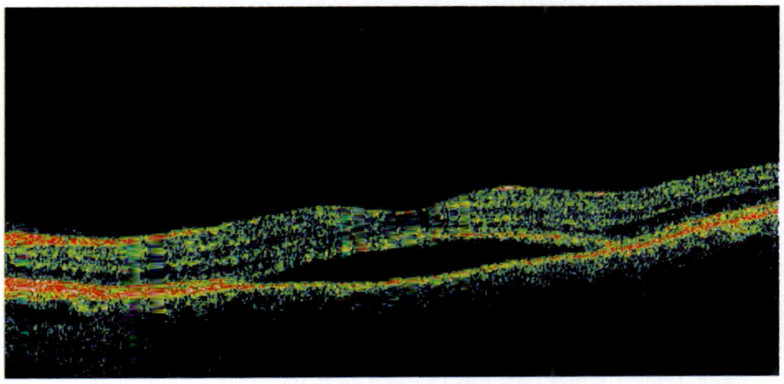

FIGURE 3.12 OCT of a patient with central serous choroidopathy showing subretinal fluid.

Pathology

- Subretinal proteinaceous fluid.
- Retinal photoreceptors normal unless serous detachment is chronic.

Disease Course

- Spontaneous resolution of subretinal fluid occurs in 3 to 4 months with improvement of VA to 20/30 or better in over 90% of patients.
- Recurrences may occur in up to 50% of patients.
- Uncommon complications include CNVM, macular edema, and peripheral chorioretinal atrophic tracts.

Treatment and Management

- Observation: Prescribing hyperopic glasses may help to temporize until ICSC resolves.
- Focal laser photocoagulation: may hasten resolution of fluid; however, final VA and recurrence rates are unaffected. Photocoagulation usually is reserved for patients in whom (a) occupational needs require hastened resolution, (b) prolonged leakage persists over 4 to 6 months, or (c) previous episode resulted in a permanent loss of vision.
- Photodynamic therapy with Verteporfin using either full fluence or half fluence has shown some promise in some small series in inducing resolution of subretinal fluid with some improvement in VA, but is still experimental.
- Corticosteroids are contraindicated, and in some instances, may exacerbate the condition.

Medications

None effective.

Differential Diagnosis

- Serous detachments in pregnancy, hypertension, or corticosteroid use: very similar in clinical appearance to ICSC.
- Age-related macular degeneration.
- Rhegmatogenous RD: Look for peripheral retinal breaks.

Reference

Gass JDM. Pathogenesis of disciform detachment of the neuroepithelium, II: idiopathic central serous choroidopathy. *Am J Ophthalmol* 1967;63:587–615.

Cystoid Macular Edema

Summary

CME is the accumulation of fluid in a petalloid pattern in the outer plexiform layer of the macula. It may be seen in many ocular diseases.

Causes of Cystoid Macular Edema

- Postsurgical:
  - Cataract extraction, especially with capsular rupture or vitreous loss.
  - Vitrectomy.
  - Cyclophotocoagulation.
  - Cryopexy.
- Uveitis.
- Vascular.
  - Vein occlusion (branch retinal vein occlusion [BRVO], CRVO).
  - Diabetes mellitus.
- Miscellaneous.
  - Epiretinal membranes.
  - RP.
  - Nicotinic acid maculopathy.
  - Juvenile X-linked retinoschisis.
  - Cytomegalovirus (CMV) retinitis.

Etiology

- Mechanism of disease is unknown. Hypotheses include the following:

Inflammation: Perifoveal capillary leakage stimulated by prostaglandins released as a result of inflammation secondary to surgery, uveitis, or other factors.

Vitreous traction: leads to retinal capillary dilation and leakage.

Ultraviolet light: may generate free radicals, leading to prostaglandin release.

Signs and Symptoms

- Unilateral decreased vision or metamorphopsia.
- Dulled foveal reflex or foveal cysts noted on slit-lamp biomicroscopy.

Demographics

- Depends on etiology.
- Has been reported to occur in a dominantly inherited pattern.

RETINA

Ophthalmic Findings

- Foveal cysts or dulled foveal reflex, usually unilateral (can be bilateral if associated with systemic disease).
- Intraocular lens; possible posterior capsule rupture or vitreous strands to wound or iris if associated with complicated cataract extraction.
- Hemorrhages, microaneurysms, cotton-wool spots, perimacular edema associated with vascular disease such as diabetic retinopathy, central or BRVO, retinal telangiectasis.
- Anterior chamber cell and flare, vitreous cells, other signs of inflammation associated with uveitic causes.
- Pigmentary retinopathy, attenuated retinal vessels, waxy pallor of optic nerve if associated with RP.
- Distortion of intraretinal vessels, contraction of macular surface secondary to epiretinal fibrosis.

Systemic Findings

- Depends on etiology.
- Diabetic patients may have nephropathy, neuropathy, or other microvascular abnormalities.
- Patients with venous occlusive disease may have signs of systemic vascular disease, hypertension, hypercholesterolemia, etc.

Special Tests

Fluorescein angiographic characteristics:

Focal areas of hyperfluorescence early.
Late pooling of dye in cystoid spaces.
OCT shows the cystic spaces and can be used as a guide to follow the response to treatment (Figure 3.12).

Pathology

Accumulation of edema in outer plexiform layer of macula.

Disease Course

- Depends on etiology.

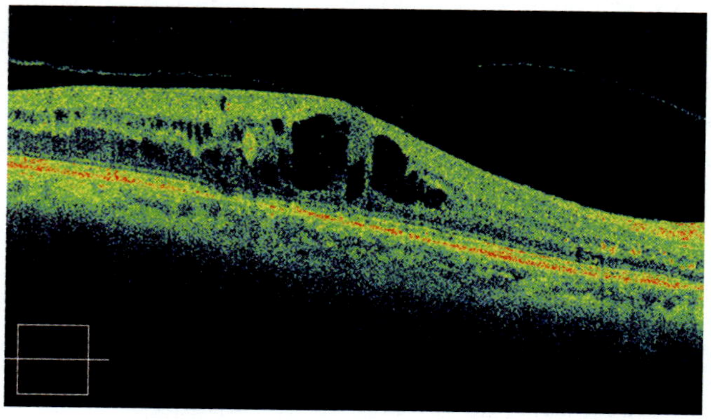

FIGURE 3.12. Cirrus SD-OCT of a patient with CME showing the intraretinal cystic spaces.

- Acute pseudophakic CME may resolve over weeks to months without treatment.
- Chronic pseudophakic CME frequently persists, ultimately resulting in chronic photoreceptor and RPE alterations.
- CME associated with diabetic retinopathy gradually progresses and can result in significant visual decline.
- CME associated with uveitis waxes and wanes with the underlying uveitis.

Treatment and Management

- Depends on etiology.
- Pseudophakic CME.

  Most common cause.

  Low frequency of occurrence (estimated at 1% to 2% of uncomplicated cataract extractions) has made the completion of a randomized, masked, controlled study difficult.

  Stepwise treatment options:

  1. Topical nonsteroidal anti-inflammatory drugs (NSAIDs) and/or topical prednisolone for at least 1 month have been shown in several pilot studies to be of benefit.
  2. Sub-Tenon corticosteroids (triamcinolone 40 mg/1 mL).
  3. Nd: YAG laser vitreolysis or anterior segment reconstruction when indicated.
  4. Pars plana vitrectomy.
- Diabetic macular edema: focal or grid laser for clinically significant macular edema (CSME).
- BRVO: focal or grid laser for persistent macular edema and vision 20/40 or worse.
- Uveitis: topical, periocular, and systemic corticosteroids; refractory cases may require immunosuppressives.

Medications

- Topical NSAIDs (nepafenac, ketorolac, diclofenac, bromfenac) and corticosteroids (prednisolone) are most commonly used for initial treatment of pseudophakic CME. Treatment is instituted at three to four times a day for at least 1 to 2 months and then tapered slowly when vision stabilizes. If topical therapy fails, one may consider sub-Tenon or intravitreal steroid or intravitreal anti-VEGF therapy.
- Systemic corticosteroids may be beneficial in the treatment of CME associated with uveitis.
- Acetazolamide has shown limited success in the treatment of CME associated with RP and CMV retinitis.

Follow-Up

- Pseudophakic CME: monthly or every other month while on treatment.
- Eight weeks after laser treatment (diabetic and vein occlusion patients).

Differential Diagnosis

Epiretinal membrane: usually see membrane overlying macula, associated with vessel straightening and tortuosity.

Macular degeneration: Exudative disease can result in CME associated with drusen, subretinal and intraretinal hemorrhage.

Juvenile X-linked retinoschisis, nicotinic retinopathy, and CME associated with RP. These diseases may have the cystoid appearance noted on slit-lamp biomicroscopy but will not leak during angiography.

References

Coscas G, Gaudric A. Natural course of nonaphakic cystoid macular edema. *Surv Ophthalmol* 1984;28(Suppl):471–484.

Hariprasad SM, Akudman, L, Clever JA, et al. Treatment of cystoid macular edema with the new-generation NSAID Nepafenac 0.1%. *Clin Ophthalmol* 2009;3(1):147–154.

Hariprasad SM, Callanan D. Topical Nepafenac 0.1% for the treatment of chronic uveitic cystoid macular edema. *Retin Cases Brief Rep* 2008;2(4):304–308.

Spaide RF, Yannuzzi LA. Cystoid macular edema after cataract surgery. *Semin Ophthalmol* 1993;8:121–129.

Macular Hole

Summary

A full-thickness round defect in the macula involving all layers from the ILM to the outer segments of the photoreceptor layer.

Etiology (Theories)

- Idiopathic macular holes are caused by tangential traction of the cortical vitreous overlying the fovea.
- Macular holes may also be seen following trauma, in high myopia, and following chronic CME.

Signs and Symptoms

Blurred vision.

Metamorphopsia.

Demographics

Women more than men.

Sixth decade or older.

Ophthalmic Findings

- Round, punched-out lesion approximately one third disk diameter in size, with a surrounding cuff of subretinal fluid (Table 3.2).
- Epiretinal fibrosis may be seen at edges, especially prevalent with traumatic holes.

Systemic Findings

None.

Table 3.2

Classification of idiopathic macular holes

Stage 1	Foveal detachment; decreased or absent foveal depression, presence of a yellow spot or ring
Stage 2	Early hole formation; enlarged yellow ring with eccentric or central dehiscence
Stage 3	Fully developed macular hole; hole with surrounding cuff of subretinal fluid; operculum may be seen within area of hole
Stage 4	Full-thickness macular hole with posterior vitreous separation

Special Tests

Watzke slit-beam test: The patient notices a break in a thin beam centered over the macular hole.

FA: early hyperfluorescence without late leakage (result of loss of xanthophyll, which is located in the inner layers of the retina).

OCT: differentiates full thickness from lamellar holes and may show vitreous attachment at edges and confirm closure postsurgery and possibly prognosis with intact outer retinal layers at baseline and follow-up (Figure 3.13).

Pathology

Full-thickness loss of retinal tissue from the ILM to the outer segment of the photoreceptor layer. The posterior cortical vitreous may be attached.

Disease Course

- Fifty percent of stage 1 holes may resolve with occurrence of a posterior vitreous detachment (PVD).
- Stage 2 holes typically progress to advanced stages.
- Progression from stage 1 to fully developed stage 3 or stage 4 hole can occur over a period of weeks or as long as several years (typically within 6 months).

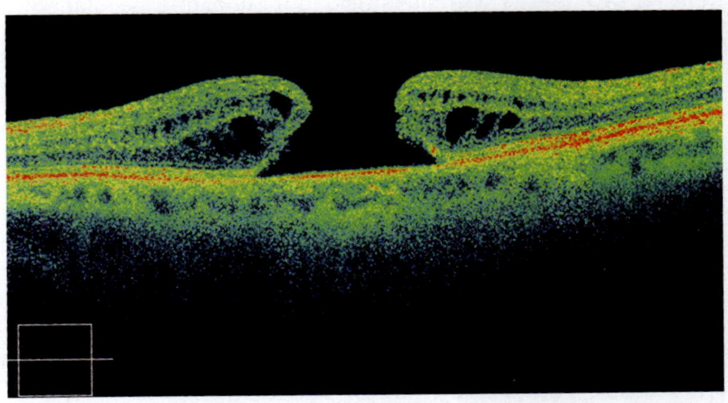

FIGURE 3.13. Cirrus SD-OCT of a patient with full-thickness macular hole.

- VA in patients with full-thickness macular holes is typically stable in the 20/80 to 20/200 range.
- Spontaneous closure of macular holes may occur but is rare. It may be seen with formation of an epiretinal membrane.
- Risk of hole development in the normal fellow eye is between 10% and 15%.

Treatment and Management

Intervention consisting of pars plana vitrectomy, stripping of the posterior hyaloid, with and without internal limiting membrane (ILM) peel, and gas tamponade with or without the adjunctive use of autologous serum or other materials can result in closure of the hole and improved vision. Visual improvement of two lines or greater has been achieved in as many as 80% of patients, and dramatic improvement has been reported. The postoperative period requires the patient to maintain a face-down position for periods of 1 to 2 weeks.

Medications

None.

Follow-Up

Without intervention, the course is relatively stable. RD from macular holes is rare and is usually seen in association with high myopia or trauma. If the patient does not desire surgery, annual follow-up is appropriate.

Differential Diagnosis

Epiretinal membrane: Fibrosis overlying macula can result in a pseudohole. May see vessel tortuosity and straightening.

Age-related macular degeneration: central atrophy with surrounding drusen.

CME: edema in petalloid pattern easily discerned on FA.

References

Gass JDM. Idiopathic senile macular hole: its early stages and pathogenesis. *Arch Ophthalmol* 1988;106:629–639.

Kelly NE, Wendel RT. Vitreous surgery for idiopathic macular hole: results of a pilot study. *Arch Ophthalmol* 1991;109:654–659.

Epiretinal Membranes

Summary

Epiretinal membranes, also referred to as *macular pucker*, *surface wrinkling retinopathy*, or *preretinal fibrosis*, are fibrotic membranes that form by cellular proliferation on the inner surface of the retina.

Etiology

Idiopathic.
Trauma.
Ocular inflammatory disease.
Ocular surgery (especially RD repair and cataract surgery).
Retinal vascular occlusive disease.

Signs and Symptoms

Asymptomatic if mild.
Metamorphopsia.
Blurred vision.
Macropsia.
Rarely diplopia.

Demographics

Most common in elderly (age group in whom PVD most likely to have occurred).

Ophthalmic Findings

- Depends on degree of contraction.
- Classified according to severity.
  Cellophane maculopathy: translucent membrane with minimal distortion.
  Macular pucker: distinct tissue easily visible on retinal surface with distortion and wrinkling of macular surface.
- PVD present in over 90%.
- Simple membranes may be visible as a mild sheen to the retina with irregular light reflex.
- May be thickened and opaque.
- Distortion of retinal vessels, with tortuosity and straightening.
- Foveal ectopia.
- Retinal striae.
- Pseudohole of macula.
- Various degrees of macular edema.
- Traction elevation of macula in severe cases.

Systemic Findings

None.

Special Tests

Fluorescein angiographic characteristics:

Vascular tortuosity and straightening.
Retinal vascular leakage if contraction significant.
OCT can identify the membrane, associated macular edema, and used to follow progression and response to vitrectomy (Figure 3.14).

Pathology

- May be composed of different cell types, including retinal pigment epithelial cells, fibrocytes, fibrous astrocytes, inflammatory cells, and macrophages.
- Interlacing network of cells and collagen adherent to ILM.

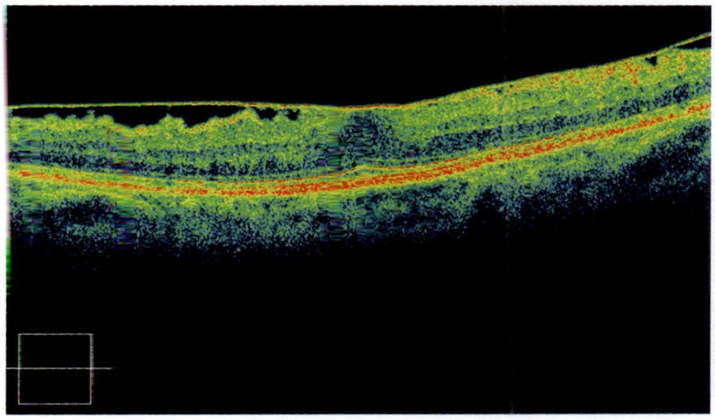

FIGURE 3.14. Cirrus SD-OCT showing epiretinal membrane and loss of foveal depression.

Disease Course

- Vision ranges from normal to worse than 20/200 (<5%).
- Most patients, 20/70 or better.
- Vision usually stable once membrane formed.

Treatment and Management

- Observation if vision minimally affected. Look carefully for retinal holes or tears on examination.
- If significant visual impairment, vitrectomy and membrane stripping should be considered.

Medications

None.

Follow-Up

Annual examination unless vision worsens.

Differential Diagnosis

Retinal vascular disease: BRVO or retinal telangiectasis can produce edema and vascular abnormalities; differentiated by FA.

Age-related macular degeneration: subretinal fibrosis versus preretinal fibrosis.

References

De Bustros S, Thompson JT, Michels RG, et al. Vitrectomy for idiopathic epiretinal membranes causing macular pucker. *Ophthalmology* 1988;72:692–695.

Smiddy WE, Maguire AM, Green WR, et al. Idiopathic epiretinal membranes: ultrastructural characteristics and clinicopathologic correlation. *Ophthalmology* 1989;96:811–821.

Pathologic Myopia

Summary

Pathologic myopia is progressive degeneration associated with myopia of –6.0 diopters or greater and excess axial elongation.

Etiology

Presumed multifactorial (e.g., genetic, environmental).

Signs and Symptoms

Blurred vision.
Scotoma.
Metamorphopsia.
Photopsias.
Floaters.

Demographics

Most common in Asians, least common in blacks.
Women more frequently than men.
Associated with higher education.

Ophthalmic Findings

- Chorioretinal atrophy, particularly in posterior pole (Figure 3.15).
- Peripapillary crescent, tilted disks.
- Lacquer cracks: breaks in Bruch membrane.
- Subretinal hemorrhages: from breaks in Bruch membrane.
- CNVM, Forster-Fuchs spot.
- Lattice degeneration, retinal tears, RD.
- Vitreous detachment, syneresis.
- Posterior staphyloma.
- Strabismus, anisometropic amblyopia.
- Glaucoma.

> A staphyloma represents an area of ectatic sclera with absent or severely atrophic overlying choroidal or retinal tissue.

Systemic Findings

None.

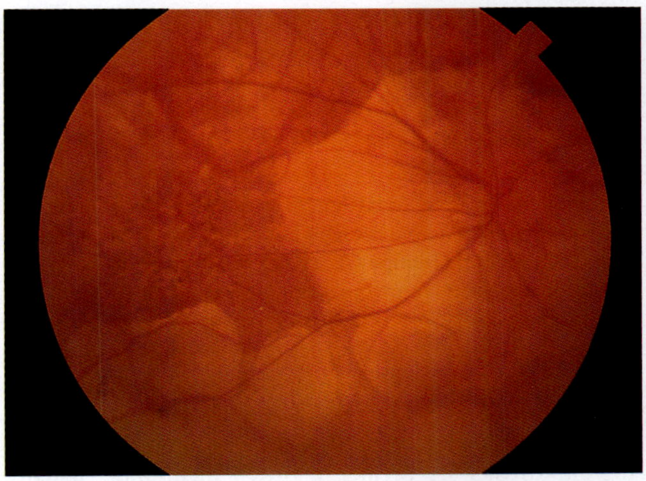

FIGURE 3.15. Multiple areas of chorioretinal atrophy due to myopic degeneration.

Special Tests

- IVFA: to determine presence of CNVM.
- A-scan ultrasonography to measure axial length.

Pathology

- Posterior staphyloma lined with atrophic choroid.
- Chorioretinal atrophy of posterior pole.
- RPE hyperpigmentation/hypopigmentation.
- Vitreous syneresis.

Disease Course

Neovascular complications tend to occur during adulthood. Some patients who develop CNVM may have spontaneous regression of the NV.

Treatment

- Laser photocoagulation of extrafoveal CNVM. Complications of laser include progressive RPE atrophy around treated area. Photodynamic therapy (PDT) with Verteporfin has shown promise in subfoveal CNV secondary to pathologic myopia (see study section, VIP study). Some pilot studies have also shown promise of anti-VEGF intravitreal injections.
- Laser photocoagulation of retinal tears.
- Scleral buckling for RD.
- Vitrectomy for posterior retinal breaks and RD.

Medications

None.

Follow-Up

Patients should monitor their central vision with Amsler grids. Patients should be educated on the symptoms of RD.

Differential Diagnosis

Choroideremia.

ARMD: See p. 106.

Presumed ocular histoplasmosis syndrome (POHS): See p. 250.

References

Curtin BJ, Karlin DB. Axial length measurements and fundus changes of the myopic eye. *Am J Ophthalmol* 1971;71:42–53.

Jalkh AE, Weiter JJ, Trempe CL, et al. Choroidal neovascularization in degenerative myopia: role of laser photocoagulation. *Ophthalmic Surg* 1987;18:721–725.

Angioid Streaks

Summary

Angioid streaks are breaks in Bruch membrane, usually radiating from the optic disk. Fifty percent are associated with systemic disorders.

Etiology

Unknown; associations with elastic tissue diseases.

Signs and Symptoms

Asymptomatic.

Blurred vision.

Scotoma.

Metamorphopsia.

Demographics (PEPSI)

Pseudoxanthoma elasticum (PXE).

Ehlers-Danlos syndrome.

Paget disease.

Sickle cell disease association.

Idiopathic.

Ophthalmic Findings

RPE changes radiating from optic disk (reddish brown or gray color) (Figure 3.16).

Nearly always bilateral.

CNVM.

Subretinal hemorrhage: may occur with minor trauma.

Macular degeneration.

"Peau d'orange" changes: with PXE; diffuse RPE mottling.

Optic disk drusen: may be seen with PXE.

Systemic Findings

PXE: elastic tissue disease causing "plucked-chicken skin," gastrointestinal (GI) tract bleeding, cardiac disease.

Paget disease: progressive connective tissue disease causing increased bony mass, high alkaline phosphatase.

Hemoglobinopathies (e.g., sickle cell disease, thalassemias). Complications such as CNVM rare with angioid streaks associated with this group of disorders.

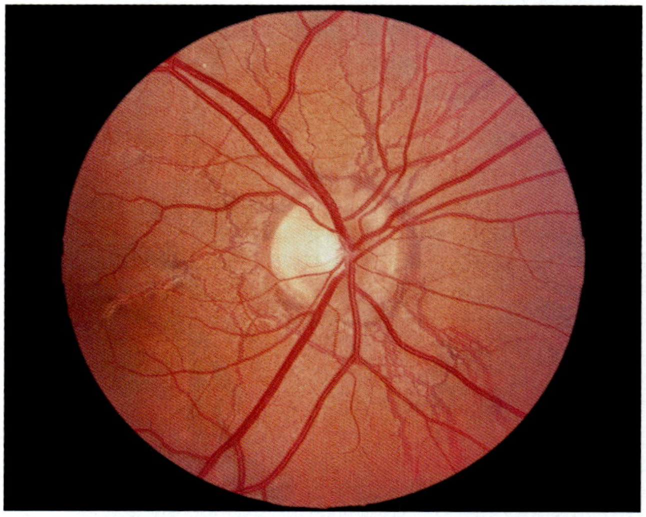

FIGURE 3.16. Angioid streaks radiating from the optic nerve.

Ehler-Danlos syndrome: connective tissue disorder, hyperextensible skin.

Systemic Associations of Angioid Streaks

- Pseudoxanthoma elasticum
- Ehlers-Danlos syndrome
- Paget disease
- Sickle cell and other hemoglobinopathies
- Idiopathic

Special Tests

IVFA shows hyperfluorescence of streaks; helps show CNVM.

Pathology

- Thickened Bruch membrane (basophilia and calcification).
- Elastic degeneration of Bruch membrane.

Disease Course

Patients may initially be asymptomatic but lose vision over time.

Treatment

Medical, dermatologic consult.
Avoid trauma.
Laser photocoagulation for CNVM: has a high recurrence rate. PDT and anti-VEGF off-label treatment may be of some benefit but have not been tested prospectively.

Medications

None.

Follow-Up

Education and Amsler grid testing.

Differential Diagnosis

- ARMD.
- Myopic degeneration: lacquer cracks.
- Presumed ocular histoplasmosis: Ohio-Mississippi River Valley, peripapillary pigment ring, peripheral punched-out chorioretinal scars.
- Choroidal rupture: history of trauma, crescent-shaped lesions radial to optic disk.

Reference

Clarkson JG, Altman RD. Angioid streaks. *Surv Ophthalmol* 1982;26:235–246.

Photic Retinopathy

Summary

Degeneration of retinal photoreceptors may occur from photochemical injury.

Etiology

- Sun gazing. May occur with direct or indirect viewing of the sun. May follow viewing of the sun after observing an eclipse.
- Ophthalmic instruments (e.g., operating microscope, fiberoptic endoilluminator). Prolonged operating time and intensity of light beam are risk factors.
- Arc welding without wearing protective eyewear.

Signs and Symptoms

Decreased vision within several hours after exposure.
Central/paracentral scotomas.
Headache.
Metamorphopsia.

Solar Retinopathy

Demographics

Sungazers.
Psychosis: drug-induced or psychiatric illness.

Ophthalmic Findings

VA 20/40 to 20/100 or worse, short term.
Usually bilateral.
Yellow spot in fovea that becomes reddish several days later.
RPE changes.
Lamellar hole.

Systemic Findings

None.

Special Tests

IVFA: Initially normal. May have central staining. Weeks later, may have only mild RPE defects.
OCT: Abnormal reflectivity in the outer foveal retina, fragmentation or interruption of the inner high reflective layer.

Pathology

Photoreceptor destruction thought due to free radical formation and tissue oxidation, RPE necrosis.

Disease Course

- VA may spontaneously improve.
- May have residual central/paracentral scotoma.

RETINA

Treatment

Observation for spontaneous improvement.

Medications

None.

Follow-Up

Education to prevent sun gazing, use of protective eyewear.

Light Toxicity From Ophthalmic Instruments

Demographics

- Patients who have undergone recent cataract surgery (high-intensity coaxial light from surgical microscope).
- Vitreoretinal surgical patients.

Ophthalmic Findings

- Round or oval retinal lesions, usually in parafoveal location.
- Lesions usually within arcade vessels.
- RPE mottling and atrophy weeks after surgery.

Systemic Findings

None.

Special Tests

IVFA: staining of acute lesion. Later in course, IVFA shows window defects in region of involvement.

Disease Course

- Vision may return to normal several months after surgery.
- May have persistent paracentral scotoma.

Treatment

Observation.

Medications

None.

Follow-Up

Minimize intraocular surgery times and direct light exposure (e.g., use of pupil occluders during surgery).

Differential Diagnosis

CNVM.
Drug toxicity.

References

Green WR, Robertson DM. Pathologic findings of photic retinopathy in the human eye. *Am J Ophthalmol* 1991;112:520–527.

Jorge R, Costa RA, Quirino LS, et al. OCT findings in patients with late solar retinopathy. *Am J Ophthalmol* 2004;137:1139–1143.

Tso MOM, Woodford BJ. Effect of photic injury on the retinal tissues. *Ophthalmology* 1983;90:952–963.

Drug Toxicity

Phenothiazines

Summary

Phenothiazine use can result in ocular toxicity, manifest by various degrees of pigmentary retinopathy. This has been most commonly seen with thioridazine (Mellaril) and chlorpromazine (Thorazine).

Etiology

- The exact cause of toxicity is unknown. Phenothiazines are absorbed by melanin, resulting in concentration in uveal tissues and RPE.
- Acute retinopathy can be seen 3 to 8 weeks after thioridazine use in doses of more than 800 mg/day.
- Chlorpromazine retinopathy is typically milder. It is usually seen after high doses for prolonged periods (2,400 mg/day for 1 year).

Signs and Symptoms

Blurred vision.
Dyschromatopsia.
Nyctalopia.

Ophthalmic Findings

Pigmentary retinopathy.
Confluent areas of RPE depigmentation.
Abnormal pigmentation of eyelids, conjunctiva, cornea, and lens capsule.

Systemic Findings

Psychotic disorders.
Manic-depressive illness.

Special Tests

- Visual-field abnormalities.
- Abnormal dark adaptation.
- IVFA may reveal a wide spectrum of RPE abnormalities ranging from mild alterations to extensive areas of RPE and choriocapillaris atrophy.
- ERG: ranges from normal (early toxicity) to attenuated (severe toxicity).

Pathology

- Atrophy of the RPE and choriocapillaris.
- Atrophy and disorganization of the photoreceptor outer segments.

Disease Course

- Early toxicity: visual complaints associated with a normal fundus picture or a fine pigmentary retinopathy.
- Immediate cessation of medication may result in reversal of visual and fundus abnormalities.
- Late toxicity: Continued use of medication can lead to widespread RPE and choriocapillaris atrophy, which may progress despite cessation of medication.
- Recovery of vision may occur slowly over time.

Treatment and Management

Immediate discontinuation of phenothiazine (retinopathy may still progress).

Medications

None.

Follow-Up

Periodic examinations to document recovery or progression after cessation.

Differential Diagnosis

RP: extensive RPE atrophy associated with attenuated vessels, optic nerve pallor.

Cancer-associated retinopathy: widespread RPE atrophy associated with underlying malignancy.

Reference

Miller FS III, Bunt-Milam AH, Kalina RE. Clinical-ultrastructural study of thioridazine retinopathy. *Ophthalmology* 1982;89: 1478–1488.

Tamoxifen

Summary

Tamoxifen, an antiestrogen that has been found to be an effective therapeutic agent in breast cancer, can cause a crystalline retinopathy, macular edema, and visual loss.

Etiology

- The exact mechanism of toxicity is unknown.
- Initial reports of toxicity were in patients who received high doses of tamoxifen (total doses > 90 g); these doses are no longer prescribed.
- Low-dosage (tamoxifen 10 mg b.i.d.) long-term therapy may cause toxicity.

Signs and Symptoms

Blurred vision.

Metamorphopsia.

Diplopia.

Demographics

- Typically in women with history of breast cancer.
- Rarely seen in men undergoing hormonal therapy.

Ophthalmic Findings

Bilateral whorl-like corneal opacities.

Refractile crystals at the level of the inner retina (Figure 3.17).

Macular edema.

RPE abnormalities.

Optic neuritis.

Systemic Findings

History of breast cancer.

Special Tests

Fluorescein angiographic characteristics:

- Pinpoint macular lesions that hyperfluoresce early and leak late.
- Crystalline lesions are hyperfluorescent.

OCT:

Foveolar cystoids space, loss of photoreceptors, and lack of macular thickening.

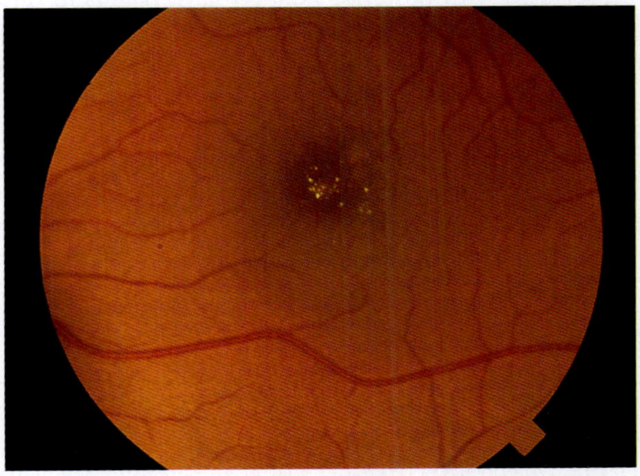

FIGURE 3.17. A 53-year-old woman with multiple crystalline deposits in inner retina after 8 years of tamoxifen treatment.

Pathology

- Refractile lesions in the nerve fiber and inner plexiform layers.
- May represent products of axonal degeneration.

Disease Course

- Toxicity usually not seen in patients receiving low-dose therapy unless long course of treatment (>7 years) with large cumulative dose (>10 g).
- Toxicity in patients receiving low-dose therapy is slowly progressive.

Treatment and Management

- Referral to oncologist for consideration of change of therapy if signs of toxicity.
- Toxicity from high-dose treatment remains stable after discontinuation of drug.
- Toxicity from low-dose treatment has shown regression of retinopathy with visual recovery after drug discontinuation.

Medications

None effective.

Follow-Up

Other crystalline maculopathies:

Canthaxanthine maculopathy: skin-tanning agent that can cause a doughnut-like pattern of superficial retinal crystals in the superficial retina.

Oxalosis: Primary or secondary oxalosis may cause a crystalline retinopathy. Diagnosis is aided by detection of urinary oxalate.

Bietti crystalline dystrophy: tapetoretinal degeneration associated with posterior pole crystals. Begins in third decade, autosomal recessive inheritance.

Autosomal dominant crystalline dystrophy: crystalline retinopathy seen predominantly in young female patients.

Calcified macular drusen: Refractile lesions are frequently accompanied by noncalcified drusen.

Talc retinopathy: refractile crystals in the retina seen in intravenous (i.v.) drug abusers who inject crushed oral medications containing talc compounds.

References

Gualino V, Cohen SY, Delyfer MN, et al. OCT findings of in tamoxifen retinopathy. *Am J Ophthalmol* 2005;140:757–758.

Heier JS, Dragoo RA, Enzenauer RW, et al. Screening for ocular toxicity in asymptomatic patients treated with tamoxifen. *Am J Ophthalmol* 1994;117:772–775.

Kaiser-Kupfer MI, Kupfer C, Rodrigues MM. Tamoxifen retinopathy: a clinicopathologic report. *Ophthalmology* 1981;88:89–93.

Chloroquine and Hydroxychloroquine

Summary

Prolonged use of chloroquine and hydroxychloroquine (Plaquenil), agents used for the treatment of rheumatoid arthritis, amebiasis, malaria, and systemic lupus erythematosus can cause degeneration of the RPE and sensory retina.

Etiology

- Mechanism of retinopathy not known.
- Toxicity seen with chronic use of chloroquine in doses greater than 250 mg/day, or hydroxychloroquine in doses greater than 6.5 mg/kg/day.
- Hydroxychloroquine is much less toxic to the eye.

Signs and Symptoms

Visual loss.
Paracentral scotoma.

Demographics

Toxicity from hydroxychloroquine is most likely in elderly, underweight patients (the toxicity is dose and duration dependent).

Ophthalmic Findings

Corneal deposits.
Bull's-eye maculopathy: Figure 3.18.
Generalized retinal pigmentary degeneration.
Retinal vessel attenuation.
Optic disk pallor.

Systemic Findings

Rheumatoid arthritis.

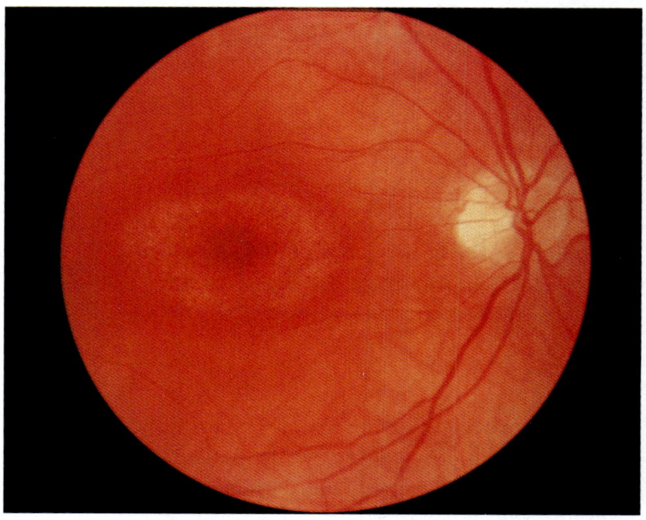

FIGURE 3.18. RPE depigmentation in bull's-eye configuration resulting from chloroquine retinopathy.

Systemic lupus erythematosus.
Amebiasis.
Malaria.

Special Tests

Amsler grid: central and paracentral abnormalities, red Amsler may be more sensitive.
Humphrey 10-2 visual field examination with a red test object: detects abnormalities in central 20 degrees.
IVFA: bull's-eye pattern of hyperfluorescence.

Pathology

- Chloroquine is concentrated in the RPE.
- RPE depigmentation, rod and cone receptor loss occurs in the macula.

Disease Course

- Early toxicity is evident in paracentral scotomas.
- Central scotoma develops with increasing toxicity.
- Early visual loss may be reversible with immediate cessation of treatment.
- If central visual loss and/or absolute scotoma is present, progressive loss may occur despite discontinuation of medication.

Treatment and Management

If toxicity detected, discontinue drug immediately.

Medications

None.

Follow-Up

- Chloroquine toxicity is rare today, since the large majority of patients previously given this medication have been converted to regimen of hydroxychloroquine.
- Patients without underlying macular disease or evidence of toxicity should be given an Amsler grid for self-monitoring and can be followed annually.
- Patients with underlying macular disease (i.e., macular degeneration) or taking more than 6.5 mg/kg/day of hydroxychloroquine should be followed more frequently.

Differential Diagnosis

Cone dystrophy: bull's-eye maculopathy similar, but central vision affected earlier, and to a greater degree. ERG would reveal greater involvement of photopic response.
Stargardt disease: bull's-eye maculopathy with retinal flecks. Florescein angiography reveals silent choroid.
ARMD: can occasionally see bilateral macular RPE atrophy, associated with surrounding drusen (see p. 106).
Benign concentric annular dystrophy: bull's-eye maculopathy in young patients with minimal central visual loss.

References

Easterbrook M. The ocular safety of hydroxychloroquine. *Semin Arthritis Rheum* 1993;23:62–67.
Weiner A, Sandberg MA, Gaudio AR, et al. Hydroxychloroquine retinopathy. *Am J Ophthalmol* 1991;112:528–534.

Methoxyflurane

Summary

Use of the nonflammable anesthetic methoxyflurane can result in secondary oxalosis being evident in the eye by crystalline deposits in the posterior pole and midperiphery.

Etiology

Prolonged general anesthesia with the inhalational anesthetic methoxyflurane, especially in the presence of underlying renal dysfunction.

Signs and Symptoms

Normal VA.

Ophthalmic Findings

- Numerous yellow-white punctate crystalline deposits scattered about the posterior pole and midperiphery.
- Deposits may course along the retinal arteries.

Systemic Findings

Renal dysfunction (may occur before or as a result of methoxyflurane anesthesia).

Pathology

- Birefringent crystalline deposits in RPE.
- Crystalline deposits composed of calcium oxalate.

Medications

None effective.

Differential Diagnosis

Canthaxanthine maculopathy: skin-tanning agent that can cause a doughnut-like pattern of superficial retinal crystals in the superficial retina.
Bietti crystalline dystrophy: tapetoretinal degeneration associated with posterior pole crystals. Begins in third decade, autosomal recessive inheritance.

Autosomal dominant crystalline dystrophy: crystalline retinopathy seen predominantly in young female patients.
Calcified macular drusen: refractile lesions are frequently accompanied by noncalcified drusen, other changes of macular degeneration.
Talc retinopathy: refractile crystals in the retina seen in i.v. drug abusers who inject crushed oral medications containing talc compounds.
Tamoxifen retinopathy: bilateral crystalline retinopathy seen in breast cancer patients undergoing hormonal therapy.

References

Bullock JD, Albert DM. Flecked retina: appearance secondary to oxalate crystals from methoxyflurane anesthesia. *Arch Ophthalmol* 1975;93:26–30.
Novak MA, Roth AS, Levine MR. Calcium oxalate retinopathy associated with methoxyflurane anesthesia. *Retina* 1988;8:230–236.

Canthaxanthine

Summary

Canthaxanthine is an oral tanning agent that may cause a bilateral crystalline retinopathy.

Etiology

May develop in patients taking canthaxanthine regularly over an extended period.

Signs and Symptoms

VA usually normal.

Ophthalmic Findings

- Symmetric doughnut-like pattern of retinal crystals in the macula.
- Crystals can be found in the superficial retinal layers.
- Patients may develop corneal crystals.

Systemic Findings

None.

Special Tests

Fluorescein angiographic characteristics:

Typically normal.
May show a bull's-eye pattern of hyperfluorescence.

Pathology

- Lipid-soluble crystals in inner retinal layers and ciliary body.
- Crystals probably represent a canthaxanthine-lipoprotein complex.

Disease Course

- Toxicity is dose dependent.
- Usually a dose of 19 g or greater is necessary to induce retinopathy.
- Retinopathy may be seen at lower doses if underlying RPE disease, ocular hypertension, beta carotene use.

Treatment and Management

- Crystals may gradually disappear after agent is discontinued.
- May take 1 year or more for crystals to disappear.

Medications

None effective.

Differential Diagnosis

Tamoxifen retinopathy: bilateral crystalline retinopathy seen in breast cancer patients undergoing hormonal therapy.
Oxalosis: Primary or secondary oxalosis may cause a crystalline retinopathy. Diagnosis is aided by detection of urinary oxalate.
Bietti crystalline dystrophy: tapetoretinal degeneration associated with posterior pole crystals. Begins in third decade, autosomal recessive inheritance.
Autosomal dominant crystalline dystrophy: crystalline retinopathy seen predominantly in young female patients.
Calcified macular drusen: refractile lesions are frequently accompanied by noncalcified drusen.
Talc retinopathy: refractile crystals in the retina seen in i.v. drug abusers who inject crushed oral medications containing talc compounds.

References

Daicker B, Schiedt K, Adnet JJ, et al. Canthaxanthin retinopathy: an investigation by light and electron microscopy and physicochemical analysis. *Graefes Arch Clin Exp Ophthalmol* 1987;225:189–197.
Harnois C, Samson J, Malenfant M, et al. Canthaxanthin retinopathy: anatomic and functional reversibility. *Arch Ophthalmol* 1989;107:538–540.

VASCULAR DISORDERS

Diabetic Retinopathy

Summary

Diabetic retinopathy correlates with pathogenetically underlying systemic diabetes mellitus.

Etiology (Theories)

- Glycosylation of tissue proteins causes cell damage.

- The polyol pathway (aldose reductase) results in an accumulation of intracellular sorbitol, which causes basement membrane thickening and damages pericytes.

Signs and Symptoms

Blurring, distortion of vision.
Decreased night vision.
Floaters.
Decreased color vision.

Demographics

- Leading cause of blindness in ages 20 to 64 years.
- Twenty-five percent of diabetics have diabetic retinopathy.

Ophthalmic Findings of Nonproliferative Diabetic Retinopathy

See Figure 3.19.

Microaneurysms.
Dilated capillaries.
Dot-blot nerve-fiber layer hemorrhages.
Hard exudates.
Retinal edema.
Cotton-wool spots.

Systemic Findings

Diabetic nephropathy.
Polyneuropathy.
Hypertension found in 2[illegible]% of type I and 58% of type II diabetics.

Special Tests

- IVFA identifies macular capillary nonperfusion, macular edema, subtle areas of NV, or capillary dropout.

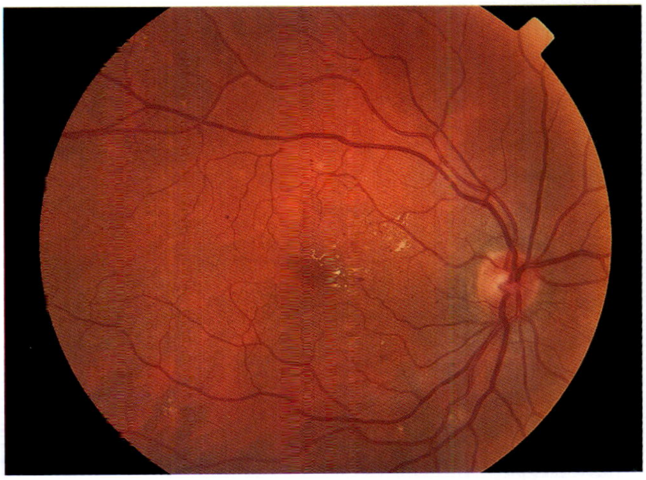

FIGURE 3.19. NPDR with hard exudates and microaneurysms.

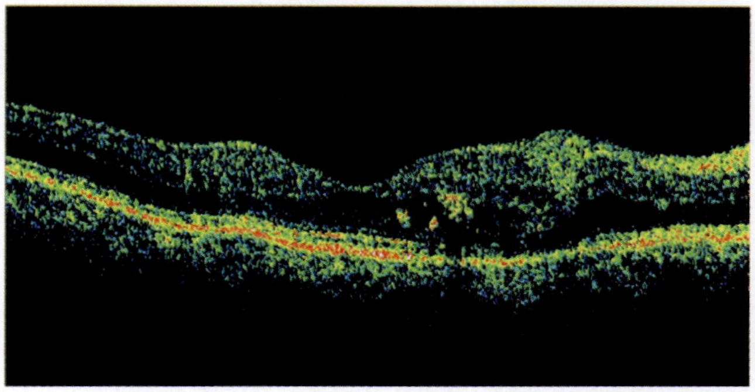

FIGURE 3.20. OCT of a patient with diabetic macular edema showing diffuse intraretinal edema and intraretinal lipid exudates.

- Ultrasonography identifies tractional retinal detachment (TRD) in eyes with opaque media.
- Color fundus photography.
  - OCT identifies macula edema, measures retinal thickness, and is reflective of the macula (Figure 3.20).

Pathology

- Thickening of the vascular basement membrane.
- Decreased number of pericytes relative to the number of endothelial cells.

Disease Course and Natural Progression

Incidence of retinopathy increases with the duration of diabetes and patient age (Table 3.3).

Treatment and Management

CSME is defined as one or more of the following features (Figure 3.21):

1. Thickening at or within 500 μm of the foveal avascular zone (FAZ).
2. Hard exudate at or within 500 μm of the FAZ with associated thickening of the adjacent retina.
3. A zone of retinal thickening 1 disk area or larger, any part of which is within 1 disk diameter of the center of the macula.

- CSME: According to the Early Treatment for Diabetic Retinopathy Study (ETDRS), focal and/or grid laser is beneficial for these eyes.
  - Intravitreal Anti-VEGF therapy.

Table 3.3

Incidence of diabetic retinopathy

Duration of insulin-dependent diabetes mellitus (years)	Incidence of retinopathy (%)
5–7	50
17–25	90

RETINA

- NPDR.
  Mild: occasional microaneurysms.
  Moderate: more microaneurysms and scattered hard exudates or cotton-wool spots.
  Severe: the presence of one of the following:
  Four quadrants of severe retinal hemorrhages.
  Two quadrants of venous beading.
  One quadrant of moderately severe IRMA. If two of these are present, this is termed *very severe NPDR*. Most patients are advised to wait until high-risk characteristics (HRCs) of proliferative diabetic retinopathy (PDR) are reached to initiate panretinal photocoagulation (PRP). If follow-up is unreliable, PRP may be initiated sooner.

Medications

Intensive insulin therapy can delay the onset of and slow the progression of diabetic retinopathy, nephropathy, and neuropathy in type I diabetics. See Diabetes Control and Complications Trial (DCCT).

Follow-Up

See Tables 3.4 and 3.5.

Differential Diagnosis

- Hypertensive retinopathy (arteriovenous [AV] nicking, copper wiring, elevated blood pressure).
- Collagen vascular disease (anti-ssA, anti-ssB, ANA, rheumatoid factor, c-ANCA, arthritis, dermatologic findings, lupus erythematous, polyarteritis nodosa, Wegener granulomatosis).
- Acquired immunodeficiency syndrome (AIDS) retinopathy (human immunodeficiency virus [HIV]–positive serology).
- Cardiac embolic disease (Hollenhorst, calcific plaques, talc).
- Sickle cell retinopathy (positive sickle cell preparation, hemoglobin electrophoresis, peripheral nonperfusion, sea-fan NV, black sunburst).
- Radiation retinopathy (history of radiation therapy).

Table 3.4

Guidelines for examinations for diabetic retinopathy

Age of onset of diabetes	First examination	Follow-up examinations
<30 y	5 y after diagnosis	Yearly
>30 y	At time of diagnosis	Yearly
Prior to pregnancy	Prior to conception or in the early first trimester	Every 3 mo

Table 3.5

Follow up guidelines for diabetic eye diseases

Disease status	Follow-up (months)
Normal or minimal NPDR	12
Moderate NPDR	6–12
Severe NPDR	3–4
Following treatment for CSME	3–4

NPDR, nonproliferative diabetic retinopathy.

- Vasculitis (sarcoidosis, toxoplasmosis, Eales disease, systemic lupus erythematosus, syphilis, vascular sheathing present).
- Leukemia (history, peripheral blood smear, bone marrow biopsy, Roth spots).

References

Diabetes Control and Complications Trial Research Group. The effect of intensive treatment of diabetes on the development and progression of long-term complications in insulin-dependent diabetes mellitus. *N Engl J Med* 1993;329:977–986.

Early Treatment Diabetic Retinopathy Study Research Group. Photocoagulation for Diabetic Macular Edema: ETDRS Report 1. *Arch Ophthalmol* 1985;103:1796–1806.

Proliferative Diabetic Retinopathy

Summary

The presence of newly formed blood vessels or fibrous tissue arising from the retina or optic disk and extending along the inner surface of the retina or disk or into the vitreous cavity.

Etiology

Closure of retinal arterioles causes nonperfusion and ischemia and stimulates the release of vasoproliferative factors stimulating NV from the retina, optic nerve, or iris.

Signs and Symptoms

Blurred vision.
Distortion.
Floaters.

Demographics

- Twenty-six percent of patients who have had diabetes for 25 to 50 years develop PDR.
- Type I diabetics have a higher risk of developing PDR than type II patients.
- There are 65,000 new cases of PDR per year and 8,000 new cases of blindness due to diabetic retinopathy per year in the United States.

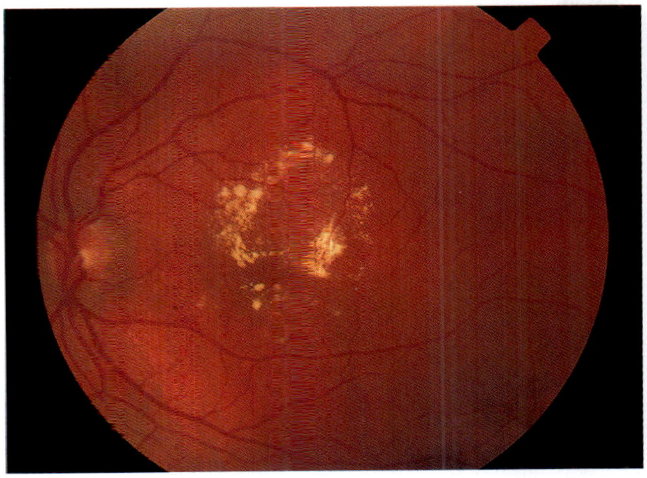

FIGURE 3.21. CSME with circinate ring of hard exudates and retinal thickening involving the fovea.

Ophthalmic Findings

Neovascularization of the disk (NVD) or elsewhere (NVE) (Figure 3.22).
Vitreous or preretinal hemorrhages.
Preretinal fibrosis.
TRD.

Systemic Findings

Nephropathy.
Polyneuropathy.
Hypertension.
Carotid occlusive disease.

Special Tests

IVFA: hyperfluorescence and leakage of dye from neovascular vessels (Figure 3.23).

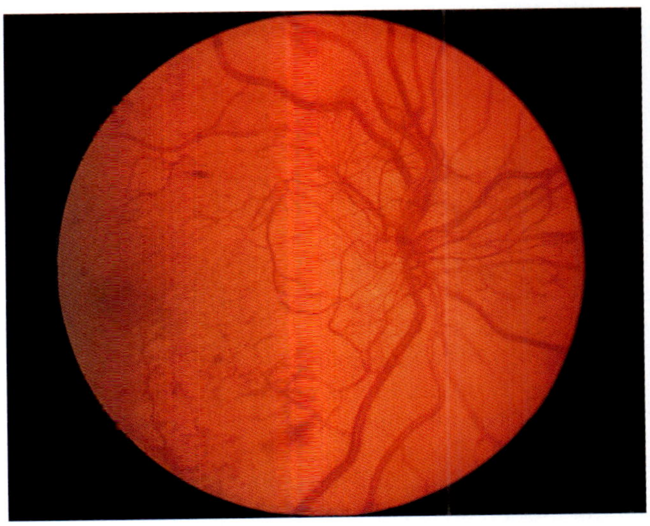

FIGURE 3.22. PDR with extensive NVD.

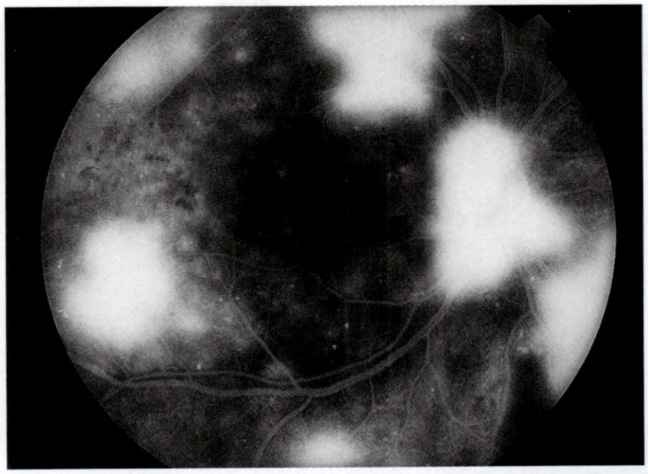

FIGURE 3.23. IVFA demonstrating multiple areas of hyperfluorescence due to leakage from neovascularization in PDR.

Ultrasonography: in cases with opaque media to evaluate underlying TRD.
Color fundus photography: helpful in following the regression or the progression of NV.
OCT: useful in following areas of macular hemorrhage or macula traction due to ERM formation.

Pathology

Growth of new vessels on retinal surface along posterior hyaloid.

Disease Course and Natural Progression

- Continued new vessel growth on the retinal surface in a cycle of proliferation and regression.
- Proliferation of fibrous tissue accompanies vascular growth.
- Regressed vessels appear sheathed.
- A partial PVD and contraction of fibrous tissue pulls neovascular vessels and creates a VH. As the partial PVD spreads in a posterior to anterior direction, it cannot be released from areas of adhesion between the vitreous and the fibrovascular proliferation.
- Fibrovascular contraction also leads to traction retinal detachment and macular dragging (Figure 3.24).
- Occasionally, vitreous separation is completed and there is involution of the abnormal vessels.

Treatment and Management

- For severe NPDR and PDR without HRCs, careful follow-up with prompt PRP if HRCs develop.
- Full-scatter PRP, which includes 1,200 to 1,600 laser burns, 500-μm, 0.1-second argon burns in two sessions, is recommended for patients with HRCs.
- Intravitreal Anti-VEGF treatment.

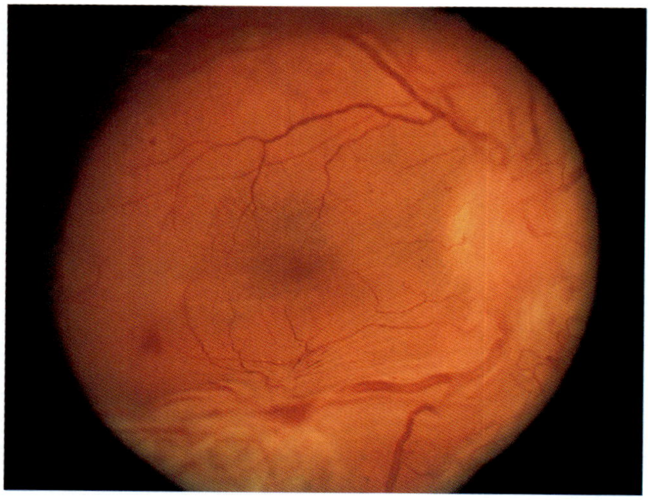

FIGURE 3.24. Fibrovascular proliferation causing TRD along inferotemporal arcade.

HRCs defined by the Diabetic Retinopathy Study:

1. NVD, at least one third of disk area.
2. NVD on or within 1 disk diameter of the disk and vitreous or preretinal hemorrhage.
3. NVE, at least half of disk area and vitreous or preretinal hemorrhage.

Panretinal Photocoagulation

- Power: 600 to 1,600 mW, increase power as needed to achieve moderate retinal burn.
- Spot size: 500 mm.
- Duration: 0.1 second.
- Comments: Divide into two sessions. Start outside of arcades, place burns one burn width apart.
- Recommended for patients who achieve HRCs.

Medical Therapy

- Intensive insulin therapy may delay and slow the progression of diabetic retinopathy (DCCT); however, patients have a higher incidence of hypoglycemic episodes.
- Aspirin treatment is not contraindicated for management of other concomitant systemic diseases (ETDRS).
- Follow-up recommended every month after treatment until vessels regress.
- Supplemental PRP is recommended for eyes with nonregressing NV, increasing NV, new VH, or new areas of NV.

Surgical Therapy

- Results of the Diabetic Vitrectomy Study showed that eyes of type I diabetics with nonclearing VH of greater than 3 months duration benefit from early vitrectomy. However, with the advent of modern-day vitrectomy technology, intervention is typically sooner.
- Other indications for vitrectomy are bilateral VH and TRD involving the macula.

Differential Diagnosis

Retinopathy of prematurity (ROP; history of prematurity, prolonged oxygenation, low birth weight, peripheral NV, macular dragging).

Sickle cell retinopathy (sea-fan NV, positive sickle cell preparation, hemoglobin electrophoresis).

Sarcoidosis (gallium scan, angiotensin-converting enzyme [ACE], abnormal chest x-ray [CXR], vasculitis, vitreous cells).

CRVO (unilateral, diffuse flame-shaped hemorrhages, venous dilation, tortuosity).

BRVO (hemorrhages involving one sector of the retina).

References

Diabetic Retinopathy Study Research Group. Indications For Photocoagulation Treatment of Diabetic Retinopathy: DRS Report 14. *Int Ophthalmol Clin* 1987;26:239–253.

Diabetic Retinopathy Vitrectomy Study Research Group. Early vitrectomy for severe vitreous hemorrhage in diabetic retinopathy: two-year results of a randomized trial—DRVS Report 2. *Arch Ophthalmol* 1985;103:1644–1652.

Radiation Retinopathy

Summary

Radiation retinopathy is characterized by a delayed-onset postradiation progressive occlusive vasculopathy that leads to capillary nonperfusion, large-vessel occlusion, retinal vascular incompetence, and retinal NV.

Etiology

Radiation-induced damage to endothelial cells of retinal vasculature.

Signs and Symptoms

Asymptomatic.

Decreased vision from macular ischemia or VHs.

Demographics

- The incidence depends on total dose and daily fraction size.
- Most studies report 30 to 35 Gy needed to produce retinopathy.
- Cobalt plaque:
  A mean of 150 Gy causes foveal damage.
  Retinopathy occurs 4 to 32 months after treatment.
- External beam radiation:
  A mean of 49 Gy causes foveal damage.
  Retinopathy occurs 7 to 36 months after treatment.
- Proton-beam radiation: A mean of 70 Gy leads to foveal damage.

Ophthalmic Findings

- Nerve fiber layer infarction (cotton-wool spots), retinal hemorrhages, microaneurysms, telangiectasis, perivascular sheathing, exudation.
- Late changes include RPE atrophy, central retinal artery occlusion (CRAO), CRVO, and NV.

Systemic Findings

None.

Special Tests

IVFA: capillary nonperfusion, microaneurysms, hyperfluorescence, telangiectasis, NV, cotton-wool spots, hard exudates, retinal hemorrhages, CME, sheathing, perivasculitis, optic disk edema, disk NV.

OCT: useful in following macular edema.

Pathology

- Focal loss of capillary endothelial cells and pericytes leading to occlusive vascular disease.
- Subsequent loss of ganglion cells, cystic changes in the outer plexiform and inner nuclear layers, and thickening of the vessel walls with preferential damage to the inner retinal layers.
- Choroidal infarction may also be seen and demonstrated on ICG angiography.

Disease Course and Natural Progression

- Widespread capillary closure and ischemia lead to retinal and disk NV and proliferation of fibrous tissue.
- Contraction of the fibroglial tissue leads to VH and TRD.
- Anterior segment NV can lead to neovascular glaucoma.

Treatment and Management

- Focal laser photocoagulation for macular edema.
- PRP for retinal ischemia and NV.
- Hyperbaric oxygen has been attempted, but effect is short lived and depends on continued treatment.
- Intravitreal Anti-VEGF therapy to assist in Neovascular regression.

Medications

None.

Follow-Up

Every 2 to 4 months.

Differential Diagnosis

- Diabetic retinopathy (diabetes; hemorrhages; microaneurysms more prominent that cotton-wool spots).
- Multiple branch retinal artery occlusions (BRAOs) (whitening along distribution of branch retinal artery; may see emboli; hemorrhages uncommon).
- Multiple venous occlusions (more hemorrhages; dilated tortuous veins).
- Ocular ischemic syndrome (midperipheral hemorrhages; low central retinal artery perfusion pressure; dilated veins).

References

Brown GC, Shields JA, Sanburn G, et al. Radiation retinopathy. *Ophthalmology* 1982;89:1494–1501.

Stollard HB. Radiant energy as a pathogenic and a therapeutic agent in ophthalmic disorders. *Br J Ophthalmol* 1933;N126(Suppl 6): 100–126.

Sickle Cell Retinopathy

Summary

Sickle cell retinopathy is characterized by retinal hemorrhages, nonperfusion, and NV as a result of arteriolar and capillary occlusion.

Etiology

Intravascular sickling, hemolysis, hemostasis, and thrombosis cause peripheral arteriolar occlusion, which leads to capillary nonperfusion and eventually to NV.

Signs and Symptoms

Asymptomatic.

Decreased vision.

Floaters secondary to VH.

Demographics

- Hemoglobin AS (HbAS) affects 8% of black Americans.
- Hemoglobin SS (HbSS) affects 0.4% of black Americans (produces the most severe systemic sickling disease).
- Hemoglobin SC (HbSC) affects 0.2% of black Americans (most common to have retinopathy).
- Hemoglobin AC (HbAC) affects 2%.
- Thalassemia (HbS-Thal) affects 0.3%.

Ophthalmic Findings

See Figure 3.25.

Salmon patch hemorrhages (intraretinal hemorrhages).

Refractile deposits (resorbed hemorrhages).

Black sunbursts (RPE hypertrophy).

Sea-fan NV.

Systemic Findings

Chronic anemia.

Aseptic necrosis of the head of the femur.

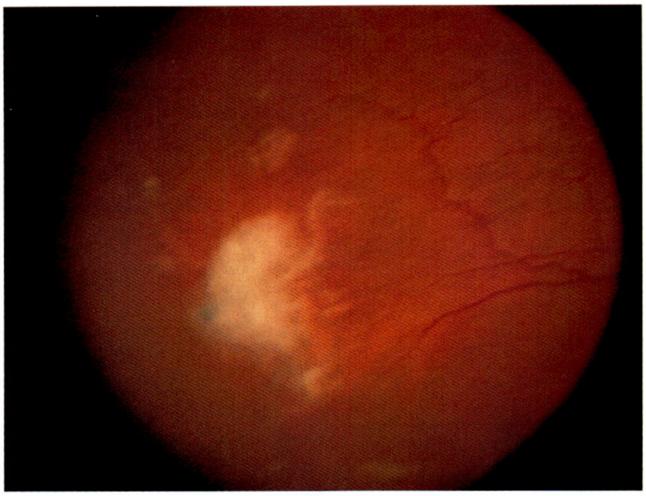

FIGURE 3.25. Sickle cell retinopathy with peripheral neovascularization.

Cerebrovascular accidents (CVAs).
Abdominal infarctions.
Bacterial infections (*Salmonella* organisms).
HbAS, HbAC: asymptomatic.
HbSC, HbS-Thal: mild anemia.

Special Tests

Sickle cell preparation.
Hemoglobin electrophoresis.
IVFA: nonperfusion, AV anastomoses at the border of perfused and nonperfused retina, sea-fan NV (Figure 3.26).
OCT: Macular Edema

Disease Course and Natural Progression

Stage I: Peripheral arterial occlusion.
Stage II: Peripheral AV anastomoses.
Stage III: Sea-fan NV.

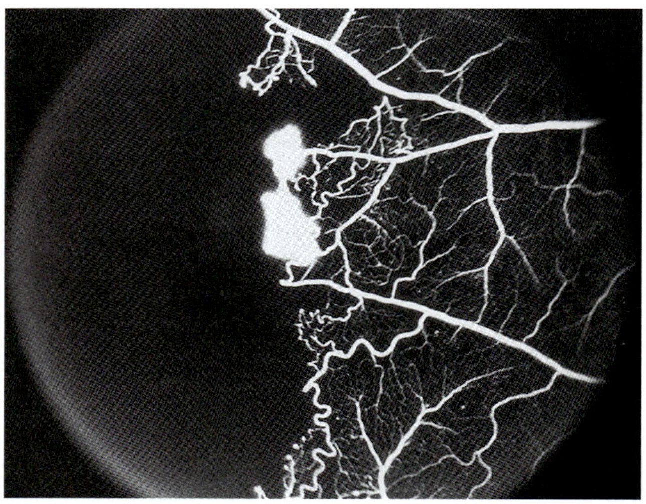

FIGURE 3.26. IVFA demonstrating peripheral nonperfusion capillary dropout and neovascularization.

Stage IV: VH.
Stage V: TRD.

Treatment and Management

- For proliferative sickle retinopathy, PRP, cryotherapy, and diathermy are available treatment modalities. Avoid treating the feeder vessel directly, since this may result in VH.
- Vitrectomy is recommended for nonclearing VH, rhegmatogenous, traction, or combined RDs.

Medications

None. Avoid carbonic anhydrase inhibitors, which can worsen sickling.

Follow-Up

Every 3 to 4 months.

Differential Diagnosis

- Eales disease (male patients, unilateral or bilateral peripheral vasculitis).
- PDR (macular ischemia, edema, posterior nonperfusion, NV along major arcades).
- BRVO (intraretinal hemorrhages along a vessel in one sector of the retina).
- BRAO (arteriole embolus, retinal edema, retinal infarction).
- ROP (prematurity, low birth weight, oxygen exposure, macular dragging).
- Familiar exudative vitreoretinopathy (FEVR) (autosomal dominant inheritance, macular dragging): hyperviscosity (leukemia, lymphoma, macroglobulinemia, polycythemia, multiple myeloma, Roth spots, serous RDs, cotton-wool spots).
- Sarcoidosis (elevated ACE, abnormal CXR, abnormal gallium scan, vascular sheathing, vitreous cells, granulomatous uveitis).
- Ocular ischemic syndrome (painful visual loss, anterior chamber cells, midperipheral microaneurysms and hemorrhages, carotid stenosis, low retinal artery perfusion pressure).

References

Cohen SB, Fletcher ME, Goldberg MS, et al. Diagnosis and management of ocular complications of sickle hemoglobinopathies, I–V. *Ophthalmic Surg* 1986;17:57–59, 110–116, 184–188, 312–315, 369–374.

Goldberg MS. Classification and pathogenesis of proliferative sickle retinopathy. *Am J Ophthalmol* 1971;71:649–665.

Hypertensive Retinopathy

Summary

Hypertensive retinopathy is a retinal vascular condition secondary to systemic hypertension. The signs range from arterial narrowing to disk swelling and retinal hemorrhages.

Etiology

Elevation of systemic blood pressure causes focal and generalized constriction of the retinal arterioles mediated by autoregulation

Signs and Symptoms

Usually asymptomatic.

Demographics

Fifty million Americans have hypertension.

Ophthalmic Findings

See Figure 3.27.

Focal or generalized constriction of retinal arterioles.
Cotton-wool spots.
Intraretinal lipid.
Intraretinal hemorrhages.
BRAO.
BRVO.
CRVO.
Retinal arterial macroaneurysms.
Microaneurysms.
Venous congestion.
Elschnig spots and Siegrist streaks (from nonperfusion of the choriocapillaris with ischemia of overlying RPE and outer retina).

Systemic Findings

Patients may have renal failure.

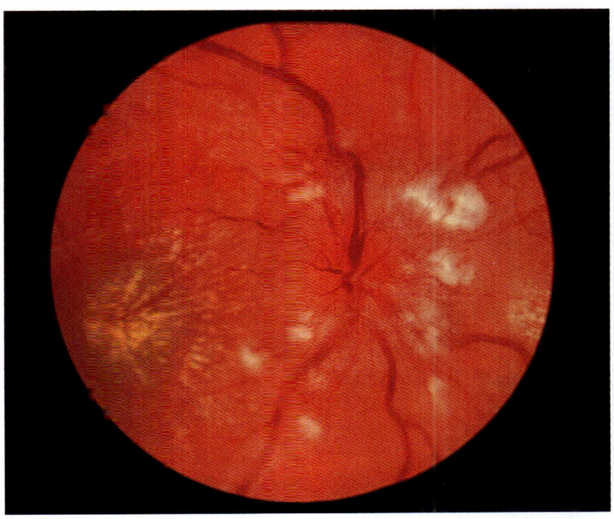

FIGURE 3.27. Malignant hypertension with disk edema, macular star, and multiple cotton-wool spots.

Myocardial infarction.
CVAs related to systemic hypertension.

Special Tests

IVFA: capillary nonperfusion, delayed venous filling, optic disk hyperfluorescence secondary to dilated capillaries, blocked fluorescence secondary to retinal hemorrhages, macular leakage.
OCT: macular edema, optic nerve head evaluation, presence of subretinal fluid.

Pathology

Constriction of the retinal arterioles, arteriosclerosis, hemorrhages, intraretinal lipid, microaneurysms, cytoid bodies.

Disease Course and Natural Progression

There are four grades:

Grade 0 is no changes.
Grade 1 is barely detectable arterial narrowing.
Grade 2 is obvious arterial narrowing with focal irregularities.
Grade 3 is grade 2 plus hemorrhages and/or exudates.
Grade 4 is grade 3 plus disk swelling.

Treatment and Management

Medical therapy to control the elevated blood pressure.

Medications

Systemic antihypertensive medications.

Follow-Up

Variable depending on severity of hypertensive retinopathy.

Differential Diagnosis

BRVO (hemorrhages along a vascular arcade, unilateral, may be bilateral).
CRVO (unilateral flame-shaped, intraretinal hemorrhages in all four quadrants, venous dilation and tortuosity).
Collagen vascular disease (history of polyarteritis nodosa, Wegener granulomatosis, rheumatoid arthritis, systemic lupus erythematosus; abnormal laboratory results may include ANA, anti–double-stranded DNA [anti-dsDNA], anti-ssA, anti-ssB, and c-ANCA).
HIV retinopathy: positive HIV serology.
Leukemia (Roth spots, abnormal peripheral smear, bone marrow biopsy).
Radiation retinopathy (history of radiation therapy).
Sickle cell retinopathy (abnormal sickle cell preparation, hemoglobin electrophoresis, sea-fan NV, peripheral nonperfusion).

Diabetic retinopathy (dot-blot hemorrhages, microaneurysms, NV).

References

Kline R, Kline BE, Moss SE, et al. Blood pressure, hypertension, retinopathy in a population. *Trans Am Ophthalmol Soc* 1993; 91:207–226.

Tso MOM, Abrams GW, Jampol LM. Hypertensive retinopathy, choroidopathy, and optic neuropathy: clinical and pathophysiological approach to classification. In: Singerman LJ, Jampol LM, eds. *Retinal and choroidal manifestations of systemic disease*. Baltimore, MD: Williams & Wilkins, 1991.

Embolic Diseases

Summary

Embolic retinal disease is a condition of visible intraretinal deposits from intravascular migration of endogenous cholesterol or calcium or transit of an injected substance.

Etiology

Intra-arterial emboli from any source:

Carotid occlusive disease.
Cardiac valvular disease.
Bone trauma.
Chronic intravenous use of talc, corn starch in drugs.
Steroid embolization after periocular injection or facial injection.

Signs and Symptoms

Asymptomatic or decreased vision.

Demographics

Hypertension.
Carotid occlusive disease.
Cardiac valve disease.
Trauma.
Patients treated for uveitis.
Drug abusers.

Ophthalmic Findings

- Intra-arterial emboli most frequently found at bifurcation of vessels.
- Refractile intravascular particles (Table 3.6).

Systemic Findings

Carotid bruit.
Cardiac murmur.
Trauma.
Needle tracks.
CVA.

Table 3.6

Features of retinal emboli

Material	Appearance	Source
Calcium	White	Cardiac valve
Cholesterol	Yellow	Carotid disease
Lipid	Yellow	Chest trauma, bone fracture, pancreatitis
Steroid	White	Steroid injection
Fibrin	Grey	Carotid disease
Talc	Refractile	Intravenous injection

Special Tests

Carotid Doppler.
IVFA: refractile intravascular and intraretinal deposits.
OCT: Initially, there is thickening of the inner retina in the region of the of the retina supplied by the obstructed artery. Eventually, the inner retina becomes severely attenuated.

Pathology

Intraretinal deposits of foreign substance.

Disease Course and Natural Progression

Release of endogenous cholesterol, calcium, or lipid; chronic use of talc or corn starch leads to deposition in the retina. Patients are asymptomatic or have decreased vision if there is macular infarction.

Treatment and Management

Send for immediate carotid or cardiac emboli workup.
Cease drug abuse.

Medications

- Cholesterol emboli may be dislodged downstream by ocular massage.
- Intraocular pressure (IOP)–lowering agents.

Follow-Up

Per internist to lower cholesterol, control diabetes, lower blood pressure, and stop smoking.

Differential Diagnosis

Platelet fibrin emboli (history of carotid disease, grayish coloration of embolus).
Cholesterol emboli (yellow; vessel bifurcations and carotid disease).
Calcium emboli (white, near disk, cardiac valve disease).
Cardiac myxoma (young patient, left eye more frequent).

Lipid emboli (history of chest trauma, bone fracture, or pancreatitis)

Retrobulbar steroid injection.

Reference

Arruga J, Sanders MD. Ophthalmologic findings in seventy patients with evidence of retinal embolism. *Ophthalmology* 1982;89:1336–1347.

Hollenhorst Plaques

Summary

Hollenhorst plaques are cholesterol emboli that usually originate from the carotid arteries or major cardiac arteries and lodge in the retinal arterial system.

Etiology

Atherosclerotic deposits in the carotid artery, cardiac arteries, or in the central retinal artery.

Signs and Symptoms

Asymptomatic, transient visual obscurations, unilateral weakness of an arm or leg, transient ischemic attacks, CVA.

Demographics

Embolus is visible in 20% of patients with CRAO.

Ophthalmic Findings

- Glistening yellow cholesterol embolus present at the arterial bifurcation (Figure 3.28).

Systemic Findings

Hypertension.

Diabetes.

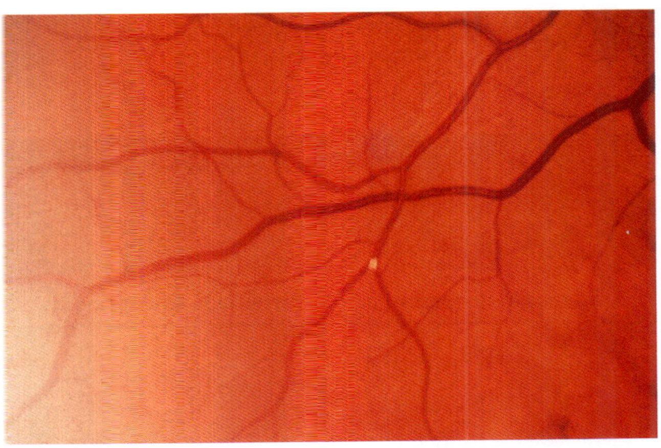

FIGURE 3.28. Hollenhorst plaque at an arteriolar bifurcation.

Special Tests

Color photographs.

Carotid auscultation reveals a bruit.

Carotid Doppler shows narrowing of the carotid artery.

Echocardiogram (transesophageal) may reveal cardiac pathology.

Pathology

Cholesterol embolus in the lumen of the arteriole.

Disease Course and Natural Progression

Fifty-six percent mortality over 9 years versus 27% for age-matched controls without emboli.

Treatment and Management

Carotid endarterectomy.

Control systemic hypertension and diabetes.

Medications

Drugs to lower cholesterol, control diabetes, lower blood pressure, and stop smoking.

Follow-Up

Variable; medical evaluation is most important.

Differential Diagnosis

Calcific emboli: cardiac valve disease, white coloration.

Talc, starch: i.v. drug abuse.

Platelet fibrin emboli: also seen in carotid disease, grayish coloration.

Cardiac myxoma: younger patient, left eye more commonly involved than right eye.

Lipid embolus: history of chest trauma, pancreatitis, or bone fracture.

Reference

Gold DH: Retinal arterial occlusions. *Trans Am Acad Ophthalmol Otolaryngol* 1977;83:392–408.

Vein Occlusion

Central Retinal Vein Occlusion

Summary

CRVO occurs in an ischemic and nonischemic variety secondary to thrombosis of the central retinal vein at the level of the lamina cribrosa.

Etiology

Thrombosis of the central retinal vein at and posterior to the level of the lamina cribrosa.

Signs and Symptoms

Decreased vision.
May have transient visual obscuration before event.

Demographics

- Ninety percent of patients are over 50 years of age.
- Association with chronic open-angle glaucoma, hypertension, diabetes, oral contraceptives, and diuretics.

Ophthalmic Findings

See Figure 3.29.

Dilated tortuous retinal veins.
Swollen optic disks.
Intraretinal hemorrhages.
Retinal edema.
Cotton-wool spots.
Ischemic CRVO may have a relative afferent pupillary defect.

Systemic Findings

Hypertension is present in 61% of patients.
Diabetes is present in 7%.
Arteriosclerosis.

Special Tests

- IVFA.
  Nonischemic CRVO:
  Diffuse capillary leakage.
  Prolongation of venous filling time.
  Ischemic CRVO:
  Widespread capillary nonperfusion.
  Pronounced prolongation of venous filling time.
- ERG: ischemic type of CRVO; there is decreased ERG bright flash, and a diminished scotopic b:a wave-amplitude ratio (photoreceptors receive nourishment from the unaffected choriocapillaris).
- Gonioscopy to evaluate for angle NV.

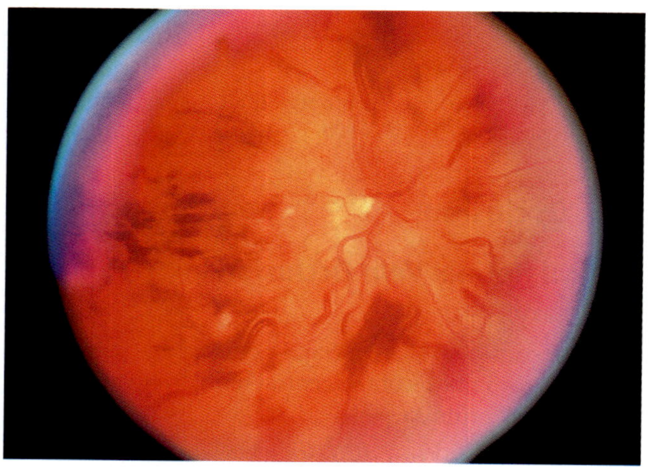

FIGURE 3.29. CRVO with multiple nerve-fiber layer hemorrhages and cotton wool spots in all quadrants, optic disk edema, and dilated tortuous vessels.

Pathology

- Thrombosis of the central retinal vein at the level of the lamina cribrosa.
- Acute occlusions present with retinal edema, focal retinal necrosis, and subretinal, intraretinal, and preretinal hemorrhages.
- Chronic CRVO is characterized by hemosiderosis, disorganization of the retinal architecture, gliosis, and fibrovascular preretinal membranes.

Disease Course

- Most cases of nonischemic CRVO (48%) completely resolve.
- Twenty-two percent progress to complete occlusion.
- Thirty percent have partial resolution.
- Prognosis is markedly worse in eyes with an ischemic CRVO:
  Ten percent of patients achieve acuity better than 20/400.
  Thirty percent develop neovascularization of the iris (NVI) usually within 3 months (Table 3.7).

Treatment and Management

- Measure IOP.
- Perform gonioscopy to see if there is angle closure or angle NV.
- Perform a dilated fundus examination.
- Initially retinal hemorrhage may preclude good IVFA assessment of extent of nonperfusion, but VA is another way to assess this.
- Initial poor VA correlates with ischemia.
- As the hemorrhage clears, an IVFA may be useful to demonstrate areas of nonperfusion.
- Consultation with an internist is important to treat associated medical conditions such as hypertension, diabetes, or elevated cholesterol.
- OCT to assess presence of macular edema

Table 3.7

Area of retinal ischemia and risk of developing NVI

Disk areas of nonperfusion	Percentage developing NVI
10–29	16
30–74	36
>75	52

NVI, neovascularization of the iris.

- Laser treatment:
  No benefit of grid photocoagulation for macular edema in older patients with CRVO.
  A trend toward improved vision in younger patients treated with focal grid laser in the CRVO study.
  PRP if iris NV is present.

Medications

Ozurdex, sustained delivery dexamethasone implant, is the first FDA-approved pharmacologic to treat macular edema secondary to RVO. Other intravitreal anti-VEGF agents and intravitreal steroids have been employed with variable success in treating macular edema secondary to RVO.

Intravitreal anti-VEGF agents can be used as an adjunct to PRP to treat rubeosis.

Follow-Up

Every 6 weeks for the first 6 months; then depending on whether macular edema is being treated.

Differential Diagnosis

Hyperviscosity retinopathy: usually bilateral, history of multiple myeloma or Waldenstrom macroglobulinemia, lymphoma, or leukemia.

Ocular ischemic syndrome: decreased retinal arterial pressure, primarily peripheral intraretinal hemorrhages; carotid occlusion.

Vasculitides: sarcoidosis (elevated ACE, abnormal gallium scan, abnormal CXR, granulomatous uveitis), systemic lupus erythematosus (positive ANA, anti-dsDNA; rheumatologic, dermatologic, pulmonary, or cardiac abnormalities), syphilis (positive result on rapid plasmin reagin [RPR] test and FTA-Abs).

Diabetic retinopathy: hemorrhages, microaneurysms concentrated in posterior pole.

Reference

Central Vein Occlusion Study Group. Baseline and early natural history report: the central vein occlusion study. *Arch Ophthalmol* 1993;111:1087–1095.

Branch Retinal Vein Occlusion

Summary

BRVOs are occlusions of the vein at the site of AV crossing.

Etiology

Occlusion of the vein at the AV crossing due to atherosclerotic arteriole compressing adjacent vein confined by common adventitial sheath.

Signs and Symptoms

Blurred vision.
May be asymptomatic.

Demographics

Age 60 to 70 years.
Association with hypertension.

Ophthalmic Findings

See Figure 3.30.

- Superficial hemorrhages.
- Retinal edema.
- Cotton-wool spots in the involved retinal sector.
- Dilated tortuous vein.
- The superotemporal quadrant is involved 63% of the time.
- Sclerosed and sheathed vessels in chronic cases.
- Collateral vessels that cross horizontal raphe.

Systemic Findings

Association with systemic hypertension.

Special Tests

IVFA: delayed venous filling in affected vessel, blocked fluorescence due to hemorrhage, nonperfusion, retinal edema, hyperfluorescence secondary to NV.

OCT: to assess presence of macular edema.

Pathology

- Common adventitia binds the branch artery and vein in a normal retina.
- Thickening of the arterial wall (atherosclerosis) compresses the adjacent vein causing turbulence of flow, endothelial damage, and thrombotic occlusion.

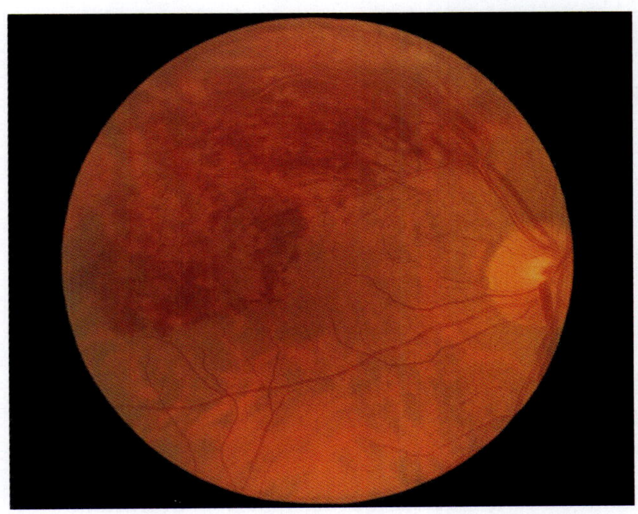

FIGURE 3.30. Superotemporal BRVO.

Disease Course

- Most spontaneously resolve with VA remaining 20/40 or better.
- Persistent macular edema may lead to decreased vision.
- Greater than five disk areas of nonperfusion at risk for NV of the retina and VH.

Treatment and Management

- As the hemorrhage clears, an IVFA may be useful to demonstrate areas of nonperfusion.
- Focal grid photocoagulation is recommended for chronic macular edema with intact perifoveal capillary perfusion after at least 3 months' delay for spontaneous resolution of macular edema. Initiate focal grid if VA is 20/40 to 20/200. Retreatment is recommended every 3 months if areas of leakage persist.
- Intravitreal steroids and intravitreal anti-VEGF agents can be used to treat macular edema.
- PRP if there is retinal or iris NV.

Medications

Same as CRVO.

Follow-Up

Depends on extent of complications such as macular edema and ischemia.

Differential Diagnosis

Diabetic retinopathy: history of diabetes mellitus, scattered hemorrhages throughout posterior pole, microaneurysms, hard exudates.

Radiation retinopathy: history of local radiation treatment, similar appearance to diabetic retinopathy.

Arteriole macroaneurysm: most common in elderly women, hyperfluorescence of macroaneurysm on IVFA, spontaneous involution of lesion.

References

Branch Vein Occlusion Study Group. Argon laser scatter photocoagulation for prevention of neovascularization and vitreous hemorrhage in branch vein occlusion: a randomized clinical trial. *Arch Ophthalmol* 1986;104:34–41.

BVOS Group. Argon laser photocoagulation for macular edema in branch vein occlusion. *Am J Ophthalmol* 1984;98: 271–282.

Central and Branch Retinal Artery Occlusion

Summary

Sudden painless visual loss secondary to occlusion of the central retinal artery or one of its branches.

Etiology

Atherosclerosis-related thrombosis at the level of the lamina cribrosa. Other etiologies include embolization, atherosclerotic plaque, spasm, dissecting aneurysm, hemorrhage under an atherosclerotic plaque, circulatory collapse. One to two percent of patients have giant cell arteritis.

Signs and Symptoms

Profound, sudden, severe painless loss of vision. Some have a history of amaurosis fugax. Sixty-six percent have vision of less than 20/400. Eighteen percent have a vision of ≥20/40 when there is a patent cilioretinal artery. No light perception is evident in patients with combined ophthalmic retinal artery occlusions and CRAOs.

Demographics

Mean age in the early 60s.
No sex predilection.
Right and left eyes affected equally.
Bilateral in 1% to 2% of patients.

Ophthalmic Findings

Afferent pupillary defect.

Opacified and edematous retina. This resolves in 4 to 6 weeks.

Optic disk pallor.

Vascular attenuation, box carring.

Macular cherry-red spot.

Visible embolus in 20% of eyes (Hollenhorst plaque: carotid; calcific plaque: cardiac valve).

Systemic Findings

- Hypertension in two thirds of patients.
- Diabetes in one fourth of patients.
- Cardiac valvular disease in one fourth of patients.
- Carotid atherosclerosis in 50% of patients.
- The leading cause of subsequent death is cardiovascular disease.

Special Tests

IVFA: Normal choroidal filling, delayed arterial filling time, and delayed AV transit time. The filling time reverts to normal over time (Figure 3.31).

Erythrocyte sedimentation rate (ESR): Elevated in giant cell arteritis.

ERG: decreased b wave.

Visual field shows a remaining temporal island. If there is a patent cilioretinal artery, the visual field may show a small central island.

Carotid Doppler examinations show carotid stenosis.

Echocardiogram may show valvular plaques.

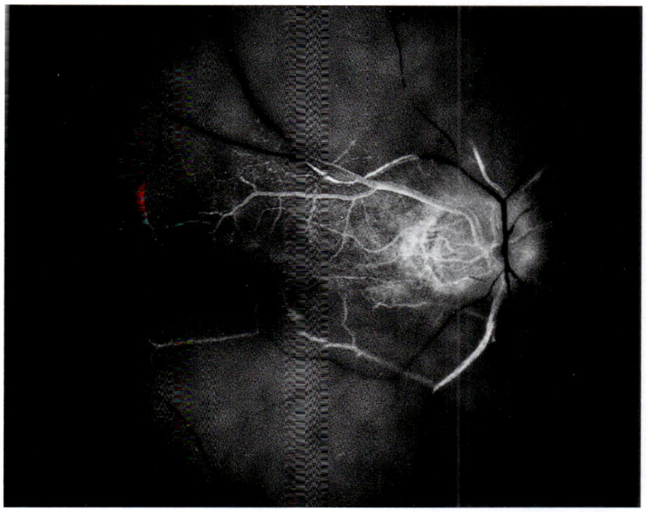

FIGURE 3.31 Late phase of intravenous fluorescein angiogram of a CRAO demonstrating severe retinal nonperfusion.

Pathology

Thrombosis at the level of the lamina scleralis, inner ischemic atrophy.

Disease Course and Natural Progression

- There may be a history of amaurosis fugax.
- Permanent visual deficit.
- Eighteen percent of patients develop NVI.

Treatment and Management

From animal studies, efforts to reverse damage following a CRAO are probably ineffective after approximately 90 minutes from the occlusive event.

- Reduce IOP by ocular massage, anterior chamber paracentesis.
- Inhalation therapy with 95% oxygen and 5% carbon dioxide 10 minutes every hour and every 4 hours through the night.
- Oral acetazolamide, aspirin.
- Intravenous steroids for patients with giant cell arteritis.

Medications

Intravenous steroids for patients with giant cell arteritis to prevent involvement of fellow eye.

Follow-Up

Every 6 weeks for the first 3 months; as needed thereafter. Administer PRP if NVI develops.

Differential Diagnosis

- Intraocular gentamicin injection.
- Arteritic anterior ischemic optic neuropathy: history of jaw claudication, scalp tenderness, weight loss, fever, elevated ESR.
- Ophthalmic artery occlusion: no cherry-red spot, entire retina white.

Reference

Hayreh SS, Kolder HE, Weingeist TA. Central retinal artery occlusion and retinal tolerance time. *Ophthalmology* 1980; 87:75–78.

Ocular Ischemic Syndrome

Summary

Ocular ischemic syndrome is a condition with ocular symptoms and signs attributable to chronic, severe carotid artery or ophthalmic artery obstruction and subsequent ocular hypoperfusion (Table 3.8).

Etiology

Atherosclerosis, giant cell arteritis.

Signs and Symptoms

Gradual visual loss over a period of weeks to months; dull, aching pain; prolonged recovery to bright light.

Demographics

- Age over 55 years with a mean of 65 years of age.
- Male more often than female patients by a ratio of 2:1, affects 7.5 per million individuals.
- Greater than 90% obstruction of carotid flow.
- Twenty percent of patients bilateral involvement.

Ophthalmic Findings

Iris NV with high or low IOP.
Anterior chamber cell and flare.
Narrow retinal arteries.
Dilated veins.
Hemorrhages.
Midperipheral microaneurysms.
NVD.
NVE.
Cotton-wool spots.
Cherry-red spot.
Spontaneous pulsations of the arteries.

Systemic Findings

Hypertension.
Diabetes.
Cardiovascular disease.
CVAs.
Peripheral atherosclerotic vascular disease.
Five-year mortality is 40%.

Table 3.8

Ophthalmic features that help to distinguish the ocular ischemic syndrome from other ocular diseases

	Ocular ischemic syndrome	Nonischemic central retinal vein obstruction	Diabetic retinopathy
Laterality	Unilateral in 80%	Unilateral	Bilateral
Age	50s–80s	50s–80s	Variable
Fundus signs			
Veins	Dilated, beaded	Dilated, tortuous	Dilated, beaded
Optic disk	Normal	Swollen	Normal
Retinal arterial perfusion pressure (ophthalmodynamometry)	Decreased	Normal	Normal
Retinal hemorrhages	Mild	Mild to severe	Mild to moderate
Microaneurysms	Midperiphery	Variable	Posterior pole
Hard exudate	Absent unless concomitant diabetic retinopathy	Rare	Common
Fluorescein angiography			
Choroidal filling	Delayed, patchy	Normal	Normal
AV transit time	Prolonged	Prolonged	Normal
Retinal vessel staining	Prominent arterial	Prominent venous	Usually absent

Special Tests

IVFA: delayed choroidal filling, delayed AV transit time, vascular staining, macular edema (15%), retinal capillary nonperfusion.

Ophthalmodynamometry: decreased retinal artery perfusion pressure.

ERG: decreased amplitude of a and b waves.

Carotid angiography: demonstrates greater than 90% stenosis.

Pathology

Atherosclerotic narrowing of the carotid arteries.

Disease Course and Natural Progression

Progressive carotid stenosis leads to gradual vision loss and dull, aching ocular pain.

Treatment and Management

Carotid endarterectomy: 25% get stabilization or improvement in vision. Surgery is recommended if there is greater than 70% stenosis and the patient is symptomatic. The 2-year CVA rate is 9% for treated versus 26% of untreated patients.

PRP: for NVI.

Medications

None.

Follow-Up

Every 6 weeks and monitor for rubeosis and pressure elevation.

Differential Diagnosis

CRVO: swollen disk, normal retinal artery perfusion pressure, normal choroidal filling, venous staining.

PDR: bilateral, variable age, normal retinal artery perfusion pressure, posterior pole microaneurysms, hard exudate, normal choroidal filling and AV transit, absent vessel staining.

Reference

North American Symptomatic Carotid Endarterectomy Trial Collaborators. Beneficial effect of carotid endarterectomy in symptomatic patients with high grade carotid stenosis. *N Engl J Med* 1991;325:445–453.

Macroaneurysms

Summary

Acquired macroaneurysms are round or fusiform dilations of the retinal arterioles occurring in the posterior pole within the first three orders of arteriolar bifurcation.

Etiology

Systemic hypertension.

Signs and Symptoms

Asymptomatic or decreased vision.

Demographics

Female more often than male patients.

Ten percent are bilateral, may be multiple.

Age range is 60 to 70 years.

Ophthalmic Findings

See Figure 3.32.

Sub-ILM, intraretinal, subretinal hemorrhages.
Macular edema.
VH.
Arteriolar emboli.
Capillary telangiectasia.

Systemic Findings

Two thirds have hypertension, arteriosclerotic cardiovascular disease.

Special Tests

IVFA: blockage by surrounding hemorrhage. In the early phase, there is arterial filling, and in the late stages, there is staining of the vessel walls due to leakage. There is also leakage of the surrounding capillaries and dilation of the arterial vessel with hyperfluorescence.
OCT: shows location of hemorrhage.

Pathology

Distension of involved retinal arteriole.
Fibroglial proliferation.
Dilated capillaries.
Extravasated blood, lipoidal exudates, hemosiderin deposits.

Disease Course and Natural Progression

- Good visual prognosis, since lesions often thrombose and undergo spontaneous involution with resolution of exudate.
- Some patients have progression of exudation with further vision loss.

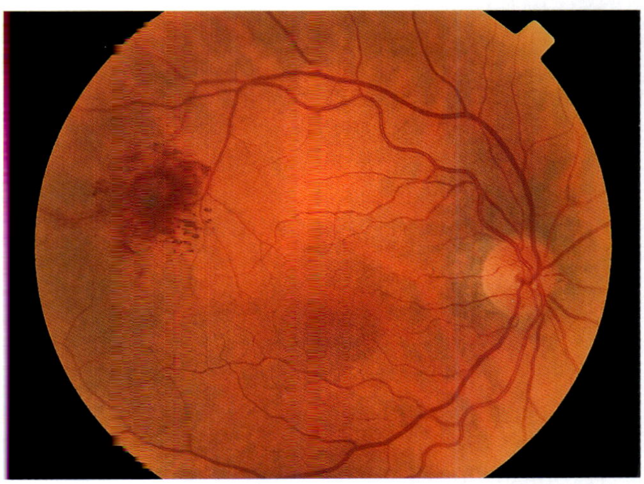

FIGURE 3.32. Macroaneurysm with surrounding retinal hemorrhage.

Treatment and Management

- Laser photocoagulation if macular edema is visually significant. Light treatment with a large spot size is recommended. One should be careful if the distal portion of the arteriole supplies the macula, since a complication of treatment is occlusion of the vessel.
- Systemic evaluation for hypertension and cardiovascular disease.

Medications

None.

Follow-Up

Variable depending on macular involvement.

Differential Diagnosis

Diabetic retinopathy: abnormal glucose tolerance test, diffuse hemorrhages, macular exudates, and NV.
Retinal telangiectasia: telangiectatic perifoveal vessels.
Capillary hemangioma: autosomal dominant inheritance, red/orange retinal mass.
Malignant melanoma: B and A scan appearance, double circulation on IVFA.
Hemorrhagic PED in ARMD: drusen, RPE changes, no capillary abnormalities.

Reference

Rabb MF, Gagliano DA, Teskee MP. Retinal arterial macroaneurysms. *Surv Ophthalmol* 1988;33:73–96.

Perifoveal Telangiectasis

Summary

Perifoveal retinal telangiectasis (PFT) is a developmental retinal vascular disorder characterized by ectasia of the retinal capillaries in which there is irregular capillary dilatation and incompetence. PFT is a condition of microaneurysmal and saccular dilation and capillary nonperfusion of the perifoveal capillaries.

Etiology

Unknown.

Signs and Symptoms

Group 1A: Vision loss is usually in the 20/25 to 20/40 range.
Group 1B: There is minimal vision loss usually in the range of 20/25.
Group 2: There is minimal vision loss with vision usually better than 20/30.
Group 3: Patients may have anywhere from minimal vision loss to legal blindness.

Demographics

PFT is divided into congenital and acquired causes:

Group 1A is unilateral congenital PFT. It occurs in men with a mean age of 40 years.

Group 1B is acquired unilateral idiopathic PFT, which occurs in men with a mean age of 40 years.

Group 2 is acquired bilateral PFT, which affects both men and women with an age range of 50 to 60 years; this is the most common type.

Group 3 is acquired bilateral PFT with capillary nonperfusion, which affects patients mostly in their fifties.

Ophthalmic Findings

- In Group 1A, the temporal half of the macula has telangiectatic vessels with macular exudate and edema.
- In Group 1B, there are telangiectatic vessels involving the 1 o'clock position at the edge of the FAZ with or without exudate.
- Group 2 has bilateral symmetric telangiectatic vessels usually less than 1 disk diameter in extent involving the temporal fovea with minimal edema, mild dilation of the retinal capillaries, and graying of the retina. There are right-angled venules present. There is RPE hyperplasia along the right-angled venules. Some cases have a yellow lesion in the FAZ. CNV is possible.
- Group 3 has telangiectatic vessels and an enlarged FAZ with disk pallor present; small gold flecks on retinal surface described by Gass.

Systemic Findings

In the older patients with bilateral involvement, a glucose tolerance test demonstrates diabetes in one third of patients.

Special Tests

IVFA: Group 1A shows leakage from the telangiectatic vessels. Group 1B has minimal leakage. In Group 2, there is perifoveal capillary leakage, dilated ectatic perifoveal capillaries, and blocked fluorescence in the areas of RPE hyperplasia. In Group 3, there is no leakage from the telangiectatic vessels, and there is an enlarged FAZ.

Pathology

Similar to diabetic microangiopathy with deposits of excess basement membrane in the retinal capillaries.

Disease Course and Natural Progression

Congenital or acquired telangiectatic vessels lead to exudation and edema in Groups 1A and 2 or to nonperfusion in Group 3, which causes vision loss.

Treatment and Management

Group 1A: Photocoagulation may be beneficial. Also, spontaneous resolution is possible.

Groups 1B, 2, and 3: No treatment is recommended. Laser photocoagulation has not been found to improve visual outcome.

Associated CNV is treated with anti-VEGF therapies, similar to other causes of CNV.

Medications

None. Intravitreal anti-VEGF and steroids have been employed with variable success to treat secondary macular edema.

Follow-Up

Variable depending on vision and amount of exudation.

Differential Diagnosis

- BRVO affects capillary bed distal to AV crossing, capillary dilation secondary to collateral pathways, venous outflow.
- Radiation retinopathy: multiple abnormal retinal areas, soft exudate, NV, and a history of radiation therapy.
- Carotid occlusive disease: iris NV, anterior chamber cell and flare, cherry-red spot, arterial narrowing, venous dilation.
- ARMD: fluorescein angiographic findings, deeper leakage, drusen, RPE changes, no retinal capillary disease.
- Foveal macular dystrophy: yellow lesions resemble PFT Group 2. No telangiectatic vessels or leakage on fluorescein.
- Focal choroiditis may be confused with PFT Group 2 secondary to RPE hyperplasia.
- Diabetic retinopathy: diffuse hemorrhages, cotton-wool spots, microaneurysms, NV.

References

Gass JD, Oyakawa RT. Idiopathic juxtafoveolar retinal telangiectasis. *Arch Ophthalmol* 1982;100:769–780.

Park DW, Schatz H, McDonald HR, et al. Grid laser photocoagulation for macular edema in bilateral juxtafoveal telangiectasis. *Ophthalmology* 1997;104:1838–1846.

Familial Exudative Vitreoretinopathy (Fevr)

Summary

FEVR is a bilateral autosomal dominant disorder of peripheral retinal vascular development often associated with retinal traction.

Etiology

It is postulated that there is a genetic defect that induces abnormal development of the hyaloid vascular system.

Signs and Symptoms

Asymptomatic.
May have decreased vision.
May present as an exotropia.

Demographics

Autosomal dominant inheritance.
Bilateral and symmetric.

Ophthalmic Findings

Bilateral involvement.
Avascular zone in the peripheral retina.
TRD.
Retinal folds.
Temporal dragging of the macula.
AV shunts at the margin of vascularized retina, peripheral NV.
VH is rare.
Other findings may include myopia, vitreous "snowflakes," vitreous bands, and retinal pigmentary changes.

Systemic Findings

None.

Special Tests

- IVFA: avascular border posterior to the ora serrata.
- AV anastomoses that leak fluorescein.

Pathology

Vitreous membranes, peripheral vascular occlusion, cholesterol crystals, intraretinal and subretinal hemorrhage, chronic subretinal fluid, contracture and thickening of the retina with dilated telangiectatic vessels.

Disease Course and Natural Progression

The majority of teenage carriers have no visual impairment.
Retinal folds may progress rapidly or slowly, or stabilize.
Rarely vision loss beyond 20 to 30 years of age, usually secondary to rhegmatogenous RD or TRD.

Treatment and Management

Examine family members.
Correct strabismus.
Cryotherapy or laser photocoagulation for NV.
Scleral buckle, pars plana vitrectomy for TRD.

Medications

None.

Follow-Up

Variable.

Differential Diagnosis

ROP: prematurity, oxygen treatment, low birth weight, progressive to the cicatricial stage, or aborts and vascularizes the periphery. The avascular zone is unchanged in FEVR.
Persistent hyperplastic primary vitreous (PHPV): retinal folds in conjunction with remnants of the hyaloid vascular system, retinal dysplasia, elongated ciliary processes, glaucoma, abnormal development in the seventh to the eighth week of gestation versus in the last month of gestation for FEVR.

Reference

Tasmin W, Augsberger JJ, Shields JA, et al. Familial exudative vitreoretinopathy. *Trans Am Ophthalmol Soc* 1981;79:211–226.

Retinopathy of Prematurity

Summary

ROP is a proliferative retinopathy of premature and low-birth-weight infants.

Etiology

- In the primary stage, oxygen exposure causes vasoconstriction of incompletely vascularized retina.
- In the secondary stage, there is endothelial proliferation.

Signs and Symptoms

Asymptomatic.
Strabismus.

Demographics

- Vision loss in 1,300 children per year in the United States.
- Sixty-six percent of infants with birth weight less than 1,250 g affected, and 82% of infants with birth weight of less than 1,000 g.
- Prematurity, low birth weight, prolonged oxygen exposure, complicated hospital course, and elevated partial pressure of CO_2 (PCO_2) are the main risk factors.

Ophthalmic Findings

See Figures 3.33 and 3.34.

Temporal dragging of the macula.
Amblyopia.
Myopia.
Strabismus.

Classification of ROP

- Stage 1: Demarcation line.
- Stage 2: Ridge.
- Stage 3: Ridge and extraretinal fibrovascular proliferation.
- Stage 4: Subtotal RD.
- Stage 5: Total RD.
- Plus disease is retinal vascular dilation and tortuosity in the posterior pole.
- Threshold disease is a disease of stage 3 or worse involving five contiguous or eight noncontiguous clock-hour positions of retina in zone 1 or 2 with Plus disease.

Systemic Findings

Low birth weight.
Cerebral palsy.
Respiratory distress syndrome.
Sepsis.
Necrotizing bowel disease.

Special Tests

IVFA: Peripheral nonperfusion, leakage of dye from neovascular vessels (rarely performed).

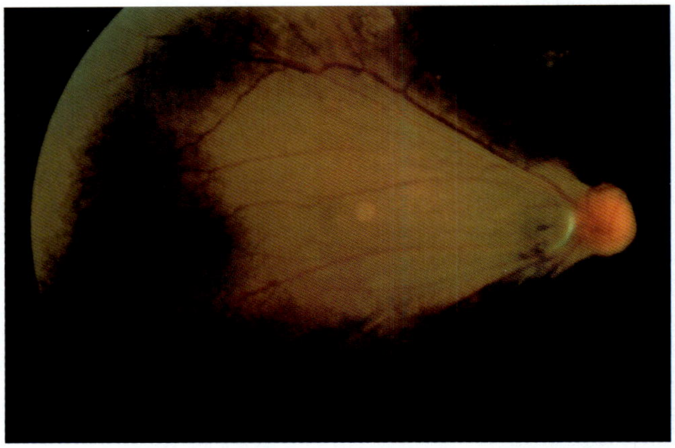

FIGURE 3.34. ROP with temporal dragging of the macula.

Pathology

Avascular retina, NV, fibrovascular proliferation in the advanced stages.

Disease Course and Natural Progression

- Eighty-five percent of infants have spontaneous regression.
- Seven percent at weight less than 1,250 g progress to threshold ROP.
- NV leads to fibrosis, which progresses to contracture of proliferative tissue causing RD and macular distortion.

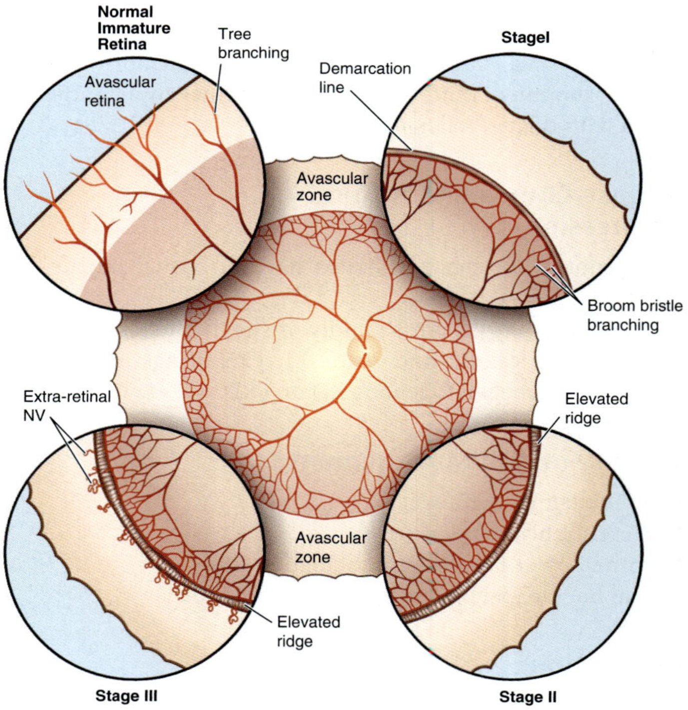

FIGURE 3.33. Diagram of the vascular pattern associated with normal immature retina and stage I to stage III ROP.

Treatment and Management

- Examine all high-risk infants, which include those of less than 36 weeks' gestation or weighing less than 2,000 g.
- Initial examination should be at 7 to 9 weeks of age, and then examination should be performed every 2 weeks until prethreshold value is reached; then examination should be performed every week.
- Treat when patient reaches threshold, which is defined as stage 3 + ROP in five contiguous or eight cumulative clock-hours of retinal involvement in zone 1 or 2. Treatment is with cryotherapy or laser photocoagulation.
- Scleral buckle or vitrectomy for stage 4, and pars plana vitrectomy for stage 5.

Medications

Anti-VEGF therapies (Investigational).

Follow-Up

Every 2 weeks until prethreshold; then every week until regression or threshold is reached, at which time treatment should be started.

Differential Diagnosis

- FEVR: no history of prematurity, family history, no history of oxygen exposure. NV may occur several years after birth.
- Retinoblastoma may resemble stage 4 or 5, calcification on computed tomography (CT).
- Congenital cataracts.
- Norrie disease.

Reference

Cryotherapy for Retinopathy of Prematurity Collaborative Group. Multicenter trial of cryotherapy for retinopathy of prematurity: preliminary results. *Arch Ophthalmol* 1988;106:471–479.

Coats Disease

Summary

Coats disease is an idiopathic condition characterized by telangiectatic and aneurysmal retinal vessels with intraretinal and subretinal exudates.

Etiology

Primary vascular etiology with breakdown of the blood–retinal barrier versus endocrinologic basis.

Signs and Symptoms

Juvenile type:

Decreased vision.
Strabismus.
Leukocoria.
Adult type:
Asymptomatic.
Decreased vision.

Demographics

Male-to-female ratio of 3:1.
Eighty percent of cases are unilateral.
No racial or ethnic predilection.

Ophthalmic Findings

See Figure 3.35.

Localized yellow/green subretinal exudates.
Serous RD.
Frequently involves macula.
Telangiectatic vessels and microaneurysms.

Systemic Findings

None.

Special Tests

IVFA: numerous localized abnormalities of the retinal vasculature. Early and persistent leakage from telangiectatic vessels and aneurysms. Capillary nonperfusion and anomalous vessels are seen.
OCT: to assess presence of macular edema.

Pathology

- Loss of the vascular endothelium and pericytes with subsequent mural disorganization from ischemia.

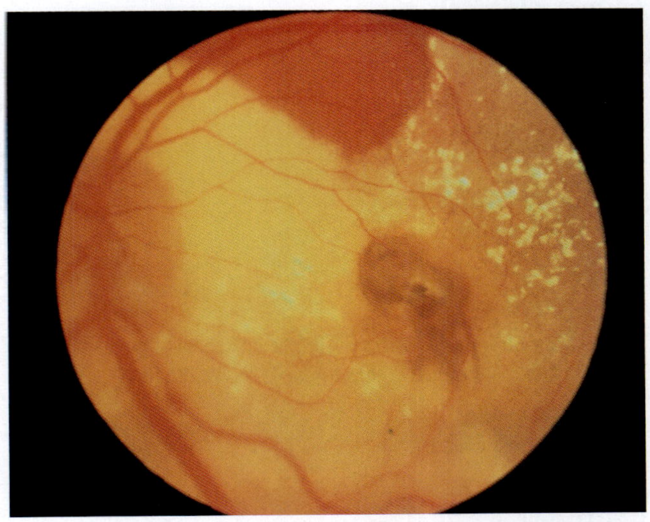

FIGURE 3.35. Coats disease with massive subretinal lipid exudation.

- Subsequent damage to the blood–retinal barrier results in telangiectasia and massive outpouring of subretinal lipid exudate.

Disease Course and Natural Progression

- Variable but progressive clinical course.
- Subretinal exudation leads to serous RD.
- CNV may develop in the area of the lipid.

Treatment and Management

- Observation if lesions are limited in extent or do not threaten the macula.
- IVFA-guided photocoagulation if macula is involved or threatened.
- Cryotherapy if exudative detachment present.
- Pars plana vitrectomy if a TRD develops.
- Prognosis is poor, and eyes may have amblyopia.
- Adjunctive intravitreal steroids or intravitreal anti-VEGF agents may be used.

Medications

None.

Follow-Up

Variable depending on macular involvement.

Differential Diagnosis

Differential diagnosis is that of leukocoria including the following:
Retinoblastoma.
RD.
PHPV.
Congenital cataract.
Norrie disease.
FEVR.
Eales disease.
Vasculitis.
Tumor with exudation.
Diabetes.
BRVO.
Juxtafoveal telangiectasis.
Radiation retinopathy.

Reference

Ridley MD, Shields JA, Brown GC, et al. Coats' disease: evaluation of management. *Ophthalmology* 1982;89:1381–1387.

Von Hippel Disease

Summary

Von Hippel disease is an isolated retinal vascular abnormality or one of many systemic abnormalities characterized by a red/orange intraretinal mass with a dilated feeder artery and draining vein.

Etiology

Isolated retinal vascular abnormality.

Signs and Symptoms

Asymptomatic.
Decreased vision.

Demographics

- Autosomal dominant inheritance with incomplete penetrance and sporadic forms occur.
- Fifty percent of cases are bilateral.

Ophthalmic Findings

See Figure 3.36.

- Spherical orange/red tumor fed by a dilated tortuous retinal artery and drained by an engorged vein with associated retinal exudation.
- Lesions are multiple or bilateral in 50% of cases and can involve the retinal or optic nerve.
- Angiomatous variant, which is peripheral and has no large feeding or draining vessel.

Systemic Findings

Von Hippel–Lindau disease (VHL)

Central nervous system (CNS) hemangioblastomas.
Cysts in kidneys, pancreas, liver, epididymis, ovaries.
Renal cell carcinoma.
Pheochromocytoma.

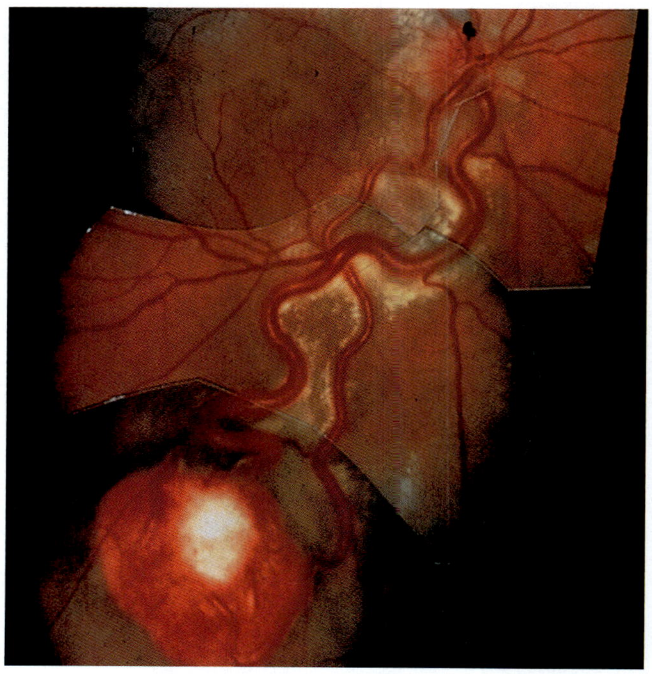

FIGURE 3.36. Von Hippel angioma with dilated feeder vessels.

Special Tests

IVFA: hyperfluorescence of tumor with prominent dilated feeding artery and draining venule (Figure 3.37).
A/B Scan: high internal reflectivity of the angioma.

Pathology

Tortuous large diameter capillaries lined by normal endothelium.

Disease Course and Natural Progression

- Enlargement with time leading to increased exudation, serous detachment, VH, or macular pucker.
- Recurrence after treatment.
- May involute spontaneously.

Treatment and Management

- Photocoagulation or cryotherapy of the lesion. This may result in increased exudation.
- Pars plana vitrectomy, scleral buckle in cases of RD.
- Systemic evaluation for CNS, pancreatic, liver, or renal involvement.

Follow-Up

Variable, depending on extent of exudation.

Differential Diagnosis

Macroaneurysm: hypertension, fusiform dilations of arterioles with surrounding hemorrhage, exudate.
Coats disease: telangiectatic aneurysmal vessels, males, unilateral.
Diabetic retinopathy: microaneurysms, dot-blot hemorrhages, concentrated in posterior pole.
Congenital retinal AV malformation.
Sickle cell retinopathy: peripheral nonperfusion, sea-fan NV, sickle preparation.
Presumed acquired retinal hemangioma.

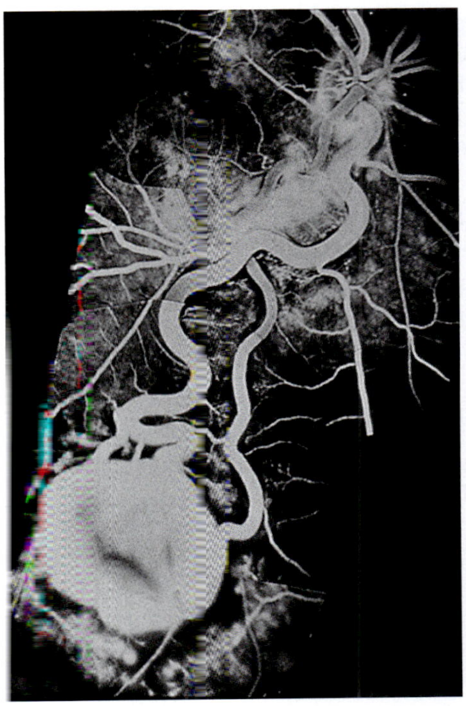

FIGURE 3.37. IVFA demonstrating hyperfluorescence of the angioma.

Reference

Hardwig P, Robertson DM. von Hippel-Lindau disease: a familial, often lethal, multisystem phakomatosis. *Ophthalmology* 1984; 91:263–270.

Wyburn-Mason Disease

Summary

Wyburn-Mason disease is a rare ocular cephalic syndrome in which abnormal retinal AV anastomoses are associated with arteriovenous malformations (AVMs) in the ipsilateral midbrain region.

Etiology

Unknown.

Signs and Symptoms

Mild proptosis.
Poor vision.

Demographics

Sporadic occurrence.

Ophthalmic Findings

See Figure 3.38.

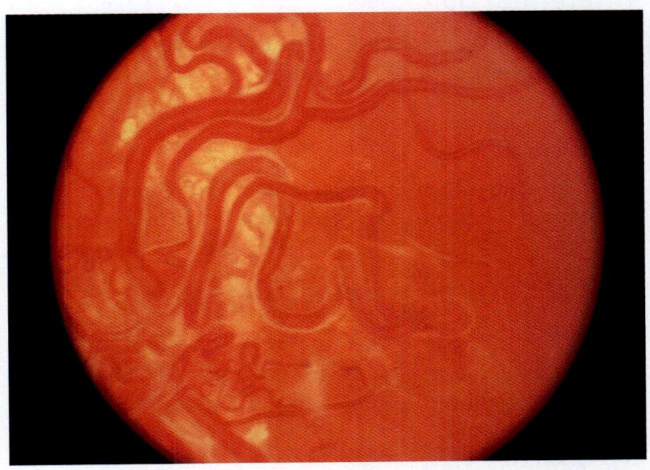

FIGURE 3.38. Racemose angioma with markedly dilated, tortuous anomalous vessels.

- Racemose lesions in the retina, which may also involve the optic nerve, chiasm, tract.
- Usually unilateral.

Systemic Findings

Ipsilateral AVMs of the brain, face, or orbit.
Cranial-nerve palsies.
Visual-field abnormalities.

Special Tests

IVFA: retinal AVM without leakage.
Magnetic resonance imaging (MRI), cerebral angiogram: CNS AVMs commonly involving the midbrain.

Pathology

- Anomalous vessels of the retina with some protruding into the vitreous.
- Thinning and thickening of vessel walls with fibromuscular medial coats of variable thickness and fibrohyalin adventitial layers.

Disease Course and Natural Progression

Usually stationary; however, can rarely cause exudation if the lesion is large.

Treatment and Management

Rarely necessary; cerebral angiography and MRI should be performed to rule out intracranial AVM.

Medications

None.

Follow-Up

Variable.

Differential Diagnosis

VHL: Exudation and exudative RD are more common, autosomal dominant in inheritance.

Reference

Archer DB, Duteman A, Ernest JT, et al. Arteriovenous communications of the retina. *Am J Ophthalmol* 1973;75:224–241.

Retinal Cavernous Hemangioma

Summary

Cavernous hemangioma is a rare vascular hamartoma composed of clumps of dark intraretinal aneurysms.

Etiology

Unknown.

Signs and Symptoms

Asymptomatic.
Unilateral.
Ten percent are symptomatic when the lesion is located near or in the macula.

Demographics

Questionable autosomal dominant with incomplete penetrance versus variable expression.

Ophthalmic Findings

- Clumps of intraretinal aneurysms, "clusters of grapes."
- Layering of red blood cells in aneurysms, "pseudohypopyon."
- Fibroglial membrane on surface.
- VH.
- Subretinal, intraretinal, preretinal hemorrhages.

Systemic Findings

May have skin or CNS hemangiomas.

Special Tests

IVFA: Aneurysms fill slowly and incompletely; fluorescein collects in the superior portion of the aneurysm with blood blocking fluorescein inferiorly.
Ultrasound: A scan: high internal reflectivity. B scan: irregular surface, large internal acoustic density, absence of choroidal excavation.

Pathology

- Multiple endothelial-lined aneurysms separated by thin fibrous septa.
- No intraretinal or subretinal exudate is found.
- Preretinal membrane can overlie the tumor that contains fibrous astrocytes with cytoplasmic filaments.

Disease Course and Natural Progression

- Usually stationary; however, visual loss may occur from growth of epiretinal membrane.
- VH is the most common cause of vision loss.

Treatment and Management

Rarely necessary; however, photocoagulation or cryotherapy if VH is present.

Medications

None.

Follow-Up

Variable.

Differential Diagnosis

Coats disease: exudative RD.
Leber miliary aneurysms: progressive course.
BRVO: telangiectatic vessels, microaneurysms, exudate.
Capillary hemangioma: feeder vessels, exudate, autosomal dominant inheritance.
Racemose hemangioma: dilation of larger vessels, AV anastomoses.
Diabetic retinopathy: microaneurysms, dot-blot hemorrhages, lipid, exudate, cotton-wool spots, NV.

Reference

Gass JDM. Cavernous hemangioma of the retina: a neuro-oculocutaneous syndrome. *Am J Ophthalmol* 1971;71:799–814.

Anemia

Summary

Anemia is a condition of decreased number of normal red blood cells or a reduction of normal hemoglobin that leads to ischemia of the retina and other tissues.

Etiology

Decreased oxygen delivery to the retina.

Signs and Symptoms

Asymptomatic.
Decreased vision.
Floaters.

Demographics

Patients with leukemia, multiple myeloma, Waldenstrom macroglobulinemia, lymphoma, or various chronic diseases can manifest anemia.

Ophthalmic Findings

Superficial flame-shaped hemorrhages.
Cotton-wool spots.
Microaneurysms.
White-centered hemorrhages (Roth spot).
Hard exudates with macular edema
Mild dilation of the arteries and veins.
Arteriolar sheathing in patients with chronic leukemia.
Exudative RD and necrotizing retinitis in patients with Hodgkin disease.
NV.

Systemic Findings

Anemia.
Painless lymph node enlargement.
Reed-Sternberg cells in patients with Hodgkin lymphoma.

Special Tests

IVFA: Capillary nonperfusion, capillary dilation, leakage.
Vitreous cytology for lymphoma cells.
Bone marrow biopsy.
Peripheral smear.
Serum protein electrophoresis (SPEP) to demonstrate plasmacytoma.

Pathology

Hemorrhages, accumulation of axoplasmic debris (cotton-wool spots, capillary occlusion, microaneurysms).

Disease Course and Natural Progression

Ischemia as evidenced by microaneurysms, hard exudate, dilated capillaries, hemorrhages, and arteriolar sheathing may lead to visual loss.

Treatment and Management

Treatment of the underlying condition and anemia.

Medications

Variable depending on condition.

Follow-Up

Medical evaluation is the mainstay of management.

Differential Diagnosis

Hypertensive retinopathy: AV nicking, disk edema.
Diabetic retinopathy: Elevated hemoglobin A1c or abnormal glucose tolerance test. Dot-blot hemorrhages, NV of disk, neovascularization of iris.
Endocarditis: blood cultures, echocardiogram.
Collagen vascular disease: Polyarteritis Nodosum, Wegener Granulomatosis, Systemic Lupus Erythematosus, Rheumatoid Arthritis: history of arthritis, skin rashes or evidence of systemic vasculitis, abnormal laboratory test results: ANA, c-ANCA, anti-ssA, anti-ssB, anti-dsDNA, rheumatoid factor.
Radiation retinopathy: history of radiation treatment, microaneurysms.
Sickle cell retinopathy: peripheral nonperfusion, sea-fan NV.

Reference

Kincaid MC, Green WR. Ocular and orbital involvement in leukemia. *Surv Ophthalmol* 1983;27:211–232.

Hyperviscocity

Summary

Increased blood viscosity causes accumulation of blood products and cells leading to vascular occlusion.

Etiology

Leukemia.
Lymphoma.
Waldenstrom macroglobulinemia.
Polycythemia vera.
Multiple myeloma.

Signs and Symptoms

Asymptomatic; patients with lymphoma may have bleeding diatheses and organomegaly.

Demographics

- Seventy-five percent of chronic leukemias have intraocular involvement.
- Eighty-two percent of acute leukemias have intraocular involvement.

Ophthalmic Findings

White-centered hemorrhages.
Choroidal infiltrates.
Serous RDs.
Hemorrhages in all retinal layers.
Cotton-wool spots.
Venous occlusion.
Microaneurysms.
NV (chronic myelogenous leukemias).
Venous dilation.
Papilledema (polycythemia vera).
Pars plana cysts (multiple myeloma).
Sea-fan NV may be present.

Systemic Findings

- CNS leukemia.
- Acute leukemia patients may have bleeding diatheses and infections.
- Vague symptoms in patients with chronic leukemias.
- Increased immunoglobulin M (IgM) fraction of plasma proteins in patients with Waldenstrom macroglobulinemia.

Special Tests

Bone marrow biopsy.
Peripheral blood smear.
Cytologic examination of the vitreous (reticulum cell carcinoma).
SPEP.

Pathology

- Hemorrhages, neurofibrillar infarcts, venous occlusions, leukemic cells.
- Neoplastic infiltrates of the retina and optic nerve in lymphoma.
- Low platelet counts are associated with intraretinal hemorrhages.

Disease Course and Natural Progression

Hyperviscosity leads to venous occlusion, microaneurysms, hemorrhages, and peripheral nonperfusion, which stimulates the development of NV.

Treatment and Management

- Chemotherapy, radiation therapy for leukemia.
- Leukopheresis for hyperleukocytic retinopathy.
- Plasmapheresis for Waldenstrom macroglobulinemia.

Medications

Medical management by a hematologist/oncologist is required.

Follow-Up

Medical evaluation and treatment are most important.

Differential Diagnosis

CRVO: unilateral flame-shaped hemorrhages, venous dilation, tortuosity.
Sickle cell retinopathy: abnormal sickle preparation, hemoglobin electrophoresis, sea-fan NV, peripheral nonperfusion.
Diabetic retinopathy: dot-blot hemorrhages, NV, abnormal glucose tolerance test result, elevated hemoglobin A1c.
Hypertensive retinopathy: AV nicking, elevated blood pressure.
Collagen vascular disease: Polyarteritis Nodosum, Wegener Granulomatosis, Systemic Lupus Erythematosus, Rheumatoid Arthritis: history of arthritis, skin rashes or evidence of systemic vasculitis, abnormal laboratory test results: ANA, c-ANCA, anti-ssA, anti-ssB, anti-dsDNA, rheumatoid factor.

Reference

Carr RE, Henkind P. Retinal findings associated with serum hyperviscosity. *Am J Ophthalmol* 1963;56:23–31.

INFLAMMATION

Toxoplasmosis

Summary

Worldwide cat-transmitted parasitic zoonosis ranging from life-threatening congenital infection to flulike acquired infection; retinochoroiditis is generally self-limited but may be recurrent, and vision loss is dependent on extent and area of involvement.

Etiology

- *Toxoplasma gondii*, an obligate intracellular parasite, exists as trophozoite, bradyzoite, or sporozoite; sporozoites (oocysts) are produced within the cat host by both asexual and sexual reproduction and shed by the millions in feces.
- Oocysts in contaminated meat, poultry, eggs, or dirt are ingested by humans leading to proliferation of the invasive tachyzoite and its destructive inflammatory sequelae
- Tachyzoite invasion of the retina leads to retinitis until the host immune response quells the infection and the parasite is encysted.

Signs and Symptoms

Unilateral floaters.
Metamorphopsia.
Decreased vision.
Ocular pain and redness.
Flulike symptoms in acquired infection.
Congenital infection: triad of convulsions, cerebral calcifications, and retinochoroiditis; also can have hydrocephalus, mental retardation, jaundice, rash, and fever.

Demographics

- Twenty to seventy percent of persons in the United States have positive titers for toxoplasma. Antibody positivity increases with age.
- Unclear if majority of cases represent reactivation of congenital infection or if they are acquired.
- Maternal infection before or during gestation leads to fetal transmission, with severe consequences in first trimester but highest transmission (40%) within the third trimester; bilateral congenital retinochoroiditis occurs in nearly 80% of patients.
- More common and virulent in immunocompromised individuals.

Ophthalmic Findings

Fine stellate endothelial keratic precipitates.
Granulomatous anterior chamber inflammatory reaction.
Cataract.
Moderate-to-severe vitritis, "headlight in fog"; precipitates on posterior hyaloid face (Figure 3.39).
Single or multiple patches of necrotizing retinitis, often adjacent to preexisting chorioretinal scar.
Optic neuritis.
CME.
Retinal vasculitis.
Papillitis.
BRVO in areas of retinitis.
Scleritis (rarely).

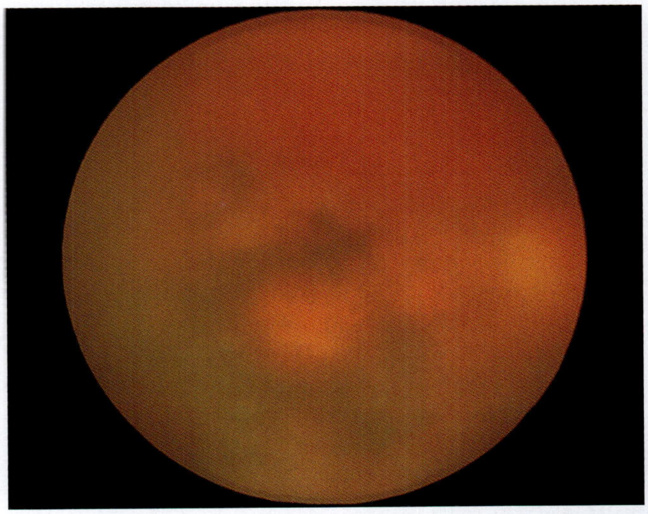

FIGURE 3.39. Acute toxoplasma retinochoroiditis with dense vitritis.

Systemic Findings

Acquired infection: See above.
Congenital infection: See above.

Special Tests

Toxoplasma immunoglobulin G (IgG) and IgM titers.
Sabin-Feldman dye test: tests ability of serum antibody to fix complement and lyse cells.
Enzyme-linked immunosorbent assay (ELISA) or indirect fluorescent antibody test.
Polymerase chain reaction (PCR) of vitreous specimen.
Other tests: FTA-Abs, purified protein derivative (PPD), ELISA for *Toxocara* organisms.

Pathology

- Retinal necrosis with mononuclear cellular infiltrate; adjacent choroidal necrosis may be seen.
- Scars bordering areas of active infection common; cysts or tachyzoites may be identified in or near affected retina.

Disease Course

- Reactivated retinitis has course of weeks to months, resolving spontaneously.
- Before resolution, necrotizing macular retinitis may cause permanent visual loss.
- Multidrug treatment of active retinitis or papillitis limits spread of infection and may prevent severe visual loss.
- Approximately 80% of patients will have recurrence within 5 years.

Treatment and Management

Medical treatment of macular-threatening lesions or cases with significant visual loss due to vitritis.

Medications

Triple therapy:

Sulfadiazine: 2 g by mouth (p.o.) × 1, then 1 g q.i.d. with high fluid intake.
Pyrimethamine (Daraprim): 50 mg p.o. Q12 × 2, then 25 mg b.i.d.
Folinic acid (leucovorin): 3 to 5 mg p.o. twice weekly.
Clindamycin, azithromycin, clarithromycin, spiramycin, minocycline, atovaquone, and trimethoprim/sulfamethoxazole are alternative/adjuvant therapies.
Prednisone: 20 to 80 mg p.o. daily can be added to reduce inflammation, only after beginning antibiotics
Infected pregnant women: sulfadiazine, clindamycin, or spiramycin.

Follow-Up

- Weekly; observe for complications of medical treatment (pseudomembranous colitis, bone marrow suppression, steroid effects).
- Biweekly complete blood cell count (CBC).

Differential Diagnosis

Syphilis.
Sarcoidosis.
Tuberculous chorioretinitis.
CMV retinitis.
Acute retinal necrosis/Progressive outer retinal necrosis (PORN).
Ocular toxocara.
Intraocular Lymphoma.
Optic neuritis.
Retinoblastoma.

Reference

Engstrom RE Jr, Holland GN, Nussenblatt RB, et al. Current practices in the management of ocular toxoplasmosis. *Am J Ophthalmol* 1991;111:601–610.

Sarcoidosis

Summary

Sarcoidosis is a multisystem, granulomatous disorder of unknown etiology with ocular involvement occurring in 15% to 25% of patients.

Etiology

Unknown.

Signs and Symptoms

Pain.
Photophobia.
Blurred vision.
Floaters.
Red Eyes.

Demographics

- Most often affects adults younger than 40 years of age.
- Increased incidence in African Americans and native Scandinavians.
- Slight female predilection.

Ophthalmic Findings

- Chronic granulomatous or nongranulomatous anterior uveitis (two third of patients).
- Mutton fat keratic precipitates.
- Koeppe and Busacca iris nodules.

Posterior involvement in 20% to 30% of patients includes the following:

- Vitritis with white cell clumping (“snowballs”).
- Exudates and sheathing along peripheral retinal vasculature (“candle-wax drippings”).
- Chorioretinal granulomas.
  CME.
  Optic nerve granulomas, disk edema.
- Occlusive retinal vasculitis with retinal NV.

Other ocular findings:

- Lacrimal infiltration with keratitis sicca.
- Extraocular muscle infiltration with motility restriction and proptosis.
- Conjunctival granulomas.
- Orbital inflammation.

Systemic Findings

- May affect lungs, musculoskeletal system, nervous system, skin, spleen, bones, CNS.
- Ninety percent with intrathoracic involvement ranging from hilar lymphadenopathy to diffuse pulmonary infiltration with fibrosis.

Special Tests

- Abnormal CXR with evidence of hilar lymphadenopathy.
- Biopsy of skin, palpable lymph nodes, lung, liver, and conjunctiva showing noncaseating granulomas is usually required for diagnosis.
- ACE detects total body granuloma content but is nonspecific.
- Gallium scan of head, neck, and mediastinum for foci of uptake.
- Serum lysozyme, SPEP, and serum calcium.
- Kveim skin test (nodule induction using a suspension of human sarcoid tissue) is no longer used.

Pathology

Characteristic noncaseating granuloma composed of epithelioid cells and multinucleated giant cells, often surrounded by a thin, incomplete rim of lymphocytes.

Disease Course

- Three characteristic courses (monophasic, relapsing, or chronic) associated with progressively worsening visual prognosis.
- Visual loss often associated with vascular occlusion, retinal NV, macular involvement, or optic nerve lesions.
- Secondary glaucoma is a poor prognostic sign.

Treatment and Management

- Steroids (topical, depot, systemic) depending on degree of inflammation and response to previous treatment.
- Cycloplegics for comfort and prevention of synechiae.
- Treatment for glaucoma depends on etiology (inflammatory, steroid induced, angle closure, or neovascular).
- Steroid-sparing agents required in those with chronic progressive disease especially with posterior involvement.

Medications

Topical steroids.
Periocular steroids.
Systemic steroids for posterior involvement or severe anterior uveitis.
Cycloplegic agents.
Steroid-sparing agents including methotrexate, cyclosporine, azathioprine, mycophenolate mofetil in those with chronic disease.

Follow-Up

- One to two times per week during acute episodes with cycloplegic and steroid taper as inflammation resolves.
- Closely follow IOP and fundus findings.
- Asymptomatic adults should be seen every 6 months.
- Asymptomatic children should be seen every 3 months.

Differential Diagnosis (Entities and Distinguishing Features)

Tuberculosis: positive PPD, abnormal CXR, acid-fast bacilli on sputum sample or bronchial washing.
Syphilis: positive FTA-Abs or RPR test result.
Idiopathic pars planitis: vitreous opacification with exudate at ora serrata; less significant anterior segment findings. Negative systemic workup and negative review of systems.
Vogt-Koyanagi-Harada disease—poliosis, vitiligo, headaches, exudative RD, pigmentary changes, negative CXR, negative laboratory findings.

Reference

Karma A, Huhti E, Poukkula A. Course and outcome of ocular sarcoidosis. *Am J Ophthalmol* 1988;106:467–472.

Birdshot Retinochoroidopathy

Summary

Birdshot retinochoroidopathy is an ocular inflammatory disease characterized by multiple, bilateral, often symmetric foci of hypopigmentation at the level of the choroid.

Etiology

Possible genetic predisposition in HLA-A29 patients.

Signs and Symptoms

Blurred vision.
Floaters.
Nyctalopia.
Dyschromotopsia.

Demographics

Occurs in third to sixth decade, average age of 50.
Men and women equally affected.
Strong association with HLA-A29 antigen.

Ophthalmic Findings

See Figure 3.40.

- Discrete, creamy, oval, hypopigmented spots less than 0.5 mm in diameter at the level of choroid that are located predominantly posteriorly and nasally.
- Vitreous inflammation varies from mild to severe. Mild anterior segment inflammation.

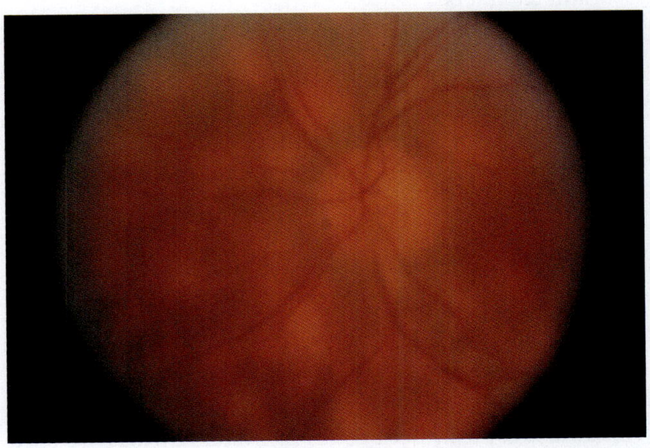

FIGURE 3.40. Birdshot retinochoroidopathy with multiple small yellow choroidal lesions and a mild vitritis.

- May have attenuation of retinal vasculature with inflammatory sheathing.
  - CME.
  - Epiretinal membrane.
  - CNVM.
- Disk edema or atrophy may be present.

Systemic Findings

None.

Special Tests

- IVFA:
  Choroidal spots show early hypofluorescence with subtle hyperfluorescence in later stages.
  Retinal vascular leakage can be significant on angiography.
  Cystoid macular leakage.
  Late leakage from optic disk.
  ICG angiography.
  Birdshot lesions appear dark and hypofluorescent.
- ERG: reduced amplitude and increased latency of the b wave.
- HLA-A29 antigen associated with 96% sensitivity and 93% specificity (incidence in normal population is 7%).

Pathology

Unknown. Pathology of patients reveals lymphoid infiltrate in middle layers of choroid with similar infiltrate around retina vessels.

Disease Course

- Chronic disease, characterized by numerous exacerbations and remissions.
- Fifty percent of patients maintain acuity of 20/60 or better after 5 years.
- Visual loss usually due to CME.
  Vision loss also occurs secondary to optic atrophy, macular pigmentary changes, CNV, epiretinal membrane and cataracts.

Treatment and Management

- CME often is often steroid responsive but may require chronic immunosuppressive therapy.
- Vision loss can also occur in those without macular edema.
  Serial visual fields and ERGs are needed to follow patients.
- Vision loss from macular edema, field loss on GVF testing or changes in ERG necessitate chronic immunosuppressive therapy.

Medications

- Steroids (topical, periocular, or systemic) may be used depending on the VA and the response to previous treatment.
- Immunosuppression (cyclosporine A, azathioprine, mycophenoloate mofetil) for those with chronic disease.

Follow-Up

- During acute exacerbations, patients are followed every 1 to 4 weeks.
- During quieter phases, patients may be seen every 3 to 6 months.

Differential Diagnosis (Entities and Distinguishing Features)

Pars planitis: vitritis with snowbanking and exudate along the ora serrata, negative HLA-A29.

Intraocular lymphoma: patients older than 50 years, negative HLA-A29, not responsive to steroid therapy, creamy elevated subretinal lesions.

Syphilis: positive FTA-Abs, negative HLA-A29.

Multiple evanescent white dot syndrome (MEWDS): unilateral, limited course following viral illness, negative HLA-A29.

Acute posterior multifocal placoid pigment epitheliopathy (APMPPE)—large plaque-like lesions, self-limiting with pigmentary changes. Negative HLA-A29.

Reference

Priem HA, Oosterhuis JA. Birdshot chorioretinopathy: clinical characteristics and evolution. *Br J Ophthalmol* 1988;72: 646–659.

Punctate Inner Choroidopathy

Summary

Multifocal choroidal lesions in young healthy myopic women.

Etiology

Unknown.

Signs and Symptoms

Diminished VA.
Central or paracentral scotomas.
Photopsias.

Demographics

- Affects young adults aged 16 to 40 years.
- Ninety percent of affected patients are women.
- Associated with myopia.

Ophthalmic Findings

- Two to six (although sometimes more) slightly fuzzy yellow lesions 100 to 300 μm in diameter located at the level of the RPE and inner choroid; clustered in the macula and the midperiphery.

- Collections of lesions can be associated with overlying subretinal fluid accumulations.
- RPE atrophy as lesions become more chronic. CNV can occur.
- No anterior segment or vitreous cells.

Systemic Findings

None.

Special Tests

- FA reveals late leakage from the RPE lesions correlating with the degree of overlying fluid.
- Central or paracentral scotoma by Amsler grid testing.

Pathology

N/A

Disease Course

- Acute fuzzy yellow lesions develop into deep cylindrical scars with overlying chorioretinal atrophy and progressive pigmentation.
- May be recurrent symptomatic episodes.
- Patients developing CNV or foveal RPE atrophy experience moderate visual loss.

Treatment and Management

- CNV can occur in many patients. Treatment varies on location from laser photocoagulation, PDT, and intravitreal anti-VEGF therapy.
- Steroids and immunosuppressive agents are used in some with chronic disease or progressive systems.

Medications

Steroids—can be used in acute phase or chronic phase when new symptoms occur. Also can be used in patients with CNV, though unknown how much benefit they provide.

Immunosuppressive therapy (cyclosporine, methotrexate, mycophenolate, azathioprine) can be used in those with chronic disease that appears progressive.

Follow-Up

Monthly.

Differential Diagnosis

- POHS: geographic exposure history, static appearance of histoplasmosis lesions.
- Multifocal choroiditis with panuveitis (MCP): may represent an alternative manifestation of the same disease but is differentiated by its relapsing nature in conjunction with ocular inflammation.
- Sarcoidosis: systemic findings, laboratory findings. Significant anterior segment and posterior segment inflammation.
- Birdshot choroidoretinopathy: characteristic cream colored lesions seen especially nasally. Vitreous inflammation, HLA-A29 positive.

Reference

Watzke RC, Packer AJ, Folk JC, et al. Punctate inner choroidopathy. *Am J Ophthalmol* 1984;98:572–584.

Acute Posterior Multifocal Placoid Pigment Epitheliopathy

Summary

APMPPE is characterized by multiple creamy plaques bilaterally, at the level of the RPE and the inner choroid.

Etiology

Pathogenesis is unclear, but APMPPE is thought to represent either an infectious (possibly viral) or an autoimmune choroidal vasculopathy with overlying RPE dysfunction and atrophy.

Signs and Symptoms

Diminished central and paracentral vision.
Visual scotomas.
Photopsias.

Demographics

Adolescents and young adults between the ages of 20 and 50 years.

Ophthalmic Findings

See Figure 3.41.

- Multiple, pale yellow, homogenous, round, discrete lesions at the level of the RPE and choriocapillaris.
- Lesions are usually less than 1 disk diameter in size.
- New lesions may develop up to 3 weeks after time of initial onset.
- Serous RDs, uveitis, retinal vasculitis, and episcleritis have all been described in association with an APMPPE-like presentation.
- CNV can occur in patients after resolution of disease.

Systemic Findings

- Antecedent flulike illness.
- Rarely associated with cerebral vasculitis, erythema nodosum, dysacusis, and tinnitus.

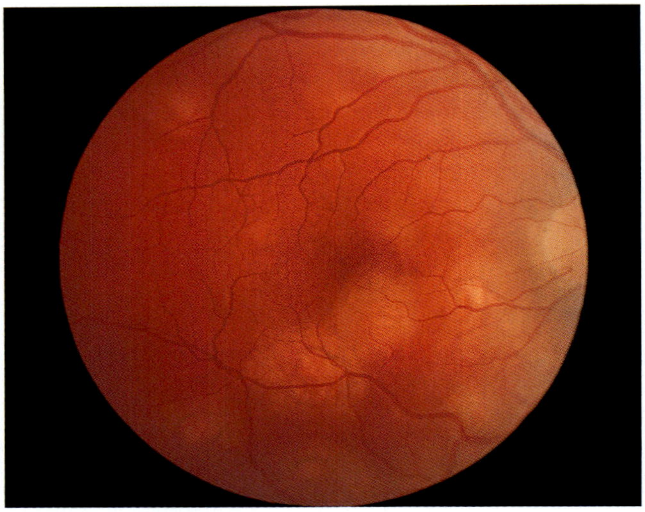

FIGURE 3.41. APMPPE with creamy infiltrates.

Special Tests

IVFA: demonstrates early hypofluorescence of the placoid lesions, with late hyperfluorescence (Figure 3.42). IVFA may also show delayed choroidal filling, with discrete lobular filling of the choriocapillaris.

Pathology

Pathology specimen from patient with associated cerebral vasculitis demonstrated choroidal vasculopathy in areas of involvement.

Disease Course

- Follows an acute course, usually without recurrence.

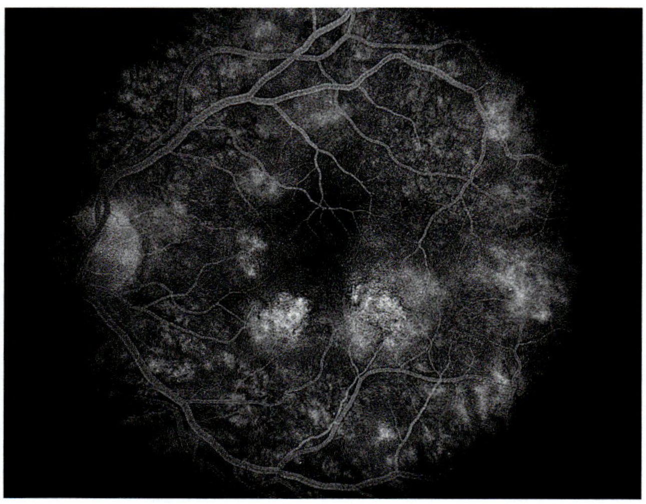

FIGURE 3.42. Late phase of intravenous fluorescein angiogram demonstrating focal areas of hyperfluorescence corresponding to placoid lesions in APMPPE.

- Most patients recover acuities of 20/40 or better as the lesions fade over 2 to 6 weeks.
- May develop sites of pigment clumping and depigmentation.
- Poorer visual prognosis with foveal involvement.
- Cerebral vasculitis can occur weeks to months after retinal involvement

Treatment and Management

No evidence that corticosteroids are of any benefit, although a short course of treatment has been proposed in patients with foveal involvement and profound visual loss.

Follow-Up

Observation for spontaneous resolution.

Differential Diagnosis

Serpiginous choroidopathy: progressive, insidious, helical shape of lesions.

Birdshot retinochoroiditis: creamy, subretinal lesions seen especially nasally. Significant vitreous inflammation and usually associated with HLA-A29.

Multifocal choroiditis: significant inflammation with multifocal lesion that variably hyperfluoresce on angiography. Usually progressive.

MEWDS: typically unilateral, affecting woman more than men with small lesions noted on exam.

References

Gass JDM. Acute posterior multifocal placoid pigment epitheliopathy. *Arch Ophthalmol* 1968;80:177–185.

Ryan SJ, Maumenee AE. Acute posterior multifocal placoid pigment epitheliopathy. *Am J Ophthalmol* 1972;74:1066–1074.

Serpiginous Choroidopathy (Geographic Helicoid Peripapillary Choroidopathy)

Summary

Serpiginous choroidopathy is chronic recurrent retinochoroiditis characterized by the helical shape of inflammation extending from the optic nerve, with adjacent atrophic scarring.

Etiology

Unknown.

Signs and Symptoms

Blurred vision.
Central or paracentral scotomas.
Photopsias.

Demographics

Ages 30 to 70 years.

Ophthalmic Findings

- Acute onset of pale yellow or gray subretinal inflammation and edema, usually bordering atrophic scar, and extending outward in a serpentine fashion from the optic nerve or the macula.
- Older lesions show scar and atrophy with adjacent pigment epithelial hyperplasia.
- Mild vitritis and/or anterior chamber inflammation.
- Vascular sheathing.
- Shallow RPE detachments.
- CNV may develop.

Systemic Findings

None.

Special Tests

IVFA: Active lesions block choroidal fluorescence but will show diffuse uptake in the later stages; inactive sites of RPE atrophy can show transmitted choroidal fluorescence or hypofluorescence depending on the degree of choriocapillaris disruption.

Amsler grid testing: may demonstrate scotoma corresponding to fundus lesions.

Pathology

- Acute lesions are thought to represent a multifocal, nongranulomatous inflammation affecting the inner choroid and the RPE.

Disease Course

- Progressive; recurrences may develop over months to years.
- Asymmetric involvement between eyes.
- CNVMs may develop at sites of older inflammation.

Treatment and Management

- Steroids in the treatment of acute lesions.
- Immunosuppressive therapy for those with chronic progressive disease.
- CNVMs treated with laser photocoagulation, PDT, or intravitreal anti-VEGF therapy.

Medications

Systemic corticosteroids or depot steroid injections may be of benefit in treatment of acute lesions.

Immunosuppressive agents usually started early in course due to progressive nature (drugs like cyclosporine, cyclophosphamide, azathioprine, mycophenoloate mofetil).

Use of systemic antivirals advocated by some, but unclear benefit.

Follow-Up

Careful follow-up is essential, especially during acute phases or after changes in Amsler grid testing, to rule out development of CNVMs.

Differential Diagnosis

Birdshot retinochoroiditis: creamy, subretinal lesions seen especially nasally. Significant vitreous inflammation and usually associated with HLA-A29.

Multifocal choroiditis: significant inflammation with multifocal lesion that variably hyperfluoresce on angiography. Usually progressive.

MEWDS: typically unilateral, affecting women more than men with small lesions noted on exam.

APMPPE—self-limited disease, sometimes can be difficult to differentiate due to similarities between diseases.

References

Chisholm IH, Gass JDM, Hutton WL. The late stage of serpiginous (geographic) choroiditis. *Am J Ophthalmol* 1976;82:343–351.

Wu JS, Lewis H, Fine SL, et al. Clinicopathologic findings in a patient with serpiginous choroiditis and treated choroidal neovascularization. *Retina* 1989;9:292–301.

Multifocal Choroiditis and Panuveitis

Summary

Multifocal choroiditis is an inflammatory disorder characterized by multiple, recurrent, circular, pale, subretinal inflammatory lesions causing visual loss.

Etiology

Unknown.

Signs and Symptoms

Decreased central vision (in most cases worse than 20/100).
Metamorphopsia.
Scotomas.
Floaters.
Photopsias.
Pain.
Photophobia.

Demographics

Usually affects young women but can occur in any age group.

May be an association with myopia.

Ophthalmic Findings

- Multiple, round, small, yellow-gray inflammatory lesions, distributed from the posterior pole to the midperiphery, at the level of the RPE and choriocapillaris. Lesions usually seen in the peripapillary area and midperiphery.

RETINA

- Anterior segment inflammation can be seen, but usually vitreous cells are noted.
- Disk edema possible, with progression to peripapillary atrophy.
- CNVMs develop in more than 25% of patients.

Systemic Findings

None.

Special Tests

- IVFA: Acute lesions demonstrate early hyperfluorescence with late leakage; older lesions may show early hyperfluorescence with fading in the later phases.
- Visual-field testing may show an enlarged blind spot or a scotoma corresponding to chorioretinal lesions.
- Subnormal ERGs may be seen.

Pathology

Unknown.

Disease Course

- MCP is a chronic, recurrent disorder lasting months to years with new lesions developing in one or both eyes, without regard to location of previous lesions.
- Lesions may become atrophic with RPE changes and subretinal fibrosis.
- One third of patients may develop macular and peripapillary CNVMs.
- Fifty percent of patients, vision remains worse than 20/200 in the more severely affected eye.

Treatment and Management

- Steroids indicated for patients with CME, severe vitreous inflammation, extensive choroiditis, and subretinal NV.
- CNVMs treated with laser photocoagulation, PDT, or intravitreal anti-VEGF therapy.
- Chronic immunosuppressive therapy indicated for patients with chronic disease.

Medications

- Steroids—usually oral therapy.
- Immunosuppressive therapy (cyclosporine, methotrexate, mycophenoalate, azathioprine) can be used in those with chronic disease that appears progressive.

Follow-Up

- Careful follow-up for development of CNVMs.
- Amsler grid testing.

Differential Diagnosis

MEWDS: Typical lesions are intraretinal and quickly fade without recurrences.

POHS: Lesions can look similar, but not accompanied by vitritis, anterior segment inflammation, or ERG changes. Usually has history of living in endemic areas

Birdshot choroidopathy: lesions usually associated with retinal vascular inflammation. HLA-A29 positive.

Sarcoidosis: characteristic CXR findings, elevated ACE, noncaseating granuloma on biopsy.

Punctate inner choroidopathy—typically myopic women. Lesions concentrated in posterior pole without any inflammation

References

Dreyer RF, Gass JDM. Multifocal choroiditis and panuveitis: a syndrome that mimics ocular histoplasmosis. *Arch Ophthalmol* 1984;102:1776–1784.

Morgan CM, Schatz H. Recurrent multifocal choroiditis. *Ophthalmology* 1986;93:1138–1147.

Multiple Evanescent White Dot Syndrome

Summary

MEWDS is a rare, self-limited disease of acute, usually unilateral visual loss, often following viral illness in young women, characterized by multiple small lesions at the level of the RPE.

Etiology

Unknown.

Signs and Symptoms

Blurred vision.
Photopsias.
Scotomas.
Enlargement of blind spot.

Demographics

Young adults.
Seventy-five percent of patients are women.

Ophthalmic Findings

- Multiple granular white dots at the level of the RPE that tend to concentrate in the macula but spare the fovea. Typically does not extend beyond arcades.
- Mild retinal vessel sheathing and blurred disk margins can be seen.
- Low-grade vitreous reaction may also be seen.

Systemic Findings

None.

Special Tests

- Visual field testing may show an enlarged blind spot.

- IVFA: The acute RPE lesions show early and late hyperfluorescence, with late staining and disk leakage.
- ERG may be severely diminished.

Pathology

Unknown.

Disease Course

- Acuity returns to normal within weeks.
- A chronic bilateral form of MEWDS with multiple recurrences has been described.
- Rarely, late CNVMs may be seen.

Treatment and Management

None.

Medications

None.

Follow-Up

Biweekly if diagnosis uncertain.

Differential Diagnosis

Acute multifocal placoid pigment epitheliopathy (AMPPE): bilateral with significant pigmentary changes and early hypofluorescence on FA.

Acute retinal pigment epitheliitis: associated with hyperpigmented lesions that exhibit central hypofluorescence with a rim of hyperfluorescence by FA; no ERG changes.

Birdshot retinochoroiditis: creamy, subretinal lesions seen especially nasally. Significant vitreous inflammation and usually associated with HLA-A29.

Multifocal choroiditis: significant inflammation with multifocal lesion that variably hyperfluoresce on angiography. Usually progressive.

Sarcoidosis: abnormal CXR and other systemic findings in conjunction with a granulomatous uveitis.

Acute idiopathic blind-spot enlargement: no visible retinal lesions.

Reference

Jampol LM, Sieving PA, Pugh D, et al. Multiple evanescent white dot syndrome, I: clinical findings. *Arch Ophthalmol* 1984; 102:671–674.

Sympathetic Ophthalmia

See p. 204.

Vogt-Koyanagi-Harada Syndrome

Summary

Bilateral diffuse granulomatous uveitis associated with leptomeningitis and dermatologic changes.

Etiology

Inflammation of melanin-containing cells of the uvea, leptomeninges of the inner ear, and dermal melanocytes.

Signs and Symptoms

Ocular pain.
Blurry vision.
Headaches.
Dysacusis/tinnitus.
Alopecia, poliosis, or vitiligo.

Demographics

- Asian, Hispanic, or Native American ancestry.
- Female patients more likely to be affected than male patients.
- Age of onset, 20 to 50 years.
- Eighty-eight percent of cases bilateral.

Ophthalmic Findings

Anterior segment involvement in 90% of eyes:

Iridocyclitis.
Keratic precipitates.
Cataracts.
Posterior and anterior synechiae.
Iris nodules.
Glaucoma.
Keratitis, scleritis.
Perilimbal vitiligo.
Posterior segment involvement in 90% eyes:
Vitritis.
Choroiditis manifesting as either serous RDs or focal areas of subretinal fluid.
Dalen-Fuchs nodules.
Hyperemia of optic disk.
Those with chronic disease may have ocular depigmentation (sunset glow fundus) or RPE migration.

Systemic Findings

Integumentary (does not precede onset of CNS or ocular disease).
Alopecia (hair loss).
Poliosis (loss of color from hair).
Vitiligo (amelanotic patches of skin).
Neurological/auditory findings (may have resolved by the time of ocular findings).
Meningismus (malaise, fever, headache, abdominal pain, stiffness of neck/back).
Tinnitus.
Cerebral spinal fluid pleocytosis.
Complete VKH disease occurs when bilateral ocular involvement as noted above occurs with both integumentary and neurological findings.

RETINA

Incomplete VKH occurs if bilateral ocular involvement occurs with either integumentary or neurological findings.

Probably VKH occurs if only bilateral ocular findings are found.

In all cases, there should not be a history of penetrating ocular injury or surgery preceding initial onset of uveitis and no clinical or laboratory findings of other ocular diseases.

Special Tests

- IVFA: early patchy filling of choroid with punctate spots of hyperfluorescence; later dye leakage, especially underlying serous RDs.
- B-scan ultrasonography: demonstrates choroidal thickening, posterior scleritis, multiple sites of serous RD.
- Lumbar puncture rarely needed to confirm diagnosis as diagnosis is typically clinical.
- ICG angiography reveals multiple hypofluorescent spots and pinpoint hyperfluorescent spots in areas of exudative RD.
- Strong association of HLA-DR4 and Japanese patients. HLA DR1 and DR4 seen in some Hispanic populations.

Pathology

- Nonnecrotizing diffuse granulomatous inflammation throughout the uvea.
- Choriocapillaris and retina destroyed by inflammatory nodules.
- Dalen-Fuchs nodules noted (focal aggregations of epithelioid cells between the retina and Bruch membrane).
- Skin shows lack of melanocytes in depigmented patches with lymphocytes at margins.

Disease Course

- Prodromal stage: headaches, meningitic symptoms, orbital pain, cranial-nerve palsies. Last only for a few days.
- Uveitic stage: bilateral panuveitis with typically serous RDs.
- Chronic or convalescent stage: depigmentation of choroid (sunset glow fundus), perilimbal vitiligo (Sugiura sign), chorioretinal pigmentary changes, dermatologic changes.
- Recurrent stage: sequelae of chronic uveitis.
- Successful taper-off of steroids may take as long as 6 months.
- Forty percent of patients retain acuities of 20/30 or better; approximately 40% of patients have vision worse than 20/200.

Treatment and Management

Systemic steroid treatment.

Chronic immunosuppressive therapy needed in majority of patients.

Medications

Systemic corticosteroids.

Topical and periocular steroids.

Immunosuppressive therapy (cyclosporine, methotrexate, mycophenoalate, azathioprine) can be used in those with chronic disease that appears progressive.

Follow-Up: twice weekly at first and then biweekly. Watch for development of steroid-induced glaucoma.

Differential Diagnosis

Sympathetic ophthalmia: associated with eye trauma or eye surgery

Primary intraocular lymphoma.

Uveal effusion syndrome—no intraocular inflammation seen.

Posterior scleritis—systemic symptoms not seen, anterior segment inflammation not found.

Sarcoidosis—abnormal appearance on CXR, abnormal lab findings.

APMPPE: lacks vitritis and anterior segment involvement; skin normal.

MEWDS: unilateral, posterior, self-limited.

References

Moorthy RS, Inomata H, Rao NA. Vogt-Koyanagi-Harada syndrome. *Surv Ophthalmol* 1995;39:265–292.

Rubsamen PE, Gass JD. Vogt-Koyanagi-Harada syndrome: clinical course, therapy, and long-term visual outcome. *Arch Ophthalmol* 1991;109:682–687.

Whipple Disease

Summary

Whipple disease is a rare multisystem disorder characterized by intestinal malabsorption and arthralgias, in conjunction with pars planitis, vitritis, retinal exudate, and hemorrhage.

Etiology

Infection with *Tropheryma whippleii*, a Gram-negative actinomycete.

Signs and Symptoms

Diarrhea and weight loss.

Arthralgias.

Fever.

Diffuse lymphadenopathy.

Cutaneous hyperpigmentation.

Nonspecific CNS changes.

Demographics

Occurs mostly in middle-aged white men.

Ophthalmic Findings

Vitreous opacification with peripheral exudate overlying the pars plana.

Retinal hemorrhage and exudate.
Cotton-wool spots.
Chorioretinitis.
Disk edema.
Retinal vasculitis.

Systemic Findings

Steatorrhea.
Lymphadenopathy.
Hyperpigmentation of the skin.
Heart murmur.
Nonspecific neurologic findings ranging from dementia to seizures.

Special Tests

- Intestinal biopsy (jejunum) revealing foamy macrophages containing periodic acid–Schiff (PAS)–positive granules.
- PCR has been used to identify the organism in vitreous aspirates.

Pathology

Foamy macrophages containing PAS-positive intercellular granules may be seen in multiple organs including the eye.

Disease Course

- Systemic findings are migratory and transient.
- Remission of symptoms and reduction of PAS-laden macrophages with antibiotics.

Treatment and Management

Long-term antibiotic therapy.

Medications

- Oral penicillin, tetracycline, or erythromycin for 1 year.
- Trimethoprim-sulfamethoxazole may be needed for CNS involvement.

Follow-Up

Weekly.

Differential Diagnosis (Entities and Distinguishing Features)

Intraocular lymphoma.
Behçet disease.
Sarcoidosis.

References

Avila MP, Jalkh AE, Feldman E, et al. Manifestations of Whipple's disease in the posterior segment of the eye. *Arch Ophthalmol* 1984;102:384–390.

Relman DA, Schmidt TM, MacDermott RP, et al. Identification of the uncultured bacillus of Whipple's disease. *N Engl J Med* 1992;327:293–301.

Acquired Immunodeficiency Syndrome

Summary

AIDS is a severe multisystem disease affecting persons with the human immunodeficiency virus. It is characterized by opportunistic infections.

Etiology

- AIDS is caused by HIV, a retrovirus that targets CD4 helper T cells and macrophages leading to immune deficiency with subsequent opportunistic infections and characteristic neoplasms.
- HIV retinopathy is thought to be a multifactorial process mediated by both hematologic disturbances and endothelial cell infection, with a progressive microvasculopathy.

Signs and Symptoms

Noninfectious retinopathy is asymptomatic.
Floaters.
Photopsias.
Blurred vision.
Visual-field defects.

Demographics

Incidence increased in high-risk groups such as homosexual men, people with multiple sexual partners, intravenous drug abusers, blood transfusion recipients, and infants born to mothers with AIDS.

Ophthalmic Findings

- Ocular findings may be seen in up to 70% of HIV-positive patients and may be the first manifestation of disseminated infection.
- HIV (noninfectious) retinopathy is the most common finding and is characterized by cotton-wool spots, microaneurysms, and hemorrhage in both the nerve-fiber layer and the inner retina; there is no associated inflammation or vitreous reaction.
- Herpes zoster ophthalmicus.
- Molluscum contagiosum.
- CMV retinitis.
- Toxoplasmosis.
- Syphilis.
- Herpes-associated retinitis (PORN/acute retinal necrosis).
- Kaposi sarcoma nodules.
- Candidal and other fungal retinitis.
- *Pneumocystis carinii* choroidopathy.
- Mycobacterial infection.

Systemic Findings

- Systemic opportunistic infections, especially *P. carinii* pneumonia, CMV colitis, mycobacterium avium intracellulare, toxoplasmosis, coccidioidomycosis.
- Lymphoma.
- Kaposi sarcoma.
- Cachexia.

Natural History

- Acute primary flulike infection following initial exposure.
- Asymptomatic period ranging from 2 to 10 years, characterized by generalized lymphadenopathy and slowly declining helper T cells.
- AIDS: symptomatic disease marked by opportunistic infection and malignancies.
- Fatigue, malaise, fever, chills, sweats, diarrhea, lymphadenopathy, and weight loss are nonspecific findings of disease progression.

Special Tests

- ELISA for HIV antibody is sensitive but not specific; Western blot following a positive ELISA to screen out false-positive results.
- IVFA: Noninfectious retinopathy is characterized by microvascular changes including microaneurysm formation, telangectasia, and capillary nonperfusion.

Pathology

- Cotton-wool spots, the most common ocular lesions in HIV, are identical to cotton-wool spots seen in other diseases and consist of multiple swollen, interrupted axons known as *cytoid bodies*.
- Microvascular changes are manifested by PAS-positive capillary-wall thickening.

Disease Course

- Most cotton-wool spots regress in 6 to 12 weeks, but progressive nerve-fiber layer infarction may lead to diminished contrast sensitivity and color vision.

Treatment and Management

- AIDS is managed by combinations of antiretroviral agents with adjunctive treatment and prophylaxis for opportunistic infections and should be handled by an internist familiar with the most current regimens.
- Infectious retinopathy is treated according to the particular inciting agent.

Medications

Multiple combinations of anti-HIV agents are commonly used.

Follow-Up

Patients with AIDS should have funduscopic examination every 3 to 4 months to evaluate for CMV retinitis and other opportunistic infectious retinopathies.

Differential Diagnosis

- The cotton-wool spots, microaneurysms, and hemorrhages of HIV retinopathy are nonspecific and may also be associated with:
  - Diabetes.
  - Hypertension.
  - Anemia.
  - Immune complex diseases (e.g., systemic lupus erythematosus, dermatomyositis, and leukemia).
- It is imperative to include AIDS in the differential diagnosis of any patient with this pattern of nonspecific retinopathy in the absence of other known systemic disease.

Reference

Freeman WR, Lerner CW, Mines JA, et al. A prospective study of the ophthalmologic findings in the acquired immunodeficiency syndrome. *Am J Ophthalmol* 1984;97:133–142.

Ocular Histoplasmosis

Summary

Ocular histoplasmosis (formerly presumed ocular histoplasmosis [POHS]) is disease of young to middle-aged adults who are likely to have been exposed to the *Histoplasma capsulatum* organism. They present with blurred and distorted vision associated with characteristic "histo spots" and subsequent CNVMs.

Etiology

Presumed to be infection with *H. capsulatum* (although this has never been confirmed by Koch postulates), which causes a focal choroiditis that resolves as an atrophic scar disrupting Bruch membrane.

Signs and Symptoms

- Decreased VA.
- Metamorphopsia.
- The presence of visual symptoms should suggest subretinal neovascular membrane or fluid accumulation, since the atrophic choroidal lesions (histo spots) are asymptomatic.

Demographics

- Patients usually live or have spent time in the Ohio-Mississippi River Valley.
- Adults between the ages of 20 and 50 years.

- Rarely affects African American or Hispanic individuals.
- There may be a genetic predisposition in patients with HLA-B7 and HLA-DRw2.

Ophthalmic Findings

See Figure 3.43.

- Characteristic histo spots are yellow-white, punched-out, round chorioretinal scars usually less than 1 mm in diameter.
- CNVMs.
- Peripapillary atrophy and chorioretinal scarring, with pigment deposition between disk and sections of visible sclera.
- Linear streaks of chorioretinal atrophy in the periphery.
- Absence of vitritis or anterior segment reaction.

Systemic Findings

- Usually asymptomatic in normal hosts, although pulmonary histoplasmosis may develop following heavy exposure.
- Patients with suboptimal host defenses may develop disseminated histoplasmosis and chronic pulmonary infection, sometimes with an exuberant fibrotic response.

Special Tests

- Amsler grid testing may demonstrate scotomas.
- Controversy exists regarding the necessity of skin testing given the possibility of reactivating an inactive lesion.

Pathology

Presenting lesion is a choroidal granuloma progressing to scar with RPE atrophy, breaks in Bruch membrane, and subsequent subretinal neovascular membrane formation.

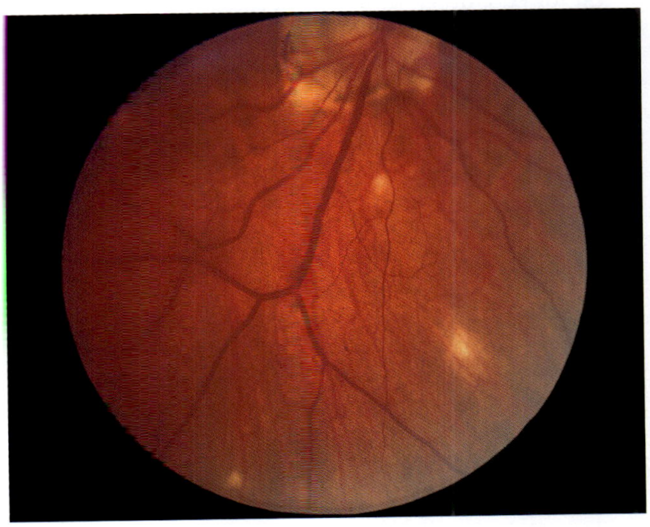

FIGURE 3.43 Punched-out chorioretinal lesions of POHS. Peripapillary ring of pigmentation is visible.

Disease Course

- One quarter of patients with macular spots develop CNVMs in the next 3 years; these patients have a 59% chance of 20/200 or worse VA if untreated.
- Patients without macular involvement have a low incidence of CNVM formation.
- With time, CNVMs may develop into a fibrovascular disciform scar.

Treatment and Management

- Extrafoveal and juxtafoveal CNVMs may be treated with laser photocoagulation according to the guidelines of the MPS.
- Corticosteroids may be of benefit during the early choroiditis and in those patients with subfoveal neovascular membranes.
- Submacular surgery to extract subfoveal CNVM.
- Additional treatments are being explored such as PDT, PDT combined with steroids, anti-VEGF agents.

Medications

Consider corticosteroids (e.g., prednisone 40 to 100 mg p.o. q.d. over 2 to 3 weeks) for subfoveal neovascular membranes.

Follow-Up

High-risk patients with macular lesions or previous visual loss should use the Amsler grid on a daily basis to detect new CNVM.

Differential Diagnosis

High myopia: Atrophic zones are pale and confined to the posterior pole; peripapillary atrophy is often associated with tilted disks, pigment ring at the periphery of the scleral crescent, and lacquer cracks.

ARMD: Patients are over age 50 years, often have drusen, and do not have characteristic histo spots.

Toxoplasmosis: associated with vitritis or anterior segment inflammation.

Angioid streaks: Radial hyperpigmented and hypopigmented streaks often emanating from the disk often associated with a variety of systemic ailments (e.g., PXE, Ehlers-Danlos syndrome, Paget disease, and sickle cell anemia). CNV associated with streaks themselves and lack histo spots.

Multifocal choroiditis and panuveitis: may have vitritis or anterior segment inflammation.

References

Hawkins BS, Bressler NM, Bressler SB, et al. Surgical removal vs observation for subfoveal choroidal neovascularization, either associated with the ocular histoplasmosis syndrome or

RETINA

idiopathic: I. Ophthalmic findings from a randomized clinical trial: Submacular Surgery Trials (SST) Group H Trial: SST Report No. 9. *Arch Ophthalmol* 2004;122:1597–1611.

Hawkins BS, Miskala PH, Bass EB, et al. Surgical removal vs observation for subfoveal choroidal neovascularization, either associated with the ocular histoplasmosis syndrome or idiopathic: II. Quality-of-life findings from a randomized clinical trial: SST Group H Trial: SST Report No. 10. *Arch Ophthalmol* 2004;122:1616–1628.

Macular Photocoagulation Study Group. Argon laser photocoagulation for neovascular maculopathy: five-year results from randomized clinical trials. *Arch Ophthalmol* 1991;109:1109–1114.

Macular Photocoagulation Study Group. Krypton laser photocoagulation for idiopathic neovascular lesions: results of a randomized clinical trial. *Arch Ophthalmol* 1990;108:832–837.

Syphilis

Summary

Syphilis is known as *the great imitator* and can present with inflammation of practically any portion of the eye. Bilateral granulomatous uveitis associated with either congenital or acquired syphilis and its systemic manifestations.

Etiology

Infection with the bacteria *Treponema pallidum* leads to primary, secondary, and tertiary syphilis; ocular symptoms develop rarely in primary stage (chancre of lids, conjunctiva, or lacrimal gland), in about 10% of secondary syphilis, and more frequent in late tertiary syphilis.

Signs and Symptoms

Blurred vision.
Ocular pain, redness, and photophobia.
Conjunctival discharge, ulceration.

Demographics

Sexually active individuals with or without high-risk activities.
Intravenous drug users.
HIV-positive individuals.
Children born to high-risk mothers.

Ophthalmic Findings

- Congenital syphilis: iridocyclitis from birth to 6 months; chorioretinitis and its sequelae after 6 months; interstitial keratitis from 2 months to adulthood.
- Ocular involvement may occur any stage of acquired syphilis.
- Dacryoadenitis, dacryocystitis, conjunctivitis.
- Scleritis, episcleritis.
- Interstitial keratitis with vascular ingrowth ("salmon patch").
- Bilateral or unilateral granulomatous uveitis.
- Roseola (iris hyperemia).
- Argyll Robertson pupil: accommodative constriction but no light reaction.
- Retinitis, chorioretinitis.
- Retinal vasculitis.
- Pigmentary retinopathy.
- Optic atrophy.

Systemic Findings

Primary: genital or oral chancre; regional lymphadenopathy.
Secondary: generalized maculopapular or pustular rash commonly on flexar or volar surfaces (palms and soles) with or without lymphadenopathy. Rash resolves with pigmentary changes and erosion of mucous membranes where involved.
Tertiary: aortitis, CNS manifestations including tabes dorsalis; Argyll Robertson pupil.
Congenital: Hutchinson teeth (peg-shaped teeth), saber shins, saddle nose, deafness, mental retardation, angular scars from angles of mouth.

Special Tests

- Venereal Disease Research Laboratory (VDRL) or RPR test detects titers against anticardiolipin antibody. Becomes positive 1 to 2 weeks after symptoms in primary syphilis, 99% of those with secondary syphilis, but only 70% with later stages. Becomes negative with treatment and shows false positive with any other disorder that elevates anticardiolipin antibody (various infectious/autoimmune disorders).
- FTA-Abs or microhemagglutination–*Treponema pallidium* (MHATP) test is more sensitive in later-stage disease and remains positive after treatment.
- Lumbar puncture with VDRL to evaluate possibility of neurosyphilis.
- Test for HIV, other sexually transmitted diseases.
- Consider serum ACE level, lysozyme, HLA-B27, CXR, PPD based upon presentation.

Pathology

Epithelioid cells, lymphocytes, and plasma cells within ocular tissue; spirochetes may be identified by dark field microscopy.

Disease Course

- Treated primary or secondary syphilis has excellent prognosis; tertiary syphilis may lead to irreparable damage.
- Ocular manifestations and activity may persist despite eradication of bacterium.

Treatment and Management

- Medical treatment.
- Sexual partners should be tested and treated as necessary.

Medications

- Exact recommendations change and vary—Consider Infectious Disease team consultation.
- Nonneurosyphilis:
  Procaine penicillin G 2.4 million units daily for 10 days
  For penicillin allergic, consider desensitization or Tetracycline 500 mg p.o. b.i.d. for 30 days *or* Erythromycin 500 mg p.o. q.i.d. for 15 days.
- Neurosyphilis: i.v. aqueous procaine penicillin G 2 to 4 million units i.v. q4 hours for 10 days.
- Topical and periocular steroids; cycloplegic agents as needed.

Follow-Up

- Biweekly until resolved.
- Repeated serologic tests should be performed if disease recurs, as patients may become reinfected.

Differential Diagnosis

T. gondii.
Rubella.
CMV.
HIV.
Herpes simplex virus (HSV), varicella-zoster virus (VZV).
HLA-B27–related uveitis.
Primary intraocular lymphoma.
Sarcoid.

References

Tamesis RR, Foster CS. Ocular syphilis. *Ophthalmology* 1990; 97:1281–1287.

Whitcup SM. Bacterial and fungal diseases. In: Nussenblatt RB, Whitcup SM, eds. *Uveitis fundamentals and clinical practice*, 3rd ed. Philadelphia, PA: Mosby, 2010;162–169.

Pneumocystis

Summary

Bilateral multiple, slowly enlarging round to oval pale yellow choroidal infiltrates without vitritis in patients with AIDS frequently receiving aerosolized pentamidine.

Etiology

P. carinii, present in up to 80% of patients with AIDS who have not had prophylaxis, leads to choroidopathy in patients receiving aerosolized pentamidine.

Signs and Symptoms

Mild visual changes but rarely symptomatic.

Ophthalmic Findings

- Yellow to pale yellow choroidal infiltrates in the posterior pole, ranging in size from 300 to >3,000 µm.
- Retinal vessels and vitreous unaffected.

Systemic Findings

Disseminated pneumocystosis.

Special Tests

- CXR.
- Bronchial washing or biopsy to establish diagnosis.
- If diagnosis unclear, test for other causes as needed.

Pathology

Eosinophilic, acellular, vacuolated lesions at level of choroid; choroidal vessels demonstrate cellular infiltration.

Disease Course

Choroidal infiltrates disappear following systemic treatment.

Treatment and Management

See below.

Medications

Intravenous pentamidine or double strength trimethoprim/sulfamethoxazole.

Follow-Up

Weekly until resolution of lesions confirms presumptive diagnosis.

Differential Diagnosis

Candidal retinitis.
Mycobacterial retinitis.
Cryptococcal choroiditis.
Primary intraocular lymphoma.
Sarcoid.
Dalen-Fuchs nodules (VKH syndrome; sympathetic ophthalmia).

Reference

Shami JF, Freeman WR, Ai E. A multicenter study of Pneumocystis choroidopathy. *Am J Ophthalmol* 1991;112:15–22.

Lyme Disease

Summary

Spirochetal infection similar to syphilis with primary, secondary, and tertiary systemic manifestations; any phase may lead to uveitic ocular involvement.

RETINA

Etiology

- Infection occurs after the tick vector, *Ixodes dammini*, transmits the spirochete *Borrelia burgdorferi* (also *Borrelia garinii* and *Borrelia afzelii* in Europe/Asia) to the accidental human host.
- *I. dammini* resides on lizards and deer in the western United States and deer in the eastern United States.

Signs and Symptoms

Inguinal rash.
Neurologic complaints.
Arthritis.
Eye pain.
Decreased vision.

Demographics

Outdoor participants in endemic areas.

Ophthalmic Findings

Conjunctivitis (11% in early-stage disease).
Keratitis.
Episcleritis.
Keratitis.
Bilateral or unilateral granulomatous uveitis.
Vitritis.
Choroiditis with exudative RDs.
Retinal vasculitis.
Optic neuritis.
Cranial-nerve palsies affecting the eye or orbit.

Systemic Findings

Rash at site of tick bite: erythema chronicum migrans.
Fever, malaise.
Neurologic deficits: facial nerve palsy(ies).
Cardiac abnormalities.
Arthritis, joint effusions.

Special Tests

ELISA for serum antibody to *Borrelia* species (Lyme titers).
IgM, IgG titers; acute and convalescent titers may be useful.
Lumbar puncture to evaluate other causes of neurologic disease.

Pathology

Epithelioid cells, lymphocytes, and plasma cells within ocular tissue.

Disease Course

Untreated disease can progress to tertiary form over course of months to years.

Treatment and Management

- Systemic treatment.
- If uveitis present, topical treatment with steroids and cycloplegics is indicated.

Medications

- Tetracycline, doxycycline, amoxicillin, erythromycin, or doxycycline for 3 to 4 weeks.
- Neurologic disease or severe Uveitis should be treated with i.v. third-generation cephalosporin (Ceftriaxone).

Follow-Up

Biweekly.

Differential Diagnosis

Syphilis.
Sarcoid.
Viral meningitis.
Other causes of uveitis.

References

Whitcup SM. Bacterial and fungal diseases. In: Nussenblatt RB, Whitcup SM, eds. *Uveitis fundamentals and clinical practice*, 3rd ed. Philadelphia, PA: Mosby, 2010;170–176.
Winterkorn JM. Lyme disease: neurologic and ophthalmic manifestations. *Surv Ophthalmol* 1990;35:191–204.

Leber Stellate Neuroretinitis/ Cat-Scratch Disease

Summary

Unilateral loss of vision associated with prodromal fever and lymphadenopathy in cat-exposed individuals.

Etiology

Bartonella (Rochalimaea) henselae, a slow-growing, Gram-negative, rod-shaped bacteria; prevalent in cats and detectable in sera of affected individuals.

Signs and Symptoms

Mild to severe central vision loss.
Fever, malaise, lymphadenopathy.

Demographics

Individuals exposed to or scratched by a cat.

Ophthalmic Findings

See Figure 3.44.

Normal to counting-finger VA.
Afferent pupillary defect may be seen.

Mild to moderate vitritis.
Optic disk swelling.
Hemimacular or macular star.
Cotton-wool spots.
Retinal hemorrhage.

Systemic Findings

Antecedent fever and flulike illness.
Unilateral or bilateral cervical, submandibular or preauricular adenopathy.
Aseptic meningitis.
Bacillary angiomatosis.

Special Tests

- Blood culture, serum immunofluorescence assay to *B. henselae*
- Lymph node biopsy/culture: Warthin-Starry stain demonstrates coccobacillary organisms.
- Consider blood culture of cat.
- Other serologic studies as suggested by examination and history.

Pathology

Noncaseating necrotizing granulomas of lymph nodes; perivascular lymphocytic infiltrate.

Disease Course

- Resolution of infection over 2 to 4 weeks with treatment.
- Visual recovery may be incomplete.

Treatment and Management

See below.

Medications

- Need for treatment debated because of self-limiting disease.

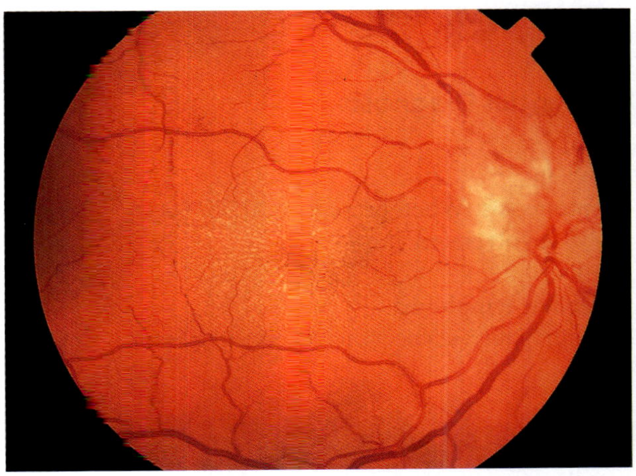

FIGURE 3-44. Neuroretinitis in a child. Note optic disk edema and macular exudates.

- Empiric courses of erythromycin, tetracycline, azithromycin, trimethoprim-sulfamethoxazole, gentamycin, or rifampin.
- Prednisone may be useful in slowly recovering neuroretinitis.

Follow-Up

Weekly while active.

Differential Diagnosis

Syphilis.
Tularemia.
Tuberculosis.
Toxoplasma infection.
Psittacosis.
Behçet disease.
Optic neuritis.
Leukemia.
Sarcoid.

References

Slater LN, Hensel D, Coody DW. A newly recognized fastidious gram-negative pathogen as a cause of fever and bacteremia. *N Engl J Med* 1990;323:1587–1593.

Wong MT, Dolan MJ, Melcher GP. Neuroretinitis, aseptic meningitis, and lymphadenitis associated with Bartonella (Rochalimaea) henselae infection in immunocompetent patients and patients infected with human immunodeficiency virus type I. *Clin Infect Dis* 1995;21:352–360.

Viral Retinitis

Cytomegalovirus

Summary

Viral retinitis of individuals with decreased cell-mediated immunity (patients with AIDS, newborns) that leads to loss of vision, and in patients with AIDS, a 30% incidence of RD.

Etiology

CMV, a double-stranded DNA virus, with nearly 80% antibody positivity in the United States population postulated to infect the retina from hematogenous spread of virus.

Signs and Symptoms

Floaters.
Decreased vision.

Demographics

Twenty-five percent of patients with AIDS, especially with CD4-positive cell counts less than 100/mm^3.

Immunosuppressed patients.
Newborns.

Ophthalmic Findings

See Figure 3.45.

- Bilateral in 30% of cases.
- Mild granulomatous iridocyclitis; hypopyon rare.
- Mild to moderate vitritis.
- Patches of granular white retinitis, especially perivascularly, leading to large geographic areas of necrosis.
- Vasculitis; vascular sheathing.
- Inactive areas of infection with atrophic retina and RPE pigmentary changes.
- Nerve-fiber layer infarcts and intraretinal hemorrhages common, especially at borders of retinitis.
- Optic neuritis, optic atrophy.
- Multiple atrophic retinal holes in areas of treated or untreated retinitis.
- RD: rhegmatogenous or exudative.
- Atypical presentations when patients have reconstituted immune systems secondary to anti-HIV medications.

Systemic Findings

- CD4-positive cell count less than 200/mm^3; average count: 50 cells/mm^3.
- CMV colitis, nephritis, pneumonitis, encephalitis, hepatitis.

Special Tests

- Fundus photos to follow course.
- Appropriate HIV workup: CMV retinitis may be AIDS-defining illness in 5% of HIV-positive patients.
- Retinal biopsy during posterior segment surgery, if diagnosis unclear.

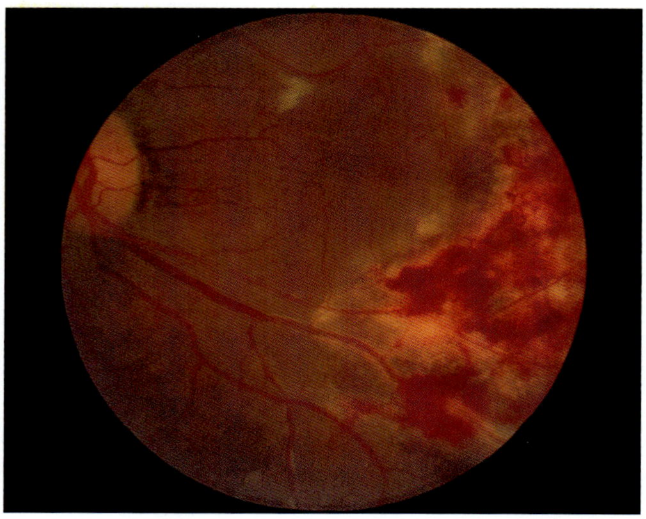

FIGURE 3.45. CMV retinitis with hemorrhagic retinal necrosis and cotton-wool spots.

- PCR of vitreous fluid.
- Consider serologic testing to rule out other causes.

Pathology

Full-thickness retinal necrosis; inclusion bodies may be seen.

Disease Course

Slowly progressive, ultimately leading to loss of vision through macular involvement, RD, or optic neuritis and optic atrophy.

Treatment and Management

- Surgical repair of RD as warranted.
- Intravitreal ganciclovir implant.

Medications

- Valganciclovir oral or Ganciclovir (DHPG) b.i.d. i.v. induction followed by daily i.v. or oral maintenance.
- Foscarnet b.i.d. i.v. induction followed by daily i.v. maintenance.
- Cidofovir (Vistide) i.v. weekly induction followed by biweekly maintenance.
- Intraocular ganciclovir sustained-release implant available for maintenance therapy.
- Intraocular injections of ganciclovir (DHPG), foscarnet, or cidofovir (HPMPC) can be used to treat resistant cases or in individuals who do not tolerate systemic therapy.
- Systemic antiretroviral medical treatment leads to improvement of CMV retinitis.

Follow-Up

- Evaluate for ganciclovir-induced bone marrow suppression.
- Evaluate for foscarnet-induced renal toxicity, seizures.
- Observation of retinitis at biweekly or monthly intervals.

Differential Diagnosis

ARN.
PORN.
Toxoplasmosis: When present in AIDS, 30% of cases have CNS involvement.
Syphilis.
Intraocular lymphoma.
HIV retinopathy: stable, non–vision-threatening retinopathy.

Reference

Gross JG, Bozzette SA, Mathews WC, et al. Longitudinal study of cytomegalovirus in acquired immune deficiency syndrome. *Ophthalmology* 1990;97:681–686.

Acute Retinal Necrosis Syndrome

Summary

Peripheral necrotizing retinitis with associated vitritis, arteritis and granulomatous uveitis, culminating in RD and profound visual loss.

Etiology

Possible VZV or HSV; rarely CMV.

Signs and Symptoms

Floaters.
Ocular pain and redness.
Decrease in peripheral vision.

Demographics

Healthy individuals.
Immunocompromised patients also at risk.
Ages 20 to 50 years (range, 3 to 89 years).

Ophthalmic Findings

- Episcleritis, scleritis.
- Moderate granulomatous anterior uveitis.
- Mild to severe vitritis.
- Patchy peripheral deep multifocal yellow-white retinal necrotic lesions, coalescing into geographic retinitis.
- Retinal and choroidal vasculitis.
- Multiple large full-thickness retinal holes seen during recovery phase.
- Retinal pigmentary hyperplasia.
- Traction and rhegmatogenous RD.
- Optic neuritis, optic nerve pallor or NV.
- VH.
- CME.
- Bilateral in greater than 30%, usually within 6 weeks, but second-eye involvement may be delayed many years.

Systemic Findings

Cerebrospinal fluid (CSF) pleocytosis.
Viral encephalitis may be observed.
Herpes simplex vesicles or herpes zoster lesions.
Vesicular eruption of ear (Ramsay Hunt syndrome).

Special Tests

Acute and convalescent titers of HSV-1, HSV-2, VZV, and CMV.
CBC, liver, and kidney function tests.
IVFA: choroidal filling defects, retinal arterial occlusion.
Ultrasound B-scan: detects RD or optic nerve edema.

Pathology

Full-thickness retinal necrosis, hemorrhage, choroiditis, and perivasculitis of retinal, choroidal, and extraocular muscle vasculature.

Disease Course

- Progresses over days to weeks, lasting 6 to 12 weeks.
- Thirty to sixty percent of eyes develop 20/200 vision or worse.
- Some cases are mild and self-limiting.

Treatment and Management

- Laser photocoagulation barrier at border of healthy, unaffected retina.
- Pars plana vitrectomy and/or repair of RD as indicated.

Medications

- Intravenous acyclovir for 5 to 7 days, followed by oral acyclovir for 6 weeks.
- Topical steroids.
- Cycloplegics.

Follow-Up

Daily until diagnosis confirmed and disease nonprogressive, then weekly during oral antiviral treatment.

Differential Diagnosis

CMV retinitis: occurs in immunocompromised patients, lacks vitritis, slow acting.
Diffuse toxoplasmosis: RD uncommon.
Behçet disease: should identify aphthous ulcers, rash, arthritis.
PORN: in immunocompromised hosts, little or no vitritis.
Sarcoid: extensive, rapidly progressive retinitis unusual.
Primary intraocular lymphoma.
Syphilitic retinitis.

Reference

Duker JS, Blumenkrantz MS. Diagnosis and management of the acute retinal necrosis syndrome (ARN). *Surv Ophthalmol* 1991;35:327–343.

Progressive Outer Retinal Necrosis

Summary

Acute, deep peripheral retinitis, caused by Herpes virus (usually VZV) in persons with AIDS or severe immunosuppression. Leads to severe visual loss; current treatments inadequate.

Etiology

Varicella zoster viral infection believed to be most common (HSV, CMV also implicated rarely).

Signs and Symptoms

Rapid loss of vision.
Systemic zoster infection.

Demographics

Persons with AIDS.
Immunocompromised individuals.

Ophthalmic Findings

- Multifocal, deep retinal lesions in peripheral retina, rapidly spreading posteriorly and leading to rhegmatogenous RD in 70% of eyes.
- Minimal vitritis or anterior chamber findings.
- Seventy percent of patients with bilateral disease.
- Fifty percent of patients progress to no light perception.

Systemic Findings

Seventy-five percent of cases with extraocular manifestations of VZV infection.
AIDS or other immunocompromised status.

Special Tests

PCR of ocular fluids.
Vitreous biopsy.
IVFA shows zonal microvascular changes, RPE destruction, and choroidal leakage.

Pathology

- Full-thickness retinal and choroidal necrosis.
- Intranuclear inclusions and viral particles in affected tissue.

Disease Course

Rapidly leads to severe visual loss or blindness in 50% of eyes.

Treatment and Management

Barrier laser retinopexy.
Vitrectomy with silicone oil.

Medications

- Intravitreal ganciclovir and foscarnet, plus systemic antiherpetic medications (usually intravenous ganciclovir and foscarnet).

Follow-Up

Twice weekly during acute infection.

Differential Diagnosis

CMV retinitis.
Toxoplasmosis retinitis.

References

Greven CM, Ford J, Slusher M. Progressive outer retinal necrosis secondary to varicella zoster virus in AIDS. *Retina* 1995;15:14–20.
Moorthy RS, Rao NA, Jampol LM. Management of varicella zoster virus retinitis in AIDS. *Br J Ophthalmol* 1997;81:189–194.

PARASITIC DISEASES

Onchocerciasis ("River Blindness")

Summary

Systemic microfilarial infection with *Onchocerca volvulus* leads to multiple skin nodules, granulomatous uveitis, and eventual blindness.

Etiology

O. volvulus, a filarial parasite transmitted by blackflies to humans in endemic areas; resides in dermis, lymph nodes, and eyes of human host; adult worm produces microfilarial offspring that can be seen microscopically in many body structures.

Signs and Symptoms

Painless or painful infected skin nodules.
"Leopard skin" dermatitis.
Blindness.

Demographics

- Endemic areas along riverbeds of sub-Saharan Africa and Latin America.
- Eighteen million persons infected, two million blinded by onchocerciasis.

Ophthalmic Findings

- Live parasites are found throughout ocular tissue; visible in the anterior chamber fluid, cornea, and retina.
- Punctate keratitis and local tissue necrosis following treatment with diethylcarbamazine (DEC).
- Sclerosing keratitis arising from interpalpebral fissure.
- Chronic granulomatous iridocyclitis.
- Retinal pigment epithelial atrophy.
- Optic neuritis and optic atrophy.

Systemic Findings

- Hard, round microfilarial subcutaneous nodules.
- Dermatitis, pruritus.

Special Tests

- IVFA may show atrophy of the RPE.
- Skin biopsy specimen demonstrates microfilaria; at least six negative skin snips needed to demonstrate absence of disease.
- Examination of bodily fluids for microfilaria.

Pathology

Identification of microfilaria, lymphocytes, plasma cells, and eosinophils in the affected tissues.

Disease Course

Chronic, recurrent disease; severity of outcome depends on duration and intensity of exposure.

Treatment and Management

- Nodulectomy has limited effect on decreasing parasitic load in humans.
- Prevention considered essential and includes appropriate hygiene, relocation away from river-breeding zones, and extermination of blackflies.

Medications

Ivermectin: Single annual oral dose effectively eliminates production of microfilaria by adult worm; does not result in systemic toxicity. Needs to be repeated yearly for 15 years until adult worms die.

DEC: Daily oral treatment for 1 to 2 weeks reduces microfilarial load for 6 to 12 months but results in systemic hypersensitivity reaction, the Mazzotti reaction, caused by massive death of microfilariae and characterized by pruritus, rash, fever, arthralgia, optic neuritis, and proteinuria.

Suramin: Intravenous preparation used before discovery of ivermectin causes exuberant inflammatory response.

Follow-Up

Yearly for ivermectin treatment.

Differential Diagnosis

In treated individuals, residual chorioretinal pigmentary changes need to be differentiated from active granulomatous uveitis.

Reference

Taylor HR. Onchocerciasis. *Int Ophthalmol* 1990;14:189–194.

Diffuse Unilateral Subacute Neuroretinopathy

Summary

Diffuse unilateral subacute neuroretinopathy (DUSN): nematode infection that can cause significant visual loss from vitritis, disk edema, retinitis (unilateral "wipe-out").

Etiology

Specific nematode has not been definitively identified. *Ancylostoma caninum* (hookworm found in dogs) suspected. *Baylisascaris procyonis*, an intestinal nematode infecting raccoons and skunks, has also been proposed as the larger nematode causing DUSN.

Signs and Symptoms

Unilateral decreased vision.

Floaters.

Mild ocular discomfort.

Demographics

Children and young adults.

Male more frequently than female patients.

Unilateral involvement.

The Southeastern United States and Caribbean: smaller nematode.

Northern Midwest: larger nematode.

Ophthalmic Findings

Vitritis.

Optic disk edema.

Evanescent outer retinal lesions.

Pigmented tracks in retina/RPE/choroid

Nematode sometimes visualized as coiled lesion or motile (pathognomic).

Retinal hemorrhages.

Systemic Findings

May be associated with visceral larval migrans.

Special Tests

Indirect ophthalmoscopy.

Serial fundus photography: Careful examination can reveal nematode.

IVFA: Abnormal fluorescence varies based on age of lesions. Early lesions leak on late frames and older lesions show window defect and blocked fluorescence from pigmentation.

ERG: decreased b-wave amplitude in the affected eye.

Pathology

Focal degeneration of RPE and outer retina.

Treatment and Management

Direct laser photocoagulation of the nematode.

Medications

Antihelminthic agents such as thiabendazole have been tried with limited success.

Follow-Up

Some patients may require multiple visits to search for the nematode. Careful review of fundus photographs helpful in identifying nematode. Once the nematode has been eradicated, the inflammatory changes resolve.

Differential Diagnosis

White dot syndromes: AMPPE, MEWDS, Serpiginous Choroiditis
Toxoplasmosis.
Sarcoidosis.
Ocular histoplasmosis, multifocal choroiditis.
Neuroretinitis.
RP (late stages).

References

Davis JL, Gass JDM, Olsen KR. Diffuse unilateral subacute neuroretinitis. In: Ryan SJ, ed. *Retina*, 4th ed, Philadelphia, PA: Elsevier, 2006:1721–1730.

Gass JD, Callanan DG, Bowman CB. Successful oral therapy for diffuse unilateral subacute neuroretinitis. *Trans Am Ophthalmol Soc* 1991;89:97–112.

Kazacos KR, Raymond LA, Kazacos EA, et al. The raccoon ascarid. A probable cause of human ocular larva migrans. *Ophthalmology* 1985;92:1735–1744.

Toxocara Retinochoroiditis

Summary

Unilateral ocular parasitosis caused by the nematode *Toxocara canis,* which gains access to the accidental human host by ingestion of contaminated soil and most often causes a subretinal macular granuloma.

Etiology

- *T. canis*, a worldwide nematode infecting 20% of adult dogs and 50% of puppies.
- Puppies infected transplacentally from mothers or by ingestion of ova.
- Ingestion of ova-laden soil by children (pica) gives parasite access to portal system and other sites including liver, lung, heart, brain, and eye.
- Thirty percent of some populations have positive ELISA titers to *T. canis*.

Signs and Symptoms

Unilateral decreased vision.
Ocular pain, headache.
Blunted red reflex, leukocoria.
Strabismus.

Demographics

Young children, 6 months to 4 years of age (mean age, 2 years).

Ophthalmic Findings

See Table 3.9. Ocular larva migrans involves the following:

Mild to severe decreased vision.

Table 3.9

Three ocular presentations of toxocariasis
Endophthalmitic
Pars plana (peripheral) granuloma: may mimic intermediate uveitis
Posterior pole granuloma

Leukocoria.
Strabismus.
Anterior chamber inflammation usually absent.
Mild to severe vitritis.
Yellow-white subretinal granuloma, most commonly in the posterior pole but may be seen in peripheral retina.
Bands of retinal traction drawn to center of granuloma.
Exudative RD may be seen.

Systemic Findings

Visceral larva migrans, a parasitic invasion involving the following organs and symptoms:

Liver: abdominal pain, nausea, vomiting, hepatomegaly.
Lung: pharyngitis, cough, wheezing, pneumonia.
Heart: lethargy, fever, congestive heart failure.
Brain: headache, behavior changes.
Striated muscle: leg or arm pain.

Special Tests

- Vitreous biopsy, Gram stain, culture: eosinophilia seen on Gram stain.
- Toxocara ELISA on undiluted serum, aqueous, or retinal biopsy tissue. Serum titers 1:8 or less are consistent with ocular involvement.
- Computerized tomography of orbit: calcium deposits suggest diagnosis of retinoblastoma.

Pathology

Hemorrhagic necrosis near areas of larval migration; eosinophils, histiocytes, and areas of granuloma formation are observed.

Disease Course

- Self-limited, but ocular inflammation and granuloma can lead to loss of central vision.
- Misdiagnosis may lead to enucleation.

Treatment and Management

- Diagnostic and therapeutic vitrectomy.
- Serum eosinophilia suggests parasitosis.
- Dogs, especially puppies, should be dewormed routinely.

Medications

Steroids: The worm is usually dead and causes a brisk inflammatory response.

Follow-Up

Daily until diagnosis.
Weekly until resolution of findings.

Differential Diagnosis

Endogenous endophthalmitis.
Retinoblastoma, endophytic form.
Medulloepithelioma.
Coats' disease.
Pars planitis: typically bilateral and present in older patients.
ROP: eyes, peripheral fibrous masses, and retinal folds.
FEVR.

Reference

Molk R. Ocular toxocariasis: a review of the literature. *Ann Ophthalmol* 1983;15:216–231.

Endophthalmitis

See p. 239.

HEREDITARY DISORDERS

Vitelliform Dystrophy (Best Disease)

Summary

Best vitelliform dystrophy is an inherited macular dystrophy in which there is slowly progressive atrophy of the RPE and defects of the sensory retina. Classically, it is characterized by an egg-yellow, round, raised cystic structure surrounded by a darker border in the macula.

Etiology

- Disease is caused by mutation in BEST1 (VMD2) gene (11q13) which encodes a chloride channel in basolateral RPE.
- Results in abnormal accumulation of lipofuscin granules within the RPE and in the subretinal space have been reported.

Signs and Symptoms

- Heterogeneous clinical expression.
- Typical yolklike disk often discovered on routine ophthalmoscopy. May be asymptomatic.
- Bilateral VA is often only mildly affected early in disease, but in later stages, some patients will have a diminution to counting fingers, which may be partially reversible.
- Loss of central visual-field sensitivity.
- Color vision is affected; usually a mild red-green dyschromatopsia.
- Patients are often hypermetropic.
- May be associated with CNVM.

Demographics

- Inheritance is autosomal dominant, mapping of genetic mutation to chromosome 11q13.
- Penetrance is incomplete and expression is variable.
- Equal incidence of disease among males and females.
- Roughly 50% of the children of affected carriers are affected. Genetic testing available through Carver Labs, Iowa City, IA.
- Vitelliform lesions are usually seen in patients 3 to 15 years old; sometimes, the lesions first appear in later life.

Ophthalmic Findings

See Figure 3.46.

Typically, bilateral fundus abnormalities are seen (Table 3.10).

Systemic Findings

None.

Special Tests

- EOG is the critical diagnostic test, in which there is severe loss of light response with an Arden ratio (light-dark ratio) of less than 1.5. The defective chloride channels result in abnormal EOG.
- EOG abnormalities serve as a marker for carriers with normal fundi.

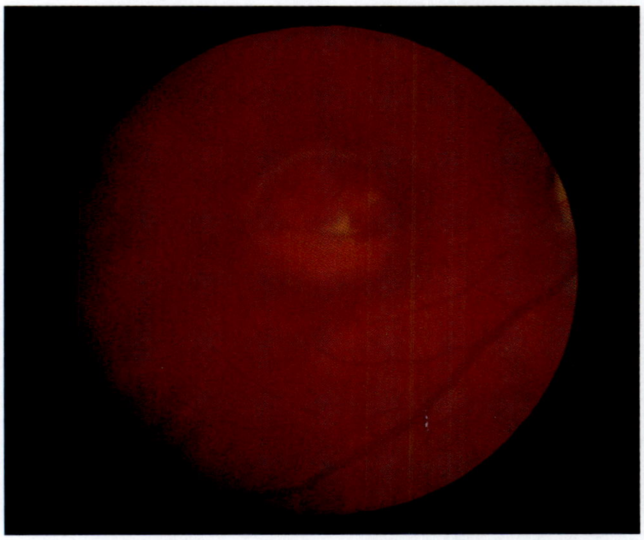

FIGURE 3.46. Best disease with pseudohypopyon stage macular lesion. Yellowish subretinal material has accumulated inferiorly.

Table 3.10

Clinical stages of Best disease

Stage		Fundus appearance
I	Previtelliform stage	Normal fundus examination
II	Vitelliform stage	Yolklike, disciform structure with a darker border in the macula, 0.5–3 disk diameters Rarely, multiple vitelliform structures in the posterior pole.
III	Pseudohypopyon stage	Over time, the disciform lesion may disappear or rupture, and the contents may disintegrate into a cystlike structure with a visible fluid level in the subretinal space.
IV	"Scrambled-egg" stage	Yellow deposits scattered throughout the posterior pole.
V	Neovascularization stage	Subretinal neovascularization may occur late in the disease, and round areas of chorioretinal atrophy are likely to develop at the macula.

Pathology

Loss of RPE and photoreceptor cells in sharply demarcated areas of the macula, with accumulation of lipofuscin in residual RPE cells.

Disease Course and Natural Progression

Visual potential is usually very good and typically remains 20/40 in the better eye; only 4% of patients have less than 20/200 vision in the better eye.

Treatment and Management

Treatment associated with CNVM.

When a sporadic case is discovered, EOG should be performed in family members to determine their carrier status.

Follow-Up

Periodic monitoring.
Genetic counseling and testing.

Differential Diagnosis

Central serous choroidopathy: may have fundus photos that resemble vitelliform macular dystrophy; EOG may be necessary to distinguish entities.
Pigment epithelial detachment in ARMD.
Pattern dystrophies.
North Carolina Macular Dystrophy.
Toxoplasma retinochoroiditis: Atrophic scar may resemble atrophy of vitelliform macular dystrophy. Positive toxoplasma titers.
Disciform macular degeneration: elderly patients, typically will have subretinal CNV.

References

Benson WE, Kilker AE, Enoch JM, et al. Best's vitelliform macular dystrophy. *Am J Ophthalmol* 1975;79:59–66.

Lotery AJ, Munier FL, Fishman GA, et al. Allelic variation in the VMD2 gene in best disease and age-related macular degeneration. *Invest Ophthalmol Vis Sci* 2000;41(6):1291–1296.

Stargardt Disease/Fundus Flavimaculatus

Summary

Stargardt disease is usually an autosomal recessive, juvenile-onset condition in which the macula is atrophic and is surrounded by discrete yellow flecks. Autosomal dominant cases have also been reported.

Etiology

Pathogenesis involves a photoreceptor cell–specific transmembrane transporter of Vitamin A (ABCR4) that is mutated and appears to allow the accumulation of lipofuscin or an acid mucopolysaccharide within the RPE. The recessive AABCA1 is located at 1p22.1. The same gene product has been implicated in some forms of cone rod degeneration and some forms of RP. The dominant form has been mapped to 4P15.32 (Protein is prominin 1) and 6q14.1 (ELOVL4) that codes for protein involved in elongation of very long fatty acids.

Signs and Symptoms

Bilateral, gradual diminution of vision.

Demographics

Typical onset between 6 and 20 years of age.
Several children in a family are often affected.
Consanguinity of parents is often found in autosomal recessive forms.
Rarely autosomal dominant. (See genetics above.)

Ophthalmic Findings

See Figure 3.47.

- Initially, ophthalmoscopy reveals no abnormalities.
- Later, disappearance of foveolar reflex.

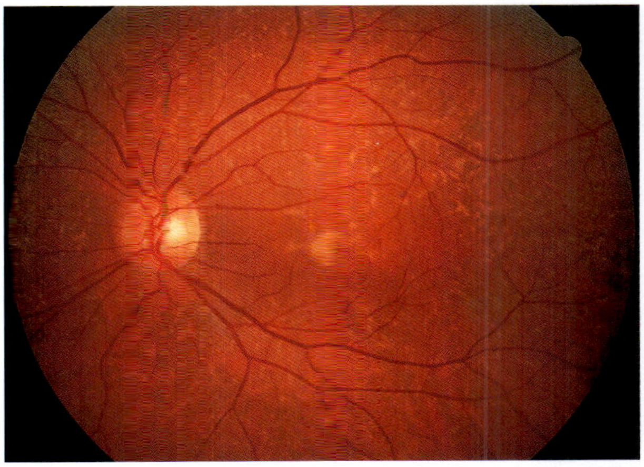

FIGURE 3.47. Fundus flavimaculatus with yellow pisciform macular flecks.

- Development of grayish yellow spots on the RPE with a pisciform (fishtail) appearance (due to lipfuscin A2E deposits).
- Fovea may appear granular and varnished.
- Yellowish perifoveal flecks beneath vessels within the RPE.
- Horizontal area of atrophic pigment epithelium may have a "beaten bronze" or a bull's eye appearance (Bull's Eye Maculopathy).
- Marked geographic atrophy.

Systemic Findings

None.

Special Tests

- IVFA characteristics (Figure 3.48):
  Parafoveal window defect.

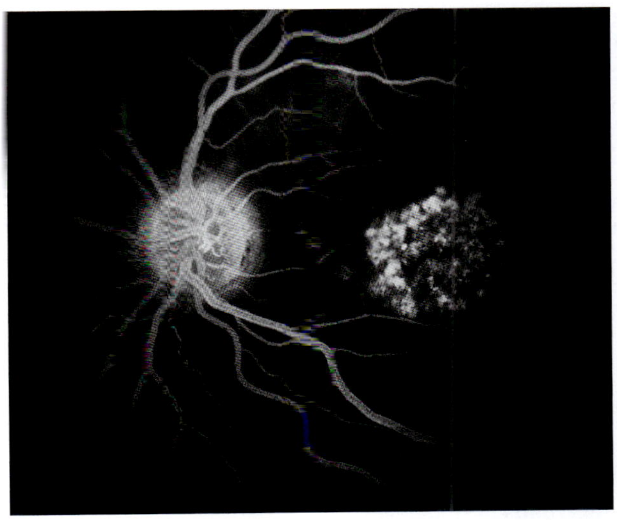

FIGURE 3.48. IVFA showing dark choroid and macular RPE window defects in Stargardt disease.

  Flecks develop as the disease progresses and may become confluent secondary to RPE atrophy: dark choroid effect, in which retinal circulation is highlighted against a hypofluorescent choroid.
  Autofluorescence may be present.
- EOG is subnormal in advanced cases.
- ERG is normal at first but becomes abnormal with progression.

Pathology

- Few nuclear remnants remain between Bruch membrane and the external limiting membrane.
- Defects in photoreceptors may be secondary to RPE abnormalities.
- Electron microscopy demonstrates enlarged RPE cells that are irregular and arranged in a pisciform configuration; surrounding RPE cells may appear normal.
- Accumulation of lipofuscin within RPE cells.

Disease Course

- Area of atrophy gradually extends and new flecks appear as far as the midperiphery.
- Eventually, extensive atrophy of the choriocapillaris may occur.

Treatment and Management

Observation.
Low-vision aids.
Genetic counseling.

Medications

None are effective.

Differential Diagnosis

Fleck retina syndromes:

Retinitis punctata albescens (RPA).
Drusen.
Fundus albipunctatus.
Chloroquine retinopathy.
Cone dystrophy.

Reference

Noble KG, Carr RE. Stargardt's disease and fundus flavimaculatus. *Arch Ophthalmol* 1979;97:1281–1285.

Leber Congenital Amaurosis

Summary

Leber congenital amaurosis (LCA) or congenital RP is a group of disorders in which there is severe visual impairment from infancy with severely affected to nonrecordable ERG.

Etiology/Genetic

Prior to 1996 was clinical diagnosis. Now have identified eleven (11) genes on seven (7) chromosomes. Gene products varied.

Signs and Symptoms

Severe visual impairment before age 1 year.
Nystagmus.
Poor pupillary reflexes.
Keratoconus may be found.
Mental retardation in less than a third of reported cases.
Often have high hyperopia.

Demographics

Onset of signs and symptoms before age 1 year.
Autosomal recessive inheritance (rarely inherited Autosomal dominant CRX gene mutation).
Consanguinity in parents not uncommon.

Ophthalmic Findings

- Nystagmus roving.
- Decreased or absent pupil reflexes.
- Normal fundus appearance in most patients.
- Some may have subtle RPE granularity and mild vessel attenuation.

*May have Coats' like response in 7% of children

Systemic Findings

None.

Special Tests

Electrophysiologic testing is essential: decreased ERG amplitudes. May be nonrecordable.

Pathology

- Selective destruction of photoreceptor outer segments.
- Macrophages near sites of photoreceptor loss.

Disease Course

Congenital occurrence.
Stable, without progression or improvement.

Treatment and Management

Observation: Consider nonprofit genetic testing (University of Iowa, Dr. Ed Stone).
Enroll patient in studies designed to define genotype-phenotype correlations.
Low-vision training.
Avoid sensory deprivation, which may be the cause of the psychomotor retardation reported in many LCA patients.

Medications

None effective.

Gene therapy restores vision in Briard canine model. Limited clinical trials in humans underway in London, United Kingdom, and Pittsburg, Pennsylvania.

Differential Diagnosis

- Infantile Refsum disease: phytanic acid storage disease, secondary to deficiency of phytanic acid oxidase:
  Deafness, RPE defects, vessel attenuation, often esotropia.
  Submaximal ERG, rods and cone.
- Congenital stationary night blindness (CSNB):
  Loss of dark adaptation.
  Several inheritance patterns.
  Fundi may appear normal.
- Batten disease: early infantile neuronal ceroid lipofuscinosis:
  Accumulation of lipopigment in neurons of retina and CNS.
  Loss of vision, dementia, seizures, eventually death.

References

Acland GM, Agquirre GD, Bennett J, et al. *Nat Genet* 2001; 28(1):92–95.
Heher KL, Traboulsi EI, Maumenee IH. The natural history of Leber's congenital amaurosis. *Ophthalmology* 1992;99:241–245.

X-Linked Juvenile Retinoschisis

Summary

X-linked juvenile retinoschisis is a vitreoretinal dystrophy characterized by a splitting of the retina within the nerve fiber layer at the fovea, occurring exclusively in boys.

Etiology/Genetics

Pathogenesis may represent a defect of Müller cells, which allows the ILM to split away from the remaining retina. RS1 gene (Xp22.2) involved in abnormal protein product that may be sequestered in cell. More than 125 mutations have been associated with the disease.

Signs and Symptoms

Central vision typically in 20/60 range.
VH.
Strabismus.
Hyperopia and astigmatism.
Nystagmus.
Symmetrical bilateral macular involvement.

Demographics

Congenital.
Exclusively occurs in male patients.
Usually diagnosed in early boyhood.

Ophthalmic Findings

See Figure 3.49.

- Frequently presents with VH from torn vessels in areas of retinoschisis.
- Foveal retinoschisis is a characteristic sign and often the only abnormality.
- Fine folds may be seen radiating from fovea.
- Round microcysts in perifoveal area.
- Vitreous veil with or without retinal vessels enclosed.
- Rarely RD.
- Peripheral schisis may or may not be present but generally develops with time, typically inferiorly
- Pigmentary deposits may develop in areas of schisis.

Special Tests

- IVFA:
  Macula may be entirely normal or have pigment epithelial atrophy.
  Delayed retinal blood flow.
  Leakage rarely occurs.
- Visual-field testing:
  Relative central scotoma.
  May have scotoma in upper peripheral nasal field.
- Color vision:
  As in other macular disorders, color vision is abnormal.
  Red-green dyschromatopsia.
- ERG:
  Selective loss of b-waves.
  ERG may be extinguished when extensive retinal damage has occurred.
- EOG and dark adaptation studies are normal.

*Genetic testing for RS1 (only known gene association)

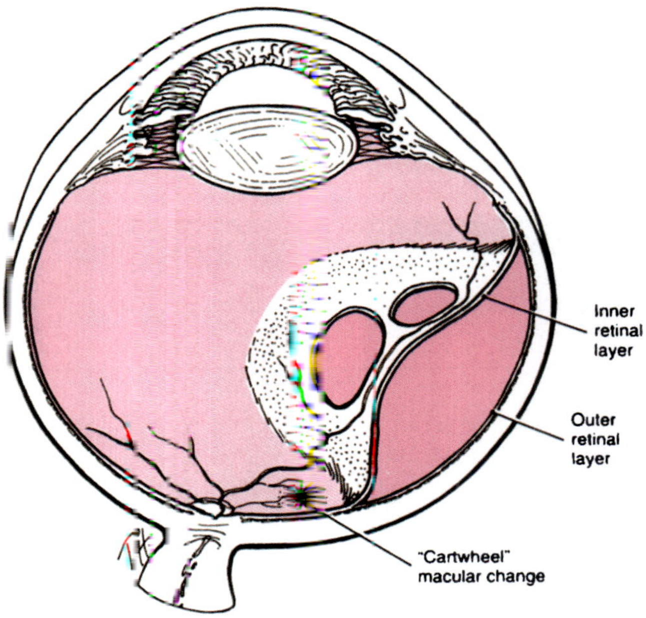

FIGURE 3.49 Drawing of X-linked retinoschiosis. The splitting occurs in the nerve-fiber layer.

Pathology

- Cleavage of retina in nerve-fiber layer.
- Atrophy of central and peripheral nerve-fiber layer.
- Extracellular, intraretinal filaments may accumulate and cause cell degeneration with schisis formation.

Disease Course

Usually, slow progression.

Treatment and Management

- Treat amblyopia with patching.
- Surgical repair of RD.

*Genetic counseling—X-linked carrier women—50% chance transmitting disease causing mutation. Affected males pass disease causing mutation to all daughters and no sons.

Medications

None effective.

Follow-Up

Every 6 months with more frequent visits if there is amblyopia or if surgical intervention is required.

Differential Diagnosis

- Goldman-Favre disease:
  Extensive vitreoretinal dystrophy with bone corpuscle pigmentation and severe night blindness.
  Macular plications are much coarser than in juvenile X-linked retinoschisis.
- Choroidal folds: Folds in choroid and in ILM may resemble focal retinoschisis.
- RP: Pigmentary changes may develop in area of schisis, and X-linked retinoschisis may be mistaken for RP.
- Rhegmatogenous RD:
  Elevation of the inner retinal layer may occur in X-linked retinoschisis and may be mistaken for rhegmatogenous RD.
  Rhegmatogenous RD extends to the ora serrata, while X-linked retinoschisis does not.

Reference

Sabates FN. Juvenile retinoschisis. *Am J Ophthalmol* 1966;62: 683–688.

Retinitis Pigmentosa

Summary

RP is a group of inherited diseases of the retina in which there is progressive photoreceptor dysfunction (rods and cones) and RPE associated with cell loss and eventual retinal atrophy. Different classification systems are used, based on inheritance pattern, gene defect, distribution of abnormal retina, and pattern of ERG abnormalities. Affected individuals first experience dark adaptation issues (night blindness) with progressive peripheral visual field constriction and in late stages some lose central acuity.

Etiology/Genetics

Pathogenesis is poorly understood.

Molecular genetics of RP is very complicated. More than 134 mutations have been associated with the disease. Identified genes with defects of encoding proteins involved in phototransduction, recycling of rhodopsin, photoreceptor structure, photoreceptor cell transcription factor, and function of many involved genes remain unidentified.

Signs and Symptoms

Night blindness (loss of rod function predominates in early disease).

Visual-field losses, especially midperipheral, which may enlarge to form a ring scotoma.

Central vision loss; severity depends on type of RP. (Central Va usually present until late stages.)

Loss of color vision may eventually occur.

Photopsias.

High-level myopia and astigmatism are common in some forms of RP.

Demographics

- Depending on type of RP, symptoms may appear in childhood or early adulthood.
- Genetic disease, but 40% have no affected relatives.
- Four inheritance patterns:
  Autosomal dominant (most common): 15% to 20%.
  Autosomal recessive: 5% to 20%.
  X-linked recessive: 5% to 15%.
  Unknown (simplex): 40% to 50% (single occurrence in a family).
- Incidence is about 1 in 4,000 in the United States. (Affects both males and females.)

Ophthalmic Findings

See Figure 3.50.

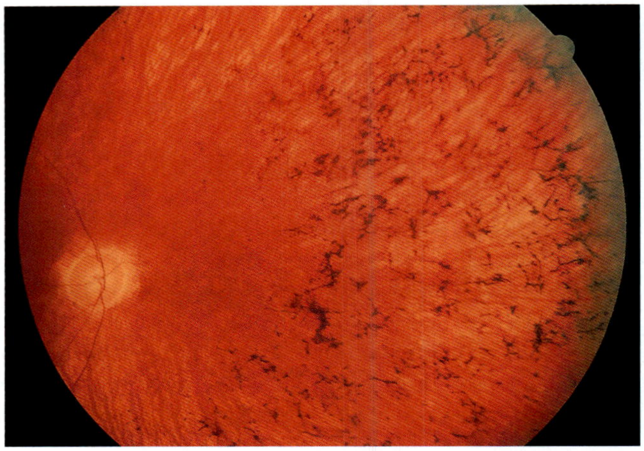

FIGURE 3.50. RP with "bone spicules," retinal vascular attenuation, and waxy disk pallor.

Narrowing of retinal vessels.

Depigmentation of the RPE.

Intraretinal "bone spicule" formation and perivascular pigmentary cuffing.

Waxy pallor of optic disks.

Vitreous cells (thought to be T lymphocytes)

Posterior subcapsular cataract.

Glaucoma.

CME.

Epiretinal membrane.

Hyaline bodies (drusen) of optic nerve head.

Rare occurrence exudative vasculopathy with telangiectatic vessels, serous RD, lipid deposition in retina (cause unknown).

Systemic Findings

Variable and may include associated disorders (Table 3.11).

Special Tests

- ERG is gold standard for diagnosis of RP:
  Marked reduction of rod and cone signals (rod loss predominates).

Table 3.11

Retinitis pigmentosa associated disorders

Syndrome	Findings
Usher syndrome	RP plus congenital deafness
Refsum disease	Autosomal recessive RP plus increased serum phytanic acid with ataxia, distal extremity weakness, deafness, anosmia, and ocular motility disturbances
Hereditary abetalipoproteinemia (Bassen-Kornzweig syndrome)	RP plus fat intolerance, diarrhea, crenated erythrocytes, ataxia, restrictive ocular motility
Laurence-Moon–Bardet-Biedl syndrome	RP and mental retardation, obesity, polydactyly, hypogenitalism, paraplegia
Kearns-Sayre syndrome	Autosomal recessive RP with normal arterioles, progressive limitation of ocular movements, ptosis, and heart block

RP, retinitis pigmentosa.

a- and b-waves are reduced; and b waves are prolonged. Late in course, ERG may become undetectable.

- Goldmann perimetry is useful:
  - Midperipheral scotomata are seen early; may coalesce into ring scotoma.
  - May have small central tunnel of VA late in course.
- Dark adaptometry is abnormal in RP:
  - Delayed rod-cone break.
  - Elevated final threshold, typically three or more log units above normal in advanced RP.
  - Prolonged recovery to final threshold.

Pathology

- Degeneration of rods, then cones, beginning in outer segments.
- Gradual depigmentation of the RPE occurs with some RPE proliferation, macrophage phagocytosis of liberated pigment, and migration of macrophages and RPE cells into the retina.
- Gliosis occurs in the photoreceptors, binding the retina to Bruch membrane and leading to sclerotic nets in the peripheral retina.
- Luminal narrowing of vessels occurs because of hyaline thickening.
- Choriocapillaris and choroid are unaffected.
- Epiretinal membrane of smooth muscle cells has been shown to form in the macular area.

Disease Course (Depends on Genetic Defect)

Highly dependent on type of RP; studies suggest relentless, slow progression of ERG findings and visual-field loss, but relative stability of central VA and dark-adaptation thresholds.

Treatment and Management

- Multitude of treatments have been attempted, including with various vitamins and minerals, vasodilators, cortisone, and placental extract: None of these treatments have been studied with randomized, double-blinded protocols with ERG end points to measure progression, and no therapy can be recommended as efficacious.
- Molecular genetic diagnostic testing can be offered to patients with some forms of the disease; while it may help identify affected family members, at present it does not lead to therapy (limited trial of Ciliary Neurotropic Growth Factor underway by NEI).
- If systemic conditions are suspected, order appropriate tests.

Medications

None proven effective, but studies continue on efficacy of Vitamin A, DHEA. Suggestion: Vitamin E ingestion may accelerate decline of ERG (Berson).

Differential Diagnosis

Ocular trauma.
Drug toxicity: phenothiazines.
Infections: syphilis, rubella, other severe uveitis.
Inflammatory: Harada disease.
Hereditary: gyrate atrophy, choroideremia, CSNB, Leber Congenital Amaurosis.
Pigmentary: paravenous retinochoroidal atrophy.
Chronic RD.
Metabolic: Refsum disease, abetalipoproteinemia.

Reference

Berson EL. Retinitis pigmentosa: the Friedenwald lecture. *Invest Ophthalmol Vis Sci* 1993;34:1659–1676.
RetNet. http://www.sph.uth.tmc.edu/Retnet/

RETINA

Cone Dystrophy

Summary

The cone dystrophies are a rare group of heterogeneous, inherited disorders of the retina in which cone photoreceptor dysfunction predominates. Pedigrees showing autosomal dominant, autosomal recessive, and X-linked inheritance have been described.

Etiology/Genetics

- Pathogenesis of dominant subtypes involves genetic defects in DOMCR (6p21.1), which encodes proteins regulating synaptic membrane exocytosis, guanylate cyclase–activating protein, and RDS-peripherin protein. Also, dominant mutations on chromosomes 17 and 19 have been identified. Recessive subtypes include mutations on chromosomes 1,2,8, 17, and 18, and some involve cGMP-gated cation channel activation. X-Linked Recessive subtypes are mapped to Xp11.4 the COD1 protein.
- Absence of macular photoreceptors with associated pigment epithelium degeneration.
- Cones may have an enzymatic or structural disorder that leads to their degeneration.

Signs and Symptoms

Loss of VA, often to 20/200 range by age 30 years.
Progressive color vision defects.
Photophobia.

Ophthalmic Findings

- Most common finding is bull's-eye maculopathy, showing a clearly defined zone of atrophic RPE surrounding a darker central zone.
- Pigment stippling and scattered, round pigment clumps in the posterior pole sometimes associated with diffuse atrophy of the posterior pole and bone corpuscles in the midperiphery.

- Occasionally, atrophy of the choriocapillaris and larger choroidal vessels.
- Rarely, yellowish, perifoveal flecks occur in the RPE and a horizontal oval of RPE atrophy may develop.

Systemic Findings

None.

Special Tests

- IVFA appearance varies with the pattern of ophthalmoscopic changes: Commonly, a horizontal ovoid zone of hyperfluorescence surrounds a nonfluorescent center.
- Color vision testing:
  - Frequent errors on Ishihara plates and Hardy-Rand-Ritter series.
  - More than 500 errors on the Farnsworth-Munsell 100 Hue test.
- Electroretinography:
  - Absent or very low recordings of components that are cone-mediated, including dark-adapted cone-mediated x wave, 30-Hz flicker, and photopic responses.
  - Slight to moderate loss of rod function is variably present.

Pathology

- Histologic examinations of affected eyes are rare.
- One case showed complete absence of the outer layer of rods and cones, with marked pigment changes of the RPE and atrophy of the optic disk.

Disease Course

- Highly variable age of onset and severity among individuals, even within same family.
- Typically, the disease manifests in the first two decades, with progressive loss of vision thereafter, sometimes to hand motion.
- Color vision is severely affected when VA reaches 20/60 range.

Treatment and Management

- No effective treatment.
- Genetic studies and visual screening may help identify affected family members. (Some forms have ABCA4 mutation. Cure may eventually come from process blocking lipofuscin buildup or advances in gene therapy.)

Medications

None proven effective.

Differential Diagnosis

- Other macular dystrophies, including Stargardt disease, in which the photopic ERG is still normal.
- Hereditary optic atrophy may require FA, color vision testing, and ERG to differentiate.
- End-stage disease may resemble RP.
- Bull's-eye maculopathy may be seen with chloroquine use.

Reference

Krill AE, Deutman AF. Dominant macular degenerations: the cone dystrophies. *Am J Ophthalmol* 1972;73:352–369.

Albinism

Summary

Oculocutaneous albinism is a hereditary pigmentary dilution of the skin, the skin and eyes, or the eyes alone in which congenitally decreased VA and nystagmus may occur.

Etiology/Genetics

All types of oculocutaneous albinism are characterized by reduction in the amount of melanin within each pigment organelle or melanosome. Gene mutations during tyrosinase production, processing, or melanosome growth and maturation. OCA2 is the most common mutation occurring in 1 in 15,000 people. X-linked mutation in GPR143 gene (G protein–coupled receptor) is mapped to Xp22.3. This is an important part of signaling pathway for growth melanosomes, and more than 60 mutations thus far have been described.

Signs and Symptoms

- Two clinical patterns are found:
  1. Congenitally subnormal VA and nystagmus (typical).
  2. Normal or minimally affected acuity without nystagmus (albinoid).
- Photophobia.
- Pink reflex through undilated pupil.
- Iris transillumination.
- Decreased pigmentation of hair and skin.

Demographics

- Most types share autosomal recessive inheritance, but some are X-linked or autosomal dominant. (See genetics, above.)
- In X-linked cases, female carriers may have partial iris transillumination or patchy retinal hypopigmentation.

Ophthalmic Findings

- Hypoplasia of the macula with abnormal vascular patterns in typical albinism.
- Normal macula may be seen in albinoidism.
- No visible foveal reflex and no macula lutea pigment.
- Choroidal vessels are easily seen.

Systemic Findings

- Decreased or absent pigmentation of eyes, skin, and hair.
- Association of oculocutaneous albinism with Chédiak-Higashi syndrome, a lysosomal defect that impairs neutrophil function and confers extreme susceptibility to bacterial infections.
- Association with Hermansky-Pudlak syndrome, characterized by a platelet defect that may cause easy bruising and excessive bleeding.

Special Tests

Bleeding time recommended before anticipated surgeries.

Pathology

- Absence of foveal differentiation without melanin pigment in all structures.
- RPE distention by lipofuscin.

Disease Course

- Congenital onset.
- Variable severity (mild form of “albinoidism” vs. typical severe pattern).

Treatment and Management

Tinted glasses may reduce photophobia.
Low-vision aids.
Genetic counseling.
If associated Chédiak-Higashi or Hermansky-Pudlak syndromes are suspected, hematology consultation should be obtained.

Medications

None effective.

Differential Diagnosis

Blond fundus (normal variant): choroidal vessels easily seen through lightly pigmented retina, but fovea is not hypoplastic, foveal reflex is intact and vision may be normal.

Reference

Witkop CJ Jr, Quevedo WC Jr, Fitzpatrick TB, et al. Albinism. In: Scriver CR, Beaudet AL, Sly WS, et al., eds. *The metabolic basis of inherited disease*, 6th ed., vol. 2. New York, NY: McGraw-Hill, 1989:2905–2947.

Oguchi Disease

Summary

Oguchi disease is a rare autosomal recessive variant of CSNB in which there is a prominent funduscopic abnormality. In the light-adapted state, the fundus is diffuse yellow or gray and changes to normal color in the dark-adapted state (the Mizuo phenomenon) thought to be caused by overstimulation of rods).

Etiology/Genetics

- Disease is related to an abnormality of the bipolar cell network.
- SAG gene (2p37.1) codes for arrestin (S-antigen) and also rhodpsin kinase gene abnormalities have been reported.

Signs and Symptoms

Night blindness.
May present with nystagmus.

Demographics

- Congenital, presents in childhood with equal sex distribution.
- More common in Japanese population.
- Parental consanguinity may be found.

Ophthalmic Findings

- Distinguished from other types of CSNB by peculiar gray-white metallic discoloration of retina in the light-adapted state.
- Vessels stand out in marked relief against the background, and the macula appears abnormally dark.
- After prolonged dark adaptation, the retina appears perfectly normal.

Systemic Findings

None.

Special Tests

- ERG shows normal cone response.
- Abortive rod response reduced in amplitude and increased in latency.
- Dark adaptation: After prolonged adaptation, most patients show a slow fall in threshold until normal levels are reached.

Pathology

- Few histologic studies have been performed in patients, but there appears to be an abnormal layer between the RPE and the photoreceptors.
- Outer segments of both rod and cone receptors have abnormal microvacuoles or tubular internal structures instead of normal lamellae.

Disease Course

Stationary, not progressive.
Loss of night vision.
VA may remain normal.

Treatment and Management

Genetic counseling.
Low-vision aids.

Medications

None effective.

Differential Diagnosis

CSNB with normal fundus.
RP.
LCA.

Reference

Mizuo G. On a new discovery in the dark adaptation on Oguchi's disease. *Acta Soc Ophthalmol Jpn* 1913;17:1148.

Congenital Stationary Night Blindness

Summary

CSNB is a group of hereditary disorders characterized by a loss of dark adaptation or a markedly prolonged adaptation capability that leaves cone function largely intact.

Etiology

- CSNB has been classified based on the following:
  - By inheritance pattern (Table 3.12).
  - By fundus appearance:
    - Normal.
    - Abnormal.
  - By characteristic ERG findings:
    - Absent scotopic ERG (type I).
    - Negative ERG (type II).
- The more common CSNB with normal fundi is described below:
  - Type I results from a defect in photoreceptor transduction, not a defect in rhodopsin or an absence of rods.
  - Type II results from abnormal neural transmission.
- Genetic locus (Table 3.13).

Table 3.12

Inheritance of CSNB

Type	Inheritance
Nougaret	Autosomal dominant
Riggs	Autosomal recessive (without myopia)
Schubert-Bornschein	Autosomal recessive or X-linked with myopia
Oguchi	Autosomal recessive
Fundus albipunctatus	Autosomal recessive

Table 3.13

Genetic locus of CSNB

Type of CSNB	Chromosome	Gene product
Autosomal dominant	4p16.3	PDE6Beta
Autosomal recessive	5p35.3	GRM6
	11q1Beta	CABP4
	13q.34	GRK1
X-linked recessive	Xp11.4	CSNB4
	Xp11.23	CACNA1F

Source: RetNet.

Signs and Symptoms

- Congenital onset of night blindness.
- VA ranges from normal to 20/200, often with myopia.
- Children may present with nystagmus.

Demographics

Varies with type of CSNB.
Congenital onset.
Young male and female patients affected.

Ophthalmic Findings

Fundus appearance of CSNB patients is normal, except in certain types (see below).

Systemic Findings

None.

Special Tests

ERG: normal or nearly normal cone responses.

Pathology

Few histologic studies, but findings indicate normal pattern and proportion of rods and cones, suggesting a functional abnormality in neural transmission and not a defect in photoreceptor structure.

Disease Course

- Disease is stationary, not progressive.
- Long-term visual prognosis is good.

Treatment and Management

- Patients should be introduced to the night vision pocket scope, which may improve vision at night.
- Low-vision consultation.
- Genetic counseling may be helpful.

Differential Diagnosis

- RP can be differentiated by abnormal funduscopic appearance, clinical course, and visual-field loss and by ERG, which shows loss of both rod and cone signals.

- LCA: Nystagmus may be similar, but ERG responses are lost from both rods and cones. Hyperopia is common. Most cases are autosomal recessive.

References

Berson EL. Retinitis pigmentosa and allied diseases. In: Albert DM, Jakobiec FA, eds. *Principles and practice of ophthalmology*, vol. 2. Philadelphia, PA: WB Saunders, 1994:1227–1232.

Carr RE. Abnormalities of cone and rod function. In: Ryan SJ, ed. *Retina*, vol. 1. St. Louis, MO: Mosby, 1994:506–508.

Fundus Albipunctatus

Summary

Fundus albipunctatus is a form of recessively inherited CSNB in which there are yellow-white deposits in the peripheral deep retina and delayed dark adaptation.

Etiology/Genetics

- Patients have a delay in rod and cone visual pigment regeneration.
- This defect is likely to be secondary to an abnormality in the relationship between the photoreceptors and the pigment epithelium.

*Candidate gene RDH5 is located on 12q13.2, and affected protein is an RPE microsomal enzyme (11 cis retinol dehydrogenase 5).

Signs and Symptoms

Night blindness.
VA is normal.

Demographics

Congenital.
Presents in childhood with equal sex distribution.
Parental consanguinity may be found.

Ophthalmic Findings

- Multiple yellow-white spots located deep in the retina, most dense in the posterior pole and more scattered toward the periphery.
- Macula is spared.
- Over time, the yellow-white flecks seen in early childhood may mature to punctate dots that increase in number.

Systemic Findings

None.

Special Tests

- Dark adaptation: Patients attain normal dark-adapted final thresholds if dark adapted for a sufficiently long period.
- ERG responses follow the course of dark adaptation: There is a delay in reaching the full amplitude of the ERG.

Pathology

No histopathologic studies have been conducted in patients with this condition.

Disease Course

Stationary, not progressive, night blindness.
VA remains normal.
Several cases of spontaneous resolution of night blindness have been reported.

Treatment and Management

- Reported association with vitamin A deficiency is controversial.
- Same as CSNB.

Medications

Not effective.

Differential Diagnosis

- RPA: The lesions of fundus albipunctatus do not appear atrophic as they do in RPA.
- Vitamin A deficiency retinopathy: small, irregular, coalescent whitish-yellow deposits, deep in midperipheral retina, associated with visual-field constriction and night blindness.

Reference

Marmor MF. Long-term follow-up of the physiologic abnormalities and fundus changes in fundus albipunctatus. *Ophthalmology* 1990;97:380–384.

Choroideremia

Summary

Choroideremia is an X-linked recessive inherited degeneration of the choriocapillaris, photoreceptors, and RPE affecting male patients, which causes night blindness and loss of vision.

Etiology

- The CHM gene is located on the long arm of the X chromosome at Xq21.2.
- The corresponding gene is expressed in the retina, choroid, and RPE. The gene product is geranylgeranyl transferase Rab-escort protein 1. Rab geranylgeranyl catalyzes the attachment of geranylgeranyl isoprenoids to Rab guanine triphosphatases, which are key regulators in vesicular transport.

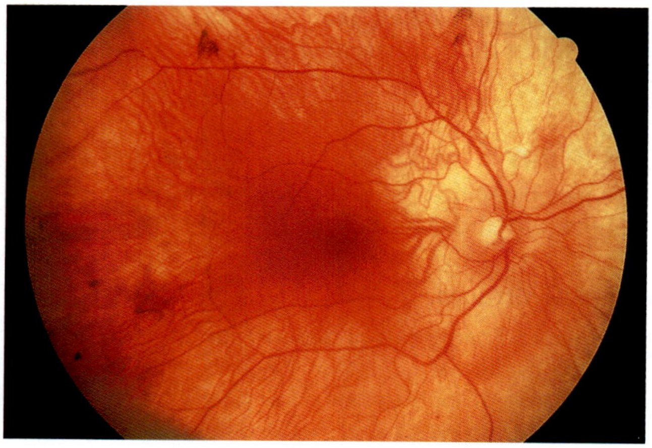

FIGURE 3.51. Choroideremia. Extensive RPE and choroidal atrophy are present.

Signs and Symptoms

- Night blindness in male patients, aged 4 to 30 years.
- Normal VA in childhood with gradual loss of central vision to hand-motion range.
- Gradual loss of peripheral vision (progression of disease continues throughout life).

Demographics

- Male children and young adults are affected.
- Female patients may be asymptomatic carriers with mild funduscopic changes.

Ophthalmic Findings

See Figure 3.51.

- At an early stage, there is granularity and deep pigmentation of the RPE in the peripheral retina.
  With loss of the RPE, choroidal vessels are at first prominent but eventually disappear.
  Macula is spared until about age 30 years.
- Later, extensive choroidal atrophy and clumped pigment appear.
- Female carriers may have midperipheral minor RPE atrophy, migration of pigment into deeper retinal layers, and peripheral radial pigment clumping.

Systemic Findings

None.

Special Tests

ERG: Both rod and cone signals are reduced in amplitude with delays in b-wave implicit time. In more advanced stages, ERGs are undetectable, and dark-adaptation thresholds are increased.

Pathology

- Studies have revealed extensive choroidal atrophy.
- Choroidal remnants are located at the macula and the ora serrata.
- RPE and photoreceptors may have diffuse atrophy.
- Bruch membrane may be disrupted, and gliosis may extend into the choroid.

Disease Course

- Night blindness is often the presenting complaint.
- Gradual, severe, peripheral vision loss follows with progressive loss of central VA.

Treatment and Management

- No effective treatment is currently available. There is genetic testing available through Dr. Ian McDonald, University of Alberta, Edmonton, Canada.
- May be helpful to wear darkly tinted sunglasses to alleviate symptoms.
- Genetic counseling may be valuable.

Medications

None effective.

Differential Diagnosis

- RP: Generally, choroid atrophy is not seen and bone spicules of pigment are found on fundus examination.
- Gyrate atrophy:
  Will see scalloped RPE and choriocapillaris atrophy.
  May have high myopia with astigmatism, posterior subcapsular cataract, and hyperornithinemia.
- Thioridazine retinopathy: pigment clumps between posterior pole and equator with areas of depigmentation and visual-field abnormalities. History of more than 800 mg/day.
- Albinism: a blond fundus without RPE clumping. Choroidal vasculature is easily seen, absent foveal reflex and iris transillumination defects may be present.

Reference

McCulloch C. Choroideremia: a clinical and pathologic review. *Trans Am Ophthalmol Soc* 1969;67:142–195.

Tan KT, Guiu-Rozas E, Bon RS, et al. Design, synthesis, and characterization of peptide-based rab geranylgeranyl transferase inhibitors. *J Med Chem* 2009;52(24):8025–8037.

Gyrate Atrophy

Summary

Gyrate atrophy of the choroid and retina is an autosomal recessive disorder caused by reduced activity of ornithine aminotransferase. Patients with gyrate atrophy have myopia, night blindness, and progressive peripheral visual-field loss.

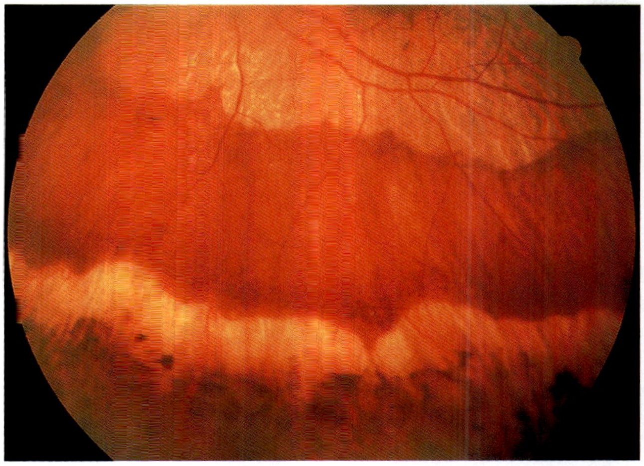

FIGURE 3.52 Peripheral scalloped areas of RPE atrophy in gyrate atrophy.

Etiology/Genetics

Autosomal recessive ornithine aminotransferase deficiency.
OAT Gene located on 10q26.13. Gene product ornithine aminotransferase.
Plasma ornithine levels are significantly increased.

Signs and Symptoms

Night blindness.
Loss of peripheral vision by age 10 years, progressing to tunnel vision and blindness by age 50 years.
Myopia.

Demographics

Presentation in childhood.
No sex predilection.

Ophthalmic Findings

See Figure 3-52.

- RPE atrophy starting in midperiphery.
- Sharply circumscribed areas of fundal atrophy with scalloped margins that enlarge and become confluent.
- Retinal vessels are markedly attenuated.
- Late in the disease, optic atrophy may ensue.

Systemic Findings

Elevation of serum ornithine levels.
Hypolysinemia.
Hyperornithinuria.
Seizures in some patients.

Special Tests

- Serum amino acid measurements for ornithine and lysine.
- Small or nondetectable full-field ERG.

Pathology

- An abrupt transition from near-normal retina to zones of near-total atrophy of retina and RPE is present.
- Mitochondrial abnormalities are seen in photoreceptors, corneal endothelium, and iris pigment epithelium.

Disease Course

Progressive loss of vision.
Blindness by age 50 years is usual.

Treatment and Management

- Supplemental vitamin B_6 (pyridoxine) may be effective in some patients.
- Low-protein, low-arginine diet may be effective in decreasing plasma ornithine levels.
- Reducing serum ornithine may improve long-term visual outcome.

Medications

Vitamin B_6 may be useful.

Follow-Up

- Frequent serum ornithine levels are obtained initially to assess response to dose of vitamin B_6 and degree and effectiveness of dietary protein restriction.
- Serum ornithine levels of 0.15 to 0.20 mmol are optimal.

Differential Diagnosis

Choroideremia.
RP.
Thioridazine retinopathy.

Reference

Kaiser-Kupfer MI, Caruso RC, Valle D. Gyrate atrophy of the choroid and retina: long-term reduction of ornithine slows retinal degeneration. *Arch Ophthalmol* 1991;109:1539–1548.

Central Areolar Choroidal Dystrophy

Summary

Central areolar choroidal dystrophy is an autosomal dominant disorder in which there is circumscribed atrophy of the RPE and choriocapillaris in the foveal region.

Etiology/Genetics

The gene CACD is mapped to 17p13. There are also reported mutations in PPH2 gene and a point mutation in the RDS peripherin 2 gene. The pathogenesis may be defect in adhesion molecule involved in stabilization and compaction of outer disk segments.

Signs and Symptoms

- VA is normal early in life.
- Starting at age 40 years, patients have loss of VA that is associated with loss of pigmentation of RPE.

Demographics

Clinical onset at middle age and equal sex ratio.

Ophthalmic Findings

- Early RPE mottling in macula.
- Gradual development of symmetric, well-defined areas of geographic atrophy of the RPE, with underlying larger choroidal vessels visible.
- No drusen, myopia, serous or hemorrhagic disciform detachment of the RPE or inflammation of the choroid.

Systemic Findings

None.

Special Tests

- IVFA shows hyperfluorescence corresponding to the areas of pigment epithelial atrophy.
- Choroidal vessels are outlined by fluorescein, and hyperfluorescence is seen at the edges of the lesion indicating dye leakage from intact choroidal capillaries.
- ERG is typically normal.

Pathology

- Well-demarcated avascular zone that is atrophic and fibrotic.
- Normal vessels.
- The outer retinal layer including the RPE is absent in areas with underlying atrophy of the choroid.

Disease Course

- As the area of atrophy increases, VA falls to count-fingers range in both eyes.
- The disease has variable expression.

Treatment and Management

No treatment is shown to be effective.

Medications

None effective.

Differential Diagnosis

Toxoplasmosis.
ARMD.
Stargardt disease.

Reference

Ferry AP, Llovera I, Shafer DM. Central areolar choroidal dystrophy. *Arch Ophthalmol* 1972;88:39–43.

Pattern Dystrophies of the RPE

Summary

This group of heritable disorders is characterized by relatively good vision in the first five decades of life, a pattern of granular or reticular yellow-white or dark pigment at the level of the RPE, and the absence of drusen.

Etiology/Genetics

- Type of inheritance varies by type of dystrophy.
- Butterfly dystrophy is autosomal dominant, characterized by pigment deposits radiating from the fovea in a pattern reminiscent of the butterfly's wings. Associated with mutation BSMD at 5q21.2 in peripherin /RDS gene.
- Sjögren reticular dystrophy is an autosomal recessive disease characterized by a network of pigmented lines surrounding the macula and extending peripherally.
- Adult Vitelliform Dystrophy reported defect in RDS gene at 6p.21.1 in peripherin 2 protein.

Signs and Symptoms

- Patients present with slightly decreased VA or mild metamorphopsia.
- Patients may be asymptomatic.

Demographics

Presents in early adulthood.
Both sexes are affected equally.

Ophthalmic Findings

- Yellowish-white or darkly pigmented, symmetric lesions often in the center of the macula.
- Sometimes the lesions are eccentric.
- May be yellowish deposits in the outer retina, often with a central area of hyperpigmentation, occasionally surrounded by a circinate pattern of hyperpigmentation (bull's-eye maculopathy).

Systemic Findings

None.

Special Tests

ERG: Cone and rods amplitudes are unaffected.

IVFA: Central blocked fluorescence on angiography corresponds to pigment clumping at the level of the RPE, surrounded by hyperfluorescence corresponding to yellowish material. There is no leakage, confirming the absence of CNV.

Pathology

No histopathologic studies have been conducted.

Disease Course

While VA may be minimally affected early in the disease course, vision loss becomes marked as atrophy ensues, usually by midlife.

Treatment and Management

No treatment has been shown to be effective.

Some place patients on antioxidants (Age-Related Eye Disease Study I) but data are lacking to support efficacy in this disorder.

Medications

None effective.

Differential Diagnosis

Stargardt disease: Clinical course is accelerated and more severe; atrophy in Stargardt's disease may be outside the macula.

ARMD: usually multifocal, preservation of the fovea until very late stage; typical occurrence at the ages of 70 to 90.

Bull's-eye maculopathy: a common finding in cone dystrophy, fundus flavimaculatus, and chloroquine maculopathy; differentiation depends on history and clinical course.

Reference

Marmor MF, McNamara JA. Pattern dystrophy of the retinal pigment epithelium and geographic atrophy of the macula. *Am J Ophthalmol* 1996;122:382–392.

Metabolic Diseases

Cherry-Red Spot

Summary

A cherry-red spot at the fovea may be observed in several hereditary metabolic diseases in which abnormal metabolic products accumulate in the ganglion cells that surround the fovea.

These disorders include Tay-Sachs disease (G_{M2} gangliosidosis type I), Sandhoff disease (G_{M2} gangliosidosis type II), generalized gangliosidosis (G_{M1} gangliosidosis type I), mucolipidosis type I, and the cherry-red spot–myoclonus syndrome.

Etiology

Each storage disease has a specific enzyme defect that leads to abnormal accumulation of material in the retinal ganglion cells which may destroy them or at least impede their normal function (Table 3 14).

Tay-Sachs disease:

- Leads to glycolipid accumulation (G_{M2} ganglioside) in the neuronal lysosomes of the retina and brain and to blindness, mental retardation, and death by age 5 years.
- Typically, affected children are of Ashkenazi Jewish or French-Canadian ancestry.

Demographics

Autosomal recessive inheritance.

Affects patients early in life.

Ophthalmic Findings

- Cherry-red spot in the fovea and the parafovea. Over time, it disappears as VA declines. Cherry-red spot is seen because of the higher density of ganglion cells in the parafoveal areas compared to fovea. In the foveola, where there are normally no ganglion cells, the reddish color of the underlying choroid is visible.
- Optic atrophy is end result.

Special Tests

- Each storage disease has a specific enzyme deficiency.
- Diagnostic testing involves serum or leukocyte enzyme assays.

Pathology

Tay-Sachs disease:

- Ganglioside material accumulates in neuronal tissues of brain and retina.
- Retinal ganglion cells are distended and stain positively for lipids.

Disease Course

Tay-Sachs disease: progressive vision loss and mental retardation; death by age 6 years.

Treatment and Management

- Genetic counseling can be useful to identify carriers of the trait.
- No treatment has been found to be effective.

Reference

Swartz M. Other diseases: drug toxicity and metabolic and nutritional conditions. In: Ryan SJ, ed. *Retina*, vol. 2. St. Louis, MO: Mosby, 1994:1762–1763.

Mucopolysaccharidosis

Summary

The mucopolysaccharidoses (MPS) are a group of inherited diseases of metabolism in which enzyme deficiencies within lysosomes result in tissue deposits of glycosaminoglycans,

RETINA

Table 3.14

Differential diagnosis and etiology of a cherry-red spot in the macula

Condition	Cause
Tay-Sachs disease	Hexosaminidase A enzyme deficiency
Sandhoff disease	Hexosaminidase A and B enzyme deficiency
Generalized gangliosidosis	Beta-galactosidase enzyme deficiency
Mucolipidosis type I	Neuraminidase enzyme deficiency
Cherry-red spot–myoclonus syndrome	Neuraminidase enzyme deficiency
Central retinal artery occlusion	Interruption of inner retinal blood supply: • Ganglion cell death causes retinal opacification • Foveola preserved choriocapillaris perfusion

an incompletely degraded type of mucopolysaccharide. Corneal clouding, retinal pigment degeneration, and optic nerve atrophy may result.

Etiology

Inborn errors of mucopolysaccharide degradation lead to accumulation of excessive quantities of incompletely metabolized acid mucopolysaccharides and complex lipids in lysosomes within various structures of the eye.

Signs and Symptoms

- Decreased vision.
- Coarse facial features.
- Mental retardation is common.
- Corneal clouding, depending on MPS subtype.

Demographics

- All MPS variants have autosomal recessive inheritance except MPS type II (Hunter syndrome), which is X-linked recessive.
- No sex predilection, except for Hunter syndrome, which exclusively affects males.

Ophthalmic Findings

- Four of the variants of mucopolysaccharidosis involve heparan sulfate storage, and only these MPS variants are associated with retinal dystrophy (pigmentary retinopathy):
  MPS I-H (Hurler syndrome).
  MPS I-S (Scheie syndrome).
  MPS II (Hunter syndrome).
  MPS III (Sanfilippo syndrome).
- Retinal pigmentary degeneration is characteristic, with RPE migration into the midperipheral retina in a perivascular location, giving the retina a bone-spicule appearance.
- Optic atrophy occurs late.

Systemic Findings

- Mental retardation is common.
- Coarse facial features.
- Short stature is common.
- Organomegaly (e.g., hepatomegaly) and heart disease, depending on type.

Special Tests

- ERG shows a pattern similar to rod-cone dystrophy in types I, II, and III.
- Electron microscopy of conjunctival biopsy specimen may be helpful in initial evaluation of patients suspected to have a systemic MPS.

Pathology

- Increased amounts of mucopolysaccharide can be seen in corneal tissue, producing variable clouding.
- Retinal pigment degeneration occurs with RPE migration into midperipheral retinal locations in a perivascular distribution pattern, giving a spiculated retinal appearance: RPE accumulation of mucopolysaccharide probably leads to photoreceptor cell death.

Disease Course

- Variable, depending on type and severity.
- Patients may have a normal lifespan or die in childhood.

Treatment and Management

Systemic: No effective treatment is known.

Ocular: For MPS variants involving corneal clouding, corneal transplant has been performed, but long-term visual success of this approach remains unknown.

Medications

Lifelong enzyme replacement therapy is available (laronidase for MPS Type I and idursulfase for MPS Type II) that may help mitigate systemic complications and corneal clouding (laronidase in MPS Type I).

Differential Diagnosis

RP: Spiculated appearance of retina may appear similar, but clinical picture, course, and pathophysiology distinguish the disease.

CRAO: This must be differentiated from the cherry-red spot appearance of the macula observed in a case of an acute CRAO, which would be very rare in the younger age group typically observed in patients with metabolic diseases with ophthalmic manifestations.

Reference

Neufeld EF, Muenzer J. The mucopolysaccharidoses. In: Schriver CR, Beaudet AL, Sly WS, et al., eds. *The metabolic basis of inherited disease*. New York, NY: McGraw Hill, 1989:1565.

Sphingolipidoses

Summary

This group of inherited disorders is characterized by various defects in sphingosine-containing glycolipid metabolism. Toxic metabolic intermediary products accumulate in neural and sometimes visceral tissues. Several diseases are briefly described below:

- Tay-Sachs disease.
- Niemann-Pick disease:
  Autosomal recessive sphingomyelinase deficiency in which sphingomyelin accumulates in various organs.
  In the eye, a cherry-red spot and subtle corneal opacity may be seen in more than 50% of patients.
- Fabry disease:
  X-linked alpha-galactosidase A deficiency.
  In the eye, leads to superficial corneal opacity, anterior lens capsular deposits, conjunctival aneurysmal dilations, and retinal vascular tortuosity in affected male patients.
- Gaucher disease:
  Autosomal recessive glucocerebrosidase deficiency.
  Produces white spots beneath the retina, probably clusters of lipid-laden histiocytes, and sometimes a cherry-red spot.

Special Tests

Each disease is diagnosed by assaying specific enzymatic activity from tissue samples.

Disease Course

Highly variable, depending on type and degree of enzyme deficiency, but ranges from severe mental retardation and death by age 5 years for a severe form of Niemann-Pick disease to relatively good health and normal VA into adulthood for less severe forms.

Treatment and Medications

None clinically effective.

Differential Diagnosis (Disorders Characterized by Cherry-Red Spot)

CRAO.
Hexosaminidase A and B deficiency (Sandhoff disease).
β-Galactosidase deficiency.
Neuraminidase deficiency.

Reference

O'Brien JS. The gangliosidoses. In: Stanbury JB, Wyngaarden JB, Fredrickson DS, et al., eds. *The metabolic basis of inherited disease*. New York, NY: McGraw-Hill, 1983.

Cystinosis

Summary

Cystinosis is an autosomal recessive disorder of lysosome storage in which cystine accumulates because of a defect in its transport mechanism out of lysosomes. The disease frequently presents in late infancy with growth retardation, progressive renal failure, hypothyroidism, and retinopathy.

Etiology

- Cystine crystals accumulate in various tissues because of defective cystine transport from lysosomes.
- Crystals have been observed in the iris, choroid, ciliary body, conjunctiva, and RPE.

Signs and Symptoms

- No significant visual disturbance.
- Mild photophobia.
- Corneal and conjunctival deposits are visible.

Demographics

There are three clinical patterns that vary in onset and severity.

1. Childhood type: most common type; characterized by onset in infancy and death before puberty.
2. Adolescent type: onset during first or second decade characterized by mild nephropathy, diminished life expectancy, and corneal and conjunctival crystal deposits.
3. Benign or adult type: onset in late teens to early fifties characterized by mild photophobia without ophthalmoscopic abnormalities and normal life expectancy.

Ophthalmic Findings

- Corneal crystals.
- Posterior synechiae.
- Patchy RPE depigmentation interspersed with pigment clumps.
- Retinal hemorrhages.

Systemic Findings (Childhood Type)

- Renal failure: Cystinois is the number one cause of Fanconi syndrome in children.
- Hypothyroidism.
- Growth retardation.
- Renal rickets.

Special Tests

- Cystine crystals may be demonstrated in frozen tissue biopsy specimens by polarized light.
- Measure free cystine content in leukocytes.

Pathology

Cystine crystals found throughout ocular tissues, rarely in neurosensory retina.

Disease Course

- Childhood type:
  Glare disability may require corneal transplantation.
  Death before puberty is typical, but visual disturbances are rare.
- Adolescent type:
  Mild nephropathy.
  Near-normal life expectancy without visual disturbances.
- Benign, adult type:
  Normal vision and life expectancy.

Treatment and Management

Disabling glare may result from corneal and lenticular deposits requiring corneal transplantation, although crystals may reaccumulate in donor graft.

Medications

- Topical cysteamine therapy reduces corneal crystals and photophobia in childhood cystinosis.
- Early systemic cysteamine reduces intracellular cystine and has been shown to improve renal function.

Reference

Cogan DG, Kuwabara T. Ocular pathology of cystinosis. *Arch Ophthalmol* 1960;63:75.

PERIPHERAL RETINAL ABNORMALITIES

Posterior Vitreous Detachment

Summary

Separation of vitreous from disk and posterior pole following vitreous liquefaction or trauma.

Etiology

Degenerative: The vitreous is composed primarily of water, collagen, and hyaluronic acid. With age or injury, the vitreous tends to liquefy and contract.

Hereditary vitreoretinal dystrophy.
Trauma: Rapid anteroposterior decompression of the eye exerts forces on the vitreoretinal interface that can induce a separation of the posterior hyaloid.
Postsurgical: Morphologic changes in the eye following cataract surgery, for example, allow the vitreous to migrate anteriorly to fill the void created by the absence of the crystalline lens.
May be seen following uveitis.
Following VH.

Signs and Symptoms

- Flashes ("lightning bolts" in the peripheral visual field).
- Floaters ("cobwebs" or "bugs" in the peripheral vision or a solitary large ring-like appearance in the central or paracentral visual field).
- May have blurred vision.

Demographics

- Age: seen more frequently after age 50 years.
- No sex predilection.
- High myopes more commonly affected.

Ophthalmic Findings

- Vitreous condensation and liquefaction.
- Weiss ring (annulus of vitreous condensation from around optic nerve).
- Intraretinal hemorrhage.
- VH: Presence with an acute PVD is highly associated with retinal breaks.

Systemic Findings

None.

Special Tests

B-scan ultrasonography: may be helpful in showing complete or partial PVD.

Pathology

Liquefaction of water-bound matrix, condensation of collagen fibril network.

Disease Course

Acute, symptomatic PVD, is associated with approximately a 15% risk of a retinal break, and this risk increases to nearly 70% if a VH is also present.

Treatment and Management

- No specific treatment for an acute PVD is indicated. The goal is to rule out the presence of a retinal break or a RD. This is achieved through evaluation of peripheral retina with scleral depression–assisted visualization to the ora serrata for 360 degrees to search for retinal tears or RD.
- Encircling laser retinopexy or cryopexy for retinal tears to reduce risk of RD.

Medications

None.

Follow-Up

Reevaluate an acute symptomatic PVD patient within several weeks if no retinal tears are found on initial examination. A chronic asymptomatic PVD that is found on routine examination in the elderly population requires no specific targeted follow-up.

Differential Diagnosis

RD: If there is significant VH obscuring views of the retina, B scan ultrasonography may help discern PVD (low to medium signal intensity on A-scan) versus RD (high signal intensity on A-scan). Migraine headache with a preceding aura (scintillating migratory scotomata) or an ocular migraine (visual aura alone without headache) can also simulate a PVD; however, they are generally not associated with persistent floaters after the aura subsides.

References

Hikichi T, Trempe CL. Relationship between floaters, light flashes, or both, and complications of posterior vitreous detachment. *Am J Ophthalmol* 1994;117:593–598.

Kakehashi A, Kado M, Akiba J, et al. Variations of posterior vitreous detachment. *Br J Ophthalmol* 1997;81:527–532.

Lattice Degeneration

Summary

Peripheral retinal degeneration with variable appearance of retinal thinning with white radial or circumferentially oriented sclerotic vessels and abnormally firm vitreoretinal attachment at these sites. Commonly observed in the asymptomatic general population but also be observed in as much as 30% of patients with RD.

Etiology

Possibly hereditary (multifactorial inheritance).

Sign and Symptoms

Asymptomatic.

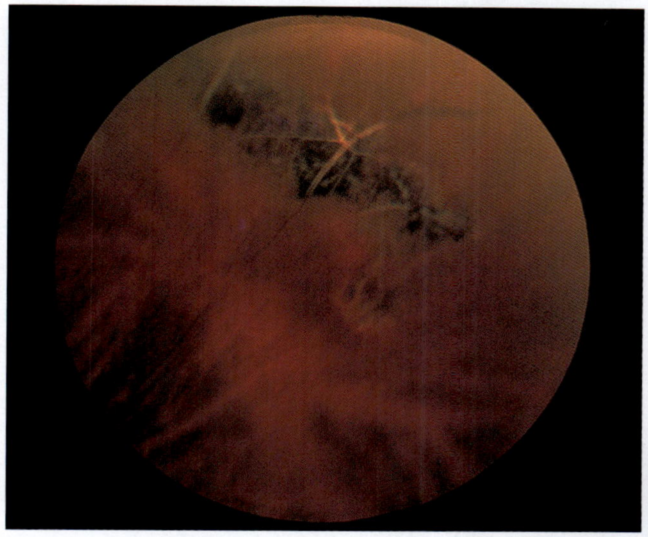

FIGURE 3.53. Lattice degeneration with sclerotic vessels forming white lattice lines.

Demographics

Present in 7% to 10% of general population.
Forty-five percent of cases have bilateral involvement.
No sex predilection.
Commonly observed in high myopes.

Ophthalmic Findings

See Figure 3.53.

- Circumferential retinal thinning with overlying vitreous liquefaction.
- Usually located anterior to equator.
- White lines branching across lesion: sclerotic vessels.
- Atrophic retinal holes are often found within or adjacent to a patch of lattice: These are not considered a great risk factor for RD and can be observed.
- Focal retinal thinning and pigment changes.

Systemic Findings

None.

Special Tests

Indirect ophthalmoscopic examination of the peripheral retina with scleral depression.

Pathology

- Lattice lines are small, thickened retinal vessels.
- Inner retinal thinning and degeneration in area of lattice.
- Liquefied vitreous overlying lesion, adherent vitreous at margins.
- Hypertrophy or hyperplasia of RPE.

Disease Course

Lesions tend to remain stable. Tractional retinal tears may develop in area of vitreoretinal adhesion along margins of lattice lesion.

Treatment and Management

- Observation: Less than 0.5% are felt to be a direct contributor to RD pathogenesis, although patches of lattice are commonly seen in eyes that have an RD.
- Prophylactic therapy not indicated for lattice with associated atrophic holes, since there is such a low risk for progression to RD and unnecessary laser may later induce a secondary epiretinal membrane.
- If patient has had prior RD, family history of RD, or aphakia, consider prophylactic photocoagulation or cryopexy.
- Prophylactic therapy if a symptomatic retinal break is also observed.
- Scleral buckling procedure with or without vitrectomy for RD.

Medications

None.

Follow-Up

Routine dilated funduscopic examination with indirect ophthalmoscopy and scleral depression.

Differential Diagnosis

Peripheral microcystic degeneration: no lattice lines, may develop schisis cavities.

Linear lesions of ocular histoplasmosis: also see peripapillary pigment ring, punched-out chorioretinal lesions.

References

Byer NE. Lattice degeneration of the retina. *Surv Ophthalmol* 1978;23:213–248.

Byer NE. Long-term natural history of lattice degeneration of the retina. *Ophthalmology* 1989;96:1396–1401.

Cobblestone Degeneration (Paving Stone Degeneration)

Summary

Age-related peripheral chorioretinal atrophy due to relative ischemia of areas of outer retina.

Etiology

Unknown.

Signs and Symptoms

Asymptomatic.

Demographics

Over age 20 years without sex predilection.

Ophthalmic Findings

- Discrete round patches of chorioretinal atrophy in the retinal periphery.
- Sharp, scalloped borders.
- May be surrounded by rim of RPE hypertrophy (a dark rim surrounding atrophy).
- Does not predispose to retinal breaks or RD.

Systemic Findings

None.

Special Tests

None.

Pathology

Outer retinal atrophy.

Underlying RPE and choriocapillaris atrophy.

Adhesion of inner retina to Bruch membrane.

Disease Course

Stable, minimally progressive lesions. Does not have any visual sequelae.

Treatment

None.

Medications

None.

Follow-Up

Routine examination.

Reference

O'Malley P, Allen RA, Straatsma BR, et al. Paving-stone degeneration of the retina. *Arch Ophthalmol* 1965;73:169.

Retinal Tears and Holes

Summary

Full-thickness retinal break (horseshoe-shaped tear or round holes) due to focal vitreoretinal traction.

Etiology

PVD.

Vitreoretinal adhesions and traction (vitreoretinal tufts).

Lattice degeneration.

Trauma, previous intraocular surgery.

YAG laser posterior capsulotomy.

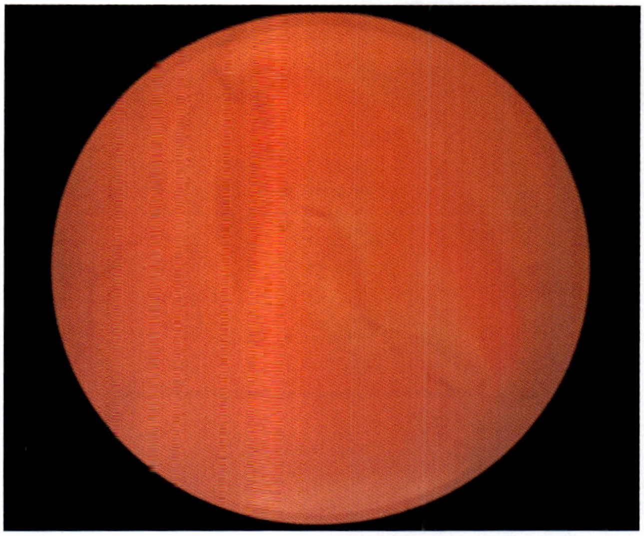

FIGURE 3.54. Horseshoe-shaped retinal tear with bridging vessel.

Demographics

- Observed in up to 15% of acute, symptomatic PVD cases at presentation.
- Patients with hereditary vitreoretinal dystrophies or family history of RD.
- Moderate to high myopia frequently associated.
- Retinal tear or detachment in fellow eye.
- Aphakia, pseudophakia, and an open posterior lens capsule are risk factors.

Signs and Symptoms

- Flashes due to vitreoretinal traction.
- Floaters due to PVD creation or VH.
- Decreased vision due to Weiss ring, VH, or RD.

Ophthalmic Findings

See Figure 3.54.

- Vitreous syneresis or PVD may cause retinal traction.
- Pigment cells in vitreous.
- Horseshoe-shaped tear (HST), round hole, operculated hole.
- May have lattice degeneration.
- May have cystic retinal tufts.
- VH, if present, indicates significant likelihood of retinal tear. In approximately 70% of cases, "tobacco dust" in the anterior vitreous is observed (also known as the *Shafer sign*). This represents RPE cells that were liberated through the break in the neurosensory retina into the preretinal space.

Systemic Findings

None.

Special Tests

- Indirect ophthalmoscopic examination of peripheral retina with scleral depression.
- B-scan ultrasonography if view is obscured by VH.

Pathology

Full-thickness defect in neurosensory retina through which fluid may travel from the vitreous cavity into the subretinal space.

Disease Course

- Acute, symptomatic retinal tears have 2% to 20% risk of progressing to RD.
- Asymptomatic retinal breaks, especially in phakic patients, have low risk of progression to RD.
- Postmortem studies show 5% to 10% incidence of retinal tears without detachment.

Management and Treatment

- Laser photocoagulation encircling the retinal break is indicated for acute, symptomatic HST.
- Cryopexy encircling the retinal break may be helpful for anterior breaks that are difficult to treat with laser.
- Treat subclinical RDs, especially if pseudophakic, aphakic, or if the fellow eye has a history of RD.
- Observation indicated for round and operculated holes: These lesions no longer have strong vitreous traction. Consider treatment if the holes are large, associated with aphakia or RD in fellow eye.
- Asymptomatic tears in phakic eyes may be observed unless patient has had prior RD. Treat if patient is going to have cataract surgery.
- Macular holes are a type of retinal break that rarely are the cause of a RD. They are managed with vitrectomy and long-acting intraocular gas tamponade.

Medications

None.

Follow-Up

Education on symptoms of retinal tears and RD. Patient should call immediately if there are any new symptoms.

References

Byer NE. The natural history of asymptomatic retinal breaks. *Ophthalmology* 1982;89:1033–1039.

Hikichi T, Trempe CL. Relationship between floaters, light flashes, or both, and complications of posterior vitreous detachment. *Am J Ophthalmol* 1994;117:593–598.

Senile Retinoschisis

Summary

Acquired splitting of the outer plexiform layer of the retina usually found in the inferotemporal quadrant as a bullous retinal elevation that mimics an RD.

Etiology

Peripheral microcystic degenerative changes of the outer plexiform layer may coalesce into cavities.

Demographics

Elderly patients; unusual to see under age 30 years.
Bilateral in 50% to 80% of cases.
May be associated with hyperopia.

Signs and Symptoms

Usually asymptomatic.

Ophthalmic Findings

- Smooth, dome-shaped cavity with "beaten metal" appearance on the retinal surface.
- Bullous retinoschisis cavities usually inferotemporally located.
- May observe small white dots (Müller cell footplate remnants) on surface of cavity:
  Normal underlying RPE.
  May develop outer schisis wall or inner schisis wall retinal holes (Figure 3.55).
  If there are both outer and inner layer holes, an RD may occur (Table 3.15).
  If just one is present, an RD is less likely to occur.

Systemic Findings

None.

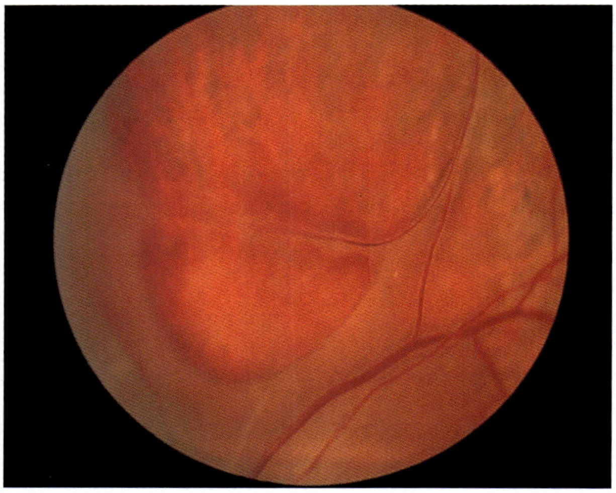

FIGURE 3.55. Retinoschisis with outer retinal holes.

Table 3.15

Comparison of x-linked and senile retinoschisis

	Juvenile X-linked retinoschisis	Senile retinoschisis
Location of schisis	Macula	Peripheral, inferotemporal most common
Retinal layer involved	Nerve-fiber layer	Outer plexiform layer

Special Tests

Visual-field testing may reveal an absolute scotoma corresponding to the area of schisis. The aiming beam of the laser photocoagulator can be focused on the suspected schisis cavity to help distinguish schisis from RD (if schisis, aiming beam not seen by patient; if RD, aiming beam may be seen by patient but less vividly than when beam shone over adjacent normal retina).

Similarly, laser photocoagulation (gray-white retinal uptake or "laser spot") will not occur over detached retina but will occur over an area of retinoschisis.

Pathology

- In bullous retinoschisis in adults, the retinal split occurs in outer plexiform layer. Not to be confused with Juvenile X-linked retinoschisis in the macula, which occurs in the nerve-fiber layer.
- Nuclear layers may become involved as schisis progresses.
- Müller fibers break down, allowing enlargement of the cystic space.

Disease Course

- Usually not progressive.
- Low incidence of RD, especially if patient develops inner and outer layer holes.
- Very rarely extends posteriorly to threaten the macula.

Treatment and Management

- Observation, indirect ophthalmoscopic examination of the peripheral retina with scleral depression.
- It is also possible in many cases to focus an OCT scan over the schisis cavity to help differentiate retinoschisis (intraretinal split on OCT) from an RD (subretinal fluid on OCT).
- If outer wall holes present with subretinal fluid, may observe, since the subretinal fluid may spontaneously regress.

- RDs with both outer and inner wall holes should be repaired, usually with vitrectomy.
- In the rare instance of posterior extension threatening the macula, one may consider photocoagulation to attempt to limit posterior extension.

Medications

None.

Follow-Up

Routine examination for asymptomatic patients.

Differential Diagnosis

RD: pigment cells in vitreous, corrugated, opacified appearance, relative scotoma, chronic RD may have RPE degeneration demarcation lines.

Reference

Byer NE. Long-term natural history study of senile retinoschisis with implications for management. *Ophthalmology* 1986;93:1127–1137.

Retinal Detachment

Summary

Separation of neurosensory retina from underlying RPE due to subretinal fluid.

Etiology

- Retinal break with leakage of liquefied vitreous into subretinal space (rhegmatogenous RD).
- Traction due to PDR, ROP, PVR (traction RD).
- Exudation of serous fluid from systemic disease, inflammation, tumor (exudative RD).

Signs and Symptoms

- Flashes, floaters, or decreased vision.
- Loss of peripheral visual field (this may fluctuate based upon body position).
- Loss of central vision if macula involved.

Rhegmatogenous Retinal Detachment: Due to Retinal Tear

Demographics

More common in patients with the following:

- An RD in the fellow eye.
- Family history of RD.
- High-level myopia.
- Aphakia, pseudophakia with or without Nd:Yag laser posterior capsulotomy.
- A history of blunt ocular or head trauma.
- Retinal necrosis (e.g., a history of CMV retinitis, ARN, PORN).

Ophthalmic Findings

- PVD, vitreous syneresis.
- Shafer sign: pigment cells in vitreous (a.k.a. "tobacco dust")
- Subretinal fluid associated with identifiable retinal break in more than 90% of cases.
- Retinal folds.
- May have low IOP compared with the fellow eye (often >5 mm Hg difference).

Systemic Findings

None for rhegmatogenous RD unless concomitant bodily trauma was present.

Special Tests

Indirect ophthalmoscopy with scleral depression to provide visualization of the peripheral retina to the ora serrata for 360 degrees.

Pathology

- Separation of the outer retinal layers from the choriocapillaris due to liquefied vitreous that has entered the subretinal space through a full-thickness retinal break.
- Photoreceptor degeneration occurs 4 to 6 weeks after RD.
- Cystoid degeneration of outer plexiform layer may lead to macrocysts.
- RPE proliferation in subretinal space.

Disease Course

- Progression to total RD without treatment.
- If the macula is attached on presentation, visual prognosis relatively good, so urgent repair (within approximately 24 hours) is indicated to prevent macular involvement of the RD.
- If the macula is already detached, there is a lower rate of both anatomic success and visual recovery. Less than 40% recover vision of 20/50 or better. Surgical repair for a macula involving RD is generally carried out within one week of presentation.
- Proliferative vitreoretinopathy (PVR) is the number one reason for failure of primary RD repair.

Treatment and Management

- Goal is to close the causative retinal break(s).
- If there is a delay between diagnosis and surgical repair, patient should remain immobile and avoid rigorous activity or reading. Bilateral eye patching can be considered to help minimize the progression of the RD.
- There are several surgical approaches that are acceptable:

Table 3.16

Characteristics of commonly used intraocular gases in vitreoretinal surgery

Gas	Amount of expansion*	Duration within eye*
Air	None	5–7 d
SF_6	Two times	10–14 d
C_3F_8	Four times	6–8 wk

*Expansion coefficients and intraocular duration refer to pure gas concentrations (e.g., 100% SF_6 or 100%C_3F_8).

- Scleral buckling procedure (anatomic success achieved in more than 90%) with or without external drainage of subretinal fluid.
- Vitrectomy, fluid-gas exchange, endolaser, and postoperative positioning to support the causative breaks (similar success rate as scleral buckling).
- Combination of scleral-buckling procedure and vitrectomy procedures.
- Office-based pneumatic retinopexy (Table 3.16) for superior RDs in phakic eyes with a single break (success rate between 70% and 85%).

Medications

None.

Follow-Up

Timing of surgical repair is important, since longstanding detachments have the worst visual prognosis.

Tractional Retinal Detachment Due to Preretinal Fibrosis and Mechanical Contraction

Not necessarily associated with retinal breaks.

Demographics

PDR.
ROP.
PVR.
RDs associated with uveitis.
Penetrating trauma.

Ophthalmic Findings

See Figure 3.56.

- Preretinal fibrovascular proliferation/membranes.
- Concave retinal surface.
- Detachment is usually localized to the region of preretinal membranes.
- Subretinal fibrosis.

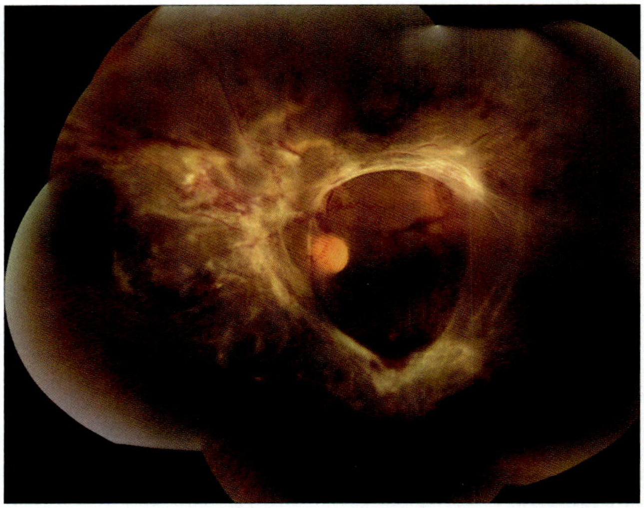

FIGURE 3.56. Tractional detachment of the macula and retina superotemporal to the optic disk in a diabetic patient with PDR.

Systemic Findings

- Traction retinal detachment is often associated with PDR with high-risk features, so systemic findings of diabetes mellitus may be observed (hyperglycemia, peripheral neuropathy, peripheral vascular disease, lower extremity ulcers).
- Prematurity.
- Other proliferative vascular disease like sickle cell disease, Eales disease, CRVO.

Special Tests

IVFA may show underlying ischemia.

Pathology

Preretinal membranes are composed of glial cells, fibroblasts, and RPE cells.

Treatment and Management

Vitrectomy with membrane dissection.

Exudative Retinal Detachment: Serous Subretinal Fluid Not Due to Primary Retinal Break or Vitreous Traction

Etiology and Risk Factors

- Inflammatory disease: posterior scleritis, Harada disease (a.k.a., "VKH"), sympathetic ophthalmia.
- Neoplasia: choroidal malignant melanoma, choroidal hemangioma, choroidal metastasis.
- Systemic diseases such as malignant hypertension, renal failure, toxemia of pregnancy.
- Idiopathic uveal effusion syndrome.
- Coats disease.

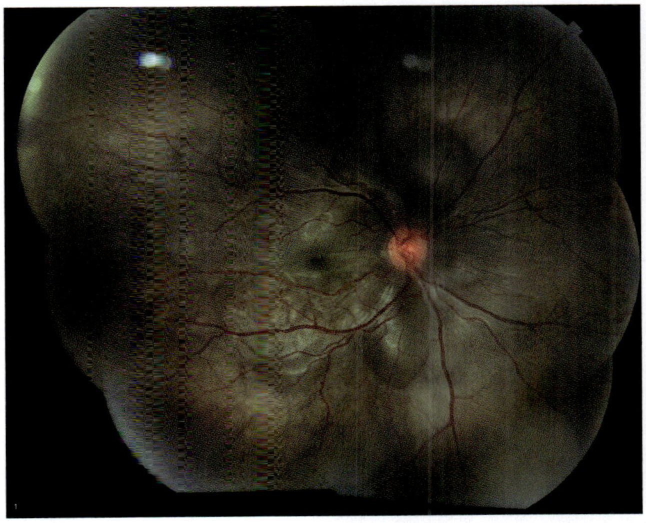

FIGURE 3.57. Exudative RD in a patient with Vogt-Koyanagi-Harada syndrome.

- Exudative ARMD
- ICSC.
- Trauma, intraocular surgery (including cryotherapy and photocoagulation).
- Nanophthalmos, thick sclera.

Ophthalmic Findings

See Figure 3.57.

- Bullous, with "shifting" subretinal fluid (this means that the ophthalmoscopic location of the RD changes with changing body position from upright to supine and vice versa).
- No primary retinal break found.
- No pigmented vitreous cells observed.
- May have underlying tumor that is supplying the exudation: melanoma, hemangioma, retinoblastoma.
- "Leopard spot" mottling of the RPE with chronic subretinal fluid.

Systemic Findings

See "Etiology and Risk Factors." Briefly, patients with exudative RDs may have signs of systemic rheumatologic or autoimmune diseases.

Special Tests

IVFA: Tumors such as malignant melanoma may show increased vascularity of the lesion, ARMD may demonstrate CNV, ICSC may have focal RPE leakage points.

B-scan ultrasonography: Posterior scleritis may show thickening of Tenon capsule; tumors may have characteristic echoes.

Treatment and Management

- Treat underlying systemic condition; comanage with internist.
- Drainage of subretinal fluid may be accomplished by creating sclerotomies, especially for cases of uveal effusion syndrome.
- Vortex vein decompression in patients with thick sclera.

Medications

Consider corticosteroids in patients with chronic inflammatory disease, in those who develop serous RD following cryopexy or laser photocoagulation. Antimetabolites and biologic agents may be used by uveitis specialists directly or in comanagement with a rheumatologist to mitigate ocular or systemic signs and symptoms.

References

Machemer R, Williams JM Sr. Pathogenesis and therapy of traction detachment in various retinal vascular diseases. *Am J Ophthalmol* 1988;105:170–181.

Michels RG, Wilkinson CP, Rice TA. *Retinal detachment*. St. Louis, MO: Mosby, 1990.

Schepens CL, Brockhurst RJ. Uveal effusion, I: clinical picture. *Arch Ophthalmol* 1963;70:189.

Proliferative Vitreoretinopathy

Summary

PVR: proliferation of RPE cells, glial cells on both retinal surfaces causing fibrosis and retinal contraction. PVR is the most common cause of failure of rhegmatogenous RD repair.

Etiology

Severe PVR may develop in patients with the following risk factors:

VH.
Preoperative PVR.
Preoperative or postoperative choroidal detachment.
Giant retinal tears.
Uveitis.

Demographics

Prior RD.
Penetrating trauma.

Signs and Symptoms

Decreased vision.
Photopsias.
Metamorphopsia.

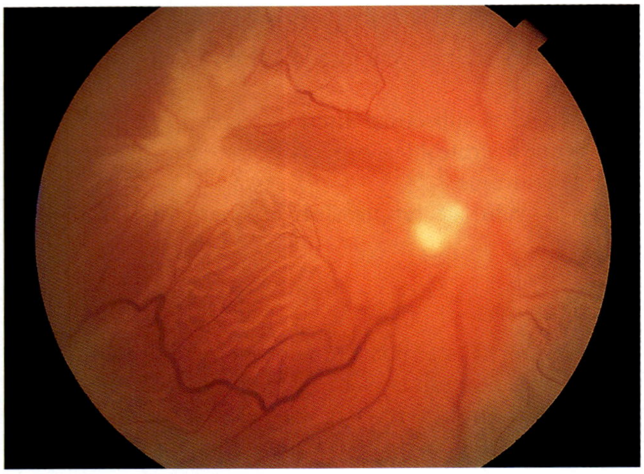

FIGURE 3.58. PVR with a star-fold causing recurrent RD in a patient who has had prior scleral buckling.

Ophthalmic Findings

See Figure 3.58.

Preretinal fibrosis.
Fixed retinal folds (star folds).
Subretinal fibrosis.
Retinal contraction and shortening.
Vitreous pigment clumps.
Vitreous condensation.

Systemic Findings

None.

Special Tests

None.

Pathology

Growth of contractile glial cells, fibroblasts, and RPE cells on retinal surface and posterior vitreous.

Disease Course

Without treatment, PVR may cause severe contraction of the retina leading to failure of surgical repair.

Treatment and Management

Scleral buckling procedure.
Vitrectomy with membrane stripping.
Silicone oil.

Medications

None available yet. Investigations are ongoing to develop drugs that inhibit cellular proliferation and collagen production.

References

Girard P, Mimoun G, Karpouzas I, et al. Clinical risk factors for proliferative vitreoretinopathy after retinal detachment surgery. *Retina* 1994;14:417–424.

Michels RG. Surgery of retinal detachment with proliferative vitreoretinopathy. *Retina* 1984;4:63–83.

VITREOUS

Developmental Abnormalities

Summary

The hyaloidal vascular system is derived from the embryonic fissure and forms the primary vitreous. In normal gestational development, this regresses and the avascular and optically clear secondary vitreous forms.

Etiology

Several congenital abnormalities may occur due to incomplete regression of the hyaloidal system.

Signs and Symptoms

Usually asymptomatic.
PFV may present with leukocoria.

Demographics

Most cases are sporadic.

Ophthalmic Findings

- Persistent pupillary membrane: Remnants of anterior tunica vasculosa lentis remain on the anterior lens surface. This is asymptomatic and benign.
- Bergmeister papilla: incomplete atrophy of the posterior hyaloidal artery sheath. May appear as gliotic membrane extending from optic disk into the midvitreous (Figure 3.59).
- Persistent Fetal Vasculature (PFV, formerly known as *persistent hyperplastic primary vitreous* or PHPV): lack of regression of the primary vitreous, especially the posterior tunica vasculosa lentis.
  Leukocoria is the most common presenting sign. This is due to a retrolental vascular membrane.
  Unilateral.
  Affected eye tends to be microphthalmic.
  Cataract formation is common.
  VH is commonly observed.
  Pupillary block glaucoma.

Systemic Findings

None.

Special Tests

None.

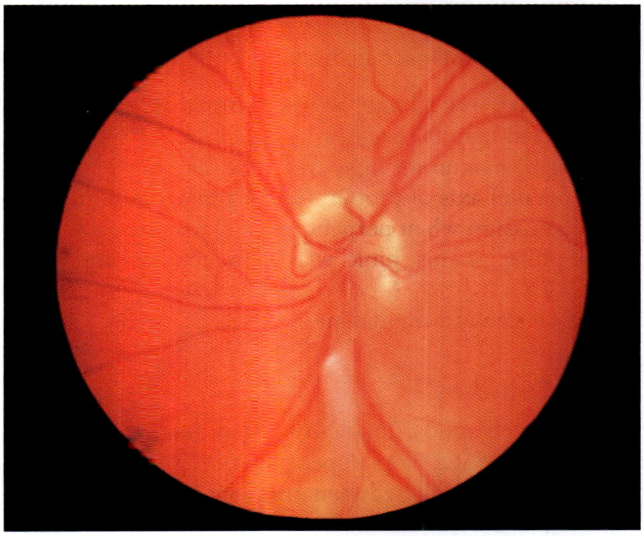

FIGURE 3.59. Bergmeister papilla extending from the optic disk.

Treatment and Management

PFV: The natural course of untreated PFV is progression to glaucoma, recurrent VHs, and phthisis. Vitrectomy and lensectomy or lens-sparing vitrectomy may help reduce the likelihood that enucleation will be necessary for advanced cases and preserve useful vision.

Medications

None.

Follow-Up

No specific follow-up is needed for persistent pupillary membranes or Bergmeister papilla. Patients with PHPV are likely to have limited visual prognosis in the affected eye.

Reference

Apple DJ, Rabb MF. Persistent hyperplastic primary vitreous. In: Apple DJ, Rabb MF, eds. *Ocular pathology*. St. Louis, MO: Mosby–Year Book, 1991;28–35.

Posterior Vitreous Detachment

See p. 184.

Asteroid Hyalosis

Summary

Calcium-lipid deposits (calcium soap crystals) seen suspended throughout the vitreous.

Etiology

Degenerative vitreous change.

Demographics

Usually unilateral.
No sex predilection.
Most commonly seen in patients over age 60 years.

Signs and Symptoms

- Usually asymptomatic.
- Decreased vision rarely.
- Floaters.

Ophthalmic Findings

Whitish vitreous opacities that may be dense enough to obscure details of the posterior pole.

Systemic Findings

None.

Pathology

PAS positive.
Stains with lipid and mucopolysaccharide stains.

Disease Course

Benign.

Special Tests

IVFA may be helpful with visualizing the fundus and evaluating for causes of decreased vision, because the opacities generally do not appear on IVFA images like they do on fundus photography and with indirect ophthalmoscopy. OCT scans may show shadowing artifacts due to overlying vitreous opacities.

Treatment and Management

- Observation.
- Vitrectomy only if patient is particularly symptomatic and other causes for symptoms have been eliminated.

Medications

None.

Follow-Up

Routine examinations.

Reference

Miller H, Miller B, Rabinowitz H. Asteroid bodies: an ultrastructural study. *Invest Ophthalmol Vis Sci* 1983;24:133–136.

Amyloidosis

Summary

Amyloidosis is a complex of diseases characterized by abnormal protein production and aberrant deposition

RETINA

in multiple tissues. It is very rare but can present as a masquerade for a variety of ophthalmic conditions.

Etiology

- Familial forms: lead to substitution errors in the genetic coding of prealbumin. Autosomal dominant.
- Nonfamilial form.

Demographics

- Autosomal dominant inheritance in hereditary forms.
- Multiple myeloma may be associated.

Signs and Symptoms

Floaters from vitreous opacities.
Eyelid hemorrhages.
Diplopia.
Dry eyes.

Ophthalmic Findings

Any part of the eye may be involved.

- Orbit:
  Ptosis: most typical presentation.
  Ophthalmoplegia.
  Proptosis.
  Sicca.
- Eyelid skin: hemorrhage linked with high probability of systemic disease.
- Glaucoma: whitish debris on iris, lens resembles pseudoexfoliation.
- Scalloped pupil: secondary to stromal infiltrate.
- Vitreous opacities: usually bilateral. May be presenting sign in familial amyloid.
- Retinal vascular occlusions.
- Cotton-wool spots.
- Retinal NV.
- Compressive optic neuropathy.

Systemic Findings

- Familial amyloid, neuropathic forms: classified into four types. Findings vary according to type, but consist of peripheral neuropathies, autonomic dysfunction, cardiomyopathies, cranial nerve palsies, and dry redundant skin.
- Nonfamilial forms:
  Acute and chronic renal failure.
  Postural hypotension.
  Waxy, maculopapular skin lesions that tend to hemorrhage.
  Polyarthralgia.
  Congestive heart failure due to infiltrates.
  GI tract bleedings.
  Pulmonary infiltrates.
- Systemic dyscrasias such as multiple myeloma, Waldenstrom macroglobulinemia.

Pathology

Characteristic microscopic findings:

Birefringence on Congo red staining: rotates plane of polarized light 90 degrees.
Dichroism: maximum light transmission when polarized on parallel axis of protein (looks green), minimal light transmission when perpendicular (looks red).
Eosinophilic, stains pink with hematoxylin and eosin (H&E).
Fluorescence with thioflavine T.

Special Studies

- Definitive diagnosis made by biopsy (e.g., conjunctival nodule, mucosal biopsy specimens).
- Laboratory: CBC, sedimentation rate, ANA, albumin, protein electrophoresis, renal and liver function studies.
- CXR.
- Electrocardiogram.

Treatment and Management

- If patient has eyelid, skin, or orbital deposits without preexisting risk factors such as multiple myeloma, systemic evaluation is needed.
- If corneal deposits of Meretoja syndrome are present, neurologic consultation is needed.
- Systemic evaluation, if any vitreoretinal findings or amyloid glaucoma.
- Orbital deposits may need debulking.
- Vitrectomy may be useful for patients visually compromised by vitreous opacities, but the recurrence rate of vitreous opacities is high.

Medications

- Steroids are indicated for multiple myeloma. However, steroids are contraindicated for primary systemic causes other than myeloma, since they can accelerate abnormal amyloid deposition.
- Dimethyl sulfoxide can be used to denature protein deposits.

Disease Course

Varies depending on etiology of amyloidosis.

Follow-Up

See "Treatment and Management."

Differential Diagnosis

- Sarcoidosis: noncaseating granulomas, positive ACE.
- Asteroid hyalosis: vitreous opacities, benign.
- Vascular occlusions from other disease such as hypertension, diabetic retinopathy.
- Pseudoexfoliation syndrome.

Reference

Knowles DM, Jakobiec FA, Rosen M, et al. Amyloidosis of the orbit and adnexae. *Surv Ophthalmol* 1975;19:367–384.

POSTERIOR SEGMENT TRAUMA

Commotio Retinae

Summary

Commotio retinae (a.k.a.: *retinal contusion*) is a temporary outer retinal whitening associated with closed-globe trauma. The visual significance is related to the proximity to the macular center. Resolution of the retinal edema may be complete or be followed by permanent chorioretinal changes.

Etiology

Blunt ocular trauma with photoreceptor stretch produced by direct linear forces in conjunction with vitreous deformation and resultant vitreoretinal tension combine to disrupt photoreceptor outer segments and cell bodies. Generally thought of as a contre-coup injury.

Signs and Symptoms

Decreased vision or asymptomatic (largely dependent on location of commotio).

Demographics

Develops in individuals after blunt ocular trauma.

Ophthalmic Findings

- Retinal whitening, often localized to the posterior pole (Berlin edema), often appearing several hours after acute injury.
- Associated findings are retinal hemorrhages, chorioretinal rupture, traumatic optic neuropathy. Retinal hemorrhages are associated rather than directly related to the retinal edema.
- With foveal involvement, there may be a cherry-red spot.

Systemic Findings

Associated head injuries.

Special Tests

Fluorescein angiographic characteristics depend on extent of injury and timing of FA in relation to injury. Window defects may develop after chronic RPE changes. Confluent areas of retinal whitening may block choroidal fluorescence.

OCT findings are dependent on severity of commotio. Increased reflectivity with small optically clear spaces in photoreceptor outer segment may be observed.

Pathology

- Both animal models and clinicopathologic correlation have demonstrated fragmentation of photoreceptors with cystic changes in the outer segments.
- Blood–retinal barrier is generally undisturbed.

Disease Course

- A self-limited disorder. Following injury, the RPE may respond with migration into the neurosensory retinal layer, resulting in variable permanent hyperpigmentation patterns.
- Concussive injuries usually clear in 3 to 4 weeks, but severe commotio retinae with contusion may be followed by a macular pigment epitheliopathy, macular hole.

Treatment and Management

FA valuable for visual prognosis.

Medications

None effective.

Follow-Up

Repeat examination in 1 to 2 weeks with a more urgent evaluation if symptoms of RD or other difficulties develop.

Differential Diagnosis

RD: elevated retinal vessels with visible retinal break; pigment visible in anterior vitreous.

BRAO: Area of whitening follows distribution of an attenuated vessel and is accompanied by edema, cotton-wool spots; cholesterol emboli may be found at bifurcation of arterioles. The retina whitening in BRAO is due to inner edema; in commotio, it is due to outer retinal edema.

White without pressure: not associated with trauma; often multifocal and bilateral affecting the peripheral retina.

References

Mansour AM, Green WR, Hogge C. Histopathology of commotio retinae. *Retina* 1992;12:24–48.

Sipperley JO, Quigley HA, Gass JDM. Traumatic retinopathy in primates: the explanation of commotio retinae. *Arch Ophthalmol* 1978;96:2267–2273.

Sony P, Venkatesh P, Gadaginamath S, Garg SP. Optical coherence tomography findings in commotio retina. *Clin Experiment Ophthalmol* 2006;34(6):621–623.

Traumatic Macular Hole

Summary

Full- or partial-thickness retinal holes developing after either blunt ocular trauma or whiplash injuries. They are associated with both distortion and decreased central vision and tend to be larger than the idiopathic subtype of macular hole.

Etiology

Unlike idiopathic macular holes that have a pathogenesis directly related to tangential vitreomacular traction, the pathogenesis of trauma-related macular holes is unclear. It is theorized that traumatic macular hole most commonly follows contusion necrosis with cystoid degeneration and cyst coalescence but may also be seen after subfoveal hemorrhage with choroidal rupture or following anteroposterior vitreous traction at the site of vitreous attachment plaques.

Signs and Symptoms

Decreased vision.
Metamorphopsia.

Demographics

Patients who sustain blunt ocular trauma are at increased risk. Unlike idiopathic macular holes seen in the elderly, they may occur at any age.

Ophthalmic Findings

See Figure 3.60.

- Round, reddish spot surrounded by a gray halo of marginally detached retina. Generally, they do not lead to development of a rhegmatogenous RD.

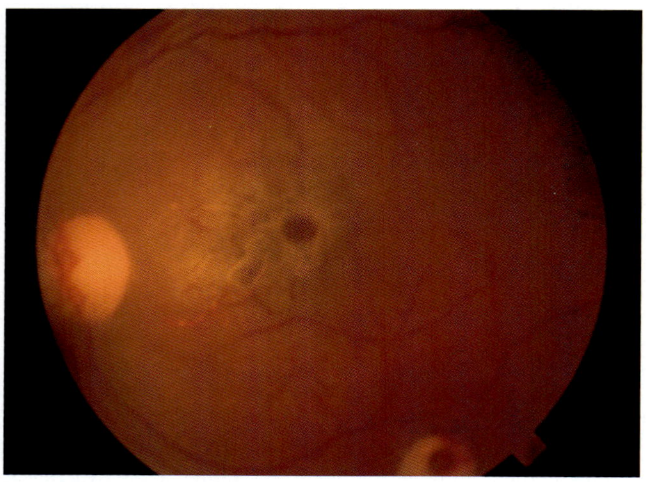

FIGURE 3.60. Traumatic macular hole in an 8-year-old boy after resolution of commotio retinae several months after blunt trauma.

- Abnormal macular depressions or pits may also be seen. Irregular margins may be observed at the hole edge.
- Occasionally, a microoperculum or a wisp of vitreoretinal tissue extending anteriorly from the hole may be noted with vitreoretinal traction–induced holes.
- Epiretinal fibrosis with retinal striae may be present.

Systemic Findings

None.

Special Tests

FA may show some vascular leakage in the presence of a coexistent severe contusion injury.

Pathology

Full-thickness retinal defect involving ILM to photoreceptor outer segments.

Disease Course

Traumatic macular holes tend to be larger, of full thickness, and associated with greater acuity losses (up to 20/200). Smaller traumatic macular holes in young patients may be associated with spontaneous closure and improved vision.

Treatment and Management

If visual function is impaired, vitrectomy and membranectomy may be of benefit. A period of observation for small macular holes in young patients may be advisable, since they may close spontaneously.

Medications

None effective.

Follow-Up

Stable macular holes may be evaluated on a yearly basis, but if severe myopia is present, more frequent evaluation is advised.

Differential Diagnosis

- Macular pucker with pseudohole: OCT imaging is valuable here. The pseudohole patients may have relatively good vision.
- Solar retinopathy: history of sun gazing or arc welding, with recovery of acuity in 3 to 6 months.

References

de Bustros S. Vitreous surgery for traumatic macular hole. *Retina* 1996;16:451–452.

Kusaka S, Fujikado T, Ikeda T, et al. Spontaneous disappearance of traumatic macular holes in young patients. *Am J Ophthalmol* 1997;123(6):837–839.

Madreperla SA, Benetz BA. Formation and treatment of a traumatic macular hole. *Arch Ophthalmol* 1997;115:1210–1211.

Retinal Tears and Dialyses

Summary

Retinal tears and dialyses may occur following blunt trauma. Dialyses represent a disinsertion of the retina from the ora serrata. In a retinal tear, there is retina anterior to the tear.

Etiology

Elongation of globe, transmission of blunt trauma forces through the vitreous produces vitreoretinal traction, which may tear the retina in a variety of patterns depending on the site of blunt impact.

Signs and Symptoms

Photopsias
Floaters
Visual-field loss
May be asymptomatic

Demographics

- Young male patients (most frequently involved in trauma).
- Myopes are more susceptible to detachment following trauma.
- Marfan and Stickler syndromes predispose patients to traumatic RDs.

Ophthalmic Findings

- Traumatic retinal dialysis is most commonly seen in the superonasal and the inferotemporal quadrants and may be accompanied by an avulsion of the vitreous base.
- Flap and operculated retinal tears may be seen at the posterior margin of the vitreous base, along meridional folds, and near the equator.

Rapid traumatic compression/decompression of globe may result in tearing of the retina along posterior vitreous base, giving rise to a "giant retinal tear" (see Figure 3.61). GRT are tears extending for more than three clock hours.

- Irregular posterior retinal tears may be seen.
- RDs may be seen in association with retinal breaks and often exhibit signs of chronicity and slow progression (demarcation lines, intraretinal cysts).
- Anterior vitreal pigmented cells, VH, or PVD.

Systemic Findings

None.

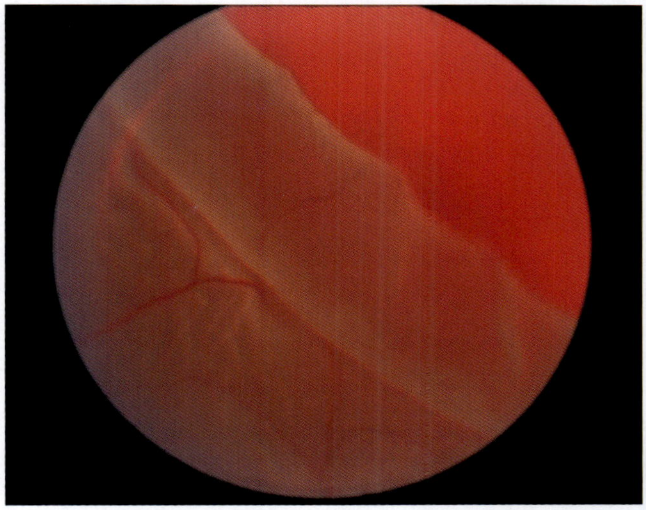

FIGURE 3.61. Giant retinal tear following blunt trauma.

Special Tests

Indirect ophthalmoscopy with scleral depression should be performed in all patients with a history of nonpenetrating blunt trauma (although a depressed examination should be deferred following traumatic hyphema).

Pathology

Retinal tear due to various etiologies.

Disease Course

- Variable: Retinal tears often times do not progress to RD; however, they occasionally can lead to severe RDs if not diagnosed and treated promptly.
- Eighty percent of RDs are diagnosed within 2 years of the injury. The RD may occur well after the time of initial injury as vitreous degeneration accelerates with trauma.

Treatment and Management

Laser retinopexy or cryotherapy.
Scleral Buckle.
Pars Plana Vitrectomy.

Medications

None effective.

Follow-Up

- Treated retinal breaks are rechecked periodically following repair to determine stability. Serial retinal exams are necessary in order to detect future breaks.
- The symptomatology of RD should be discussed, with clear instructions to seek immediate attention should they develop.

Differential Diagnosis

Choroidal effusion: accumulation of fluid in suprachoroidal space.
Commotio retinae.
White without pressure.

References

Cox MS. Retinal breaks caused by blunt nonperforating trauma at the point of impact. *Trans Am Ophthalmol Soc* 1980;78:414–465.

Johnston PB. Traumatic retinal detachment. *Br J Ophthalmol* 1991;75:18–21.

Stoffelns BM, Richard G. Is Buckle Surgery still the state of the art for retinal detachments due to retinal dialysis? *J Pediatr Ophthalmol Strabismus* 2009:1–7. doi: 10.3928/01913913-20091019-10.

Suprachoroidal Hemorrhage

Summary

Acute hemorrhagic expansion of suprachoroidal space. May result in the expulsion of ocular contents following penetrating ocular injuries: "Suprachoroidal expulsive hemorrhage."

Etiology

Rupture of posterior ciliary arteries within the suprachoroidal lamina following intraocular decompression.

Signs and Symptoms

Sudden massive loss of vision.

Demographics

Risk factors include glaucoma, advanced age, myopia, aphakia, hypertension, high myopia, and increased axial length. Risk factors are atherosclerosis, glaucoma, hypertension, and tachycardia.

Ophthalmic Findings

- Hypotony caused by ocular surgery, ruptured globe or infectious, inflammatory, or degenerative corneal perforation.
- Shallow anterior chamber.
- Prolapse of iris, lens, or vitreous, or combination of these.
- Loss or darkening of red reflex.

Systemic Findings

Often complain of headache or ocular pain.
Atherosclerosis.

Special Tests

B scan to confirm location and extent of hemorrhage.

Pathology

- Rupture of posterior ciliary artery as it passes into choroidal space.
- Blood between sclera and choroid with expulsion of retina and anterior ocular structures depending on volume of hemorrhage.

Disease Course

Extremely poor visual prognosis unless wound is closed promptly and hemorrhage is evacuated; better outcome if uveal prolapse avoided.

Treatment and Management

- Prompt surgical closure of surgical, traumatic, or infectious wound.
- Posterior sclerotomies 9 mm posterior to limbus to relieve hemorrhage.
- Possible delayed evacuation of blood after liquefaction has occurred, typically 10 to 14 days.

Medications

Intravenous acetazolamide, mannitol, labetalol, or other intravenous hypotensive agents.

Follow-Up

Postoperatively to consider draining sclerotomy.

Differential Diagnosis

- Positive posterior segment pressure related to obesity, table positioning, lid speculum, large-volume retrobulbar or peribulbar injection.
- Acute intraoperative choroidal effusion.

References

Reynolds MG, Haimovici R, Flynn HW, et al. Suprachoroidal hemorrhage: clinical features and results of secondary surgical management. *Ophthalmology* 1993;100:460–465.

Speaker MG, Guerriero PN, Marmor M. A case-control study of risk factors for intraoperative suprachoroidal expulsive hemorrhage. *Ophthalmology* 1991;98:202–210.

Choroidal Rupture

Summary

Tear(s) in Bruch membrane and underlying choriocapillaris, typically concentric to the optic nerve. Visual prognosis is dependent on location of the rupture.

Etiology

- Compression and lateral expansion of the globe leads to rupture(s) of the inelastic Bruch membrane.

- Choriocapillaris may tear producing hemorrhage, but large choroidal vessels remain intact, as does overlying retina.

Signs and Symptoms

- Normal vision to severe visual loss, depending on location of rupture.
- Evidence of orbital or ocular trauma.

Demographics

- Persons exposed to traumatic globe injuries.
- Patients with angioid streaks generally require less forceful injury to develop this finding.

Ophthalmic Findings

See Figure 3.62.

- Subretinal hemorrhage, which may obscure the underlying rupture.
- When healed and blood is resolved, white subretinal streak(s) concentric to the optic nerve in areas of previous subretinal hemorrhage may be present.
- Retina and nerve fiber layer usually intact.
- Chorioretinal vascular anastomoses may be seen after healing.
- Macular hole may develop late.

Systemic Findings

None.

Special Tests

FA shows absence of choriocapillaris and late hyperfluorescence of sclera through rupture.

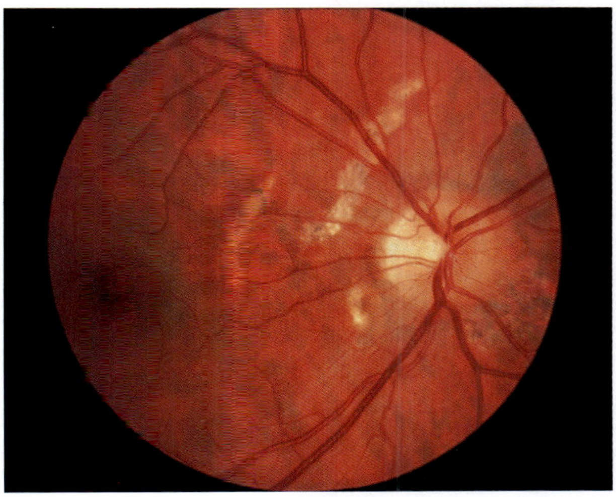

FIGURE 3.62. Choroidal rupture concentric to optic nerve following blunt trauma.

Pathology

- Bruch membrane and choriocapillaris are ruptured, as may be the underlying choroidal vessels.
- Fibrovascular ingrowth may develop during healing phase or years later.

Disease Course

- If fovea is uninvolved, visual prognosis is good.
- Late loss of central vision possible from CNV at site of choroidal rupture.

Treatment and Management

- Amsler grid monitoring.
- If CNVMs develop, laser treatment may be indicated.

Medications

None.

Follow-Up

- Biweekly during the first few months, then every 3 to 6 months.
- Long-term follow-up to detect NV.

Differential Diagnosis

- Chorioretinal scars: may be related to old infectious processes such as toxoplasmosis or histoplasmosis.
- Angioid streaks: brown or red irregular lesions that radiate from the optic nerve (rather than concentric with the nerve).
- RPE tear: typically seen without history of trauma in patients with ARMD.

References

Williams DF, Mieler WF, Williams GA. Posterior segment manifestations of ocular trauma. *Retina* 1990;10(Suppl):S35–S44.

Wood CM, Richardson J. Indirect choroidal ruptures: aetiological factors, patterns of ocular damage, and final visual outcome. *Br J Ophthalmol* 1990;74:208–211.

Chorioretinitis Sclopetaria

Summary

Rupture of choroid and retina associated with high-velocity orbital missile; a closed globe trauma. Fibrous proliferation into vitreous may develop.

Etiology

Blunt trauma ruptures choroid and overlying retina as single unit and causes hemorrhage under an intact hyaloid face; chorioretinal complex retracts exposing bare sclera.

Signs and Symptoms

Mild to profound visual loss, depending on site of rupture.

Demographics

Individuals exposed to gunshot wounds or other head trauma.

Ophthalmic Findings

Mild to severe loss of vision.
Full-thickness chorioretinal break with adjacent accordion-like retinal folds and edema, often concentric with optic nerve.
Bare sclera visible within margins of break.
Preretinal or VH.
Commotio retinae.
RD.
Afferent pupillary defect, if optic nerve injured.
Late fibrous proliferation into vitreous without RD.

Systemic Findings

Missile injury to head or other head trauma.

Special Tests

- CT scan of head and orbit to assess ruptured globe or IOFB.
- B scan of globe and orbit.

Pathology

Interruptions in Bruch membrane, retina, and choroid; fibrovascular tissue extending from choroid to retina.

Disease Course

Largely dependent on extent of damage and other associated ocular findings.

Treatment and Management

Nonsurgical management with periodic observation.
Vitrectomy for nonclearing VH.
Repair of RD.

Medications

None effective.

Follow-Up

Weekly at first and then extending follow-up interval if doing well.

Differential Diagnosis

Ruptured globe: Entrance wound may be visible; head-imaging scan may reveal full extent of injury.
VH: secondary to damage to retinal or ciliary body vessels, without extensive tissue damage. Close observation reveals source.
Large peripheral CNV complex. No bare sclera or history of trauma is present, may have ARMD features in fellow eye or posteriorly in same eye.

References

Hart JC, Natsikos VE, Raistrick ER, et al. Chorioretinitis sclopetaria. *Trans Ophthalmol Soc UK* 1980;100:276–281.
Martin DF, Awh CC, McCuen BW II. Treatment and pathogenesis of traumatic chorioretinal rupture (sclopetaria). *Am J Ophthalmol* 1994;117:190–200.

Purtscher Retinopathy

Summary

Hemorrhagic retinal angiopathy and decreased vision associated with nonocular crushing bodily trauma, especially chest compression.

Etiology (Theories)

- Fat embolization from long bone fractures.
- Air embolization from chest compression.
- Capillary dilation from venous engorgement of upper body.
- Severe angioplastic response from sudden increase in venous pressure.
- Complement-induced granulocytic aggregation following endothelial damage.

Signs and Symptoms

Bilateral or unilateral decreased vision (20/200 to counting fingers).

Demographics

Individuals with severe compressive bodily trauma.

Ophthalmic Findings

See Figure 3.63.

Peripapillary cotton-wool spots, often not involving macula.
Hard exudates.
Striate retinal hemorrhages.
Arterial spasm.
Mild retinal edema.
Cherry-red spot of macula.

Systemic Findings

Long bone fractures.
Compressive chest fractures.

Special Tests

- X-ray of long bones, chest.

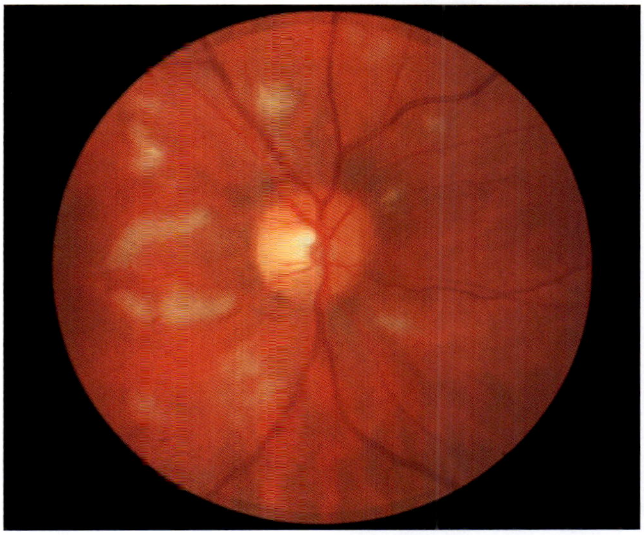

FIGURE 3.63 Purtscher retinopathy following severe compressive injury to chest. Cotton-wool spots and intraretinal hemorrhages surround optic disk.

- FA shows leakage of dye from retinal arterioles, capillaries, and venules in areas of infarct. Nonperfusion with closure of vessels or leakage in areas of infarct.

Pathology

Cytoid bodies and intraretinal hemorrhages; inner retinal atrophy from loss of retinal capillary perfusion.

Disease Course

Visual improvement to range of 20/30 to 20/200, but limited by optic atrophy and inner retinal atrophy in areas of infarct.

Treatment and Management

None.

Medications

None effective.

Differential Diagnosis

- Acute pancreatitis: no associated trauma.
- Collagen vascular diseases: may be limited to posterior pole or associated with vasculitis.
- Amniotic fluid emboli.
- Fat emboli: white infarcts, which may be smaller and more peripheral.
- Malignant hypertension: look for exudate and macular star.
- Leukemia: appropriate laboratory evaluation necessary.
- Cardiac valvular disease: symptoms of heart disease; cardiac studies reveal disease.
- High-dose alkylating chemotherapeutic agents and autologous bone marrow transplantation.

Reference

Roden D, Fitzpatrick GH, Phelan D. Purtscher's retinopathy and fat embolism. *Br J Ophthalmol* 1989;73:677–679.

Terson Syndrome

Summary

Unilateral or bilateral peripapillary VH caused by acute increased intracranial pressure. Subarachnoid hemorrhage and head trauma are primary causes.

Etiology

- Peripapillary capillary rupture caused by sudden increase in venous pressure.
- Compression of central retinal vein and rupture of chorioretinal anastomoses.

Signs and Symptoms

- Acute-onset severe headache with altered mental status.
- In aneurysmal rupture, other neurologic signs depending on location of ruptured aneurysm.
- Decreased vision may be present.

Demographics

Aneurysm patients.
Head trauma victims.

Ophthalmic Findings

- Vision may be normal or decreased from VH.
- Peripapillary preretinal, sub-ILM hemorrhages; can later form cystlike elevation of nerve-fiber layer and ILM of retina.
- VH.
- Optic disk edema.

Systemic Findings

Head trauma.
Altered mental status; coma.
Third-nerve palsy, frontal lobe dysfunction, aphasia.

Special Tests

- B scan to search for RD, IOFB, etc.
- CT scan of brain.
- Cerebral angiogram.
- Lumbar puncture; check for xanthochromia.

Pathology

Rupture of peripapillary capillaries.

Disease Course

- Terson syndrome is associated with higher fatality rate than subarachnoid hemorrhage without Terson.
- In survivors, VH and vision generally recover.

Treatment and Management

- Neurosurgery consultation.
- Head elevation, bed rest to assist clearing VH.
- Vitrectomy for nonclearing VH.

Medications

None effective.

Follow-Up

Monthly until hemorrhage clears or vitrectomy performed.

Differential Diagnosis

- Diabetic retinopathy: signs of proliferative disease.
- Traumatic retinal tear: unilateral VH associated with retinal tear.
- Vitreous detachment: unilateral VH associated with acute vitreous separation; may see Weiss ring.
- Retinal vein occlusion: unilateral optic nerve head edema associated with retinal hemorrhages in all four quadrants in CRVOs; VH more common in BRVOs.
- Sickle cell disease: bilateral disease with peripheral NV; laboratory evaluation mandatory.
  Valsalva retinopathy.

References

Pfausler B, Belcl R, Metzler R. Terson's syndrome in spontaneous subarachnoid hemorrhage: a prospective study in 60 consecutive patients. *J Neurosurg* 1996;85:392–394.

Schultz PN, Sobol WM, Weingeist TA. Long-term visual outcome in Terson syndrome. *Ophthalmology* 1991;98:1814–1819.

Intraocular Foreign Body

Summary

Posttraumatic retention of foreign material increasing risk of endophthalmitis, as well as acute and chronic toxic inflammatory reactions to the specific material.

Etiology

Traumatic penetration of globe and secondary foreign body implantation.

Signs and Symptoms

- Evidence of apparent or occult ruptured globe.
- Decreased vision from VH, hyphema, corneal laceration.
- Decreased vision from toxic inflammatory or infectious effects of IOFB.

Demographics

Persons with penetrating ocular injury.

Ophthalmic Findings

- Apparent or occult penetrating ocular injury.
- IOFB identified by direct visualization, indirect ophthalmoscopy, or imaging studies; object may by hidden by hemorrhage.
- Anterior chamber cells, cataract, vitritis, retinal necrosis, VH, siderosis bulbi, chalcosis, endophthalmitis, iris heterochromia, Kayser-Fleischer ring.
- Corneal edema inferiorly suggests foreign body in inferior angle.
- Traumatic optic neuropathy.

Systemic Findings

- Associated head, orbital, or ocular trauma.
- Glass, metal, or other foreign fragments within skin lacerations.

Special Tests

- X-rays (Caldwell or Waters view) reveal radiopaque materials.
- Thin-cut orbital CT detects radiopaque and radiolucent materials.
- B scan demonstrates foreign body and associated ocular damage.
- MRI is contraindicated unless foreign material is known to be nonmetallic.
- Culture of removed foreign object to determine bacterial or fungal exposure.

Pathology

- Inflammatory cells, necrosis; evidence of ocular trauma.
- Prussian blue iron stain is positive in iris dilator and sphincter muscles, sensory retina, trabecular meshwork.

Disease Course

- Intraocular iron fragments lead to siderosis bulbi, an accumulation of ionized iron in the epithelial tissues of the eye.
- Pure copper leads to acute chalcosis; copper alloyed to other metals in concentrations less than 85% leads to chronic chalcosis.
- Lead and zinc cause mild nongranulomatous ocular inflammation, generally well tolerated by eye.
- Glass, aluminum, gold, silver, and platinum are almost inert substances in eye.
- Organic materials tend to retain infectious agents within the eye and should be removed.
- Cilia are generally well tolerated within the eye.

Treatment and Management

- All foreign material should be removed at the time of initial surgical repair of ruptured globe to prevent endophthalmitis and toxic reactions.
- A pulsed electromagnet may be used to remove magnetic substances.
- IOFBs identified after wound healing may be observed serially to evaluate inflammatory response; ERGs may be obtained to assess development of siderosis bulbi.

  Patients may benefit from intravitreal antibiotic prophylaxis.

Medications

Intraocular antibiotics may be necessary to prevent infection due to the IOFB.

Follow-Up

Daily, looking for signs of endophthalmitis or inflammation.

Differential Diagnosis

Endophthalmitis: Presentation may be similar. Head-imaging scan may reveal IOFB.

Traumatic VH

References

Coleman DJ, Lucas BC, Rondeau MJ, et al. Management of intraocular foreign bodies. *Ophthalmology* 1987;94:1647–1653.

Slusher MM. Intraretinal foreign bodies: management and observations. *Retina* 1990;10(Suppl):S50–S54.

Traumatic Endophthalmitis

Summary

Intraocular infection secondary to penetrating ocular trauma or surgery leading to severe ocular injury, if not treated promptly. Traumatic endophthalmitis is generally more aggressive and devastating than postoperative surgical endophthalmitis and must be treated more aggressively.

Etiology

Trauma: *Bacillus cereus*, *Staphylococcus epidermidis*, Gram-negative organisms, *Streptococcus* species, fungi.

Postoperative: 2 to 7 days after surgery; *S. epidermidis*, *S. aureus*, *Streptococcus viridans*, *Proteus* species, *Pseudomonas aeruginosa*, *Haemophilus influenzae*, fungi; *Propionibacterium acnes* develops after 3 to 6 weeks.

Bleb related: 2 to 10 years after surgery; *Streptococcus* species, *H. influenzae*, *Staphylococcus* species.

Endogenous: associated with debility, hyperalimentation; *Candida* species, *H. influenzae*, *Klebsiella* species.

Signs and Symptoms

Subacute or acute loss of vision.

Red, painful eye.

Demographics

Postsurgical or posttraumatic eyes; eyes with filtering blebs.

Patients with chronic illness, diabetes.

Eyes after cataract surgery with ruptured posterior capsule.

Intravenous drug abusers.

Ophthalmic Findings

Vision from 20/20 to bare light perception.

Conjunctival chemosis, hyperemia.

Inflamed bleb, bleb leak, or purulence within bleb.

Cloudy cornea with anterior chamber inflammation or hypopyon.

Signs of ocular surgery (trabeculectomy, cataract removal).

Signs of eye trauma.

Vitreous cells; poor view of retina.

Retinal hemorrhages, cotton-wool spots.

Yellow-white retinal lesions.

Diminished red reflex.

Systemic Findings

Indwelling i.v. catheter.

Evidence of head trauma.

Special Tests

Anterior chamber paracentesis may be performed, though generally does not provide clinically useful information.

Vitreous biopsy, Gram stain, culture.

Biopsy and culture of any exposed areas of ruptured globe.

Pathology

Infectious and inflammatory cellular infiltrate within the anterior chamber and vitreous.

Disease Course

- Untreated endophthalmitis can rapidly lead to blindness.
- Visual recovery is directly related to prompt intervention and correct diagnosis of infectious agent.

Treatment and Management

- Traumatic endophthalmitis:

  Culture of draining sites in traumatic ruptured globe.

  Prompt vitrectomy, sending vitreous samples for Gram stain, fungal and bacterial cultures.

  Instill intravitreal antibiotics (discussed below).
- Postoperative endophthalmitis:

Prompt anterior chamber paracentesis and vitreous biopsy specimen for Gram stain and culture.
Instill intravitreal antibiotics, discussed below.
Immediate vitrectomy of postoperative eyes if initial vision is worse than hand motions has shown to be of benefit.

Medications

- Postoperative:
  Postoperative endophthalmitis: intravitreal amikacin (0.4 mg/0.1 mL) plus vancomycin (1.0 mg/0.1 mL) at time of vitreous biopsy (ceftazidime, 2.25 mg/0.1 mL, may be substituted for amikacin); subconjunctival ceftazidime (100 mg/0.5 mL) plus vancomycin (25 mg/0.5 mL) and dexamethasone (steroid also may be given intravitreally).
  Vitreous biopsy and antibiotic dosing may be repeated at 36 to 60 hours if not improved.
  Fortified topical antibiotics employed (ceftazidime plus vancomycin).
  Intravenous antibiotics were not shown to be beneficial in the Endophthalmitis Vitrectomy Study (EVS) for early postcataract extraction endophthalmitis, but their utility in traumatic or late postoperative endophthalmitis remains unclear.
  Late postoperative endophthalmitis: amphotericin may be substituted for ceftazidime, but all other medications as above.
- Traumatic:
  Intravitreal amikacin (0.4 mg/0.1 mL) plus vancomycin (1.0 mg/0.1 mL) at time of vitrectomy; amphotericin (0.005 mg/0.1 mL) may be added if fungal elements seen on Gram stain or in culture results; steroids avoided initially.
  Fortified topical antibiotics as above.
  Consider i.v. antibiotics (vancomycin, amikacin, ketoconazole), although no prospective studies support or contend their use.
- Oral antibiotics and antifungals:
  Given the high rate of endophthalmitis in this demographic, oral antibiotics such as Moxifloxacin 400 mg PO or i.v. are commonly employed to theoretically decrease the incidence of intraocular infections. In situations where there is a concern for fungal inoculation (plant matter/stick injuries), one may consider endophthalmitis prophylaxis with Voriconazole PO or i.v.

Follow-Up

Daily.

Differential Diagnosis

- Phacoanaphylactic uveitis: following cataract surgery or penetrating ocular trauma. Lens material may be visible.
- Postoperative inflammation due to surgical trauma (sterile endophthalmitis).
- IOFB, especially copper.
- Retinoblastoma: seeding of tumor cells in infant or young child.
- Reticulum cell sarcoma: chronic uveitis, may be responsive to steroids, in elderly patients.
- Panuveitis (sarcoid, VKH, pars planitis).

References

Hariprasad SM, Shah GK, Mieler WF, et al. Vitreous and aqueous penetration of orally administered moxifloxacin in humans. *Arch Ophthalmol* 2006;124(2):178–182.
Hariprasad SM, Mieler WF, Lin TK, et al. Voriconazole in the treatment of fungal eye infections: a review of current literature. *Br J Ophthalmol* 2008;92:871–878.
Affeldt JC, Flynn HW Jr, Forster RK, et al. Microbial endophthalmitis resulting from ocular trauma. *Ophthalmology* 1996;103:390–397.
Reynolds DS, Flynn HW, Jr. Endophthalmitis after penetrating ocular trauma. *Curr Opin Ophthalmol* 1997;8:32–38.

Sympathetic Ophthalmia

Summary

Painful red eye with decreased vision and photophobia in a person in whom the contralateral eye recently experienced a penetrating ocular injury 4 to 8 weeks (but up to several decades) earlier.

Etiology

Either involves an autoimmune attack on uveal-retinal antigen of injured eye and subsequent immune attack on the uninjured "sympathizing" eye or is in response to a viral or infectious stimulus.

Signs and Symptoms

- Decreased vision in injured eye because of trauma and inflammation, and in the "sympathizing" eye as a result of the inflammation and its sequelae.
- Bilateral eye pain and redness.

Demographics

- Persons with penetrating ocular trauma (more commonly men) or surgery involving the uveal tract (ruptured globe, laser photocoagulation, cryotherapy, intraocular surgery, radiation therapy to globe).
- Incidence approximately 1 in 15,000 following intraocular surgery, and as high as 1 in 500 following penetrating ocular trauma.

Ophthalmic Findings

- Bilateral granulomatous panuveitis: mutton fat keratic precipitates, anterior chamber cells, iris nodules, vitritis, Dalen-Fuchs nodules (sites of RPE depigmentation).

- Loss of accommodation.
- Signs of chronic uveitis: peripheral anterior synechiae, iris NV, posterior synechiae, occlusio pupillae, cataract, glaucoma, cyclitic membrane, exudative RD, retinitis, vasculitis, optic atrophy.

Systemic Findings

Chronic cases may develop vitiligo, alopecia, dysacusis, and meningeal symptoms similar to VKH.

Special Tests

FTA-Abs, MHATP.

Serum ACE levels, serum lysozyme, CXR, gallium scan to rule out sarcoid.

Pathology

- Infiltration of uveal tract with T cells, other inflammatory cells.
- Macrophages, lymphocytes, and epithelioid cells along the uveal tract, sparing the retina and the choroid in early cases; aggregations of epithelioid cells between the retina and Bruch membrane.

Disease Course

- Chronic slow-acting uveitis with periods of exacerbation.
- Following treatment, 65% of eyes have 20/60 vision or better.

Treatment and Management

Strong consideration of early enucleation in blind eyes with penetrating ocular injury within first 2 weeks may prevent sympathetic ophthalmia. After the sympathetic response begins, enucleation of the injured eye may still benefit the remaining eye.

Medications

- Topical and periocular steroids.
- Systemic steroids may be used in conjunction with histamine H_2 blocker.
- Topical cycloplegics.
- Systemic immunosuppressive medications may be needed in severe cases where steroids are contraindicated.

Follow-Up

Frequent follow-up may be lengthened as course stabilizes.

Differential Diagnosis

VKH: similar etiology and course, but no history of eye injury; VKH includes symptoms of meningitis as well as vitiligo, poliosis, and alopecia; certain racial groups including native Americans and Asians have higher rates of VKH.

Syphilis: may masquerade as sympathetic ophthalmia; laboratory evaluation diagnostic.

Posttraumatic endophthalmitis: rapidly increasing inflammation usually within days of injury.

Phacoanaphylaxis: traumatic or surgical disruption of lens resulting in intense inflammation.

References

Chan CC, Roberge RG, Whitcup SM, et al. Thirty-two cases of sympathetic ophthalmia: a retrospective study at the National Eye Institute, Bethesda, MD, from 1982 to 1992. *Arch Ophthalmol* 1995;113:597–600.

Towler HM, Lightman S. Sympathetic ophthalmia. *Int Ophthalmol Clin* 1995;35:31–42.

RETINAL AND CHOROIDAL TUMORS

Malignant Melanoma of the Choroid and the Ciliary Body

Summary

Uveal tract melanoma is the most common primary intraocular tumor in adults. The highest incidence is in the choroid (85%), followed by ciliary body (10%); tumors may overlap both sites as well. Despite excellent options for local tumor control, systemic metastasis limits long-term survival in up to 50% of patients, and overall survival rates have remained stable. Ciliary body melanomas tend to be asymptomatic, harder to detect on routine examination, and are maybe larger at presentation than choroidal melanomas. Uveal melanomas are biologically different than cutaneous melanomas and should not be considered an ocular metastasis from cutaneous melanoma.

Etiology

- No established risk factors, but greater association with light skin color. No clear association with sun exposure or UV radiation.
- Typically arise from preexisting choroidal nevus or atypical melanocytic proliferation.
- Patients with oculodermal melanosis and dysplastic nevus syndrome are at increased risk.

Signs and Symptoms

- Commonly asymptomatic unless local effects exerted onto retina or lens.
- Blurred vision or metamorphopsia may be caused by the following:
  - Exudative RD.
  - Secondary cataract or induced lenticular astigmatism from anterior choroidal or ciliary body melanomas.
  - Breakthrough vitreous or subretinal hemorrhage.

- Peripheral field loss may be caused by a tumor mass or by a peripheral RD.
- Photopsias.
- Infrequently, floaters as a result of a VH or inflammatory cells may be noted.
- Rarely, eye pain from secondary elevated IOP or inflammation.

Demographics

Melanoma occurs most frequently in Caucasians aged 55 to 75. Incidence is approximately 6 per 1,000,000. Less common in pigmented races.

Ophthalmic Findings

See Figure 3.64.

- Focal conjunctival or episcleral vascular dilation in quadrant of tumor (sentinel vessel) typically in longstanding anterior choroid or ciliary body melanomas (Figure 3.65).
- Transscleral erosion of ciliary body or anterior uveal melanoma.
- Anterior chamber invasion or ciliary body melanoma into iris or drainage angle.
- Elevated dome-shaped choroidal lesion, typically greater than 2.0 mm in height.
- Variable pigmentation: typically pigmented (brown or tan) but may be amelanotic with clear visualization of choroidal vasculature.
- Tumor surface may have drusen and variable RPE changes that may suggest chronicity. The presence of lipofuscin orange pigment suggests more active tumor.
- Exudative RD may be localized over the surface of the tumor or more extensive and remote from the tumor mass in larger melanomas.

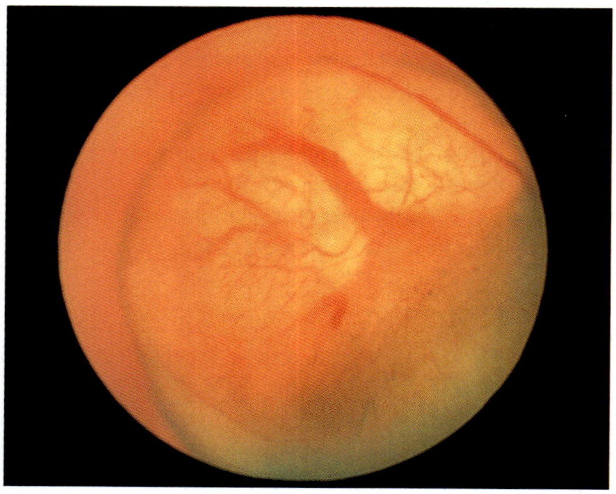

FIGURE 3.64. A pigmented medium-sized choroidal melanoma is present. The maximal thickness measured is 3.7 mm.

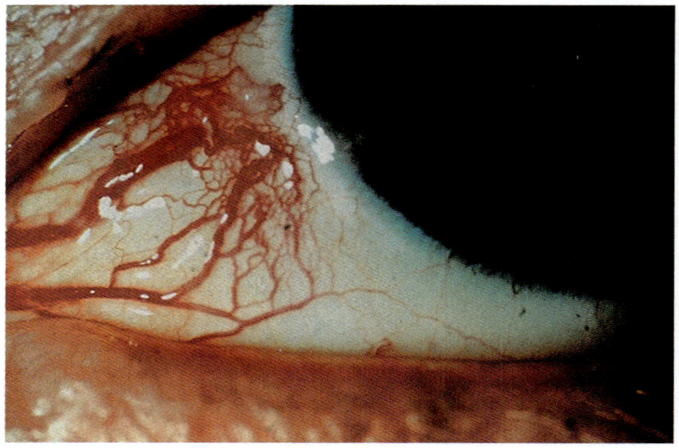

FIGURE 3.65. Dilated episcleral, "sentinel" vessels are present.

- Apical tumor growth through Bruch membrane produces classic "collar-button" or "mushroom" shape, but not typically in tumors less than 5 mm in height.
- Subretinal hemorrhage may be noted but typically occurs when Bruch membrane ruptures. Should subretinal hemorrhage occur in the absence of a "collar-button" tumor, an alternative diagnosis such as subretinal NV should be considered.

Systemic Findings

The liver is the predominant site of metastasis, followed by the lungs. At the time of diagnosis, systemic screening for metastatic disease is recommended. Most patients will not have systemic metastases at the time of ocular tumor diagnosis.

Special Tests

- Color fundus photography
  - To document the location and appearance of the tumor for future follow-up.
- IVFA:
  1. Mostly helpful in excluding other diagnoses such as subretinal hemorrhage.
  2. Angiographic findings may include the following:
     i. Double circulation: Visualization of tumor vessels and retinal vessels (Figure 3.66) occurs in elevated and predominantly amelanotic tumors.
     ii. Punctate or pinpoint hyperfluoresence.
- Ultrasonography:
  1. A scan: accurately measures tumor height and reflectivity pattern. Usually, a low-to-medium reflectivity occurs because of the homogeneous nature of melanomas (Figure 3.67).
  2. B scan: determines shape and contour (Figure 3.68), particularly in the presence of a collar-button configuration. It is also helpful in determining the presence of extrascleral extension and adjacent RD.

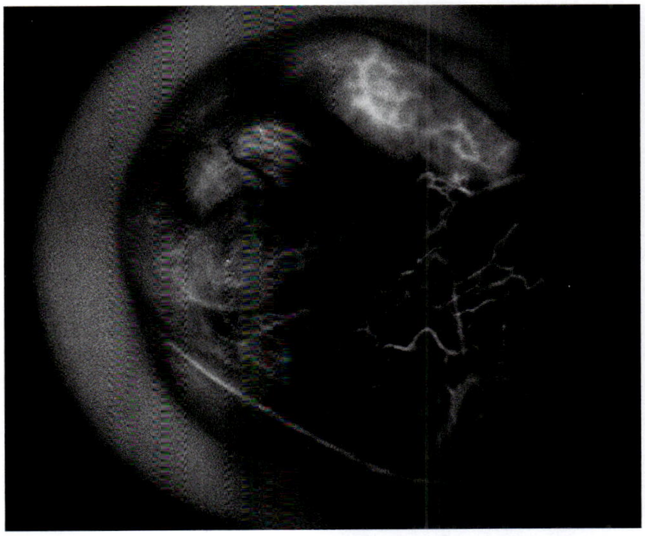

FIGURE 3.66. An AV-phase angiogram shows filling of the retinal vessels overlying the mass, as well as filling of vessels within the tumor. This is referred to as a *double circulation.*

- Fine-needle aspiration biopsy:
  1. For cases with diagnostic uncertainty and for prognostic testing.
  2. Tumors anterior to the equator are sampled through a transscleral approach, which those posterior to the equator are accessed through a transvitreal, pars plana approach.
  3. Fine needle aspirates from the tumors are submitted to experienced cytopathologists for diagnosis.
- CT and MRI:
  1. Orbital studies may confirm the intraocular tumor and associated RD, but not diagnostic of melanoma.

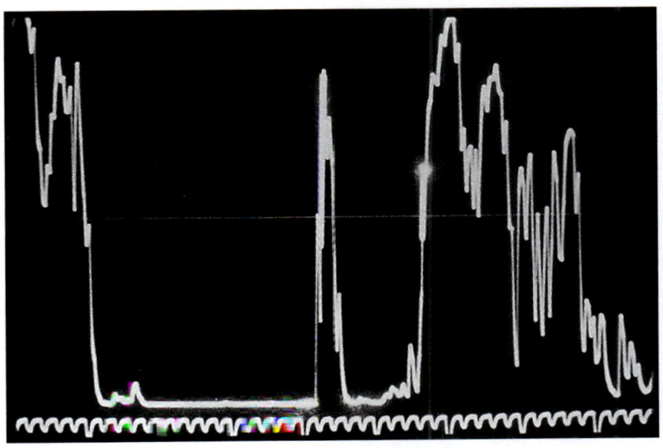

FIGURE 3.67. An A-scan ultrasound is shown. Going from left to right, the highest peaks at the left side are from the corneal surface. The next highest peak is from the tumor-retinal interface, and the next highest peak is from the sclera. The height of the echoes within the tumor is evaluated to determine the reflectivity pattern. In this case, the reflectivity is low and regular.

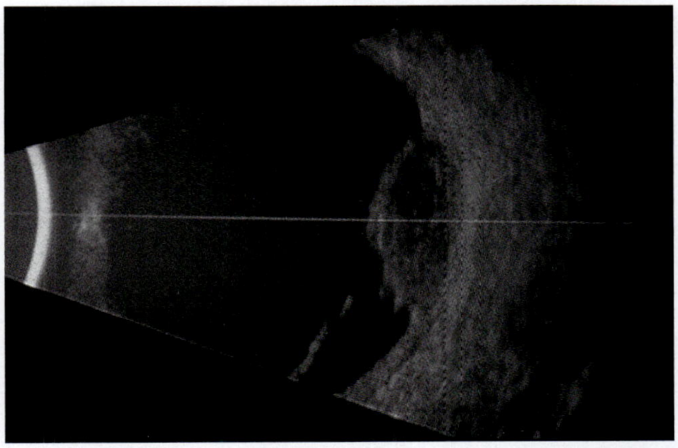

FIGURE 3.68. A B-scan ultrasound is shown. A dome-shaped mass is present with a RD below.

  Greater utility in determining extraocular extension or extension along optic nerve.
  2. Abdominal studies are indicated to assess extent of metastasis, if melanoma is confirmed.
- X-ray: CXRs are indicated if melanoma is confirmed as part of the metastatic workup.
- Blood work: Liver enzyme studies are indicated, if melanoma is confirmed.

Pathology

See Table 3.17.

Disease Course

- Poor prognostic factors:
  1. Large tumor size (largest tumor diameter, >16 mm, or height, >10 mm).
  2. Anterior tumors.
  3. Older age (not in all series).
  4. Extrascleral extension.
  5. Diffuse tumor growth pattern.
  6. Epithelioid cell type.
  7. Cytogenetic alterations (monosomy 3) and gene expression profile abnormalities.
- The 5-year survival for medium-sized melanomas (10 to 16 mm basal diameter and 2.5 to 10 mm maximal thickness) ranges between 60% and 85% depending on many of the above factors. The 5-year survival for large melanomas ranges from 50% to 75%.

Treatment and Management

- Overview:
  1. Goals of treatment:
     a. Local control of intraocular tumor.
     b. Prevention of subsequent metastases.
     c. Globe-sparing therapies when appropriate.
     d. Preservation of vision when possible.

Table 3.17

Malignant melanoma cell types and prognosis

Cell type	Description	Prognosis
Spindle A	Cells are slender with flattened nuclei and a basophilic nuclear line caused by infolding of the nuclear membrane. The nucleus is devoid of nucleolus.	Best
Spindle B	Cells are slightly larger than spindle A cells and have a round or an oval nucleus and prominent nucleolus. These cells tend to merge to form a syncytium.	Intermediate
Epithelioid	Cells are large, round, and have well-demarcated cell membranes, eosinophilic cytoplasm, and round nuclei with prominent nucleoli. They are polymorphic and have variable amounts of pigment.	Worst
Mixed	Most common presentation. Cell types from two or more of the above types are present.	Intermediate

2. Micrometastatic disease: It is theorized that subclinical metastases likely have occurred months to years prior to diagnosis of intraocular melanoma in tumors with high malignant potential. Clinical metastases may occur at a peak incidence of 3 to 5 years after diagnosis of ocular melanoma, despite successful treatment of intraocular tumor.
3. No survival benefit to local globe-sparing therapies (e.g., plaque brachytherapy) compared to enucleation for medium-sized tumors per the COMS study.

- Enucleation:
  1. Local tumor control in eyes harboring melanomas whose size (either base or apical height) is not amenable to globe-sparing radiotherapy.
  2. Treatment of eyes with choroidal or ciliary body melanoma and features incompatible with long-term health of the eye including neovascular glaucoma, advanced secondary glaucoma, extensive extraocular extension, optic nerve infiltration.
  3. Patient preference in lieu of globe-sparing therapies.
  4. No evidence that enucleation procedure itself increases risk of metastatic seeding.
     a. COMS Large Tumor study demonstrated no survival benefit in patients receiving pre-enucleation external beam radiotherapy compared to enucleation alone.
- Radiation treatment: The goal of this globe-sparing treatment is to destroy or inactivate tumor cells, prevent future metastatic spread, and preserve vision.
  1. Episcleral plaque radiotherapy (brachytherapy).
     a. Radioactive seeds are secured into a specially designed carrier that is then secured to the sclera directly over the tumor. The plaque is kept in place for 3 to 5 days, delivering a radiation dose of approximately 85 Gy to the tumor apex.
     b. Most common radioisotopes used are iodine 125 (^{125}I) and ruthenium 106 (^{106}Ru). Palladium 103 (^{103}Pl), Cobalt 60 (^{60}Co), and iridium 192 (^{192}Ir) have also been reported.
     c. Local tumor control rates exceed 90% at 10 years and depend on tumor size, location, radiation dose utilized, and preexisting systemic factors including diabetic retinopathy.
     d. Common side effects include vision loss from cataract and radiation retinopathy, radiation optic neuropathy, neovascular glaucoma
  2. Charged particle: external beam radiotherapy with proton or helium ions. Small tantalum rings are surgically secured to the sclera to mark the margins of melanoma. This allows later radiologic localization of the tumor margins to guide the radiation treatment. Benefit reported as less collateral damage to surrounding structures due to focused delivery of radiation. May be more beneficial.
  3. Laser photocoagulation: A slit-lamp or an indirect ophthalmoscope-mounted 810-nm diode transpupillary thermotherapy to raise internal temperature within tumor by 4°C has been used as primary therapy in tumors up to 4.0 mm in thickness or as adjuvant treatment following plaque radiotherapy. Local tumor control by laser alone is inferior to plaque radiotherapy and is not considered first-line therapy except in rare cases.
  4. Local resection: anterior melanomas involving the ciliary body and/or anterior choroid; there are several different approaches, but typically a partial-thickness scleral flap is produced over the area of melanoma, which is then excised with a portion of the remaining layer of sclera. Some authors have expressed concern about intrascleral spread of the melanoma and potentially inadequate resection of the entire tumor.

Medications

None effective.

Follow-Up

- Small melanomas should be reassessed every 4 to 6 months for growth, with ophthalmic examination, ultrasonic and photographs.
- Follow-up of medium-sized and large melanomas varies with treatment modality employed.

Differential Diagnosis of Choroidal Melanoma

Pigmented Lesions

Choroidal nevus: typically less than 2.5 mm in thickness, may be melanotic or amelanotic, may be associated with localized features that may be predictive of future growth or malignant transformation including subretinal fluid and orange pigment on the tumor surface (lipofuscin).

Congenital hypertrophy of the RPE: flat, black lesions; may be surrounded by a halo of depigmentation; well-defined borders; depigmented foci within the lesion (lacunae).

Melanocytoma: dark black lesions commonly seen near or on the optic nerve; slow growing with rare risk of malignant transformation into uveal melanoma.

Peripheral exudative hemorrhagic chorioretinopathy: nonmacular CNVM with elevated subretinal hemorrhage and disciform scarring. Not always associated with ARMD; typically with subretinal hemorrhage of various ages, which resolves over time.

Reactive hyperplasia of the RPE secondary to trauma or inflammation: prior history of trauma or inflammation and these lesions are flat and can be associated with gliosis.

Choroidal detachments: associated with ocular surgery trauma, hypotony, etc. They are multilobular. Transillumination and IVFA can be used to differentiate from malignant melanoma.

Nonpigmented Lesions

Choroidal hemangioma: reddish-orange, slightly elevated, and can be differentiated from a malignant melanoma with ultrasonography.

Choroidal osteoma: yellowish-orange, occurs near the optic nerve, has pseudopod-like formations, and occurs more frequently in young women.

Metastatic carcinoma: history of lung or breast cancer, the lesions are flat and have a creamy brown color. Subretinal fluid is frequently associated, and these lesions are typically multifocal and can be bilateral.

Posterior scleritis: Choroidal folds are present along with intense pain and possibly a history of systemic inflammatory disease. A nodular inflammatory lesion may be seen in the choroid. Choroidal thickening with sub-Tenon fluid (T sign) may be seen on B scan ultrasonography.

Other inflammatory masses.

References

The Collaborative Ocular Melanoma Study (COMS) Group. The COMS randomized trial of pre-enucleation radiation of large choroidal melanomas: IV. Ten year mortality findings and prognostic factors. COMS report 24. *Am J Ophthalmol* 2004;138:936–951.

The Collaborative Ocular Melanoma Study (COMS) Group. The COMS randomized trial of iodine 125 brachytherapy for choroidal melanoma: V. Twelve-year mortality rates and prognostic factors: COMS report No. 28. *Arch Ophthalmol* 2006;124(12):1684–1693.

Shields CL, Cater J, Shields JA, et al. Combination of clinical factors predictive of growth of small choroidal melanocytic tumors. *Arch Ophthalmol* 2000;118:360–364.

Shields JA, Mashayekhi A, Ra S, et al. Pseudomelanomas of the posterior uveal tract: the 2006 Taylor R. Smith Lecture. *Retina* 2005;25(6):767–771.

Choroidal Osteoma

Summary

Choroidal osteomas are benign bony tumors generally located in the juxtapapillary choroid.

Etiology

These are osseous choristomas (histologically normal tissue in an abnormal location). The origin is unknown, although they have been described following inflammation and can progress or disappear during observation or following laser photocoagulation.

Signs and Symptoms

Blurred or distorted vision, particularly if the macula is involved and CNVMs are present.

Demographics

- Prevalence and incidence data are not available, but osteoma is considered to be rare.
- Young adult women are most commonly affected.

Ophthalmic Findings

- Usually occurs in the juxtapapillary and macular areas and appears orangish, whitish, or a whitish-yellow (Figure 3.69).
- Bilateral in 20% of cases.
- Small, vascular "spiders" may be seen over the surface.
- CNVM is a frequent complication.

RETINA

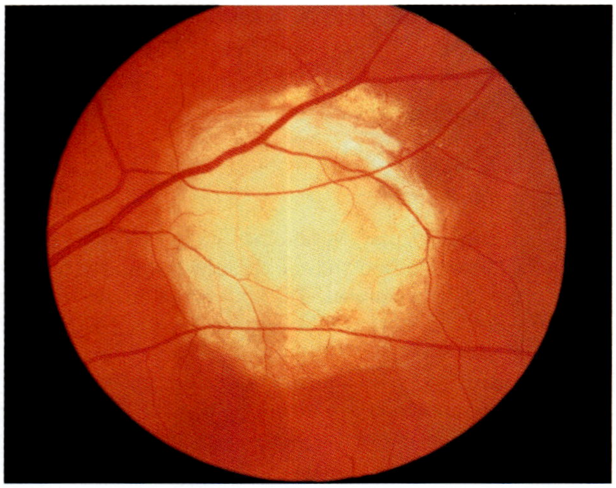

FIGURE 3.69. A choroidal osteoma is present involving much of the posterior pole. The VA was 20/40.

Systemic Findings

None.

Special Tests

- IVFA

  Early relative hyperfluorescence reflects disturbance and attenuation of the RPE. The hyperfluorescence is usually more diffuse as compared with a hemangioma or a melanoma.

  Late focal staining occurs in patients with serous detachment of the retina with or without CNVM.
- Ultrasonography.

The presence of hyperreflectivity suggestive of calcification can be confirmed.

Pathology

- Histologic examination shows presence of bone formation, with bony trabeculae with endothelial-lined cavernous spaces and capillary blood vessels.
- Osteoblasts, osteocytes, and osteoclasts are present.

Disease Course

- Typically enlarge slowly, usually over many years.
- Visual impairment occurs with macular involvement or with development of CNVM. Other patients may lose vision because of degeneration of photoreceptors overlying the osteoma.

Treatment and Management

- In most cases, no treatment is necessary.
- In cases with CNVM formation affecting or threatening vision, treatment options may include laser photocoagulation, verteporfin photodynamic therapy, submacular surgery, and anti-VEGF therapy.

Medications

None necessary.

Follow-Up

Yearly, sooner if assessment and treatment of CNVM is required.

Differential Diagnosis of Choroidal Osteoma

1. Conditions associated with intraocular calcifications occurring in sclerochoroidal calcifications:
   a. Hyperparathyroidism.
   b. Chronic renal failure.
   c. Vitamin D intoxication.
2. Conditions associated with CNVM formation (these conditions demonstrate leakage on IVFA along with lacy filling pattern).
3. Amelanotic melanoma (ultrasonography shows typical pattern along with elevation and reflectivity).
4. Retinoblastoma (children, elevated retinal mass).

Reference

Shields CL, Sun H, Demirci H, et al. Factors predictive of tumor growth, tumor decalification, choroidal neovascularization and visual outcome in 74 eyes with choroidal osteoma. *Arch Ophthalmol* 2005;123(12):1658–1666.

Vascular Tumors of the Retina and the Choroid

Retinal Capillary Hemangioma

Summary

Retinal capillary hemangioma (also known as *von Hippel tumor*, *angiomatosis retinae*, *capillary hemangioblastoma*) appears as a red to orange tumor located within the retina with large tortuous feeding and draining blood vessels.

Etiology

- This lesion is a hamartoma resulting from abnormal proliferation of retinal capillaries.
- Capillary hemangioma of the retina is a defining feature of systemic VHL disease, which is inherited as an autosomal dominant trait with complete penetrance by the sixth and seventh decades. The gene is located on the short arm of chromosome 3 and functions as a recessive tumor suppressor gene.

Signs and Symptoms

Blurred vision.
Distorted vision.

Demographics

- Asymptomatic lesions can be detected from the first to the eighth decades of life.
- Ocular symptoms usually begin in young adulthood.

Ophthalmic Findings

- Initially they appear as red or gray dots (the size of small microaneurysms), which enlarge slowly.
- Afferent and efferent vessels are of normal size initially, but slowly enlarge with time.
- Prominent retinal vessels emerging from the optic disk may suggest peripheral hemangioma.
- Eventually multiple angiomas can be found in the same eye.
  Bilateral in 50% of cases.
  Red-orange intraretinal mass protruding inward with an enlarged, tortuous feeder artery and an enlarged and tortuous draining vein.
  AV shunting is present within the lesion.
- Incompetence of capillary walls leads retinal edema and rarely to intraretinal and subretinal exudation.
- Exudative RD can occur.
- Epiretinal membrane leading to vitreoretinal traction and traction retinal detachment.
- VH.

Systemic Findings (Associated with von Hippel–Lindau Disease)

- VHL disease refers to the following:
  Retinal hemangioma or CNS angioma *and*
  One or more visceral cysts or tumors (pancreatic, ovarian, testicular, renal cysts) or when a single lesion of the VHL complex is found in a relative.
- All patients with multiple capillary hemangiomas of the retina should be considered to have VHL disease: Most patients who present with a solitary retinal angioma and a negative family history suggesting VHL disease fail to manifest other evidence of the disease.
- Ocular manifestations of VHL disease are usually the first to appear.
- Twenty percent of patients with angiomatosis retinae have hemangioblastomas of the cerebellum, medulla, pons and spinal cord. Retinal capillary hemangiomas occur in over 50% of patients with VHL disease.
- Visceral cysts of the liver, kidney, pancreas, epididymis and ovary.
- Neoplastic associations: meningiomas, bilateral hypernephromas (25% of patients), and pheochromocytomas (10% of patients).
- Unlike other phacomatoses, there are no skin findings.
- Polycythemia in 15% of patients.

Special Tests

A complete workup is indicated when capillary hemangiomas that are multiple or bilateral are found or when there is a unilateral capillary hemangioma with characteristic systemic findings or with a positive family history (some physicians advocate a full systemic workup in all patients with a diagnosis of retina capillary hemangioma).

- Laboratory: urine tests for levels of epinephrine and norepinephrine (for pheochromocytoma).
- IVFA is a good way to monitor patients for possible developing angiomas:
  Enlarged retinal vessels are seen connected to this hyperfluorescent tumor.
  The passage of fluorescein from the afferent artery through the tumor into the efferent vein is extremely rapid because of the presence of an AV shunt within the tumor.
  There is profuse leakage from the angioma as the angiogram progresses. Surrounding the tumor, capillary nonperfusion can occur.
- MRI of the brain to look for cerebellar angiomas.
- Abdominal CT scan looking for pancreatic cysts, pheochromocytomas, etc.
- Genetic testing for VHL gene abnormality.

Pathology

- Light microscopy demonstrates that the center of the angioma consists of tortuous capillaries with normal endothelium, basement membrane, and pericytes.
- Fenestrations are noted between endothelial cells at the time intraretinal exudation develops, but not before this.
- The capillary channels are separated by interstitial cells with foamy lipid-filled vacuoles.
- Two types of capillary hemangiomas have been identified: the endophytic type, which arises from the superficial retina, and the exophytic type, which arises from the outer layers.

Disease Course

- The clinical course is one of progression, recurrence, or development of new lesions: Spontaneous regression has been reported.
- Early detection and treatment are essential. The prognosis is excellent for tumors up to 1 disk diameter in size.

Treatment and Management

- Treatment of peripheral capillary angioma should be undertaken when the lesion is first detected.
- Transscleral cryotherapy is used for large lesions or lesions located anterior to the equator. A triple freeze-thaw cycle is effective.
- Argon laser photocoagulation should be applied directly to the surface to eradicate small lesions and can be used as an adjunct to cryotherapy for large lesions. A large

spot size, a low intensity, and a long duration are used. Complications of laser treatment include hemorrhage and increased exudation.

- Plaque radiotherapy or external beam radiotherapy can be used for localized tumors with exudation.
- VEGF inhibition may help mediate macular edema and fluid exudation, though tumor regression is less likely to be achieved.
- Surgical resection of tumor with diathermy or ligation of feeding and draining vessels.
- Genetic counseling.
- Appropriate systemic therapy.
- Complications of capillary retinal hemangiomas include massive RDs attributable to tumor exudation or vitreous traction. In these cases, pars plana vitrectomy, scleral buckling, and endolaser may be necessary.

Medications

None effective.

Follow-Up

- Every 3 to 6 months.
- A multidisciplinary surveillance approach to surveillance of families with VHL disease is essential for detection of potentially blinding or lethal complications.
- Annual indirect ophthalmoscopy starting at age 6 should years be carried out for all affected patients and relatives.

Differential Diagnosis

1. Macular exudation:
   a. Retinal arterial macroaneurysm (generally seen in older people, unilateral and usually single, associated hypertension or arteriosclerosis. Lesion is centered along arteriole without a draining venule).
   b. Coats disease (no tumefaction, "lightbulb" aneurysms, and characteristic fluorescein angiogram).
   c. Diabetic retinopathy (microaneurysms, dot-blot hemorrhages, characteristic appearance on IVFA).
   d. Retinal vasoproliferative tumor: non familial, inferiorly located globular pale appearing mass. No vascular anomalies accompany this lesion and may be associated with exudation, subretinal fluid and fibrosis.
2. Peripheral AV shunts producing dilated feeder vessels:
   a. Racemose aneurysm (Wyburn-Mason syndrome): no tumefaction; large, tortuous, dilated vessels.
   b. AV aneurysm.
   c. Anastomosis between tumor vessels and retinal vessels in retinoblastoma or malignant melanoma.
3. Surface fibroglial proliferation:
   a. Sea fans of sickle retinopathy (sclerosed peripheral blood vessels, a gray peripheral fundus, tortuous retinal veins, black sunbursts, retinal hemorrhages, refractile deposits, angioid streaks, VHs, RD, and the like are associated).
   b. Presumed acquired retinal hemangiomas seen in the elderly.

References

Singh AD, Nouri M, Shields CL, et al. Treatment of retinal capillary hemangioma. *Ophthalmology* 2002;109:1799–1806.

Singh AD, Shields CL, Shields JA. Von-Hippel-Lindau disease. *Surv Ophthalmol* 2001;46(2):117–142.

Cavernous Hemangioma of the Choroid

Summary

Choroidal hemangiomas are of two varieties: (a) localized type in patients with no systemic disorders and (b) diffuse type in patients with Sturge-Weber syndrome (encephalofacial hemangiomatosis).

Etiology

- Circumscribed hemangiomas are typically unifocal, sporadic and not associated with Sturge-Weber syndrome.
- Sturge-Weber syndrome (sporadic inheritance) is associated with diffuse choroidal hemangiomas.

Signs and Symptoms

Blurred or distorted vision.
A diffuse hemangioma is usually associated with a facial nevus.
Seizures if meningeal involvement.

Demographics

Localized cavernous hemangiomas of the choroid are rarely detected before the third decade of life.

Ophthalmic Findings

- The solitary variety is usually an amelanotic, reddish-orange mass in the posterior pole (Figure 3.70):
  In some cases, the color may make it difficult to distinguish from the surrounding choroid; therefore it is important to perform a color comparison with the fellow eye.
  Clumping of the RPE overlying the tumor may be present. This is a sign of existing or prior subretinal fluid.
- The diffuse variety (occurring in 40% of patients with Sturge-Weber syndrome) usually produces a diffuse reddish-orange thickening of the choroid and is more easily recognized because of the frequent association with facial angioma. The retinal blood vessels are frequently dilated and tortuous in the presence of a diffuse choroidal hemangioma. Glaucoma often occurs in eyes with this lesion.
- Sensory retinal elevation and cystic retinal changes overlying the tumor are frequent.

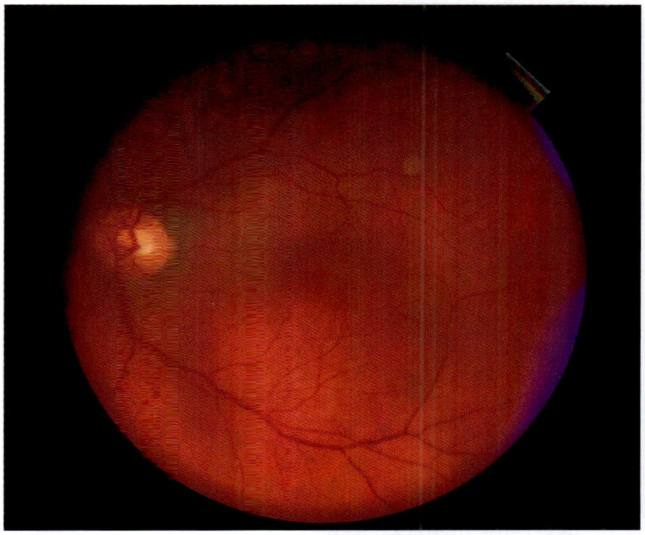

FIGURE 3.70. A reddish-orange solitary choroidal hemangioma is present inferior to the macula.

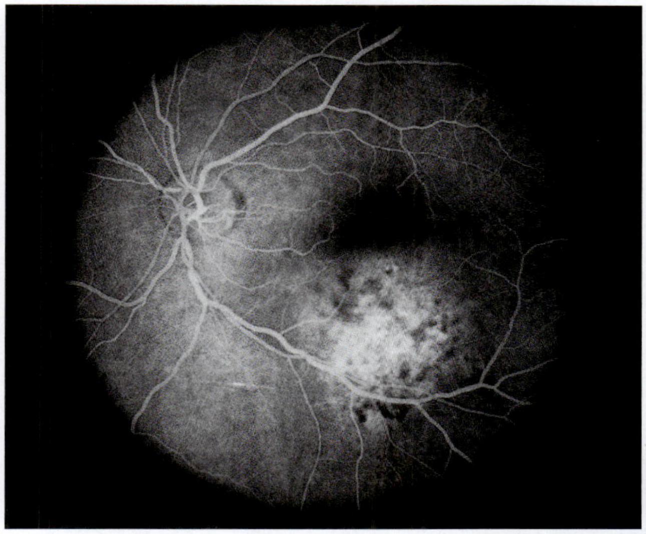

FIGURE 3.71. IVFA shows the lobular filling pattern of the hemangioma.

Systemic Findings of Sturge-Weber Syndrome

- Cutaneous angioma (nevus flammeus):
  Present at birth and involves the area of distribution of the first and second divisions of the trigeminal nerve.
  May be associated with hypertrophy of the involved areas of the face.
- Meningeal angioma:
  Ipsilateral angioma of the brain is frequently found.
  Accompanying jacksonian-type epilepsy, hemianopia, and hemiparesis can occur.
  Atrophy of the neighboring cerebral cortex can lead to variable mental deficiency.

Special Tests

- IVFA shows early hyperfluorescence of large choroidal vessels or a lobular filling pattern (Figure 3.71).
- ICG angiography demonstrates early choroidal filling and intrinsic vasculature of localized hemangiomas.
- Ultrasonography: marked vascularity of a choroidal hemangioma produces a characteristic high internal reflectivity on A-scan echography (Figure 3.72). B-scan echography usually shows a dome- or placoid-shaped mass.
- CT scan or MRI of the brain are indicated if Sturge-Weber syndrome is suspected.
- Electroencephalogram is indicated if Sturge-Weber syndrome is suspected.

Pathology

- This tumor consists of large congested choroidal vessels with thin intervascular septa.
- Overlying alterations of the RPE and cystic retinal degeneration are common.

Disease Course

- Localized choroidal hemangioma: Prognosis for life is excellent.
- Diffuse choroidal hemangioma: survival variable with systemic associations.
- Management of glaucoma with diffuse choroidal hemangiomas may be challenging as incisional surgery is associated with exudative RD or choroidal detachment.

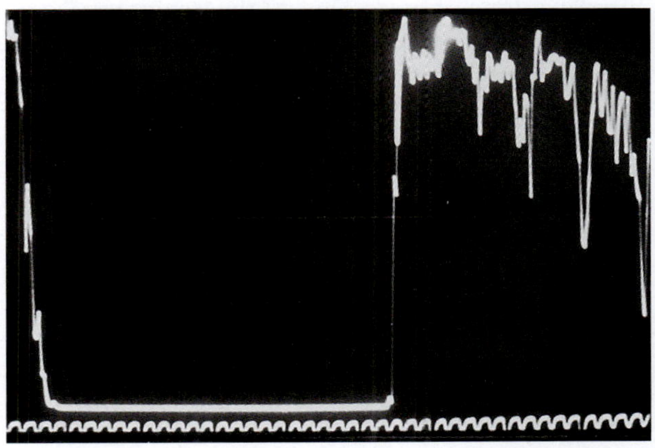

FIGURE 3.72. An A-scan ultrasound of a choroidal hemangioma. From left to right, the high peak at the far left side is from the corneal surface. The vitreous cavity is acoustically quiet and produces essentially no echoes. The next highest peak is from the retinal surface overlying the hemangioma. The reflectivity pattern of the hemangioma underlying the retina is characteristically very high.

- Recurrent exudative RDs can occur, and the visual prognosis in patients with macular detachment or macular edema is poor.

Treatment and Management

This is a benign tumor and can typically be observed. Management issues arise in symptomatic cases that are either vision threatening or have extensive serous RD:
Treatment options include the following:

1. Thermal laser photocoagulation.
2. Verteporfin photodynamic therapy demonstrates rapid resolution of subretinal fluid and often impressive tumor regression.
3. Radiotherapy (typically localized plaque brachytherapy, but external beam and proton beam may be considered) for large solitary lesions.

Medications

Aqueous suppressants to treat glaucoma.
Anticonvulsants.

Follow-Up

At least every 6 months, and sooner if glaucoma or macular detachment develops.

Differential Diagnosis of Localized Choroidal Hemangioma

- Amelanotic choroidal melanoma (ultrasonography shows typical pattern along with elevation).
- Choroidal osteomas (these are flat yellowish-orange, occur near the optic nerve, have pseudopod-like formations, and occur more frequently in young women).
- Carcinoma metastatic to the choroid (patients have a history of lung or breast cancer; the lesions are flat and have a creamy brown color. Subretinal fluid is frequently associated, and these lesions are typically bilateral).
- Inflammatory mass.
- Ocular lymphoma (abundant bilateral vitreous cells and debris are seen in patients older than 40 years of age. There is poor response to steroids. Yellow chorioretinal lesions are evident, and neurologic changes may occur).

References

Singh AD, Kaiser PK, Sears JE, et al. Photodynamic therapy of circumscribed choroidal haemangioma. *Br J Ophthalmol* 2004;88(11):1414–1418.

Shields CL, Honovar SG, Shields JE, et al. Circumscribed choroidal hemangioma: clinical manifestations and factors predictive of visual outcome in 200 consecutive cases. *Ophthalmology* 2001;108:2237–2248.

Sullivan TJ, Clarke MP, Morin JD. The ocular manifestations of Sturge-Weber syndrome. *J Pediatr Ophthalmol Strabismus* 1992;29:349–356.

Astrocytic Tumors of the Retina (Astrocytic Hamartoma, Acquired Retinal Astrocytoma)

Summary

Retinal astrocytic hamartomas are benign lesions associated with the tuberous sclerosis complex. Acquired retinal astrocytomas are rare, non-hereditary lesions with no systemic association.

Etiology

- A hamartoma (benign lesion of disorganized but mature cells native to the organ) resulting from abnormal proliferation of astrocytes.
- Inheritance: spontaneous, autosomal dominant in association with tuberous sclerosis (chromosome 9) or neurofibromatosis (type 1, chromosome 17; type 2, chromosome 22).

Signs and Symptoms

Typically visually asymptomatic, but can develop vision loss if lesion is in posterior pole.

- Leukocoria.
- Strabismus.
- Secondary amblyopia.

Seizures if tuberous sclerosis.

Demographics

- Gender: Male-to-female ratio is 1:1.
- Age of detection: infancy and childhood.
- Retinal astrocytoma is seen in about 50% of patients diagnosed with tuberous sclerosis. It is less frequently seen in patients with neurofibromatosis.
- If associated with autosomal dominant condition, the risk of recurrence is 50% per offspring.

Ophthalmic Findings

See Figure 3.73.

- Retinal and optic disk astrocytic hamartomas can occur as a solitary finding in normal patients. Most retinal astrocytomas occur near the disk and posterior pole. They may be bilateral and multifocal in patients with dominantly inherited tuberous sclerosis and, rarely, neurofibromatosis.
- Three distinct manifestations:
  1. Flat, round semitranslucent lesion.
  2. Elevated, calcific, "mulberry" lesion.
  3. Mixed type with typically central calcific core and peripherally flat with translucent edge.
- Rare findings include retinal gliosis, exudation, and documented growth. More severe retinal effects in patients with tuberous sclerosis.

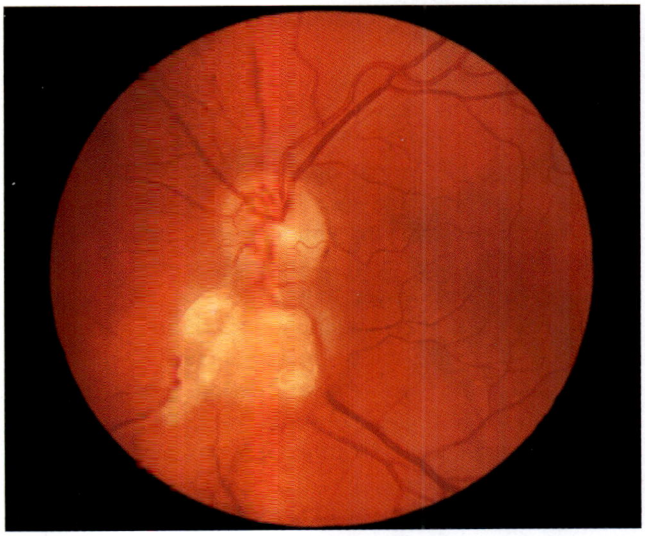

FIGURE 3.73 Late in life, astrocytic hamartomas become more opacified and develop nodular areas of calcification (mulberry appearance).

Systemic Findings of Tuberous Sclerosis

- Clinical findings generally appear during the first 3 years of life. Classic triad of seizure (93%), mental deficiency (60% of cases), and sebaceous adenoma (fibroangiomas) present in 83% of cases. Seventy-five percent of patients die by 20 years of age.
- Skin manifestations: seagreen patches, vitiligo, subungual fibromas, café-au-lait patches, and white ash-leaf spots (pathognomonic for tuberous sclerosis).
- Neurologic manifestations:
  Seizures.
  Mental retardation
  Intracranial calcification of astrocytic hamartomas.
  Subependymal hamartomas may appear as "candle-wax drippings." Intracranial astrocytomas may give the appearance of "cortical tubers."
  Glioblastomas.
  Papilledema secondary to elevated intracranial pressure.
- Other lesions: cardiac rhabdomyomas, renal angiomyolipoma ([illegible]0% of cases) cystic bony lesions, and parenchymal pulmonary cysts which may rupture resulting in pneumothorax
- Other ocular findings:
  Lids: adenoma sebaceum (angiofibroma).
  Retina: astrocytic hamartoma present in 53% of cases.

Systemic Findings of Neurofibromatosis

- Symptoms generally occur in late childhood.
- Skin findings: café-au-lait patches (99%), axillary freckling, fibroma molluscum, neurofibromas (nodular or plexiform), periungual fibromas.
- CNS findings: astrocytomas, neurilemomas (schwannomas), neurofibromas, acoustic neuromas, and optic nerve gliomas and meningiomas. Mental retardation occurs in 5% of individuals.
- Peripheral nervous system: Hamartomas of peripheral nerves, the sympathetic nervous system, the GI tract, and other viscera may occur.
- Other systemic findings: hypertension secondary to pheochromocytoma and renal artery fibroma.
- Other ocular findings:
  1. Iris: Lisch nodules (100% of affected adults), nevi, ectropion uvea.
  2. Enlarged corneal nerves.
  3. Eyelids: S-shaped plexiform neurofibromas ("bag of worms" consistency). Fifty percent of patients with such upper lid involvement have associated glaucoma.
  4. Ptosis and facial hemihypertrophy.
  5. Glaucoma: secondary to hamartomas in the anterior chamber angle, congenitally abnormal angle and closure of the angle due to tumors of the ciliary body.
  6. Occasionally, astrocytic hamartomas (ophthalmoscopically and pathologically identical to those seen in tuberous sclerosis) located within the retina are seen. Sectorial retinal pigmentation and yellow-white choroidal neural or glial hamartomas may be seen.
  7. Proptosis: secondary to optic nerve tumor or due to the absence of the greater wing of the sphenoid bone with resultant pulsating encephalocele.

Special Tests

- IVFA: varying degrees of vascularization, which are more evident angiographically than ophthalmoscopically. The tumor's blood vessels are permeable to fluorescein with evidence of late leakage. IVFA is not helpful in differentiating astrocytic hamartomas from solitary retinoblastoma.
- Echography.
- Radiologic studies:
  1. Tuberous sclerosis.
     Intracranial:
     a. These lesions are benign subependymal hamartomas. The term "brain stones" refers to the radiologic appearance of calcified astrocytic hamartomas. Larger cortical masses ("tubers") have also been described.
     b. Glioblastomas.
        Chest: pulmonary parenchymal cysts.
        Bone.
        Cystic parenchymal cysts.
        Sclerotic calcified areas are seen in the skull and spine.
  2. Neurofibromatosis.
     Intracranial:
     Optic nerve gliomas and meningiomas.
     Astrocytomas.

RETINA

Neurilemomas (schwannomas).
Acoustic neuromas.
Abdominal:
Wilms tumor.
Pheochromocytoma.

- Electroencephalogram, intelligence quotient testing.
- Twenty-four-hour urine test for epinephrine and norepinephrine.

Disease Course

Variable depending on extent of retinal astrocytic hamartoma and systemic manifestations present in association with the phakomatoses.

Treatment and Management

- These lesions show minimal evidence of growth, and no treatment is indicated.
- Should nonresolving exudation occur, laser photocoagulation to the tumor may be required.
- Genetic counseling.

Medications

Anticonvulsants, if seizures.

Follow-Up

- Patients at risk for developing astrocytic hamartoma should maintain genetic, ophthalmic, and medical surveillance every 6 to 12 months.
- Particular attention should be paid to the development of ocular, ocular adnexal, and systemic malignancies.

Differential Diagnosis of Retinal Astrocytic Hamartoma

- Retinoblastoma/retinoma (these may be endophytic, exophytic, or diffuse infiltrating simulating uveitis; iris NV, cataract, vitreous seeding, and pseudohypopyon may occur; a positive family history may be present; both may lack calcification early, retinoblastomas has a brighter white appearance to the calcified portion of the tumor, whereas in astrocytic hamartomas the calcified portions tend to be yellow and lobular. The vascular pattern in retinoblastoma tends to be more prominent, whereas angiography may be required to note the reticular vascular pattern in astrocytic hamartomas).
- Amelanotic melanoma (ultrasonography shows typical pattern with elevation and high internal reflectivity).
- Neurofibromatosis (will have systemic findings and family history).
- Combined hamartoma of the retina and RPE (juxtapapillary location in most cases, dark and minimally elevated with retinal traction and tortuous vessels and occurs in young men between the ages of 20 and 45 years).
- *T. canis* (nematode infestation consisting of a localized white granuloma located in the peripheral retina or posterior pole. Inflammation, traction bands with macular dragging and RD can occur. ELISA for toxocara will be positive).
- Myelinated nerve fibers (white lesions located along the nerve-fiber layer, occurring around the optic nerve and having indistinct borders).
- Coats disease (no tumefaction, "lightbulb" aneurysms, and characteristic fluorescein angiogram).
- Retinal telangiectasis (coarse dilation of the capillary bed confined to the juxtafoveolar region of one or both eyes; occurs in adults of either sex, no known ocular or systemic associations).
- Retinal capillary hemangioma (spherical orange or red tumor with a dilated tortuous retinal artery and an efferent engorged vein).
- Coloboma (enlargement of the papillary area with a deep central excavation with retinal blood vessel crossing the edge).
- Localized retinal edema secondary to inflammation, trauma, or vascular lesions.
- Toxoplasmosis (unilateral white/yellow retinal lesions associated with vitreous cells. An adjacent chorioretinal scar may be present).

Reference

Williams R, Taylor D. Tuberous sclerosis. *Surv Ophthalmol* 1985;30:143–154.

Intraocular Lymphoma

Summary

Primary CNS lymphoma (PCNSL) can manifest as a diffuse large B cell lymphoma in the eye as a vitreoretinal lymphoma. This is highly associated with concurrent CNS lymphoma and has a poor prognosis. Uveal lymphoma is an extranodal marginal zone B cell lymphoma that has an indolent course and does not have CNS involvement.

Etiology

Two types of ocular involvement have been described. In vitreoretinal lymphoma, patients present at 60 to 70 years and the ocular disease manifests in the vitreous and/or retina and may present before or concurrent to CNS lymphoma. The course of vision loss may be rapid and often systemic survival is poor. Uveal lymphoma presents in a younger population (ages 50 to 60) and may be associated with systemic (non-CNS) lymphoma. Vision loss is slow and prolonged. Systemic survival is better than in PCNSL but depends on degree of systemic involvement. Risk factors for this neoplasm are unclear.

Signs and Symptoms

Painless, blurred vision.

Demographics

- Affects older adults.
- No racial or sexual predilection.
- No good data exist concerning epidemiology, although in one study, only 5.6% of patients with lymphoma had ocular involvement noted during postmortem examination.

Ophthalmic Findings

Vitreoretinal lymphoma subtype:

1. Posterior or panuveitis picture with aqueous cells, CME.
2. Large vitreous cells often clumped.
3. Focal or diffuse retinal or subretinal infiltration. Typically yellow-white in color with RPE alterations.
4. Subretinal fluid may be present.
5. Optic nerve swelling in setting of CNS disease or optic nerve infiltration.
6. Retinal vasculitis.

Uveal lymphoma subtype:

1. Rare vitreous cells.
2. Slow growth of solitary choroidal mass. Typically dome-shaped with choroidal elevation and secondary RD.
3. Thickened choroid with small nummular yellow/white choroidal lesions.
4. Overlying RPE hyperpigmentation.

Systemic Findings

Vitreoretinal lymphoma: CNS signs and symptoms if CNS involvement.

Uveal lymphoma: fevers, night sweats, weight loss, peripheral lymphadenopathy.

Special Tests and Diagnostic Procedures

- Photography and IVFA provide documentation of the extent of the disease. Multiple sub-RPE focal lesions can simulate choroiditis. Angiography can show evidence of RPE changes, as well as staining in the area of infiltrate.
- Thoracic and abdominal imaging.
- MRI of the brain.
- Lumbar puncture for CSF.
- Biopsy typically required for definitive diagnosis.
  1. Vitreoretinal lymphomas diagnosed by diagnostic pars plana vitrectomy with careful cytopathology evaluation. Helps to exclude other simulating conditions such as infections or other inflammatory conditions.
  2. Predominantly retinal or uveal lymphoma: A retinal or chorioretinal biopsy may be required through a pars plana approach. Fine needle aspiration biopsy may also be used for more anterior or elevated lesions.

Pathology

- Vitreoretinal lymphoma:
  1. Large B cell lymphoma.
  2. Medium-to-large cells with minimal cytoplasm.
  3. Admixed macrophages.
  4. Chromosomal translocations (50%).
- Uveal lymphoma:
  1. Marginal zone B cells.
  2. Small cells with variable degrees of differentiation.
  3. Rare reactive macrophages and rarely necrotic.

Disease Course

Vitreoretinal lymphoma:

1. Visual outcome depends on degree of ocular involvement and CNS status.
2. Poor prognosis for long term survival.

Uveal lymphoma:

1. Favorable visual outcome if nonmacular involvement.
2. Systemic survival is good based on response to systemic lymphoma therapy.

Treatment and Management

Vitreoretinal lymphoma:

1. Coordination with medical oncologist.
2. Treatment of ocular disease:
   a. Corticosteroid therapy.
   b. Intravitreal methotrexate.
   c. External beam radiotherapy.
   d. High-dose systemic chemotherapy (ARA-c, high-dose methotrexate).
3. Treatment of CNS disease: Many oncologists will consider treating for CNS lymphoma when vitreoretinal lymphoma is diagnosed due to the high incidence of both diseases occurring concurrently.
   a. Whole-brain radiotherapy.
   b. High-dose methotrexate.
   c. Ara-C.
   d. Intrathecal chemotherapy.

Choroidal lymphoma

1. Coordination with medical oncologist to determine presence of systemic lymphoma.
2. Treatment of ocular disease: external beam radiotherapy.
3. Treatment of systemic disease: systemic chemotherapy based on histological subtype.

Follow-Up

Ocular assessment every 3 months, with more frequent visits following surgical diagnostic techniques.

Thoracic and abdominal imaging, CSF examination, and MRI of the brain repeated every 3 months.

Differential Diagnosis

Multifocal choroiditis: unilateral, occurs in young female patients. Small, round creamy lesions at the level of the RPE. Vitreous cells are present, and CNVMs may form.

MEWDS: unilateral, acute condition occurring in young women following viral illness. It can be bilateral with many creamy lesions occurring at the level of the RPE. Vision returns to normal in a few weeks without treatment.

Acute retinitis of any etiology.

Acute retinal necrosis: decreased vision associated with floaters, pain, photophobia. Multiple white opaque patches of necrotic retina gradually enlarge and merge, forming a definite border with normal retina. Many vitreous cells. Bilateral in one third of cases. RD occurs in two thirds of cases.

POHS: triad of white punched-out lesions deep in the retina, macular CNVM, and peripapillary atrophy.

Toxoplasmosis: unilateral white-yellow retinal lesions associated with vitreous cells. An adjacent chorioretinal scar may be present.

Endophthalmitis: decreased vision, anterior chamber/vitreous cells, hypopyon, increasing redness and pain.

Choroidal granuloma: mimics uveal lymphoma with domed-shaped lesion with signs of inflammation

References

Coupland SE, Damato B. Understanding intraocular lymphomas. *Clin Exper Ophthalmol* 2008;36(6):564–578.

Grimm SA, Pulido JS, Jahnke K, et al. Primary intraocular lymphoma: an International Primary Central Nervous System Lymphoma Collaborative Group Report. *Ann Oncol* 2007;18(11):1851–1855.

Ridley ME, McDonald HR, Sternberg P, et al. Retinal manifestations of ocular lymphoma (reticulum cell sarcoma). *Ophthalmology* 1992;99:1153–1161.

MAJOR STUDIES

Diabetic Retinopathy Study (DRS)

Summary

DRS evaluated the benefit of xenon arc and argon laser PRP for patients with severe NPDR and PDR.

Study Population and Entry Criteria

Patients were required to have VA of 20/100 or better and either severe NPDR in both eyes or PDR with active NV in at least one eye.

Major Study Variables

VA.

Retinopathy risk factors.

Study Design

- Multicenter, randomized clinical trial.
- Patients randomly assigned to either argon or xenon treatment group.
- One eye was randomly assigned to photocoagulation and the other to indefinite deferral of treatment.

Study Conclusions

- Patients treated with either xenon arc or argon laser PRP had an overall reduction of 50% in the rate of severe visual loss (<5/200).
- Four HRCs were identified:
  1. Vitreous or preretinal hemorrhage.
  2. NV.
  3. NV on or within 1 disk diameter of the optic disk.
  4. Moderate or severe neovascularization (NVD > one third of disk area or NVE > one half the disk area).
- Eyes with three or more HRCs were at a significantly greater risk of developing severe visual loss.
- Patients with three or more HRCs should receive PRP; eyes with two or less HRCs still benefit from PRP, but the 2-year risk of severe visual loss without treatment was so small in this group that the risks of treatment (small reductions in VA or visual field) must be given more weight.
- Harmful effects of argon laser treatment were less than those observed with xenon arc treatment.

References

The Diabetic Retinopathy Study Research Group. Four risk factors for severe visual loss in diabetic retinopathy: the third report from the Diabetic Retinopathy Study. *Arch Ophthalmol* 1979;97:654–655.

The Diabetic Retinopathy Study Research Group. Indications for photocoagulation treatment of diabetic retinopathy: Diabetic Retinopathy Study report 14. *Int Ophthalmol Clin* 1987;27:239–253.

Diabetic Retinopathy Vitrectomy Study

Summary

Evaluated the risks and benefits of performing early vitrectomy in eyes with severe PDR.

Study Population and Entry Criteria

Recent diabetic VH reducing VA to 5/200 or less for at least 1 month.

Major Study Variables

- Type of diabetes.
- VA.
- Untoward events.

Study Design

- Multicenter, randomized clinical trial.
- Patients randomized to early (1 to 6 months) versus deferred (12 months) vitrectomy.

Study Conclusions

- At 3 months after onset of VH, early vitrectomy offered a greater likelihood of recovery of 10/100 or better VA.
- At 2 years, early vitrectomy offered a greater likelihood of recovery of 10/20 or better VA.
- Early vitrectomy had better anatomic results.
- The long-term benefit of early vitrectomy was most apparent in type I diabetics.

Reference

The Diabetic Retinopathy Vitrectomy Study Research Group. Early vitrectomy for severe vitreous hemorrhage in diabetic retinopathy: two-year results of a randomized trial—Diabetic Retinopathy Study report 2. *Arch Ophthalmol* 1985;103:1644–1652.

Early Treatment Diabetic Retinopathy Study (ETDRS)

Summary

The ETDRS evaluated photocoagulation and aspirin treatment in the management of patients with nonproliferative and early PDR.

Study Population and Entry Criteria

Diabetic patients with early proliferative, moderate to severe nonproliferative and/or diabetic macular edema in each eye.

Major Study Variables

- VA.
- Progression of retinopathy.
- Occurrence of VH.

Study Design

- Multicenter, randomized clinical trial.
- Defined CSME:
  1. Thickening of the retina at or within 500 μm of the center of the macula.
  2. Hard exudate at or within 500 μm of the center of the macula associated with thickening of adjacent retina.
  3. A zone of retinal thickening equal to or larger than 1 disk area, any part of which is within 1 disk diameter of the center of the macula.
- Eyes that had macular edema and mild to moderate diabetic retinopathy were randomly assigned to the following:
  1. Immediate or delayed focal macular laser treatment.
  2. Immediate or delayed scatter laser treatment (which was further randomized to mild or full scatter).
- Eyes that had macular edema and more severe retinopathy had scatter treatment immediately and were then randomly assigned to immediate or delayed macular treatment.
- Patients randomized to receive aspirin (650 mg/day) or placebo.

Study Conclusions

- Eyes with CSME benefited from prompt focal argon laser treatment (reduced the risk of visual loss, increased the likelihood of visual improvement).
- Eyes with macular edema that is not clinically significant should generally be observed without treatment.
- Focal macular laser treatment should be performed before scatter treatment for HRCs.
- Systemic aspirin did not prevent progression to HRCs or reduce the risk of visual loss, nor did it increase the risk of VH.

References

Early Treatment of Diabetic Retinopathy Study Research Group. Photocoagulation for diabetic macular edema. *Arch Ophthalmol* 1985;103:1796–1806.

Early Treatment of Diabetic Retinopathy Study Research Group. Effects of aspirin treatment on diabetic retinopathy: ETDRS report 8. *Ophthalmology* 1991:98(Suppl):766–785.

Endophthalmitis Vitrectomy Study (EVS)

Summary

The EVS compared the role of vitreous tap versus vitrectomy, and the use of i.v. antibiotics in the treatment of patients with acute postoperative endophthalmitis.

Study Population and Entry Criteria

Acute postoperative endophthalmitis within 6 weeks following cataract surgery.

Major Study Variables

VA on presentation.
Final VA.
Organism.

Study Design

- Multicenter, randomized trial.
- Patients randomly assigned to vitreous tap versus vitrectomy.
- Patients randomly assigned to i.v. antibiotics (ceftazidime and amikacin) versus no i.v. antibiotics.
- All patients received intravitreal antibiotics.

Study Conclusions

- Intravenous antibiotics did not affect outcome.
- For patients with VA of hand motions or better, vitreous tap and injection of intravitreal antibiotics was equivalent to vitrectomy and injection of intravitreal antibiotics.
- For patients with VA of less than hand motion, vitrectomy resulted in superior outcomes than tap and inject alone.

Reference

Results of Endophthalmitis Vitrectomy Study: a randomized trial of immediate vitrectomy and of intravenous antibiotics for the treatment of postoperative bacterial endophthalmitis. *Arch Ophthalmol* 1995;113:1479–1496.

Macular Photocoagulation Study (MPS)

MPS: Laser Photocoagulation of Subfoveal CNVM

Summary

Randomized, controlled clinical studies to determine effectiveness of laser photocoagulation for treating subfoveal CNVM attributable to ARMD.

Study Population and Entry Criteria

- FA that documented fluorescein leakage from choroidal neovascular lesion with well-demarcated boundaries, no larger than 3.5 standard disk areas, under the center of FAZ.
- Best corrected VA in study eye of no better than 20/40 but no worse than 20/320 (Snellen equivalents).
- Age greater than 50 years.
- No prior photocoagulation in macula of study eye.
- No current or past use of systemic steroids.

Study Design

- Randomized, controlled clinical trial. Patients were randomized to laser photocoagulation versus observation.
- Variables studied included VA, reading speed, contrast sensitivity, laser wavelength, and lesion size.

Study Conclusions

- Compared to observation laser photocoagulation was beneficial for new subfoveal CNVM, although there was an immediate decrease in VA following treatment. Patient must be informed of this.
- From 6 months to 2 years following treatment, a larger number of untreated eyes had subsequent visual loss greater than six lines compared with treated eyes.
- Treated eyes retained greater contrast sensitivity than untreated eyes throughout 48 months of follow-up.
- Note: As PDT and new pharmacologic therapies have been developed with improved outcomes, laser of subfoveal CNV is no longer recommended.

References

Macular Photocoagulation Study Group. Laser photocoagulation of subfoveal neovascular lesions in age-related macular degeneration: results of a randomized clinical trial. *Arch Ophthalmol* 1991;109:1220–1231.

Macular Photocoagulation Study Group. Visual outcome after laser photocoagulation for subfoveal choroidal neovascularization secondary to age-related macular degeneration: the influence of initial lesion size and initial visual acuity. *Arch Ophthalmol* 1994;112:480–488.

MPS: Laser Photocoagulation of Recurrent Subfoveal CNVM

Summary

Study to determine benefit of additional laser photocoagulation for recurrent CNVM attributable to ARMD.

Study Population and Entry Criteria

- FA that documented either leaking choroidal neovascular lesion under the center of FAZ contiguous with scar from earlier treatment or CNVM within 150 μm of FAZ center contiguous to scar from earlier laser treatment that had expanded under fovea.
- No prior laser treatment to FAZ center.
- Size of CNVM and old treatment scar such that some portion of retina within 1 disk diameter of FAZ center would remain untreated and old, and new treated area would not exceed 6 disk areas, if treatment were applied according to protocol.
- Best corrected VA in study eye no better than 20/40 and no worse than 20/320.
- Age greater than 50 years.
- No current or past use of systemic steroids.

Study Design

- Randomized clinical trial.
- Patients were assigned to laser photocoagulation versus no treatment.

Study Conclusions

- Laser photocoagulation was recommended for patients who meet study entry criteria.
- Effects of treatment on VA, contrast sensitivity were similar to new subfoveal CNVM.
- Nearly 50% of treated eyes showed persistent or recurrent CNVM within 3 years.

Note: As noted above, "hot" laser of subfoveal CNV is no longer recommended as PDT and pharmacologic therapies have much improved outcomes.

References

Macular Photocoagulation Study Group. Laser photocoagulation of subfoveal recurrent neovascular lesions in age-related macular degeneration: results of a randomized clinical trial. *Arch Ophthalmol* 1991;109:1232–1241.

Macular Photocoagulation Study Group. Persistent and recurrent neovascularization after laser photocoagulation for subfoveal choroidal neovascularization of age-related macular degeneration. *Arch Ophthalmol* 1994;112:489–499.

MPS: Laser Photocoagulation for Extrafoveal Choroidal Neovascular Membrane

Summary

Multicenter controlled clinical trial to determine benefit of argon laser photocoagulation for extrafoveal CNVM in ARMD.

Study Population and Entry Criteria

- Drusen.
- Angiographic evidence of CNVM at distance of 200 to 2,500 μm from center of FAZ.
- Best corrected VA of 20/100 or better.
- Symptoms related to neovascular membrane (e.g., decreased acuity, metamorphopsia, uniocular diplopia).
- No prior photocoagulation in the study eye.
- No other ocular disease that could affect VA.
- Age greater than 50 years.
- Informed consent.

Study Design

- Randomized controlled clinical trial.
- Patients were assigned to argon laser photocoagulation versus no treatment.

Study Conclusions

- Laser photocoagulation was significantly better than no treatment in preventing or delaying large losses in VA for at least 5 years.
- Recurrences occurred in 34% of treated eyes by 5 years.

References

Macular Photocoagulation Study Group. Argon laser photocoagulation for senile macular degeneration: results of a randomized clinical trial. *Arch Ophthalmol* 1982;100:912–918.

Macular Photocoagulation Study Group. Argon laser photocoagulation for neovascular maculopathy: five-year results from randomized clinical trials. *Arch Ophthalmol* 1991;109:1109–1114.

Central Vein Occlusion Study

Summary

The central vein occlusion (CVO) study was designed to evaluate the natural history of CVO, the benefit of PRP for ischemic CVO, and the effect of laser for macular edema secondary to CVO.

Study Population and Entry Criteria

Patients with CRVO were enrolled into four groups:

Group P: perfused CVO.
Group N: nonperfused CVO.
Group I: indeterminate perfusion.
Group M: reduced VA of 20/50 or worse attributable to angiographically proven macular edema.

Major Study Variables

- VA.
- Iris NV.
- Neovascular glaucoma.

Study Design

- Multicenter, randomized controlled clinical trial.
- Eyes with ischemic CVO were randomly assigned to immediate prophylactic PRP or frequent close observation. If 2 o' clock-hour positions of iris NV or any angle NV developed, PRP was performed.
- Eyes with macular edema were randomly assigned to macular grid laser or no treatment.
- Eyes with indeterminate perfusion were followed monthly until they became eligible for group N or P.

Study Conclusions

- One third of patients with indeterminate perfusion progressed to an ischemic CVO.
- Prophylactic PRP did not totally prevent iris or angle NV, and prompt regression of NV was more likely to occur in eyes that did not undergo prophylactic laser.
- Although macular grid laser did reduce angiographic evidence of macular edema, no difference in VA was noted between treated and untreated patients.

References

The Central Vein Occlusion Study Group. Evaluation of grid pattern photocoagulation for macular edema in central vein occlusion: The Central Vein Occlusion Study Group M Report. *Ophthalmology* 1995;102:1425–1433.

The Central Vein Occlusion Study Group. A randomized clinical trial of early panretinal photocoagulation for ischemic central vein occlusion: The Central Vein Occlusion Study Group N Report. *Ophthalmology* 1995;102:1434–1444.

Branch Vein Occlusion Study

Summary

The following questions are addressed:

1. Is argon laser photocoagulation useful in improving VA in eyes with BRVO and macular edema?
2. Can peripheral scatter laser prevent the development of NV?
3. Can peripheral scatter laser prevent VH?

RETINA

Study Population and Entry Criteria

Recent BRVO (3 to 18 months since onset) divided into four groups:

Group I: eyes at risk for the development of NV (BRVO involving a retinal area of at least five disk areas).

Group II: eyes at risk for development of VH attributable to presence of disk and/or peripheral NV.

Group X: eyes at high risk for development of NV (capillary nonperfusion involving a retinal area of at least 5 disk areas).

Group III: eyes at risk for vision loss from macular edema (VA reduced at least to 20/40).

Major Study Variables

VA.

Development of NV.

Occurrence of VH.

Study Design

Multicenter, randomized controlled clinical trial:

Group I randomly assigned to peripheral scatter laser versus no laser.

Group II randomly assigned to peripheral scatter laser versus no laser.

Group X followed, entered into Group II if appropriate.

Group III randomly assigned either to grid pattern of laser within involved macular region or no laser.

Study Conclusions

- Patients receiving peripheral scatter laser are less likely to develop NV or VH than untreated controls. However, the study suggests that peripheral scatter treatment should be applied after the development of NV rather than before.
- Patients with visual loss of 20/40 or worse secondary to macular edema who undergo macular grid photocoagulation are more likely to gain two or more lines of VA (65%) than untreated controls (37%).

References

Branch Vein Occlusion Study Group. Argon laser scatter photocoagulation for prevention of neovascularization and vitreous hemorrhage in branch vein occlusion. *Arch Ophthalmol* 1986;104:34–41.

Branch Vein Occlusion Study Group. Argon laser photocoagulation for macular edema in branch vein occlusion. *Am J Ophthalmol* 1984;98:271–282.

Anchor—Ranibizumab (Lucentis)

Summary

- The Anti-VEGF Antibody for the Treatment of Predominantly Classic Choroidal Neovascularization in Age-Related Macular Degeneration (ANCHOR) study compared ranibizumab (Lucentis) with PDT with verteporfin for the treatment of neovascular ARMD.
- Ranibizumab (Lucentis) is a recombinant, humanized, monoclonal antibody Fab (fragment antigen binding) that neutralizes all active forms of VEGF-A.

Study Population and Entry Criteria

- Entry Criteria:
  - Age ≥ 50 years.
  - VA (Snellen equivalent) 20/40 to 20/320.
  - Subfoveal CNV lesion secondary to ARMD.
  - No prior verteporfin therapy (PDT).
  - Classic CNV ≥ 50% of the total lesion area (predominantly classic lesion).
  - Total lesion ≤ 5,400 5m in greatest linear dimension.
- Patients were randomly assigned to one of three groups.
  - Group 1: monthly intravitreal injections of ranibizumab 0.3 mg with sham PDT.
  - Group 2: monthly intravitreal injections of ranibizumab 0.5 mg with sham PDT.
  - Group 3: monthly sham injections with active verteporfin therapy.

Study Design

- ANCHOR was an international, multicenter, 2-year, randomized, double-blind, active-treatment-controlled study.
- Comparison of efficacy and safety of ranibizumab with verteporfin (PDT) in subjects with predominantly classic, subfoveal CNV due to ARMD.
- The primary end point was the proportion of patients losing <15 letters from baseline VA at 12 months.

Study Conclusions

- Ninety-four percent of those given 0.3 mg ranibizumab and 96% of those given 0.5 mg ranibizumab lost <15 letters compared with 64% of patients given verteporfin therapy ($p < 0.001$ for each comparison).
- VA improved by ≥15 letters in 36% of patients given 0.3 mg ranibizumab and in 40% of patients given 0.5 mg ranibizumab compared with 6% of patients given verteporfin therapy ($p < 0.001$ for each comparison).
- Severe loss of VA (loss of ≥ 30 letters) occurred in 13% of patients given verteporfin therapy but did not occur in any of the patients treated with ranibizumab ($p < 0.001$ for each comparison).
- Mean VA increased by 8.5 letters in the 0.3-mg ranibizumab group and by 11.3 letters in the 0.5-mg ranibizumab group compared with a decrease by 9.5 letters in the verteporfin therapy group ($p < 0.001$ for each comparison).
- Of the patients given 0.5 mg ranibizumab, presumed endophthalmitis occurred in 1.4% of the patients and serious uveitis in 0.7% of the patients.

- In conclusion, ranibizumab (Lucentis) was superior to verteporfin therapy (PDT) in the treatment of patients with predominantly classic neovascular ARMD.

Reference

Brown DM, Kaiser PK, Michels M, et al. Ranibizumab versus verteporfin for neovascular age-related macular degeneration. *N Engl J Med* 2006;355(14):1432–1444.

Marina—Ranibizumab (Lucentis)

Summary

- The Minimally Classic/Occult Trial of the Anti-VEGF Antibody Ranibizumab (Lucentis) in the Treatment of Neovascular Age-Related Macular Degeneration (MARINA) is a phase 3 study that evaluated ranibizumab (Lucentis) for the treatment of minimally classic or occult with no classic CNV associated with ARMD.
- MARINA was a multicenter, prospective, 2-year, double-blind, sham-controlled study of the efficacy and safety of ranibizumab.

Study Population and Entry Criteria

- The study enrolled patients with subfoveal minimally classic or occult with no classic choroidal neovascularization (CNV).
- Entry Criteria:
  - Age ≥ 50 years
  - VA (Snellen equivalent) 20/40 to 20/320.
  - Progressive subfoveal CNV secondary to ARMD.
  - No prior PDT.
  - Area of CNV must be ≥ 50% of total lesion.
  - CNV must be minimally classic or occult with no classic.
  - Lesion size ≤ 12 disk areas (DA).
- Eligible patients were randomly assigned to one of three groups:
- Group 1: receive 24 monthly intravitreal injections of ranibizumab 0.3 mg
- Group 2: receive 24 monthly intravitreal injections of ranibizumab 0.5 mg
- Group 3: receive 24 monthly sham injections.
- The primary end point was the proportion of patients losing <15 letters from baseline VA at 12 months.

Study Design

- MARINA was a multicenter, 2-year, randomized, double-blind, active-treatment-controlled study.
- Evaluation of the efficacy and safety of Ranibizumab in subjects with minimally classic or occult with no classic subfoveal CNV secondary to ARMD.
- The primary end point was the proportion of patients losing <15 letters from baseline VA at 12 months.

Study Conclusions

- VA at 12 months; 95% of patients given 0.3 mg ranibizumab and 95% of patients given 0.5 mg ranibizumab lost <15 letters compared with 62% of patients given sham injections ($p < 0.001$).
- The benefit in VA from treatment with ranibizumab was maintained at 24 months.
- VA improved by ≥15 letters in 25% of patients given 0.3 mg ranibizumab and in 34% of patients given 0.5 mg ranibizumab compared with 5% of patients given sham injections ($p < 0.001$).
- The mean increases in VA were 6.5 letters in the 0.3-mg group and 7.2 letters in the 0.5-mg group compared with a decrease of 10.4 letters in the sham-injected group ($p < 0.001$ for comparison of each dose with the sham injection group).
- The VA benefit of ranibizumab (Lucentis) was independent of baseline lesion size, lesion type, or baseline VA.
- During the study, presumed endophthalamitis was identified in 1% of patients and serious uveitis was identified in 1.3% of patients given ranibizumab.
- In conclusion, intravitreal injection of ranibizumab for 2 years prevented vision loss and improved mean VA in patients with minimally classic or occult with no classic CNV secondary to ARMD.
- Ranibizumab showed an acceptable safety profile with a small number of adverse events.

Reference

Rosenfeld PJ, Brown DM, Heier JS, et al. Ranibizumab for neovascular age-related macular degeneration. *N Engl J Med* 2006;355(14):1419–1431.

DRCR.NET—Laser Versus Intravitreal Triamcinolone

Summary

This study compared the safety and efficacy of preservative-free intravitreal triamcinolone (1 and 4 mg) to standard of care therapy of focal macular laser for the treatment of clinical significant diabetic macular edema.

Study Population and Entry Criteria

- Major eligibility criteria:
  - Age ≥ 18 years.
  - Study eye with best-corrected VA > 24 letters (20/320 or better) and <73 letters (worse than 20/40).
  - Study eye with central macular DME present on clinical exam and on OCT.
  - Mean central macular thickness on two OCT measurements >250 µm.
  - Fellow eye either eligible or has acuity >19 letters (20/400 or better) and has not been previously treated with intravitreal corticosteroids.

Study Design

- Randomized, multicenter clinical trial with 3-year follow-up
- Patients who had one study eye were randomly assigned to one of the three treatment groups:
  1. Laser photocoagulation.
  2. 1-mg intravitreal preservative-free triamcinolone acetonide injection.
  3. 4-mg intravitreal preservative-free triamcinolone acetonide injection.
- For patients with two study eyes, the right eye was randomly assigned to one of the three treatment groups. The left eye was assigned to the alternative treatment (laser or triamcinolone). If the left eye was assigned to triamcinolone, then the dose (1 or 4 mg) was randomly assigned to the left eye.
- Main efficacy outcomes:
  - Primary: ≥15-letter improvement in VA over the 3 years.
  - Secondary: change in retinal thickening (measured on OCT).
- Main safety outcomes:
  - i. Elevated IOP/glaucoma.
  - ii. Cataract/cataract surgery.
  - iii. Endophthalmitis (bacterial or inflammatory).
  - iv. RD.

Study Conclusions

- MAIN conclusions:
  - At 4 months, mean VA was better in the 4-mg triamcinolone group than in either the laser group ($p < 0.001$) or the 1-mg triamcinolone group ($p = 0.001$).
  - By 1 year, there were no significant differences among groups in mean VA.
  - At 2 years, mean VA was better in the laser group than in the other 2 groups.
  - The 3-year follow-up results are consistent with 2-year results.
  - Therefore, over a 3-year period, focal/grid photocoagulation is more effective and has fewer side effects than 1- or 4-mg doses of preservative-free intravitreal triamcinolone for most patients with DME (who have characteristics similar to the cohort in this clinical trial).
  - Focal/grid photocoagulation currently remains the benchmark against which other treatments are compared in clinical trials of DME.
- NOTE:
  - OCT results generally paralleled the VA results.
  - IOP increased from baseline in the triamcinolone groups, but most significantly the 4-mg group.
  - Treatment group differences in the VA outcome could not be attributed solely to cataract formation.
  - Most eyes receiving 4 mg of triamcinolone as given in this study are likely to require cataract surgery by the 3-year follow-up.

References

Randomized Trial Comparing Intravitreal Triamcinolone Acetonide and Focal/Grid Photocoagulation for Diabetic Macular Edema. *Ophthalmology* 2008;115(9):1447–1459.e10

DRCR.net, Beck RW, Edwards AR, et al. Three-year follow up of a randomized trial comparing focal/grid photocoagulation and intravitreal triamcinolone for diabetic macular edema. *Arch Ophthalmol* 2009;127(3):245–251.

Age-Related Eye Disease Study

Summary

The goal of AREDS was to assess the clinical course of ARMD and age-related cataract, and included a placebo-controlled randomized prevention trial of high-dose vitamin and mineral supplements for patients at risk of age-related macular degeneration and of high-dose vitamin supplement for patients at risk of age-related cataract.

Study Population and Entry Criteria

- AREDS was designed as both a study of the clinical course of age-related lens opacity and ARMD as well as a randomized, controlled trial of high-dose antioxidants and zinc to reduce progression of eye diseases common in the elderly.
- Entry Criteria: patients with ARMD who had either extensive small drusen, intermediate drusen, large drusen, noncentral geographic atrophy, or pigment abnormalities in one or both eyes, or advanced ARMD or vision loss due to ARMD in one eye. At least one eye had best-corrected VA of 20/32 or better.
- Participants with ARMD were defined as follows:
  - Category 2: mild ARMD, having small drusen (<63 μm) and few intermediate drusen (≥63 μm and <125 μm).
  - Category 3: intermediate ARMD, having extensive intermediate drusen or large drusen (≥125 μm).
  - Category 4: advanced ARMD in one eye, either geographic atrophy in the center or neovascular ARMD.

Study Design

- Double-masked, multicenter prospective study of 4,757 persons aged 55 to 80 years.
- Participants were randomly assigned to receive daily oral tablets containing:
  - Group 1: antioxidants (vitamin C, 500 mg; vitamin E, 400 IU; and beta carotene, 15 mg).
  - Group 2: zinc, 80 mg, as zinc oxide and copper, 2 mg, as cupric oxide.
  - Group 3: antioxidants plus zinc.
  - Group 4: placebo.
- Outcome measured by two methods:
  - Photographic assessment of progression to or treatment for advanced ARMD.
  - VA—moderate loss from baseline (≥15 letters).

Study Conclusions

- AREDS demonstrated a statistically significant benefit for the combination of high-dose antioxidant vitamins and zinc in providing a moderate reduction in the risk of developing advanced ARMD (over a median of 6.3 years) in persons at high risk.
- Specifically, the risk for progression was reduced by 25% for the entire study population (Categories 2 to 4) and 34% for the population of patients with Category 3 or 4 ARMD.
- The overall risk for moderate vision loss (decrease of 15 or more letters on the logarithmic chart compared with baseline) was reduced by 19% at 5 years.
- Both zinc and antioxidants plus zinc significantly reduced the odds of developing advanced ARMD in this higher-risk group.
- Smoking and hypertension were associated with the presence of large drusen and neovascular age-related macular degeneration among AREDS participants.
- Note: During the course of AREDS, supplementation of beta-carotene was demonstrated to increase the risk for lung cancer and its associated mortality in smokers.
- All-cause mortality was reduced among participants assigned to zinc alone or zinc in combination with antioxidants in comparison to participants who were not assigned to a zinc-containing supplement.

References

Age-Related Eye Disease Study Research Group. Risk factors associated with age-related macular degeneration. A case-control study in the Age-Related Eye Disease Study: Age-Related Eye Disease Study report number 3. *Ophthalmology* 2000;107:2224–2232.

Age-Related Eye Disease Study Research Group. A randomized placebo-controlled clinical trial of high-dose supplementation with vitamins C and E, beta carotene, and zinc for age-related macular degeneration and vision loss. AREDS report no. 8. *Arch Ophthalmol* 2001;119:1417–1436.

Age-Related Eye Disease Study Research Group. Associations of mortality with ocular disorders and an intervention of high-dose antioxidants and zinc in the Age-Related Eye Disease Study. AREDS report no. 13. *Arch Ophthalmol* 2004;122:716–726.

The Standard Care Versus Corticosteroid for Retinal Vein Occlusion (SCORE) Study

SCORE-BRVO Trial

Summary

- To compare the efficacy and safety of 1- and 4-mg doses of preservative-free intravitreal triamcinolone with standard care (grid photocoagulation) for eyes with vision loss associated with macular edema secondary to BRVO.

Study Population and Entry Criteria

- Inclusion criteria:
  - Participants must have central macular edema secondary to either CRVO or BRVO.
  - Eyes may be enrolled from 0 to 24 months after diagnosis.
  - VA of ≥19 letters (approximately 20/400) and ≤73 letters (approximately 20/40).
  - Mean retinal thickness on two OCT measurements ≥250 μm (central subfield).

Study Design

- Multicenter, prospective, randomized clinical trial.
- Main outcome measure gain in VA letter score of 15 or more from baseline to month 12.
- Patients randomly assigned to one of three groups:
  - Group 1: 1 mg of preservative-free intravitreal triamcinolone.
  - Group 2: 4 mg of preservative-free intravitreal triamcinolone.
  - Group 3: macular grid photocoagulation.

Study Conclusions

- There was no difference detected in VA at 12 months for the macular grid laser (standard of care) group compared with either of the triamcinolone groups.
- Rates of adverse events (particularly elevated IOP and cataract) were highest in the 4-mg group.
- Grid photocoagulation continues to be the benchmark against which other treatments are compared in clinical trials for eyes with vision loss associated with macular edema secondary to BRVO.
- Note: a clinical trial (named *BRAVO*) with promising early results, compares randibizumab (Lucentis) to macular laser (standard of care) for macular edema secondary to BRVO.

Reference

Scott IU, Ip MS, VanVeldhuisen PC, et al. A randomized trial comparing the efficacy and safety of intravitreal triamcinolone with standard care to treat vision loss associated with macular Edema secondary to branch retinal vein occlusion: the Standard Care vs Corticosteroid for Retinal Vein Occlusion (SCORE) study report 6. *Arch Ophthalmol* 2009;127(9):1115–1128.

SCORE-CRVO Trial

Summary

- To compare the efficacy and safety of 1- and 4-mg doses of preservative-free intravitreal triamcinolone with standard care (observation) for eyes with vision loss associated with macular edema secondary to CRVO.

Study Population and Entry Criteria

- Same Inclusion criteria as the SCORE-BRVO trial (see above).

Study Design

- Main outcome measure gain in VA letter score of 15 or more from baseline to month 12.
- Multicenter, randomized, clinical trial of 271 participants.
- Patients randomly assigned to one of three groups:
  - Group 1: 1 mg of preservative-free intravitreal triamcinolone.
  - Group 2: 4 mg of preservative-free intravitreal triamcinolone.
  - Group 3: observation.

Study Conclusions

- The odds of achieving the primary outcome were 5.0 times greater in the 1-mg group than the observation group (odds ratio [OR], 5.0; 95% confidence interval [CI], 1.8 to 14.1; $p = 0.001$) and 5.0 times greater in the 4-mg group than the observation group (OR, 5.0; 95% CI, 1.8 to 14.4; $p = 0.001$); there was no difference identified between the 1- and the 4-mg groups (OR, 1.0; 95% CI, 0.5 to 2.1; $p = 0.97$).
- The rates of elevated IOP and cataract were similar for the observation and the 1-mg groups, but higher in the 4-mg group.
- Intravitreal triamcinolone is superior to observation for treating vision loss associated with macular edema and secondary to CRVO in patients who have characteristics similar to those in the SCORE-CRVO trial.
- The 1-mg dose has a safety profile superior to that of the 4-mg dose.
- Note: Clinical trials (named *CRUISE*) with promising early results compared randibizumab to observation (standard of care) for macular edema secondary to CRVO.

Reference

Ip MS, Scott IU, VanVeldhuisen PC, et al. A randomized trial comparing the efficacy and safety of intravitreal triamcinolone with observation to treat vision loss associated with macular edema secondary to central retinal vein occlusion: the Standard Care vs Corticosteroid for Retinal Vein Occlusion (SCORE) study report 5. *Arch Ophthalmol* 2009;127(9):1101–1114.

Verteporfin and PDT for Exudative ARMD (TAP/VIP)

Treatment of ARMD with Photodynamic Therapy

Summary

Treatment of ARMD with photodynamic therapy (TAP) established the safety and efficacy of verteporfin therapy for neovascular ARMD and found it to be specifically most beneficial for classic CNV lesions.

Study Population and Entry Criteria

Multicenter randomized clinical trials of verteporfin were initiated in 1996 to evaluate the safety and efficacy for treating subfoveal CNV secondary to age-related macular degeneration.

Study Conclusions

- After 2 years, 59% of eyes with predominantly classic subfoveal lesions treated with PDT had lost fewer than 15 letters of VA from baseline compared with 31% of eyes assigned to placebo.
- Verteporfin therapy (PDT) significantly reduced the risk of moderate and severe vision loss, with greater benefit in the absence of occult CNV.

Note: Many trials are now underway to determine if PDT with anti-VEGF therapies is superior to anti-VEGF therapy alone.

Reference

Treatment of Age-Related Macular Degeneration with Photodynamic Therapy (TAP) Study Group. Photodynamic therapy of subfoveal choroidal neovascularization in age-related macular degeneration with verteporfin: two-year results of 2 randomized clinical trials - TAP report 2. *Arch Ophthalmol* 2001;119:198–207.

Verteporfin in Photodynamic Therapy

Summary

Verteporfin in Photodynamic Therapy (VIP) established the safety and efficacy of verteporfin therapy for subfoveal CNV from pathologic myopia.

Study Population and Entry Criteria

The VIP trial also investigated the use of verteporfin for subfoveal CNV secondary to pathologic myopia.

Study Conclusions

- After 2 years of follow-up, 36% of verteporfin-treated eyes compared with 51% of placebo-treated eyes lost at least eight letters on a logMAR VA chart.
- On the other hand, 40% of PDT treated eyes versus 13% of placebo treated eye gained at least five letters.
- Lesion size was a more important predictive factor for magnitude of treatment benefit than either lesion composition or VA for both TAP and VIP.

Reference

Verteporfin in Photodynamic Therapy (VIP) Study Group. Verteporfin therapy of subfoveal choroidal NV in pathologic myopia: 2-year results of a randomized clinical trial — VIP report no. 3. *Ophthalmology* 2003;110:667–673.

Appendix

Commonly used abbreviations in Chapter 3

ARMD	Age-related macular degeneration.
BRAO	Branch retinal artery occlusion.
BRVO	Branch retinal vein occlusion.
CME	Cystoid macular edema.
CMV	Cytomegalovirus.
CNVM	Choroidal neovascular membrane.
CRAO	Central retinal artery occlusion.
CRVO	Central retinal vein occlusion.
EOG	Electrooculogram.
ERG	Electroretinogram.
ETDRS	Early Treatment for Diabetic Retinopathy Study.
ICG	Indocyanine green (angiography).
IVFA	Intravenous fluorescein angiography.
MPS	Macular Photocoagulation Study.
NVD	Neovascularization of the disk.
NVE	Neovascularization elsewhere.
NVI	Neovascularization of the iris.
PDR	Proliferative diabetic retinopathy.
PED	Pigment epithelial detachment.
POHS	Presumed ocular histoplasmosis syndrome.
PRP	Panretinal photocoagulation.
RD	Retinal detachment.
ROP	Retinopathy of prematurity.
RPE	Retinal pigment epithelium.
TRD	Tractional retinal detachment.

CHAPTER

4

Intraocular Inflammation and Uveitis

David Hinkle

See Tables 4.1 and 4.2.

Table 4.1

Classification of uveitis entities

Anterior

Nongranulomatous	*Granulomatous*[a]
HLA-B27 associated	Sarcoid
Traumatic	TB
Fuchs	Syphilis
UGH syndrome	Herpes simplex
Posner-Schlossman	Leptospirosis
JRA	Brucellosis
IBD	
Drug induced	

Intermediate

Idiopathic/pars planitis
Multiple sclerosis
TB
Syphilis
Lyme disease
Sarcoidosis

Posterior

Vitritis	Retinitis: *Focal*	Retinitis: *Multifocal*	**Choroiditis**: *Focal*	**Choroiditis**: *Multifocal*
Idiopathic (senile vitritis)	Toxoplasmosis	Syphilis	TB	PCP
Toxoplasmosis	CMV retinitis	ARN	Toxocara	POHS
Endophthalmitis		PORN		Serpiginous choroidpathy
Lymphoma		MEWDS		Birdshot
		DUSN		Lymphoma
		Eales disease		APMPPE
				ARPE
				Whipple
				MFC/Panuveitis
				Cryptococcus
				Mycobacterium

Panuveitis

Sympathetic ophthalmia
VKH syndrome
Behçet syndrome
Endophthalmitis
Sarcoidosis
Phacoanaphylactic
Lyme disease
Masquerades

[a]Granulomatous uveitis can always present with nongranulomatous findings initially.

APMPPE, acute posterior multifocal placoid pigment epitheliopathy; ARN, acute retinal necrosis; ARPE, acute retinal pigment retinopathy; CMV, cytomegalovirus; DUSN, diffuse unilateral subacute neuroretinitis; IBD, inflammatory bowel disease; JRA, juvenile rheumatoid arthritis; MEWDS, multiple evanescent white dot syndrome; MFC, multifocal choroiditis; PCP, pneumocystis pneumoniae choroiditis; PORN, progressive outer retinal necrosis; POHS, presumed ocular histoplasmosis syndrome; TB, tuberculosis; UGH, uveitis-glaucoma-hyphema; VKH, Vogt-Koyanagi-Harada.

Table 4.2

Grading of anterior chamber cell and flare and vitreous activity

	Grade	Definition (wide beam, narrow slit)
Anterior chamber[a]	0	No cells/field
Cells	Trace	0–5 cells/field
	1+	5–10 cells/field
	2+	10–20 cells/field
	3+	20–50 cells/field
	4+	>50 cells/field
Flare	0	Complete absence
	1+	Faint/barely detectable
	2+	Moderate—iris details visible
	3+	Marked—iris details hazy
	4+	Intense—coagulated aqueous and fibrin
Vitreous[b]		
Cells/opacities	0	No opacities
	1+	Few fine and coarse opacities Fundus details clear
	2+	Scattered opacities Fundus details slightly obscured
	3+	Many opacities Fundus details markedly obscured
	4+	Dense opacities Fundus—no view

[a]From Kimura SJ, Thygeson P, Hogan MJ. Signs and symptoms of uveitis, I: anterior Uveitis. *Am J Ophthalmol* 1959;47:155–170, with permission.
[b]From Kimura SJ, Thygeson P, Hogan MJ. Signs and symptoms of uveitis, II: classification of the posterior manifestations of uveitis. *Am J Ophthalmol* 1959;47:171–176, with permission.

ANTERIOR UVEITIS

Hla-B27–Associated Diseases

Summary

The HLA-B27 antigen is associated with a number of systemic and ocular inflammatory conditions including Reiter syndrome, ankylosing spondylitis, psoriatic arthritis, and inflammatory bowel disease (Table 4.3; Figure 4.1).

Signs and Symptoms

Photophobia.
Sudden onset.
Unilateral (can alternate between eyes).

Demographics

Caucasian men.

Ophthalmic Findings

Recurrent episodes of iridocyclitis; can be severe with fibrin, hypopyon (Figure 4.1).

Posterior synechiae.
Nongranulomatous keratic precipitates.
Decreased intraocular pressure (IOP).
Macular edema common.

Disease Course

May spontaneously resolve.
Recurrent episodes common.

Treatment and Management

Intensive topical corticosteroids.
In severe cases, periocular or oral steroids may be needed.
Cycloplegics.

Etiology

- Unknown.
- Cross-reactivity of the HLA-B27 antigen and bacterial antigens (molecular mimicry).

References

Rodriguez A, Akova YA, Pedroza-Seres M, et al. Posterior segment ocular manifestations in patients with HLA-B27-associated uveitis. *Ophthalmology* 1994;101:1267–1274.

Table 4.3

HLA-B27 Associated systemic diseases

	Reiter syndrome	Ankylosing spondylitis	Psoriatic arthritis	Inflammatory bowel disease
Systemic findings	Seronegative arthritis, psoriasiform rash (keratodermia), aphthous stomatitis, balanitis, urethritis, onycholysis, enthesopathy (inflammation of tendinous insertion)	Sacroiliitis and vertebral inflammation, peripheral arthritis	Psoriasis, spondyloarthritis	Crohn disease or ulcerative colitis
Special tests	HLA-B27–positive in 60% of patients	HLA-B27–positive in 90% of patients X-rays of sacroiliac joints		Colonoscopy

Tay-Kearney ML, Schwam BL, Lowder C, et al. Clinical features and associated systemic diseases of HLA-B27 uveitis. *Am J Ophthalmol* 1996;121:47–56.

Wakefield D, Montanaro A, McCluskey P. Acute anterior uveitis and HLA-B27. *Surv Ophthalmol* 1991;36:223–233.

Plasmoid (or plastic) aqueous: descriptive term for anterior chamber fluid containing so much protein that the cells are suspended and do not move with the normal convection currents. HLA-B27–associated uveitis is one of the most common causes.

Posner-Schlossman Syndrome

Other name: glaucomatocyclitic crisis.

Summary

Posner-Schlossman syndrome is a rare condition characterized by recurrent episodes of high IOP with mild iridocyclitis.

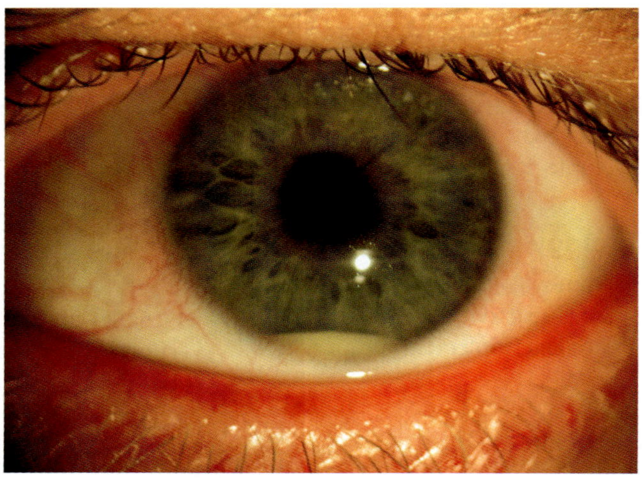

FIGURE 4.1. Severe HLA-B27–associated iridocyclitis with a plasmoid aqueous and hypopyon. (Courtesy of David Hinkle, MD.)

Etiology

Unknown.

Signs and Symptoms

Mild blurred vision.
Mild discomfort.
Many patients have very few symptoms.

Demographics

Ages, 20 to 40 years; rare in elderly individuals.
Men more often than women.

Ophthalmic Findings

Usually unilateral, acute attacks.
IOP greater than 40 mm Hg with accompanying corneal edema.
Few small, nongranulomatous keratic precipitates.
Mild anterior chamber inflammation.
Open-angle glaucoma.
No posterior synechiae.

Systemic Findings

None.

Special Tests

None.

Pathology

None.

Disease Course

- Resolution in 1 to 3 weeks with or without treatment.
- Complications: glaucomatous damage to optic nerve.

Treatment and Management

Antiglaucoma medications.
Topical corticosteroids.
Glaucoma surgery in rare cases.

Differential Diagnosis

- Acute angle-closure glaucoma (closed angle, corneal edema, and severe pain).
- Fuchs heterochromic iridocyclitis (mild IOP elevation, iris heterochromia, stellate keratic precipitates).
- Herpetic uveitis (decreased corneal sensation, increased IOP, keratitis, iris atrophy).

Reference

Harstad HK, Ringvold A. Glaucomatocyclitic crises (Posner-Schlossman syndrome): a case report. *Acta Ophthalmol Scand Suppl* 1986;64:146–151.

Phacoantigenic Uveitis

Other names: phacoanaphylactic endophthalmitis, phacoanaphylactic uveitis.

Summary

Phacoantigenic uveitis is a granulomatous reaction to lens proteins occurring following injury to the lens capsule and leakage of lens proteins into the anterior chamber.

Etiology

- Autoimmunity to lens proteins that are normally sequestered and unrecognized by the immune system.
- May have history of penetrating lens injury, rupture of the lens capsule, or retained lens fragments following cataract surgery.

Ophthalmic Findings

Chronic granulomatous anterior uveitis.
Lens capsular disruption or retained lens material.

Systemic Findings

None.

Special Tests

Anterior chamber aspirate for cultures and smears to exclude an intraocular infection.

Pathology

Zonal granuloma:

Inner zone of neutrophils adjacent to lens material.
Middle zone of monocytes, macrophages, giant cells.
Outer zone of granulation tissue with plasma cells.

Disease Course

Chronic smoldering inflammation, may resemble a low-grade endophthalmitis.

Treatment and Management

- Topical, periocular corticosteroids: temporizing measure to decrease inflammation.
- Surgical removal of lens fragments: definitive treatment.

Differential Diagnosis

Phacolytic glaucoma: caused by leakage of lens proteins from hypermature lens.
Chronic endophthalmitis: consider organisms such as *Propionibacterium acnes* and other indolent bacteria and fungi.

References

Filipe JC, Palmares J, Delgado L, et al. Phacolytic glaucoma and lens-induced uveitis. *Int Ophthalmol* 1993;17:289–293.
Thach AB, Marak GE Jr, McLean IW, et al. Phacoanaphylactic endophthalmitis: a clinicopathologic review. *Int Ophthalmol* 1991;15:271–279.

Uveitis-Glaucoma-Hyphema Syndrome

Summary

Uveitis-glaucoma-hyphema (UGH) syndrome is a rare condition related to ill-fitting intraocular lenses (IOLs) causing uveal irritation.

Etiology

Chronic uveal irritation caused by a poorly fitting IOL.

Signs and Symptoms

Ocular tenderness.
Decreased vision.

Ophthalmic Findings

Anterior uveitis, rarely with a hypopyon.
Hyphema.
Glaucoma.

IOL (usually poorly fitting anterior chamber lens, iris-fixated IOL, single-piece IOL placed in ciliary sulcus, or IOL within capsular bag with zonular laxity).
Iridodenesis, transillumination frequently seen if posterior chamber IOL.

Systemic Findings

None.

Special Tests

None.

Disease Course

Chronic, recurrent episodes of inflammation.

Treatment and Management

Medical management occasionally is sufficient.
IOL explant/exchange/repositioning.

Medications

Antiglaucoma medications.
Anti-inflammatory medications.

Differential Diagnosis

Endophthalmitis.
Lens-induced uveitis.
HLA-B27–associated uveitis.

References

Beehler CC. UGH syndrome with the 91Z lens. *J Am Intraocul Implant Soc* 1983;9:459.

Choyce DP. Complications of the AC implants of the early 1950's and the UGH or Ellingson syndrome of the late 1970's. *J Am Intraocul Implant Soc* 1978;4:22–29.

Percival SP, Das SK. UGH syndrome after posterior chamber lens implantation. *J Am Intraocul Implant Soc* 1983;9:200–201.

Causes of Uveitis with Hyphema

- HLA-B27–associated uveitis.
- Varicella-zoster virus (VZV).
- Herpes simplex virus (HSV).
- Postoperative endophthalmitis.
- UGH syndrome.
- Behçet syndrome.
- Fuchs heterochromic iridocyclitis.

Viral Diseases

Summary

The most common viral origins causing iridocyclitis are HSV and VZV. These frequently have other signs indicative of a concurrent or prior herpes virus infection.

Signs and Symptoms

Unilateral pain, photophobia, redness, decreased vision.

Ophthalmic Findings

- Granulomatous, nongranulomatous, or stellate keratic precipitates.

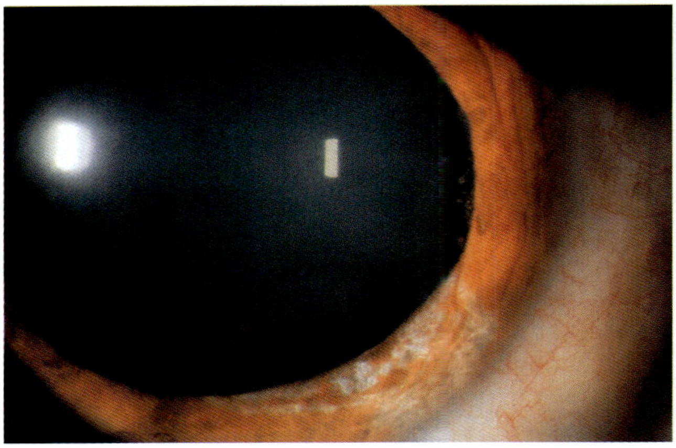

FIGURE 4.2. Varicella zoster can cause an occlusive vasculitis resulting in segmental iris atrophy.

- Diffuse distribution of keratic precipitates or concentrated under area of keratitis.
- Hypopyon.
- Elevated IOP.
- Evidence of previous ocular herpes infections:
  Epithelial dendrite.
  Stromal keratitis or scarring.
  Corneal hypoesthesia.
  Iris atrophy (Figure 4.2).
  Irregular pupil.
  Anterior uveitis.

Systemic Findings

- Skin rash affecting V1 dermatome (Hutchinson sign) (varicella zoster).
- Periocular blisters, cold sores (herpes simplex).

Treatment and Management

- Topical corticosteroid drops.
- Cycloplegia.
- Acyclovir: the use of antivirals in isolated iridocyclitis is controversial. The Herpetic Eye Disease Study showed a trend toward improvement with acyclovir, but did not recruit enough patients in this subgroup to show statistical significance.

References

The Herpetic Eye Disease Study Group. A controlled trial of oral acyclovir for iridocyclitis caused by herpes simplex virus. *Arch Ophthalmol* 1996;114:1065–1072.

Wilhelmus KR, Dawson CR, Barron BA, et al. Risk factors for herpes simplex virus epithelial keratitis recurring during treatment of stromal keratitis or iridocyclitis: Herpetic Eye Disease Study Group. *Br J Ophthalmol* 1996;80: 969–972.

Uveitis with Elevated IOP

- HSV.
- VZV.
- Posner-Schlossman syndrome.
- Sarcoidosis
- Fuchs heterochromic iridocyclitis.

Uveitis with Diffusely Distributed Keratic Precipitates

- HSV.
- VZV.
- Sarcoidosis
- Fuchs heterochromic iridocyclitis.
- Toxoplasmosis.

Juvenile Idiopathic Arthritis (Chronic Arthritis of Children)

Summary

Juvenile idiopathic arthritis (JIA) encompasses several forms of childhood arthritis. Young girls with pauciarticular arthritis most frequently develop iridocyclitis.

Etiology

Unknown.

Signs and Symptoms

Usually asymptomatic

Demographics

Young girls predominantly, onset usually less than 16 years of age.

Ophthalmic Findings

- Bilateral chronic, nongranulomatous iridocyclitis.
- Frequently develop band keratopathy (Figure 4.3), posterior synechiae, cataracts, and glaucoma.

Systemic Findings

Monoarticular or pauciarticular arthritis more common than polyarticular arthritis.

Special Tests

Rheumatoid factor negative.
Antinuclear antibody (ANA) positive (60%).

Disease Course

Chronic smoldering inflammation leading to complications such as band keratopathy, cataracts, glaucoma, and hypotony.

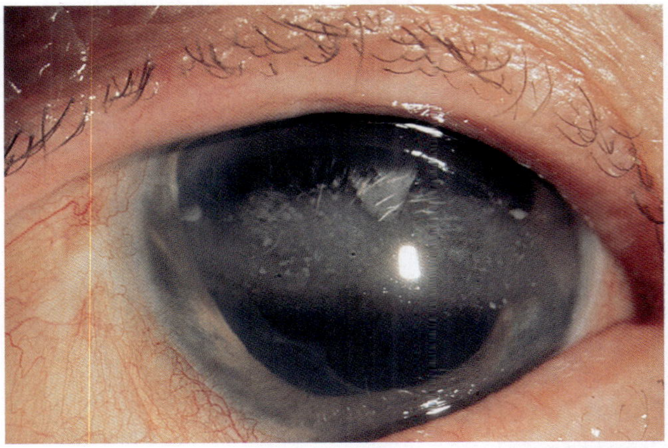

FIGURE 4.3. Chronic ocular inflammation resulting in band keratopathy in a patient with juvenile rheumatoid arthritis. (From Tasman W, Jaeger E. *The Wills Eye Hospital atlas of clinical ophthalmology,* 2nd ed. Lippincott Williams & Wilkins, 2001.)

Treatment and Management

- Topical, periocular, or systemic corticosteroids, cycloplegia, immunosuppressive agents.
- Surgical removal of cataracts, lens implantation is controversial and historically contraindicated.

Medications

- Topical and periocular corticosteroids.
- Immunosuppression if intolerant or resistant to steroids.

References

Giannini EH, Malagon CN, Van Kerckhove C, et al. Longitudinal analysis of HLA associated risks for iridocyclitis in juvenile rheumatoid arthritis. *J Rheumatol* 1991;18:1394–1397.

Wolf MD, Lichter PR, Ragsdale CG. Prognostic factors in the uveitis of juvenile rheumatoid arthritis. *Ophthalmology* 1987;94:1242–1248.

Traumatic Iritis

Summary

Blunt trauma to the eye can disrupt the blood–ocular barrier causing an anterior iridocyclitis.

Signs and Symptoms

Pain, redness, photophobia immediately or several days following blunt injury to the eye.

Ophthalmic Findings

Mild iridocyclitis.
Hypopyon (rare).
Middilated, sluggish pupil.
Decreased IOP.

UVEITIS

Disease Course

- Usually resolves quickly.

Treatment and Management

- Rule out ruptured globe and corneal abrasion.
- Topical corticosteroids (may not be needed in mild cases).
- Cycloplegia.
- Check for angle recession, iridodialysis, or cyclodialysis on subsequent visits.

Fuchs Heterochromic Iridocyclitis

Summary

Fuchs heterochromic iridocyclitis is a unilateral, chronic low-grade inflammatory condition characterized by stellate keratic precipitates, cataract formation, glaucoma, and iris heterochromia.

Etiology

Unknown.
Syndrome likely related to multiple infectious agents including toxoplasmosis and rubella, among others.

Signs and Symptoms

Usually none.

Ophthalmic Findings

- Iris heterochromia: lighter iris color in brown eyes; darker blue in blue eyes (Figure 4.4).
- Stellate keratic precipitates, diffusely distributed over cornea.
- Cataracts.
- Mild, low-grade iritis, anterior vitreous cells, and opacities.
- Abnormal-angle vessels, predisposed to bleeding and hyphema formation (Amsler sign) during ocular surgery.
- Glaucoma.
- Usually unilateral, but rarely bilateral.

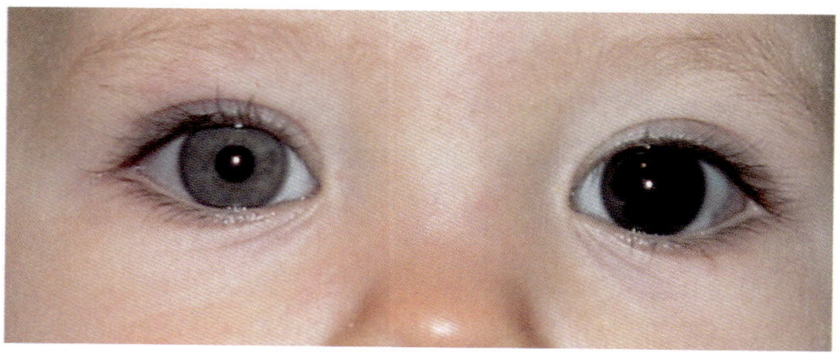

FIGURE 4.4. Iris heterochromia in the affected right eye. Loss of iris stroma results in a deeper blue. (Courtesy of Brian Forbes, MD.)

Disease Course

Chronic, low-grade inflammation.
Development of cataracts and glaucoma.

Treatment and Management

Steroids of limited use.

Differential Diagnosis

Herpetic iridocyclitis.
Posner-Schlossman syndrome.
Neovascular glaucoma.

References

Jones NP. Fuchs' heterochromic uveitis: an update. *Surv Ophthalmol* 1993;37:253–272.

La Hey E, de Jong PT, Kijlstra A. Fuchs' heterochromic cyclitis: review of the literature on the pathogenetic mechanisms. *Br J Ophthalmol* 1994;78:307–312.

Quentin CD, Reiber H. Fuchs heterochromic cyclitis: rubella virus antibodies and genome in aqueous humor. *Am J Ophthalmol* 2004;138:46–54.

INTERMEDIATE UVEITIS

Summary

Intermediate uveitis is a broad descriptive term for inflammation primarily affecting the vitreous and peripheral retina. A number of diseases can cause findings consistent with intermediate uveitis.

Etiology

- Pars planitis: idiopathic.
- Inflammatory:
  Sarcoidosis.
  Inflammatory bowel disease.
  Multiple sclerosis.
  Autoimmune (associated with HLA-DR locus).
- Infectious:
  Lyme disease.
  Toxocariasis (unilateral disease).
  Whipple disease.
  Syphilis.
  Tuberculosis (TB).

Signs and Symptoms

Floaters.
Decreased vision.

Ophthalmic Findings

Diffuse vitreous cells.
Peripheral vascular sheathing.
Pars plana "snowballs" or "snowbanks" (Figure 4.5).

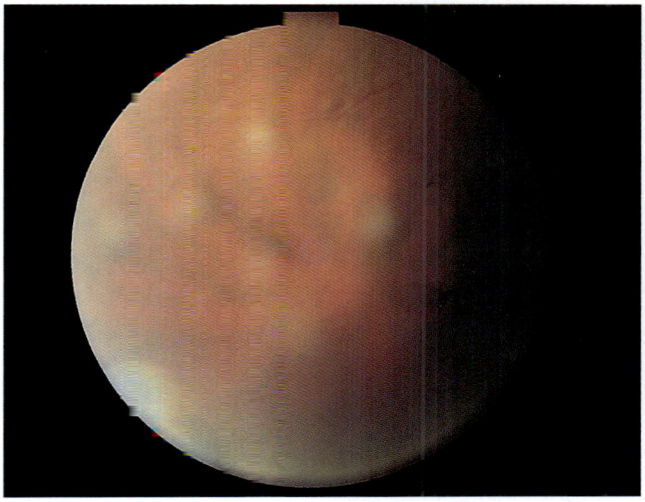

FIGURE 4.5. Gliosis and inflammatory exudate are present inferiorly as peripheral snowbanks in pars planitis. (From Tasman W, Jaeger E. *The Wills Eye Hospital atlas of clinical ophthalmology*, 2nd ed. Lippincott Williams & Wilkins, 2001.)

Vitreous hemorrhage.
Cystoid macular edema.
Cataracts.
Retinal neovascularization.

Disease Course

- Extremely variable course: Some patients may have smoldering inflammation and retain good vision.
- Others progress to cyclitic membranes, retinal detachment (RD), and phthisis.

Treatment and Management

Cryotherapy or peripheral laser photocoagulation.
Periocular and oral corticosteroids.
Immunosuppression (cyclosporine, azathioprine, methotrexate) if patient fails therapy or becomes intolerant to steroids.

Sarcoidosis

Summary

Sarcoidosis is an inflammatory condition characterized by noncaseating granulomas in multiple tissues. Ocular involvement is most frequently evident as granulomatous anterior uveitis or intermediate uveitis.

Demographics

- Sarcoid is more common in African Americans.
- Ocular inflammatory disease occurs in 25% to 50% of patients with systemic sarcoid.
- Ages, 20 to 50 years.

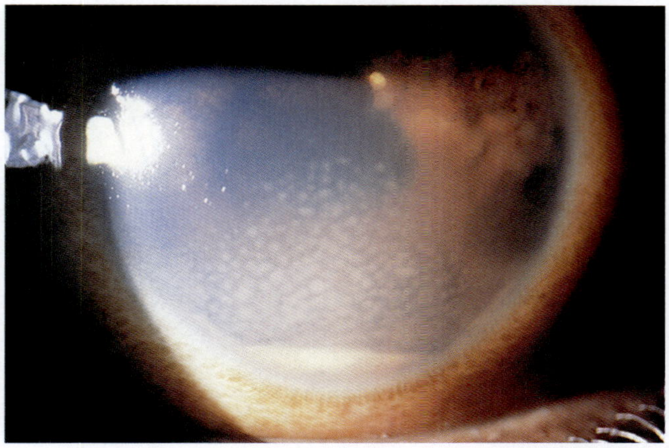

FIGURE 4.6. In granulomatous uveitis, large, greasy-appearing keratic precipitates can frequently be found in Arlt's triangle. (From Tasman W, Jaeger E. *The Wills Eye Hospital atlas of clinical ophthalmology*, 2nd ed. Lippincott Williams & Wilkins, 2001.)

Signs and Symptoms

Blurry vision, aching.

Ocular Findings

- Lid, orbit granuloma, conjunctival nodules, lacrimal gland infiltration with dry eye.
- Classic signs:
  Chronic granulomatous iridocyclitis.
  Mutton fat keratic precipitates (Figure 4.6).
  Koeppe/Busacca nodules (Figure 4.7).
  Posterior synechiae.
- Posterior:
  Granulomas (retinal or choroidal).
  Candlewax drippings (granulomas along vessels).

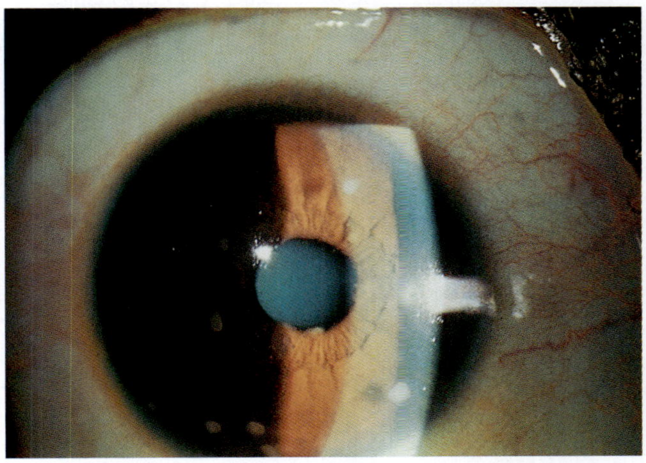

FIGURE 4.7. Koeppe nodules along the iris border at the 1, 4, and 8 o'clock positions. (From Tasman W, Jaeger E. *The Wills Eye Hospital atlas of clinical ophthalmology*, 2nd ed. Lippincott Williams & Wilkins, 2001.)

Periphlebitis.
Cystoid macular edema.
Peripheral neovascularization.
Optic nerve edema.
Optic nerve granulomas.
Snowbanks, snowballs.

Systemic Findings

Hilar lymphadenopathy.
Erythema nodosum.
Skin granulomas.
Firm, painless lymphadenopathy.
Neurologic symptoms.

Special Tests

- Elevated angiotensin-converting enzyme (ACE) and/or lysozyme levels.
- Chest radiograph (hilar adenopathy).
- Gallium scan (uptake in hilum, parotid gland, lacrimal gland).
- Biopsy of skin, conjunctival, lacrimal gland lesions.

Treatment

Topical or periocular steroids.
Cycloplegia.
Immunosuppressives in refractory cases.

Pathology

Noncaseating epithelioid granulomas or tubercles.
Langhans giant cells, Schaumann or asteroid bodies.

References

Dana MR, Merayo-Lloves J, Schaumberg DA, et al. Prognosticators for visual outcome in sarcoid uveitis. *Ophthalmology* 1996;103:1846–1853.

Jabs DA, Johns CJ. Ocular involvement in chronic sarcoidosis. *Am J Ophthalmol* 1986;102:297–301.

Karma A, Huhti E, Poukkula A. Course and outcome of ocular sarcoidosis. *Am J Ophthalmol* 1988;106:467–472.

Power WJ, Neves RA, Rodriguez A, et al. The value of combined serum angiotensin-converting enzyme and gallium scan in diagnosing ocular sarcoidosis. *Ophthalmology* 1995;102:2007–2011.

Tuberculosis

Summary

Ocular inflammation attributed to *Mycobacterium tuberculosis* can present in many different forms and should be considered on every differential for uveitis.

Etiology

Infection attributable to *M. tuberculosis* or inflammatory reaction related to distant *M. tuberculosis* infection.

Epidemiology

- Approximately 1% to 2% of patients with TB develop ocular disease.
- Can affect any age; equal sex distribution.
- Any race, but more common in developing world.

Ocular Findings

Can involve orbital adnexa, orbit, anterior and posterior segments.
Granulomatous or nongranulomatous uveitis.
Tubercle formation of eyelids and conjunctiva.
Corneal phlyctenule.
Conjunctivitis.
Scleritis.
Interstitial keratitis.
Anterior uveitis.
Vitritis.
Posterior uveitis.
Retinal vasculitis.
Choroidal granulomas.
Panuveitis.

Systemic Findings

- Can affect any organ system, lung most commonly affected.
- Fever, fatigue, weight loss, and night sweats.

Special Tests

- Tuberculin skin test (purified protein derivative [PPD]).
- Gamma interferon release assay (Quantiferon-Gold).
- Chest x-ray: can be normal in 50% of patients with ocular TB.
- Sputum cultures and smears for acid-fast bacilli.
- If possible, may culture or obtain pathologic examination of ocular specimen (nodules, granulomas).
- Serum ACE and lysozyme levels may be elevated during active disease.
- Human immunodeficiency virus (HIV) test: higher incidence in TB patients.

Pathology

- Caseating granulomatous inflammation consisting of fibroblasts lymphocytes.
- Langhans giant cells, macrophages.

Differential Diagnosis

- Sarcoidosis (increased ACE and lysozyme, anergic to PPD and other common antigens).
- Syphilis (rapid plasmin reagin [RPR], *microhemagglutination-Treponema pallidium* [MHA-TP]).

Treatment

- Consult infectious disease specialist.
- Schlaegel test (of historical interest, no longer valid).
- Multiple antituberculous drug therapy used to prevent formation of resistant strains:
  Isoniazid.
  Rifampin.
  Ethambutol.
  Streptomycin.
  Pyrazinamide.
- Topical and periocular steroids and cycloplegics are used for control of ocular inflammation.
- Oral steroids contraindicated in patients with systemic TB without concomitant antituberculous therapy.

Reference

Helm CJ, Holland GN. Ocular tuberculosis. *Surv Ophthalmol* 1993;38:229–256.

Syphilis

Summary

The ocular manifestations of syphilis are varied and protean. Almost every differential for uveitis contains syphilis.

Epidemiology

Acquired: young sexually active adults.

Etiology

Congenital infection with spirochete *Treponema pallidum*.

Transmission

Congenital: transplacental.
Acquired: sexual.

Ocular Findings

- Congenital: salt-and-pepper retinopathy, chorioretinal scarring, cataract, glaucoma interstitial keratitis, optic atrophy.
- Acquired:
  Primary: usually none.
  Secondary: acute, chronic, or recurrent granulomatous uveitis; scleritis; choroiditis; vitritis; papillitis; optic neuritis; vasculitis; keratitis linearis migrans (migrating deep stromal inflammation).
  Tertiary: Argyll-Robertson pupils (light-near dissociation), iris gumma.

Systemic Findings

- Congenital: maculopapular rash, notched incisors (Hutchinson teeth), frontal bossing, saddle nose deformity.
- Acquired:
  Primary: skin/mucus membrane lesions (painless chancre), lymphadenopathy.
  Secondary: maculopapular rash, alopecia areata, fever, fatigue, sore throat, generalized lymphadenopathy.
  Tertiary: gumma throughout body, aortic dilation, neurosyphilis (tabes dorsalis).

Diagnostic Tests

- RPR/Venereal Disease Research Laboratory (VDRL): nonspecific tests, reverts to negative result following treatment.
- Fluorescent treponemal antibody, absorbed (FTA-Abs)/ MHA-TP: specific for prior exposure to syphilis.
- Lumbar puncture VDRL and FTA-Abs: to look for neurosyphilis.
- HIV testing: higher incidence of other concomitant sexually transmitted diseases (STDs).

Treatment

- Consult with infectious disease specialist for antibiotic guidelines (usually penicillin for 10 to 14 days).
- Acute IK: topical steroids.
- Corneal transplantation may be required for corneal scarring related to IK.
- Uveitis associated with syphilis: topical, periocular, and systemic steroids following adequate antibiotic prescription.

Reference

Margo CE, Hamed LM. Ocular syphilis. *Surv Ophthalmol* 1992; 37:203–220.

Pars Planitis

Summary

At some centers, the terms *pars planitis* and *intermediate uveitis* are used interchangeably; however, in this context, pars planitis refers to intermediate uveitis of unknown etiology.

Epidemiology

Most commonly in second to fourth decades of life; 80% of cases are bilateral.

Signs and Symptoms

Blurry vision, floaters.

Ophthalmic Findings

Cystoid macular edema (CME, predominant cause of decreased vision).
Low-grade anterior chamber reaction.
Posterior synechiae (rare).

Band keratopathy.
Posterior subcapsular cataract.
Subretinal and preretinal neovascular membranes.
Vitreous hemorrhage.
Retinal phlebitis.
Snowballs: cellular aggregates in vitreous.
Snowbank: fibrovascular exudative changes of the inferior pars plana.

Etiology

Unknown; possible association with the HLA-DR locus.

Disease Course

- Seventy-five percent have benign or mild chronic disease.
- Twenty-five percent have severe chronic or relentlessly progressive inflammation leading to cyclitic membranes, RD, and phthisis.

Treatment

Stepladder treatment approach strongly recommended if CME or vasculitis present, regardless of visual acuity.

Smoking cessation; smoking correlates with vision loss.
Periocular steroid injections with topical steroids for anterior segment inflammation.
Oral nonsteroidal anti-inflammatory drugs (NSAIDs) for recurrent inflammation.
Systemic steroids for persistent or recurrent inflammation.
Cryotherapy or peripheral laser photocoagulation.
Immunosuppression (cyclosporine, azathioprine, methotrexate) if patient fails therapy or becomes intolerant to steroids.
Pars plana vitrectomy if refractory.

References

Brockhurst R, Schepens C. Uveitis IV. Peripheral uveitis: the complications of retinal detachment. *Arch Ophthalmol* 1968;80:747–753.
Donaldson MJ, Pulido JS, Herman DC, et al. Pars planitis: a 20-year study of incidence, clinical features, and outcomes. *Am J Ophthalmol* 2007;144:812–817.
Kaplan HJ. In: Saari KM, ed. *Uveitis update*. Amsterdam, The Netherlands: Excerpta Medical, 1984:169–172.
Malinowski SM, Pulido JS, Goeken NE, et al. The association of HLA-B8, B51, DR2, and multiple sclerosis in pars planitis. *Ophthalmology* 1993;100:1199–1205.

Lyme Disease

Summary

Lyme disease is a multisystem disorder caused by the spirochete *Borrelia burgdorferi* with ophthalmic, dermatologic, rheumatologic, neurologic, and cardiac manifestations (see Table 4.4).

Table 4.4
Stages of Lyme disease

	Early (stage I)	Late (stages II and III)
Systemic disease	Flulike symptoms: malaise, fever, headache myalgia, arthralgia Erythema chronicum migrans skin rash at the site of the tick bite (present in 60%–80% of patients) Lymphadenopathy	Stage II (several months after initial tick bite): cardiac and neurologic symptoms (e.g., ventricular conduction block, meningitis, cranial and peripheral nerve palsies) Stage III (months to years after initial tick bite): severe arthritis and chronic neurologic problems
Ocular disease	Conjunctivitis Episcleritis	Chronic conjunctivitis Orbital myositis Stromal keratitis Granulomatous iridocyclitis Intermediate uveitis Diffuse choroiditis Optic disk edema and neuroretinitis Retinal vasculitis Exudative retinal detachment Neuroophthalmic involvement: Bell palsy, optic neuritis, cranial nerve palsies

Etiology

Infection by the spirochete *B. burgdorferi* transmitted by Ixodes deer ticks.

Epidemiology

- Residents of tick-endemic areas: eastern coastal states, northern California, and the northern Midwest.
- History of hiking, camping.

Special Tests

Serologic testing (ELISA most sensitive, Western blot for confirmation) for IgM and IgG against *B. burgdorferi*.

In endemic areas, baseline positive serology may be present in up to 15% of patients. Positive serology plus erythema chronicum migrans or one organ system involvement is diagnostic.

In nonendemic areas, involvement of two or more organ systems is needed for the diagnosis.

Serology will cross-react with other spirochetes such as *T. pallidum*.

Lumbar puncture: CSF pleocytosis.

Disease Course

Frequent recurrences.

Differential Diagnosis

Sarcoidosis, syphilis, and TB.

Treatment

Early (stage I):

1. Doxycycline.
2. Amoxicillin.
3. Erythromycin.

Late (stages II and III):

1. Ceftriaxone.
2. Penicillin G.
3. Doxycycline (may be less effective).

References

Copeland RA Jr. Lyme uveitis. *Int Ophthalmol Clin* 1990;30:291–293.

Winward KE, Smith JL, Culbertson WW, et al. Ocular Lyme borreliosis. *Am J Ophthalmol* 1989;108:651–657.

Zaidman GW. The ocular manifestations of Lyme disease. *Int Ophthalmol Clin* 1997;37:13–28.

ENDOPHTHALMITIS

Summary

Endophthalmitis describes infectious intraocular inflammation (anterior chamber and vitreous) (Table 4.5).

Table 4.5

Organisms most often responsible for exogenous endophthalmitis

Acute postoperative endophthalmitis (onset within 2 wk of surgery)	
Mild	*Staphylococcus epidermidis*
Severe	*Staphylococcus aureus*
	Streptococcus sp.
	Gram-negative bacteria (Serratia, Pseudomonas, etc.)
Chronic postoperative (onset weeks to months after surgery)	*Propionibacterium acnes*
	S. epidermidis
	Fungi
	Achromobacter
Bleb associated	*Haemophilus influenzae*
	Streptococcus sp.
Posttraumatic	*Bacillus* sp.
	Streptococcus sp.
	Fungi
	Staphylococcus sp.

Acute Postoperative Endophthalmitis

Summary

Intraocular inflammation within days following ocular surgery is a rare complication usually secondary to bacterial infection.

Etiology

Organisms from the periocular field gaining entry into the eye, usually through wound.

Signs and Symptoms

Decreased vision.
Pain, photophobia.
Redness.

Demographics

Incidence less than 0.1% in large series of cataract extractions.

Ophthalmic Findings

Severe: rapid, fulminant course, 3 to 7 days after surgery.
Mild: slow, indolent course; onset within 2 weeks of surgery.
Anterior chamber and vitreous inflammation.
Hypopyon.
Decreased visual acuity.

Systemic Findings

None.

Special Tests

Anterior chamber and vitreous tap to determine causative organism.

Treatment and Management

Vitrectomy.
Intravitreal antibiotics.
Corticosteroids.
Fortified topical antibiotics.

References

Endophthalmitis Vitrectomy Study Group. Microbiologic factors and visual outcome in the endophthalmitis vitrectomy study: the Endophthalmitis Vitrectomy Study. *Am J Ophthalmol* 1996; 122:830–846.

Endophthalmitis Vitrectomy Study Group. Results of the Endophthalmitis Vitrectomy Study: a randomized trial of immediate vitrectomy and of intravenous antibiotics for the treatment of postoperative bacterial endophthalmitis. *Arch Ophthalmol* 1995;113:1479–1496.

Chronic Postoperative Endophthalmitis

Summary

Chronic postoperative endophthalmitis is an indolent inflammatory condition caused by less virulent organisms such as *P. acnes* and fungi.

Etiology

Low-grade infection caused by organisms such as *P. acnes*, fungi, *Staphylococcus epidermidis*, and *Achromobacter*.

Signs and Symptoms

Decreased vision.
Mild pain or photophobia.

Ophthalmic Findings

Low-grade anterior chamber or diffuse inflammation.
Keratic precipitates.
Waxing and waning course.
Capsular plaque or retained lens material.

Systemic Findings

None.

Special Tests

Vitreous tap and anaerobic cultures.
Capsular biopsy.

Pathology

Propionibacterium acnes: Gram-positive rods sequestered in capsular bag and in lens fragments.

Disease Course

- Fluctuating, low-grade iridocyclitis.
- May initially respond to topical corticosteroids.

Treatment and Management

Capsulectomy.
Removal of retained lens material.
Intravitreal antibiotics.
Cure rate is 7% with intravitreal antibiotics, 50% with intravitreal antibiotics + vitrectomy, 75% with intravitreal antibiotics + vitrectomy + partial capsulectomy, 100% with intravitreal antibiotics + vitrectomy + IOL removal and total capsulectomy.

Differential Diagnosis

Phacoantigenic uveitis.
UGH syndrome.

Reference

Mandelbaum S, Meisler DM. Postoperative chronic microbial endophthalmitis. *Int Ophthalmol Clin* 1993;33:71–79.

Bleb-Associated Endophthalmitis

Summary

Thin avascular glaucoma-filtering blebs may predispose patients to an increased risk of endophthalmitis. The most common organisms isolated are *Streptococcus* species and *Haemophilus influenzae*.

Etiology

- Hole in bleb → infection → endophthalmitis.
- Thin avascular blebs (such as after the use of antimetabolites) may be at higher risk.
- Inferior blebs are also at higher risk for infection.

Signs and Symptoms

Redness, tearing, and discharge.
Decreased vision.
Pain.

Demographics

Glaucoma patients following trabeculectomy; incidence varies from 1% to 18%.

Ophthalmic Findings

Infiltrated bleb filled with purulent material (Figure 4.8).

Hypopyon.
Anterior chamber and vitreous inflammation.
Hypotony.

Systemic Findings

None.

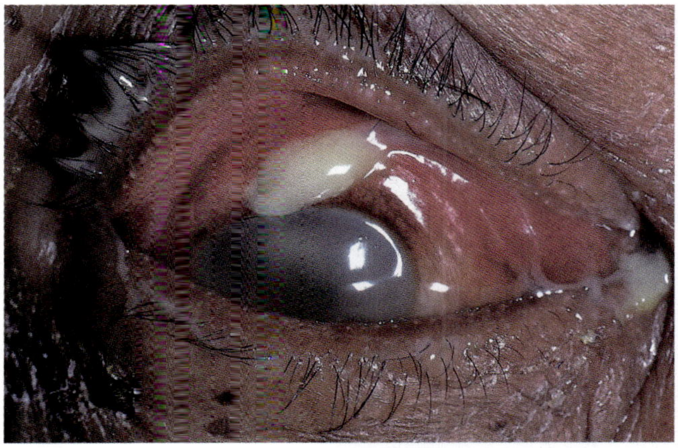

FIGURE 4.8. Infiltrated filtering bleb and severe anterior iridocyclitis in bleb-associated endophthalmitis caused by *Streptococcus pneumoniae.*

Special Tests

- Anterior chamber and vitreous tap to identify organism.
- *H. influenzae* and *Streptococcus pneumoniae* most commonly isolated.

Treatment and Management

Topical and subconjunctival antibiotics may be sufficient for localized bleb infection.
If endophthalmitis is present, treat with intravitreal antibiotics; obtain vitreous aspirate.
Repair of bleb leak.

Posttraumatic Endophthalmitis

Summary

Posttraumatic endophthalmitis is a potentially severe intraocular infection following a penetrating ocular injury.

Etiology

Penetrating ocular trauma with or without a retained intraocular foreign body allowing access of bacteria into the eye.

Signs and Symptoms

Pain.
Redness.
Decreased vision.

Demographics

Incidence up to 30% following penetrating ocular injury.

Ophthalmic Findings

Hypopyon.
Hyphema.
Vitreous hemorrhage.
Severe intraocular inflammation.
Retained intraocular foreign bodies.
Incarceration of uvea or vitreous in wound.
Leaking or gaping wound.

Systemic Findings

None.

Special Tests

- Anterior chamber and vitreous taps to determine organism responsible for infection.
- Ultrasound, computed tomography (CT), or x-ray imaging to rule out foreign bodies.

Disease Course

- Bacillus cereus infection: rapidly progressive infection. Often results in extensive ocular damage and poor acuity (Figure 4.9).
- Fungi: suspect in trauma with organic material (e.g., wood, straw).

Treatment and Management

Broad spectrum antibiotics (topical, subconjunctival, intravitreal, and i.v.).
Antifungals.
Steroids.
Vitrectomy.

Endogenous Endophthalmitis

Summary

Endogenous endophthalmitis is caused by intraocular spread of blood-borne organisms and requires systemic therapy.

Etiology

Disseminated systemic microbial infection spread to the eye.

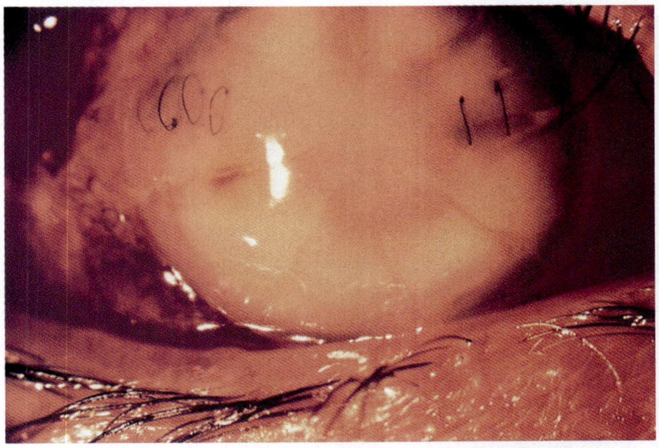

FIGURE 4.9. Severe intraocular infection caused by *Bacillus cereus* following a penetrating fish-hook injury in a patient with previous radial keratotomy.

Signs and Symptoms

Blurred vision.

Demographics

Immunosuppressed patients.
Intravenous drug abusers.
Intravenous and indwelling lines.
Chronic tissue infections (e.g., osteomyelitis).

Ophthalmic Findings

Elevated choroidal mass.
Vitritis.
Retinitis.

Systemic Findings

Infected i.v. lines.
Abscesses.
Disseminated fungal infection.
Signs of systemic infection.

Special Tests

Vitreous biopsy.
Blood cultures.
Urine cultures.

Treatment and Management

Vitrectomy.
Systemic antimicrobial treatment.

Differential Diagnosis

Intraocular lymphoma.
See Table 4.6.

Table 4.6

Organisms responsible for endogenous endophthalmitis

Organism	Source and risk factors
Candida	Systemic candidiasis i.v. drug abuse, AIDS
Aspergillus	Immunosuppression, i.v. drug abuse
Fusarium	Infected surgical wounds
Cryptococcus	AIDS patients, CNS cryptococcal infection
Staphylococcus aureus	i.v. drug abuse
Klebsiella	Hepatic abscess
Bacillus cereus	i.v. drug abuse
Streptococcus sp.	Endocarditis
Gram-negative bacilli	Enteric infections Urosepsis

AIDS, acquired immunodeficiency syndrome; CNS, central nervous system; i.v., intravenous.

MAJOR STUDY

Endophthalmitis Vitrectomy Study

Study Population

Patients with endophthalmitis after cataract surgery.

Entry Criteria

- Endophthalmitis within 6 weeks of cataract surgery or secondary IOL placement (acute postoperative endophthalmitis).
- Acuity between 20/50 and LP.

Study Design

- Multicenter randomized clinical trial.
- Four subgroups:
  1. Initial vitrectomy and i.v. antibiotics.
  2. Initial vitrectomy without i.v. antibiotics.
  3. Initial vitreous tap and i.v. antibiotics.
  4. Initial vitreous tap without i.v. antibiotics.
- All patients received intravitreal antibiotics.

Conclusions

1. Patients with acuity of hand motions (HM) or better at presentation did not benefit from immediate vitrectomy in comparison to vitreous tap and intravitreal antibiotics.
2. Immediate vitrectomy is indicated for visual acuity worse than HM at presentation.
3. No difference in final acuity or media clarity with the use of intravenous antibiotics.

References

Endophthalmitis Vitrectomy Study Group. Microbiologic factors and visual outcome in the endophthalmitis vitrectomy study. The Endophthalmitis Vitrectomy Study. *Am J Ophthalmol* 1996;122:830–846.

Endophthalmitis Vitrectomy Study Group. Results of the Endophthalmitis Vitrectomy Study: a randomized trial of immediate vitrectomy and of intravenous antibiotics for the treatment of postoperative bacterial endophthalmitis. *Arch Ophthalmol* 1995;113:1479–1496.

POSTERIOR UVEITIS

Senile Vitritis

Summary

A mild vitritis in elderly patients with a negative laboratory workup. This is a diagnosis of exclusion, and workup of possible causes should be undertaken.

Signs and Symptoms

Blurred vision or normal acuity.
Floaters.

Demographics

White, women more common than men.
Ages, 40 to 70 years (average, 52 years).

Ophthalmic Findings

Bilateral vitritis (77%).
Mild anterior chamber inflammation (33%).
Cystoid macular edema.
Epiretinal membranes.

Disease Course

Chronic smoldering vitritis.

Treatment

Steroids: limited, temporary effect.

Differential Diagnosis

- Birdshot retinochoroidopathy: multifocal ovoid choroidal lesions.
- Intraocular lymphoma.

Reference

Brinton GS, Osher RH, Gass JD. Idiopathic vitritis. *Retina* 1983; 3:95–98.

White dot syndromes

Multiple Evanescent White Dot Syndrome

Summary

Multiple evanescent white dot syndrome (MEWDS) is an acute unilateral inflammatory condition predominantly affecting young women with 100- to 200-µm discrete white spots in the retina and retinal pigment epithelium (RPE) that appear and disappear over several days' time.

Epidemiology

Women more frequently affected than men.
Average age is 25 years.
Preceding flulike illness in half of patients.

Etiology

Possible viral association.

Signs and Symptoms

Sudden onset of decreased or blurry vision.
Scotomas centrally or in periphery.
Photopsias.

Ophthalmic Findings

- Usually unilateral.
- Variable vision, occasional mild iritis.
- Multiple, discrete clusters of 100- to 200-µm white spots at the level of the RPE or deep retina, usually in the posterior pole region, that are migratory over days (Figure 4.10).
- Granular pigment changes in the macula.
- Few vitreous cells.
- Mild blurring the optic disk.
- Isolated vascular sheathing.

Differential Diagnosis

- Other white dot syndromes (acute posterior multifocal placoid pigment epitheliopathy [APMPPE], ARPE, multifocal choroiditis [MFC], diffuse unilateral subacute neuroretinitis [DUSN], AMN, punctate inner choroidopathy [PIC]).
- Birdshot retinochoroidopathy.
- Toxoplasmosis.

Special Tests

- Visual field (variable results):
  Normal.
  Generalized depression.
  Enlarged blind spots.
  Paracentral or peripheral scotomas.
- Intravenous fluorescein angiography (IVFA):
  Early: punctate hyperfluorescence at the level of the RPE in wreathlike configuration.
  Late: staining of the spots and the optic nerve.
- Electroretinogram (ERG)/electrooculogram (EOG): decreased amplitudes.

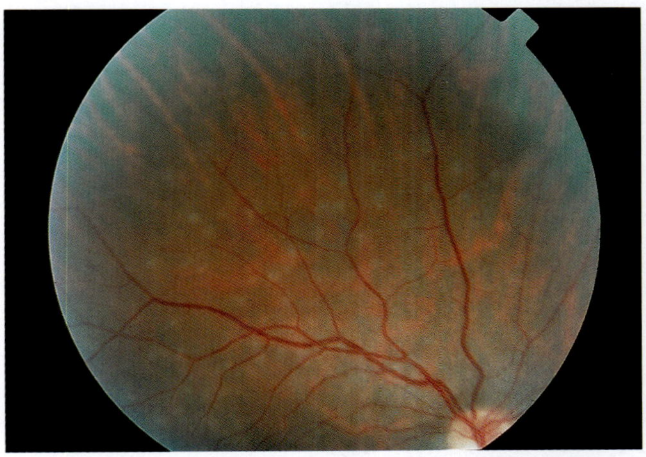

FIGURE 4.10. Multiple clusters of small white dots found in multiple evanescent white dot syndrome.

Disease Course

- Spontaneous visual recovery usually occurs in 2 to 10 weeks.
- White spots disappear with persistent macular RPE granularity.
- Photopsias may persist.
- Rarely recurs.

Treatment

None.

References

Jampol LM, Sieving PA, Pugh D, et al. Multiple evanescent white dot syndrome, I: clinical findings. *Arch Ophthalmol* 1984;102:671–674.

Sieving PA, Fishman GA, Jampol LM, et al. Multiple evanescent white dot syndrome, II: electrophysiology of the photoreceptors during retinal pigment epithelial disease. *Arch Ophthalmol* 1984;102:675–679.

Acute Posterior Multifocal Placoid Pigment Epitheliopathy

Summary

APMPPE is an inflammatory condition characterized by bilateral placoid lesions in the posterior pole, most frequently affecting young, healthy adults.

Epidemiology

Young, healthy adults.
Male and female patients equally affected.
Age, 20 to 50 years; average, 25 years.

Etiology

Possibly viral.
May be associated with HLA-B7 and HLA-DR2.

Signs and Symptoms

Rapid loss of central vision.

Ophthalmic Findings

- Often bilateral but asymmetric.
- Multiple large discrete, white-yellow, flat placoid lesions, usually in the posterior pole at the level of the RPE.

Associated Findings

Episcleritis, papillitis, vasculitis.

Systemic Findings

- Preceding flulike illness in 50%: upper respiratory tract infection, headache, erythema nodosa.
- May have serious central nervous system (CNS) involvement (headaches, meningismus, neurologic deficits); if severe headache and/or neurologic signs, should get a neurology consult.

Differential Diagnosis

Serpiginous, DUSN, MEWDS, birdshot, sarcoid, syphilis, toxoplasmosis (PORT), TB, acute retinal necrosis (ARN), intraocular lymphoma.

Special Tests

- IVFA:
  During active disease: early blockage, late diffuse hyperfluorescence.
  During inactive disease: window defects.
- Urinanalysis: casts.
- Lumbar puncture: CSF pleocytosis.
- ERG/EOG: decreased amplitudes.

Pathogenesis

Unknown.

Treatment

- None; self-limiting process.
- Consider systemic steroids if severe with bilateral decreased vision.

Disease Course

Spontaneous resolution in 10 to 14 days.
Lesions fade in 1 week.
Recovery of vision in weeks to months.
Leaves pigment epithelial mottling.
Usually does not recur.

References

Gass JD. Acute posterior multifocal placoid pigment epitheliopathy. *Arch Ophthalmol* 1968;80:177–185.

Jones NP. Acute posterior multifocal placoid pigment epitheliopathy. *Br J Ophthalmol* 1995;79:384–389.

Diffuse Unilateral Subacute Neuroretinitis

Summary

Subretinal infestation and migration of nematode larvae can cause insidious, unilateral, widespread inflammatory destruction of the neurosensory retina.

Epidemiology

- Ages, 7 to 65 years; no sex or race predilection.
- Southeastern United States and Caribbean.
- Developing countries.

Etiology

- Nematodal infection: *Baylisascaris procyonis* or *Ancylostoma caninum*. *Alaria mesocercaviae* have been associated with this syndrome.

Signs and Symptoms

Loss of vision.

Ophthalmic Findings

- Early:
- Afferent pupillary defect.

  Optic nerve swelling

  Mild vitritis.

  May see a motile subretinal worm in an area of active inflammation.

  Multiple gray-white outer retinal dots (400 to 1,500 μm).

  Serous RD

  Anterior chamber quiet.
- Late:
- RPE atrophy.

  Vision worse than 20/200.

  Decreased visual field.

  Diffuse pigment epithelial wipeout.

  Relative sparing of macula.

  Optic atrophy.

  Narrowed vessels.

  Afferent pupillary defect.

Systemic Findings

Dermatologic and other systemic signs of nematode infection.

Pathogenesis

- Toxic effect on the outer retina by the worm.
- Inflammatory reaction to worm.

Differential Diagnosis

- Optic neuritis.
- Retinitis pigmentosa: in late stages with pigment clumping and optic atrophy.

Special Tests

Abnormal ERG: loss of B wave with preservation of the A wave.

Treatment

- Laser photocoagulation of worm, causes minimal inflammatory response.
- Thiabendazole 22 mg/kg p.o. for 2 to 4 days has been used.
- Ivermectin.

Prognosis

- No recurrence or progression, once worm is killed.
- Fellow eye not affected.
- Poor final visual acuity if not treated in early phase.

References

Gass JD, Braunstein RA. Further observations concerning the diffuse unilateral subacute neuroretinitis syndrome. *Arch Ophthalmol* 1983;101:1689–1697.

Kazacos KR, Raymond LA, Kazacos EA, et al. The raccoon ascarid: a probable cause of human ocular larva migrans. *Ophthalmology* 1985;92:1735–1744.

Multifocal Choroiditis and Subretinal fibrosis

Other names:

Punctate inner choroiditis (PIC).

Multifocal choroiditis and panuveitis.

Progressive subretinal fibrosis and uveitis.

Chorioretinopathy with anterior uveitis.

Summary

Multifocal choroiditis and subretinal fibrosis encompasses a spectrum of conditions that presents with multifocal yellowish choroidal lesions with progressive subretinal fibrosis.

Epidemiology

Young women.

Average age, 27 years; most patients younger than 35 years.

Etiology

Unknown.

Signs and Symptoms

Decreased vision.

Metamorphopsia.

Photopsia.

Ophthalmic Findings

- Moderate to high myopia (between −3.00 and −10.00 diopters [D] reported).
- Bilateral.
- Early:

  Minimal or absent anterior segment inflammation and vitritis.

  Multiple punctate, yellow, inner choroidal lesions 100 to 300 μm in diameter, located in the posterior pole or midperiphery.

- Late:
  Lesions can rarely coalesce to create regions of subretinal fibrosis.
  Peripapillary pigment changes.

Systemic Findings

None.

Disease Course

- Lesions may heal within a month, leaving an atrophic scar.
- Progressive enlargement of areas of subretinal fibrosis.
- Complications:
  Serous RD.
  Cystoid macular edema.
  Choroidal neovascular membrane (CNVM) (30% to 60%).

Differential Diagnosis

Presumed ocular histoplasmosis syndrome.
MEWDS.
Birdshot retinochoroidopathy.
DUSN.
Toxoplasmosis.

Special Tests

IVFA:

Early: blockage by the lesions.
Late: staining of the lesions.

Treatment

- No definitive treatment.
- Steroids ineffective.
- Laser photocoagulation of CNVM.

Prognosis

Spontaneous resolution.

References

Dreyer RF, Gass JDM. Multifocal choroiditis and panuveitis: a syndrome that mimics ocular histoplasmosis. *Arch Ophthalmol* 1984;102:1776–1784.
Nozik RA, Dorsch W. A new chorioretinopathy associated with anterior uveitis. *Am J Ophthalmol* 1973;76:758–762.
Watzke RC, Packer AJ, Folk JC, et al. Punctate inner choroidopathy. *Am J Ophthalmol* 1984;98:572–584.

Serpiginous Choroiditis

Other names: geographic choroiditis, geographic helicoid peripapillary choroidopathy.

Summary

Serpiginous choroiditis characterized by chronic, recurrent, bilateral choroidal inflammation spreading centrifugally in a pseudopoidal fashion.

Epidemiology

Male and female patients approximately equally affected; 30- to 70-year-olds.
Usually bilateral.
Whites.

Etiology

Unknown.

Signs and Symptoms

Painless blurring or loss of vision.
Progressive and recurrent disease.
Permanent scotomas.

Ophthalmic Findings

- Anterior chamber usually quiet, but occasionally, nongranulomatous inflammation.
- Acute findings:
  Peripapillary geographic lesions, gray or gray-yellow at the level of the RPE.
  Inflammation along borders of lesions.
  Fingerlike projections usually radiating from the optic nerve.
  Macular or peripheral serpiginous lesions may occur.
  Retinal vasculitis.
  Vitritis in 20% to 30% of cases.
- Late findings:
  Atrophy and clumping of RPE with exposure of underlying choroidal vasculature (Figure 4.11).
  Subretinal choroidal neovascular membranes.

Systemic Findings

None.

Disease Course

- Progressive centrifugal extension over weeks to months, resolving with pigmentary loss, mottling, or atrophy.
- Recurrent attacks over many years.
- Marked asymmetry in progression between eyes.
- Development of CNVM at border of old scar in 20% of cases.

Differential Diagnosis

- APMPPE: viral prodrome, large round lesions, recurrences rare.

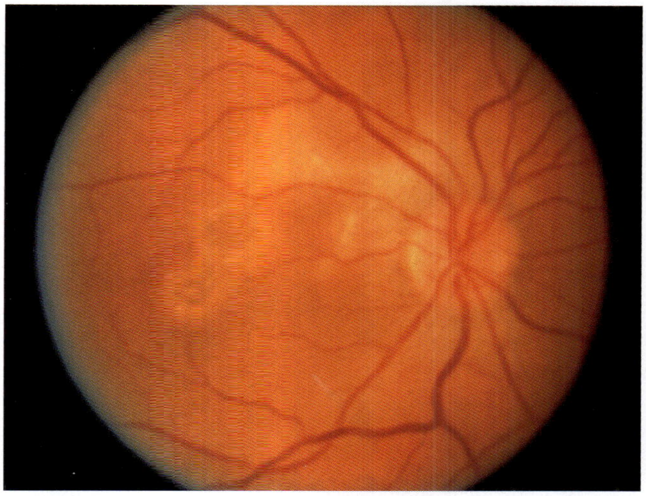

FIGURE 4.11. Serpiginous choroiditis extending from the optic nerve toward the macula.

- Toxoplasmosis: more severe vitritis, usually adjacent to typical toxoplasmosis scar.
- Choroidal ischemia TB, sarcoid, regional choroidal dystrophies

Special Tests

- IVFA:
  Early:
    Hypofluorescence with hyperfluorescent border.
    Window defect corresponding to central atrophic areas.
  Late: staining of lesions.
- Visual fields: absolute scotoma corresponding to acute lesions, relative scotomas when quiescent.

Pathology

- Atrophy of choriocapillaris, photoreceptors, and RPE.
- Choroidal lymphocytic infiltration.

Treatment

- Posterior sub-Tenon steroid injection/systemic steroids: controversial. Unknown whether better than natural history without treatment.
- Combination prednisone, azathioprine, cyclosporine A: no good studies regarding effectiveness of different regimens, although small series suggest better visual outcomes with immunomodulatory therapy.
- Laser for CNVM outside fovea.

Prognosis

- Permanent scotoma; decreased visual acuity if macula involved.
- Recurs months to years in centrifugal pattern from disk moving toward macula often contiguous with previous scar.

References

Hardy RA, Schatz H. Macular geographic helicoid choroidopathy. *Arch Ophthalmol* 1987;105:1237–1242.

Weiss H, Annesley WH Jr, Shields JA, et al. The clinical course of serpiginous choroidopathy. *Am J Ophthalmol* 1979;87:133–142.

Ocular Toxoplasmosis

Summary

Ocular toxoplasmosis is caused by *Toxoplasma gondii* infection resulting in vitritis and retinitis adjacent to previous chorioretinal scars. Atypical presentations of Toxoplasma retinochoroiditis in AIDS patients are to be distinguished from the self-limited disease in immunocompetent individuals (Table 4.7).

Etiology

Infection or recurrence of infection caused by the parasite *T. gondii*; natural host is the cat; human is the intermediate host.

Table 4.7

Differences in toxoplasmosis infection in immunocompetent and incompetent patients

	Competent	Incompetent
Laterality	Unilateral	Bilateral
Disease transmission	Congenital or acquired	Acquired
Presentation	Unifocal, adjacent to previous scar	Multifocal, can arise *de novo*
Inflammation	Moderate to severe	Mild to moderate
CNS disease	Rare	Common
Disease course	Self-limited within 6 wk	May need long-term treatment

CNS, central nervous system.

Epidemiology

- Congenital infection:
  - Most common.
  - Most severe disease if contracted in the first trimester.
  - Transmission is the greatest in the third trimester, with multisystem involvement and usually bilateral ocular disease.
- Acquired infection:
  - Ingestion of oocytes or tissue cysts in previously unexposed host.
  - Cysts found in undercooked meat, poorly cleaned vegetables from contaminated soil.
  - Transmitted from fecal-oral contamination.
- Cyst forms:
  - Tachyzoite: infectious form.
  - Bradyzoite: tissue cyst.
  - Sporozoite: oocyst of the young cat.

Signs and Symptoms

Blurred vision.
Photophobia.

Demographics

- Otherwise healthy patients.
- AIDS patients.

Ophthalmic Findings

- Congenital:
  - Microphthalmia.
  - Nystagmus.
  - Coloboma.
  - Strabismus.
  - Ptosis.
  - Macular scars.
- Acquired or reactivation:
  - Granulomatous iridocyclitis.
  - Necrotizing retinitis adjacent to large, atrophic yellow-white, unevenly pigmented chorioretinal scar.
  - Severe vitritis, "headlight in the fog" (Figure 4.12).
  - Periphlebitis.
  - Papillitis.
  - Branch retinal vein occlusion (BRVO).
  - Diffuse retinitis.
  - Gray-white punctate lesions in the outer retina and RPE.
  - More than one third of cases have macular involvement.
- Immunosuppressed patients:
  - May have atypical presentations that may resemble CMV retinitis.
  - Multiple active lesions, massive retinal necrosis.
  - Bilateral, multifocal full-thickness retinitis; may be perivascular.
  - May not have previous chorioretinal scars.
  - Mild to moderate vitritis.

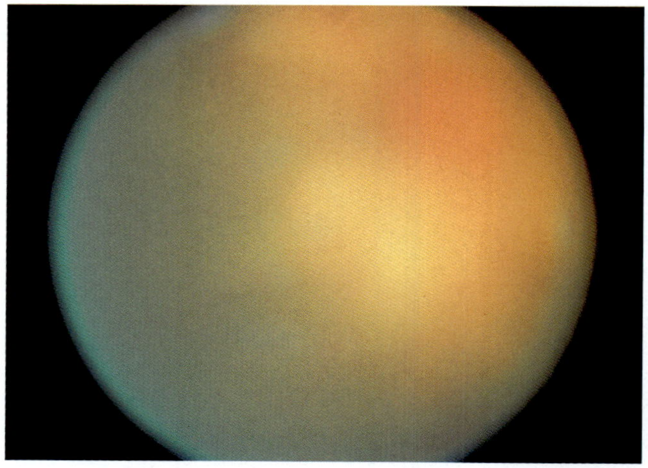

FIGURE 4.12. Severe vitritis and focal retinitis in ocular toxoplasmosis.

Systemic Findings

CNS toxoplasmosis.

Special Tests

CT scan: to look for calcified CNS toxoplasmosis lesions.
Vitreous biopsy: Polymerase chain reaction (PCR)-based assays may detect the DNA of the toxoplasma organism (not widely available).
Serologic testing: serum sample with immunoglobulin M (IgM) to toxoplasmosis, or threefold rise in immunoglobulin G (IgG); often negative in ocular disease.
IVFA: diffuse retinal vasculitis, active retinitis blocks fluorescence early, stains late.

Disease Course

- Recurrence after cessation of treatment may occur and maintenance prophylaxis recommended in AIDS patients.
- Complications: CNVM, branch retinal artery occlusion (BRAO), glaucoma, cystoid macular edema, cataracts, tractional retinal detachment (TRD), optic atrophy, epiretinal membrane (ERM), serous RD.

Treatment

- Small active peripheral lesion:
  - Observation.
  - Treatment has not been shown to hasten resolution, but may limit extent of scarring.
- Macula or optic nerve threatened or significant vitritis:
  - Pyrimethamine (Daraprim).
  - Sulfadiazine or Bactrim DS.
  - Folinic acid (leucovorin).
    - Check complete blood cell count (CBC) and platelet counts weekly.
  - *or*
  - Clindamycin (Cleocin).

Sulfadiazine
Treat for 3 to 4 weeks.
or
Trimethoprim/sulfamethoxazole (Bactrim DS or Septra).
Add clindamycin for lesions in the posterior pole.
Combination intravitreal clindamycin and dexamethasone in refractory cases or if intolerant of systemic therapy.

- May add oral steroids (prednisone) 24 to 48 hours after starting antibiotics; steroids contraindicated in immunocompromised patients.

Differential Diagnosis

- Cytomegalovirus (CMV) retinitis: hemorrhages, less vitritis.
- Focal infectious retinochoroiditis (TB, syphilis).
- Sarcoidosis
- Lymphoma

References

Holland GN, Engstrom RE Jr, Glasgow BJ, et al. Ocular toxoplasmosis in patients with the acquired immunodeficiency syndrome. *Am J Ophthalmol* 1988;106:653–667.

Parke DW, Font RL. Diffuse toxoplasmic retinochoroiditis in a patient with AIDS. *Arch Ophthalmol* 1986;104:571–575.

Rothova A. Ocular involvement in toxoplasmosis. *Br J Ophthalmol* 1993;77:371–377

Toxocariasis

Summary

Ocular toxocariasis is infection of the eye with the larva of Toxocara. Most of the damage to the eye is a consequence of the inflammatory response to the dead larva.

Etiology

Intraocular infection with nematode larva of *Toxocara* sp.

Signs and Symptoms

Can be asymptomatic in children.

Demographics

- Children; average age of presentation, 8 years.
- Exposure to puppies, contaminated soil.

Ophthalmic Findings

Three presentations:

1. Peripheral snowbanks: massive localized peripheral snowbanks, dragging of optic nerve or macula by traction bands (Figure 4.13).
2. Posterior-pole granuloma: various sizes and locations. Can have extensive retinal fibrosis.
3. Endophthalmitis: diffuse vitritis; may also have posterior-pole granuloma or peripheral snowbanks.

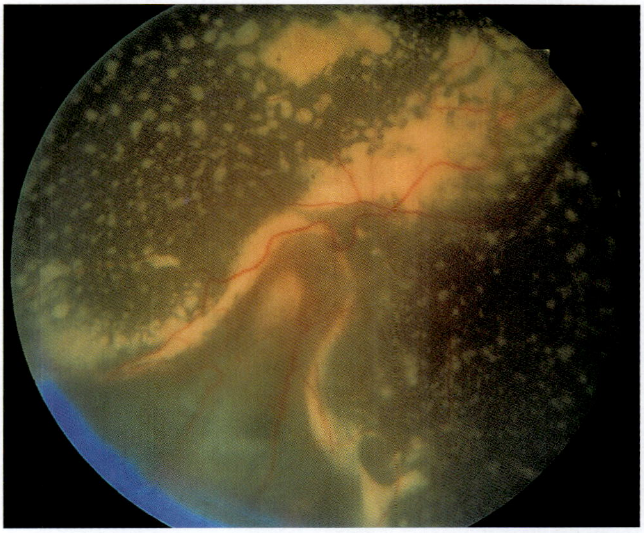

FIGURE 4.13. Traction retinal detachment and subretinal exudates associated with a peripheral toxocara granuloma.

Systemic Findings

Systemic larval infection (visceral larva migrans): rarely occurs with ocular toxocariasis.

Special Tests

- Eosinophilia (more common with visceral larva migrans).
- Elevated Toxocara IgG, IgM, and immunoglobulin E (IgE) titers.

Treatment and Management

- Corticosteroids to decrease the inflammatory response.
- Antihelminthics: not effective, since larva is already dead.
- Vitrectomy to remove traction on retina and repair breaks and detachments.

Differential Diagnosis

ROP.
Pars planitis.
Endophthalmitis.

References

Molk R. Ocular toxocariasis: a review of the literature. *Ann Ophthalmol* 1983;15:216–219, 222–227, 230–231.

Shields JA. Ocular toxocariasis: a review. *Surv Ophthalmol* 1984;28:361–381.

Acute Retinal Necrosis

Summary

Acute retinal necrosis (ARN) is a unilateral or bilateral necrotizing vaso-occlusive retinitis.

Epidemiology

Slight male preponderance.

Typically immunocompetent young adults although children and elderly may be afflicted.

Etiology

- HSV or VZV, less commonly cytomegalovirus.

Pathology

- Lymphocytic retinal and choroidal infiltrates, retinal arteritis, and sharp demarcation between normal and necrotic retina.

Signs and Symptoms

Pain.

Redness.

Floaters.

Decreased vision.

Ophthalmic Findings

American Uveitis Society Criteria for Diagnosis of ARN:

- One or more foci of retinal necrosis with discrete borders in the peripheral retina.
- Rapid progression of disease if antiviral therapy has not been given.
- Circumferential spread of disease.
- Evidence of occlusive vasculopathy with arteriolar involvement.
- A prominent inflammatory reaction in the vitreous and anterior chamber.
- Optic nerve involvement, scleritis, and pain support but are not required for the diagnosis.

Systemic Findings

Usually, none.

Differential Diagnosis

Bacterial or fungal endophthalmitis, Behçet disease, pars planitis, syphilis, cytomegalovirus retinitis, intraocular lymphoma, sarcoidosis, toxoplasmosis.

Special Tests

- PCR of aqueous or vitreous.

Treatment

- Intravenous acyclovir for 14 days, followed by oral acyclovir 800 mg five times daily for an additional 6 weeks.
- Laser barricade may prevent RD.
- Intravitreal ganciclovir or foscarnet.
- Systemic corticosteroids 24 to 48 hours after initiation of acyclovir therapy.

Prognosis

- Involvement of fellow eye is 13% and 65% with and without antiviral therapy, respectively.
- Optic neuropathy and RD associated with poor visual outcome.

Reference

Macular Photocoagulation Study Group. Laser photocoagulation for neovascular lesions nasal to the fovea: results from clinical trials for lesions secondary to ocular histoplasmosis or idiopathic causes. *Arch Ophthalmol* 1995;113:56–61.

Presumed Ocular Histoplasmosis Syndrome

Summary

Presumed ocular histoplasmosis syndrome (POHS) is a multifocal choroiditis without vitritis that is found frequently in patients residing in the Ohio and Mississippi River valley. Resolution of the choroiditis leaves characteristic atrophic chorioretinal scars. Late complications include macular CNVMS.

Epidemiology

Temperate environments, endemic in the Ohio and Mississippi River valley.

Average patient is 40 years old.

Male and female patients equally affected.

Associated with HLA-B7 and HLA-DR22.

Less common in dark-skinned races.

Etiology

- Dimorphic fungus: *Histoplasma capsulatum*.
- Spores can be found in the excreta of bats, pigeons, chickens, and birds.

Pathology

- Focal choroidal granulomas lead to atrophic scars (punched-out "histo spots"); peripapillary pigment loss.
- Variable degree of associated lymphocytic choroiditis.
- Choroidal neovascular membranes.

Signs and Symptoms

Bilateral in 60% of cases.

Asymptomatic.

May have mild flulike symptoms during initial infection.

Metamorphopsia, blurry vision, loss of central vision.

Ophthalmic Findings

- Quiet eye, no iritis, no vitritis (consider another diagnosis if inflammation present).
- Peripheral punched-out atrophic lesions; bilateral in 60% of cases.

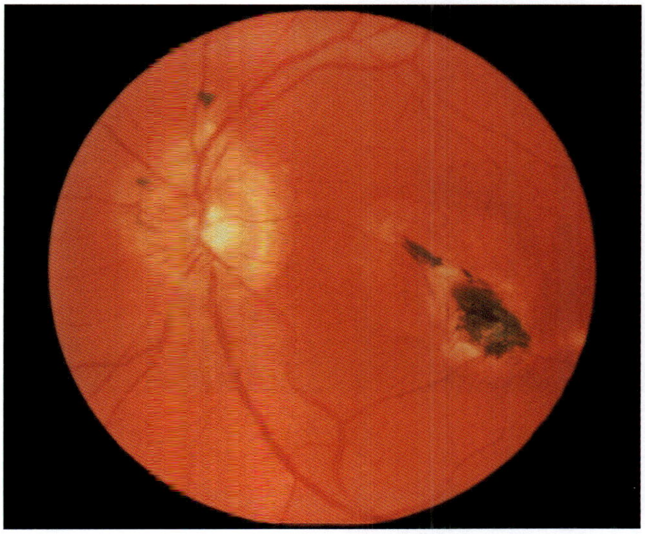

FIGURE 4.14. Macular chorioretinal scar and peripapillary atrophy in a patient with ocular histoplasmosis syndrome.

- Peripapillary atrophy in 30% to 80% (Figure 4.14).
- Macular CNVM/disciform lesions.

Systemic Findings

Usually, none.

Differential Diagnosis

Multifocal choroiditis, TB, sarcoidosis, outer toxoplasmosis.

Special Tests

- No definitive tests
- Chest x-ray: calcific granuloma from primary infection).
- IVFA: lesions block early and stain late, may have peripapillary CNVM or CNVM adjacent to prior scars.
- Skin test for histoplasmosis may exacerbate the disease.

Treatment

- Peripheral atrophic scar: none.
- Laser for CNVM if extrafoveal or juxtafoveal; questionable benefit if subfoveal.
- Possible submacular surgery for subfoveal neovascular membrane
- May use systemic or sub-Tenon steroids for active choroiditis
- No role for antifungal agents.

Prognosis

- If subfoveal CNVM develops, 75% of patients have acuity worse than 20/200.
- Involvement of second eye is 10% at 5 years, 20% at 10 years.
- Macular scar in fellow eye is a bad prognostic sign.

Reference

Macular Photocoagulation Study Group. Laser photocoagulation for neovascular lesions nasal to the fovea: results from clinical trials for lesions secondary to ocular histoplasmosis or idiopathic causes. *Arch Ophthalmol* 1995;113:56–61.

Behçet Disease

Summary

Behçet disease is a multisystem syndrome consisting of an occlusive vasculitis, oral and genital ulceration, and arthritis predominantly affecting Mediterranean and Japanese patients.

Etiology

- Unknown. Associated with HLA-B5, HLA-B51 (ocular), HLA-B12 (oral and skin), HLA-B27 (joint).

Epidemiology

- Highest prevalence in Asia (Japan) and Middle East (Turkey).
- Male patients affected more often than female patients.
- Peak age, 25 to 40 years.

Signs and Symptoms

Decreased vision, photophobia.

Ocular Findings

- Found in 70% to 90% of patients, usually follows systemic disease.
- Bilateral uveitis in 80%.
- Anterior uveitis:
  Bilateral nongranulomatous iridocyclitis.
  Hypopyon, shifts with gravity (Figure 4.15A).
  Posterior synechiae.
  Iris atrophy.
  Peripheral anterior synechiae.
- Posterior uveitis:
  Occlusive retinal vasculitis (Figure 4.15B).
  Recurrent vascular occlusions.
  Cotton-wool spots.
  Optic nerve edema.
  Neovascularization.
  Vitreous hemorrhage.

Systemic Findings

Oral or mucous membrane ulcers (Figure 4.15C).
Erythema nodosum.
Thrombophlebitis.
Arthritis.
Large vessel vaso-occlusion ("angio-Behçet").
CNS-Behçet disease: Most patients do not have ocular disease.

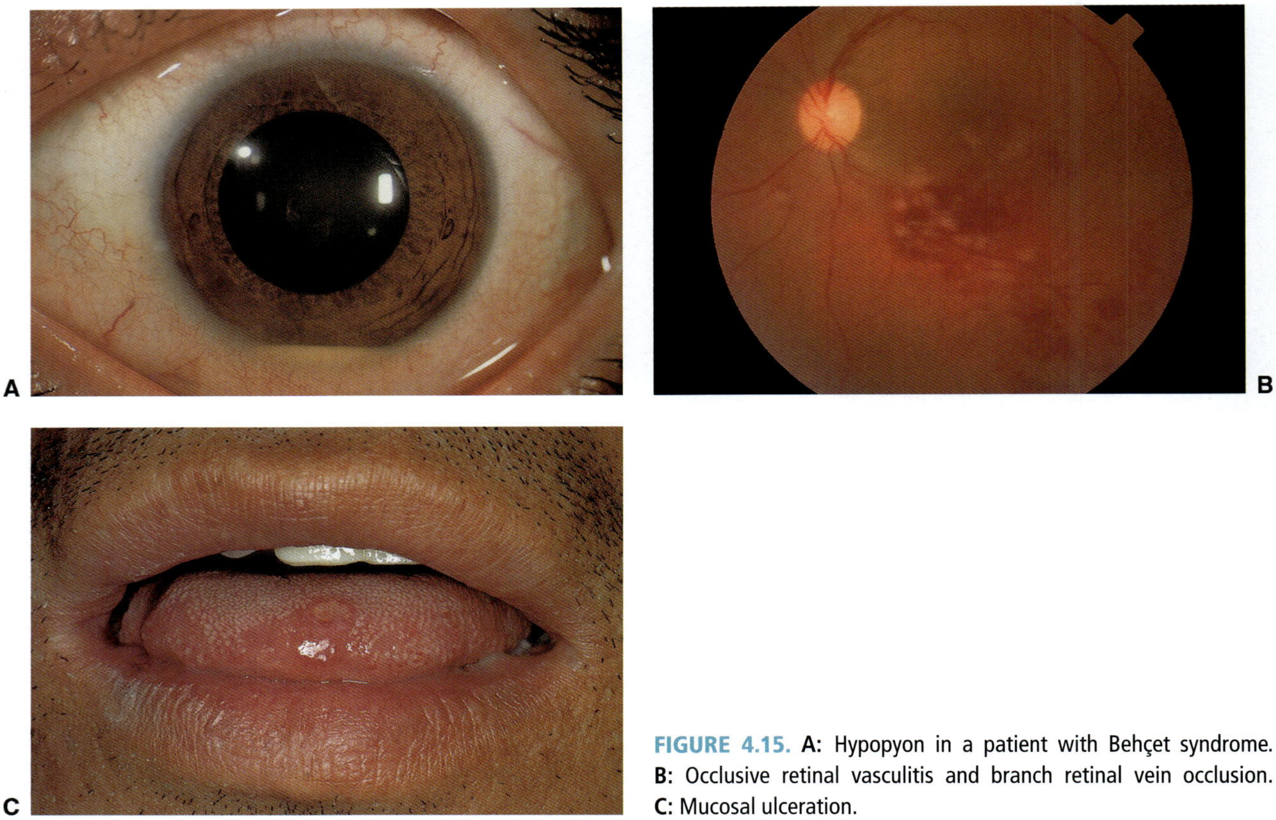

FIGURE 4.15. A: Hypopyon in a patient with Behçet syndrome. B: Occlusive retinal vasculitis and branch retinal vein occlusion. C: Mucosal ulceration.

Japanese Classification and Signs: Criteria for the Diagnosis of Behçet Disease

- Major findings:
  - Aphthous stomatitis.
  - Cutaneous lesions: dermal vasculitis, erythema nodosa, folliculitis, cutaneous hypersensitivity.
  - Genital ulcers.
  - Iridocyclitis with hypopyon.
- Minor findings:
  - Arthritis.
  - Epididymitis.
  - Intestinal tract symptoms.
  - Vascular symptoms: obliterative thrombophlebitis, arterial occlusion, aneurysm.
  - CNS involvement.
- Complete form: four major symptoms.
- Incomplete form: three major symptoms *or* one major symptom plus uveitis:
  - Suspect: two nonocular major symptoms.
  - Possible: one major symptom.

Differential Diagnosis

Sarcoidosis: oral ulcers, arthralgia, retinal vasculitis.

Reiter syndrome: HLA-B27 positivity, anterior uveitis, conjunctivitis, oral ulcers, arthritis, urethritis.

Viral, Whipple disease, Crohn disease, collagen-vascular diseases (SLE, PAN, relapsing polychondritis).

Special Tests

- HLA typing:
  - May be helpful in incomplete, suspect, and possible forms.
- Erythrocyte sedimentation rate (ESR), C-reactive protein (CRP), lysozyme level, ANA: abnormal in some cases.
- IVFA:
  - Ischemic retinal vasculitis.
  - Choroid may be involved: delayed filling or localized nonperfusion.
  - Dilated and occluded vessels.
  - Diffuse leakage from vessels.
  - Cystoid macular edema.
- Pathergy: skin-prick test with formation of blister after 24 to 48 hours.

Pathology

- Necrotizing leukocytoclastic obliterative vasculitis, complement and immunoglobulin deposits may be seen in vessel walls.
- Neutrophilic hypopyon.

Treatment

Topical and systemic steroids.

Low threshold for systemic immunosuppression with agents such as cyclosporine A, chlorambucil, cyclophosphamide, when retinal vasculitis present.

Interferon, TNF alpha–blocking biologic agents effective.
Posterior sub-Tenon steroid injections for cystoid macular edema.

Follow-Up

IVFA to monitor extent of vascular damage.

Complications

Cataracts, glaucoma, optic atrophy, RD, cystoid macular edema.

Disease Course and Prognosis

- Symptoms recur every 1 to 2 months with exacerbations and remissions.
- Poor prognosis if posterior segment involved, with 25% to 50% of patients legally blind in 4 years.
- Good prognosis if solely anterior uveitis.
- With CNS involvement, up to 40% mortality.

Reference

Michelson JB, Chisari FV. Behcet's disease. *Surv Ophthalmol* 1982; 26:190–203.

Sympathetic Ophthalmia

Summary

Sympathetic ophthalmia is a bilateral nonnecrotizing granulomatous panuveitis that may occur following penetrating ocular trauma or intraocular surgery.

Terminology

Inciting eye: eye sustaining penetrating trauma.
Sympathizing eye: fellow, uninjured eye, which develops inflammation.

Epidemiology

- Less than ten cases per year in the United States.
- Interval from insult to disease is 65% within 2 months, 80% within 3 months, and 90% within 1 year; range is 5 days to 50 years.
- Occurs in approximately 1.9/1,000 cases of penetrating ocular trauma and 1/10,000 cases of intraocular surgery.

Pathogenesis

Uveal pigment serves as an antigen for cell-mediated immune response.

Signs and Symptoms

Blurred vision.
Redness.
Photophobia in the sympathizing eye.
Decreased accommodation.

Ophthalmic Findings

Persistent granulomatous inflammatory reaction.
Mutton fat keratic precipitates.
Vitritis.
Choroidal infiltrates.
Papillitis.
Dalen-Fuchs nodules (60- to 700-µm yellowish infiltrates at the level of the RPE/Bruch membrane) in 25% to 40% of cases.
Chronic inflammation of the inciting eye.

Differential Diagnosis

Lens-induced uveitis.
Occult perforation.
Endophthalmitis in the early posttraumatic or postsurgical setting.
Sarcoidosis.
Vogt-Koyanagi-Harada (VKH) syndrome: usually has associated systemic symptoms (Table 4.8).

Special Tests

- IVFA. Early:
  Hyperfluorescence of RPE pinpoint leaks.
  Hypofluorescence at site of Dalen-Fuchs nodules.
  Patchy choroidal filling.
- Late:
  Multiple sites of leakage into sensory detachments.
  Optic nerve hyperemia.
  Hyperfluorescence of Dalen-Fuchs nodules.

Pathology

- Thickened uvea.
- Nonnecrotizing granulomatous inflammation of epithelioid cells with pigment phagocytosis, lymphocytic infiltration of choroid and iris.

Table 4.8

Comparison of VKH and sympathetic ophthalmia[a]

	VKH	Sympathetic ophthalmia
Previous ocular trauma or surgery	No	Yes
Vitiligo, poliosis, alopecia	Yes	Yes/No
Choriocapillaris involved	Yes	No

[a]The differences between these conditions have become less distinct recently; however, these are features of historical interest.
VKH, Vogt-Koyanagi-Harada syndrome.

- RPE metaplasia into epithelioid cells on Bruch membrane (Dalen-Fuchs nodules).
- Relative sparing of retina and choriocapillaris.

Treatment

- Classic teaching: Enucleation of the traumatized eye within 2 weeks after the injury (if there is no vision or there is irreparable damage) may prevent the onset of sympathetic ophthalmia.
- Enucleation of the inciting eye in delayed-onset cases of no benefit and should be avoided (as the inciting eye may ultimately have better vision).
- Systemic steroids (prednisone 1 to 1.5 mg/kg/day).
- For refractory cases use cyclosporine A or chlorambucil.

Prognosis

Sixty-five percent achieve acuity better than 20/60 in sympathizing eye following treatment.

References

Albert DM, Diaz-Rohena R. A historical review of sympathetic ophthalmia and its epidemiology. *Surv Ophthalmol* 1989; 34:1–14.

Marak GE Jr. Recent advances in sympathetic ophthalmia. *Surv Ophthalmol* 1979;24:141–156.

Vogt-Koyanagi-Harada Syndrome

Summary

VKH syndrome is characterized by bilateral severe diffuse granulomatous uveitis with serous RDs and associated CNS, dermatologic, and vestibuloauditory manifestations.

Epidemiology

- Twenty- to fifty-year-olds, usually in their thirties.
- Women affected more frequently than men.
- More prevalent in pigmented races: Asians, American Indians, Hispanics, African Americans.
- HLA-DR4 (88%).

Etiology

- Uncertain; possibly an autoimmune hypersensitivity response to melanin or other pigment.

Signs and Symptoms

Decreased vision, photophobia.

Ophthalmic Findings

- Bilateral granulomatous iridocyclitis.
- Mutton fat keratic precipitates.
- Anterior vitritis.
- Posterior synechiae.

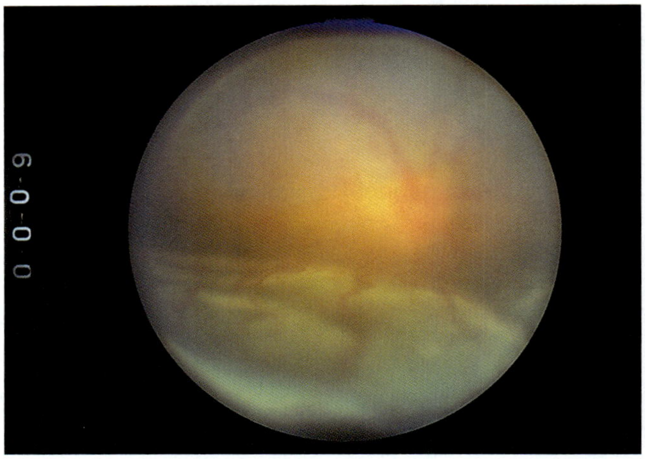

FIGURE 4.16. Multiple serous RDs in Vogt-Koyanagi-Harada syndrome. (From Tasman W, Jaeger E. *The Wills Eye Hospital atlas of clinical ophthalmology*, 2nd ed. Lippincott Williams & Wilkins, 2001.)

- Cataracts.
- Iris nodules.
- Perilimbal vitiligo (Sugiura sign).
- Optic nerve edema.
- Choroidal nodules.
- Exudative RD (Figure 4.16).
- With resolution of exudative RD, widespread RPE disruption and depigmentation: "sunset-glow" fundus.
- Dalen-Fuchs nodules.

American Uveitis Society Criteria for Diagnosis of VKH:

- No history of ocular trauma or surgery.
- Three of the following four signs:
- Bilateral chronic iridocyclitis.
- Posterior uveitis, exudative RD, sunset-glow fundus.
- Neurologic signs: neck stiffness, tinnitus, cranial nerve or CNS problems, CSF pleocytosis.
- Cutaneous findings: alopecia, poliosis, vitiligo.

Systemic Findings

Vestibuloauditory: high-frequency hearing loss (insidious onset), tinnitus, vertigo.

Dermatologic: alopecia, poliosis, vitiligo (Figure 4.17).

CNS: meningitis, headache, cranial-nerve palsies, hemiparesis.

Differential Diagnosis

- Exudative RD and uveitis.
- Syphilis.
- Posterior scleritis.
- Central serous chorioretinopathy: no inflammation. Usually one or two areas of RPE leakage on IVFA.

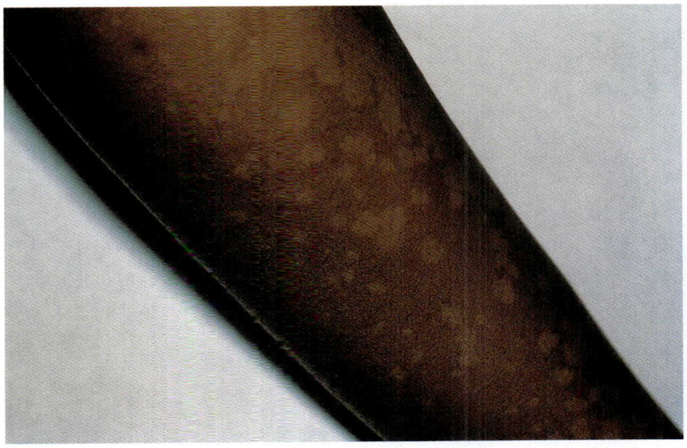

FIGURE 4.17. Depigmented vitiliginous patches in a patient with Vogt-Koyanagi-Harada syndrome.

- Uveal effusion syndrome: no inflammation or systemic manifestations.
- Sympathetic ophthalmia: rarely causes exudative RD. History of prior trauma.
- Intraocular lymphoma: older patients, no leakage on IVFA, check cytologic findings on vitreous biopsy.
- Sarcoidosis: vasculitis, choroidal granulomata.

Special Tests

- IVFA:
  Patchy delay of choroidal perfusion.
  Multiple pinpoint leaks and serous RDs.
  CNVM.
- Lumbar puncture: CSF pleocytosis in early stages.

Pathology

Lymphocyte, macrophage, and plasma cell infiltration of the choriocapillaris, chorioretinal scars, vitreal inflammatory cells, RPE changes.

Treatment

- Steroids: topical, posterior sub-Tenon steroid injection, systemic (prednisone 1 to 2 mg/kg/day with slow taper over 3 to 6 months).
- For refractory cases, use cyclosporine, azathioprine, cyclophosphamide, chlorambucil.

Disease Course

- Fifty percent of patients retain acuity better than 20/50.
- Serous RDs resolve in 2 to 3 months.
- Chronic anterior chamber reaction, glaucoma.

Reference

Moorthy RS, Inomata H, Rao NA. Vogt-Koyanagi-Harada syndrome. *Surv Ophthalmol* 1995;39:265–292.

Eales Disease

Summary

Eales disease is an idiopathic obliterative peripheral retinal vasculopathy with vitreous hemorrhage, often found in association with a positive PPD skin test result.

Epidemiology

Usually bilateral.
All ages but usually young to middle-aged adults.
Higher incidence in southeast Asia, India.
Men more frequently affected than women.

Etiology

- Idiopathic.
- High proportion of patients have a positive PPD test result (majority of patients are also found in TB-endemic areas).

Signs and Symptoms

Floaters, decreased vision.

Ophthalmic Findings

Vascular sheathing.
Focal occlusion of peripheral retinal vessels.
Cystoid macular edema.
Peripheral retinal nonperfusion and neovascularization.
Vitreous hemorrhage.
BRVO.

Special Tests

- IVFA: vascular staining, hyperfluorescence, cystoid macular edema, peripheral retinal nonperfusion.
- May have positive PPD test result

Treatment

For neovascularization: laser photocoagulation.
For persistent vitreous hemorrhage: vitrectomy.

Prognosis

- Usually retain good vision.
- Vitreous hemorrhage: most common cause of decreased vision.

References

Renie WA, Murphy RP, Anderson KC, et al. The evaluation of patients with Eales' disease. *Retina* 1983;3:243–248.
Walsh AW, Magargal LE, Robb-Doyle E. Diagnosis and treatment of Eales' disease. *Trans Pa Acad Ophthalmol Otolaryngol* 1986;38:511–514.

Birdshot Chorioretinopathy

Other name: vitiliginous choroiditis.

Summary

Birdshot chorioretinopathy is a chronic, progressive, painless nongranulomatous uveitis characterized by multifocal ovoid cream-colored choroidal lesions and vitritis strongly associated with HLA-A29.

Etiology

Unknown.

Epidemiology

- Age, 35 to 70 years; average, 50 years of age.
- More frequently seen in patients of northern European descent.
- Fifty percent to 70% of patients are women.
- Ninety-six percent of patients are HLA-A29–positive (in particular, HLA-A29.2).
- Usually bilateral but asymmetric.
- Less common in heavily pigmented patients.

Signs and Symptoms

Gradual, painless blurring of vision.
Decreased color vision.
Floaters.
Difficulty with changes in lighting conditions, nyctalopia.

Ophthalmic Findings

- Diagnostic criteria for birdshot chorioretinopathy:
  - Discrete, cream-colored choroidal spots scattered throughout the postequatorial fundus.
  - White, nonpainful eye.
  - Minimal anterior segment inflammation.
  - Vitritis without snowballs or snowbanks.
  - Retinal vascular leakage (cystoid macular edema, optic nerve edema).
- Ovoid, cream-colored lesions (Figure 4.18).
  - Size, 500 to 1,200 μm at the level of the choroid or RPE.
  - Located in the postequatorial fundus.
  - Radial distribution.
- Common findings:
  - Mild nongranulomatous iritis.
  - Diffuse vitritis with precipitates on the vitreous face.
  - Optic nerve edema.
  - Cystoid macular edema.
- Rare findings:
  - Retinitis.
  - Vasculitis.
  - Attenuated retinal vessels.
- Late findings:
  - Optic atrophy.
  - Subretinal CNVM.
  - Epiretinal membranes.
  - RPE atrophy.

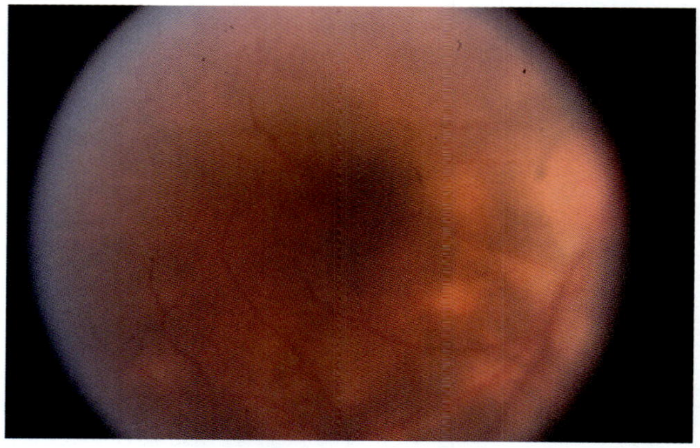

FIGURE 4.18. Multiple discrete yellowish spots at the level of the retinal pigment epithelium in a patient with birdshot retinochoroidopathy.

Systemic Findings

None.

Pathology

Diffuse chronic granulomatous inflammation with giant cells, epithelioid cells, plasma cells in outer retina, choroid, and optic nerve.

Differential Diagnosis

Sarcoid: granulomatous keratic precipitates, larger choroidal granulomas, elevated ACE and lysozyme levels.
TB: granulomatous inflammation, positive PPD test result.
Syphilis: can mimic birdshot; check RPR/VDRL and MHA-TP/FTA-Abs.
VKH syndrome: serous RDs, extraocular manifestations (alopecia, vitiligo, poliosis, tinnitus, meningismus).
Pars planitis: younger patients, peripheral snowbanks, vasculitis.
White dot syndromes: viral prodrome, different distribution or size of dots.
Intraocular lymphoma: elderly patients, magnetic resonance imaging (MRI) or LP evidence of lymphoma.

Special Tests

- HLA-A29–positive in more than 90% of patients.
- Exclude sarcoidosis, TB, and so forth.
- IVFA:
  - Early:
    - Blockage of choroidal filling pattern attributable to diffuse retinal and macular edema.
    - No blocking defect from the retinal lesions, mild hyperfluorescence.
  - Late:
    - Leakage from retinal vessels and capillaries.
    - Late staining from the retinal lesions.
    - Late leakage from optic nerve.

- ERG: decreased amplitudes.
- EOG: normal or decreased.

Disease Course

- Exacerbations and remissions of vitritis.
- Chronic progressive decrease in vision secondary to cystoid macular edema and optic nerve damage.

Treatment

Asymptomatic or mild inflammation: observe.
Cystoid macular edema: posterior sub-Tenon steroids.
Moderate: posterior sub-Tenon steroid injection or systemic prednisone.
Unresponsive: cyclosporine A, 2 to 5 mg/kg/day, other immunomodulators as needed.

Prognosis

- An exacerbating and remitting chronic disease.
- Forty percent of patients lose useful vision in one or both eyes as a result of cystoid macular edema.

References

LeHoang P, Ozdemir N, Benhamou A, et al. HLA-A29.2 subtype associated with birdshot retinochoroidopathy. *Am J Ophthalmol* 1992;113:33–35.

Priem HA, Oosterhuis JA. Birdshot chorioretinopathy: clinical characteristics and evolution. *Br J Ophthalmol* 1988;72:646–659.

Ryan SJ, Maumenee AE. Birdshot retinochoroidopathy. *Am J Ophthalmol* 1980;89:31–45.

MAJOR STUDY

Systemic Immunosuppressive Therapy for Eye Diseases (SITE)

Study Population

7,957 US residents with noninfectious ocular inflammation; 2,340 received immunosuppressive drugs.

Study Design

- Multicenter retrospective cohort study.
- Individuals receiving immunosuppressive drugs were compared to the general US population and individuals with ocular inflammation not receiving immunosuppressive drugs.

Conclusions

1. Methotrexate, azathioprine, mycophenolate mofetil, cyclosporine, dapsone and systemic corticosteroids do not appear to increase overall or cancer mortality.
2. Tumor necrosis factor inhibitors may increase overall and cancer mortality.
3. Chlorambucil and cyclophosphamide use was not associated with overall mortality, although cancer-related mortality was nonsignificantly increased.

References

Kempen JH, Daniel E, Dunn JP, et al. Overall and cancer related mortality among patients with ocular inflammation treated with immunosuppressive drugs: retrospective cohort study. *Br Med J* 2009;339:b2480.

MAJOR STUDY

Multicenter Uveitis Steroid Treatment Trial (MUST)

Study Population

255 patients with noninfectious intermediate, posterior, or panuveitis.

Study Design

- Multicenter randomized parallel treatment design clinical trial.
- Individuals randomized to systemic therapy or fluocinolone acetonide implant.

Will compare fluocinolone acetonide implant versus systemic therapy and contrast local side effects of implant (cataracts, glaucoma, RD, endophthalmitis) with the risks and complications of systemic prednisone and immunosuppressives.

Reference

Kempen JH, Daniel E, Altaweel MM, et al. The multicenter uveitis steroid treatment trial: rationale, design, and baseline characteristics. *Am J Ophthalmol* 2010;149:550–561.

UVEITIS MASQUERADES

Masquerades of uveitis:

Retinoblastoma (in children).
Leukemia.
Uveal melanoma.
Metastatic disease.
Paraneoplastic syndromes.
Lymphoma.
Occult intraocular foreign body.
Juvenile xanthogranuloma.
Pigment dispersion syndrome.

Intraocular Lymphoma

Other names: large B-cell lymphoma, reticulum cell sarcoma.

Table 4.9

Ocular disease in acquired immunodeficiency syndrome

Common	Uncommon (<5%)	Rare (<1%)
HIV retinopathy CMV retinitis	Herpes zoster ophthalmicus Kaposi sarcoma of conjunctiva or eyelids Toxoplasmic retinochoroiditis Molluscum contagiosum Bacterial or fungal corneal ulcer	PORN Cryptococcal choroiditis or papilledema Microsporidiosis Atypical mycobacterial infection Fungal choroiditis or endophthalmitis Pneumocystis choroiditis Syphilitic ocular disease TB

CMV, cytomegalovirus; HIV, human immunodeficiency virus; PORN, progressive outer retinal necrosis; TB, tuberculosis.

Summary

Intraocular lymphoma can masquerade as a chronic infection and may be a sign of CNS malignancy.

Etiology

Malignant infiltration of choroid by lymphomatous cells.

Signs and Symptoms

Blurred vision.
Floaters.

Demographics

Fifty to sixty years of age.

Ophthalmic Findings

Subretinal infiltrates.
Vitritis.
Bilateral ocular inflammation.
Visual field defects related to optic nerve or postchiasmal visual pathways.

Systemic Findings

CNS lymphoma.

Special Tests

MRI.
Lumbar puncture.
Vitreous biopsy for cytology, flow cytometry, interleukin-6 and -10, immunoglobulin heavy chain gene rearrangement.

Treatment and Management

Radiation therapy.
Chemotherapy (intrathecal methotrexate or cytosine arabinoside [ara-C]).
Initial workup may be negative, but maintain a high clinical suspicion in uveitis refractory to treatment.

Differential Diagnosis

Endophthalmitis.
Senile vitritis.

ACQUIRED IMMUNODEFICIENCY SYNDROME

See Table 4.9.

Human Immunodeficiency Virus Retinopathy

Summary

The cotton-wool spots, retinal hemorrhages, and microangiopathy seen with HIV retinopathy are the most common ocular manifestation of HIV infection.

Etiology

Exact etiology unknown. Postulates include the following:

Microvasculopathy.
Immune complex deposition.
HIV infection of endothelium.

Signs and Symptoms

None.

Demographics

HIV-positive patients; prevalence increases with degree of immunosuppression.

Ophthalmic Findings

Cotton-wool spots (Figure 4.19).
Blot hemorrhages.

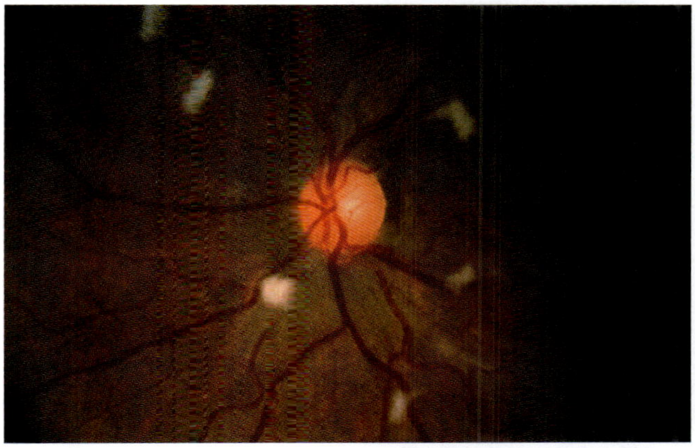

FIGURE 4.19. Cotton-wool spots may be the earliest manifestation of the microvascular abnormalities associated with acquired immunodeficiency syndrome.

Disease Course

- Lesions appear and disappear with time.
- Usually do not enlarge.

Treatment and Management

Since HIV is a marker for decreased CD4 counts, antiretroviral therapy should be instituted or modified.

Differential Diagnosis

CMV retinitis.
Diabetic retinopathy.
BRVO.

Reference

Jabs DA, Green WR, Fox R, et al. Ocular manifestations of acquired immune deficiency syndrome. *Ophthalmology* 1989;96:1092–1099.

Cytomegalovirus Retinitis

Summary

CMV retinitis is one of the most common opportunistic ocular infections in patients with AIDS, particularly when their CD4 cell counts fall below 50 cells/mm^3. CMV causes a progressive full-thickness necrotizing retinitis with hemorrhage and an overlying vitritis.

Epidemiology and Pathogenesis

- Forty percent to 100% of the general population are seropositive for CMV.
- Hematogenous seeding of the retina by infected monocytes.

Signs and Symptoms

- May be asymptomatic.
- Paracentral scotoma, decreased vision, metamorphopsia, floaters.
- Patients with AIDS and low CD4 cell counts are at higher risk.

Ophthalmic Findings

- Hemorrhagic form: crumbled cheese (thick white retinal necrosis) and ketchup (large areas of retinal hemorrhage) appearance.
- Granular form: lesions spread out from a central focus with a yellow, granular advancing border with or without hemorrhage (Figure 4.20); behind the border, there is atrophic and thinned retina with a brush-fire appearance.

Differential Diagnosis

Cotton-wool spots/HIV retinopathy.
Toxoplasmosis.
Syphilis.
HSV (ARN).
VZV (PORN).
Lymphoma.

Treatment

- May observe small peripheral lesions without treatment.
- Ganciclovir:
  Can cause leukopenia.
  Intravitreal injection weekly.
  Sustained-release intraocular implant also available.
- Foscarnet:
  Intravitreal injection weekly.
  Can cause renal toxicity and electrolyte problems.
- Cidofovir:
  Newer agent; not recommended as first-line therapy.
  Side effects (occur with i.v. or intravitreal use): uveitis, hypotony, renal failure.
  Valgancyclovir obviates the need for IV induction therapy.
- Institution of multidrug anti-HIV therapy (protease inhibitors plus nucleoside analogues).

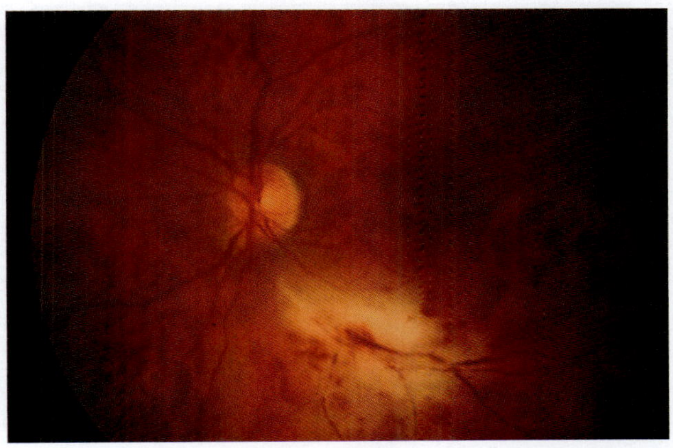

FIGURE 4.20. Wedge-shaped area of cytomegalovirus retinitis with multiple cotton-wool spots and retinal hemorrhages.

Disease Course and Prognosis

- Spreads over weeks to months with loss of vision if not treated.
- Survival once diagnosed is 5 months to 2 years but improving with new therapies.
- Poor prognosis for vision if optic nerve involved.
- Reactivation of disease can occur if not treated with maintenance therapy.
- Treatment in evolution with newer medications to treat AIDS and possible immune reconstitution.

References

Dhillon B. Combination foscarnet and ganciclovir therapy vs monotherapy for the treatment of relapsed cytomegalovirus retinitis in patients with AIDS. The Cytomegalovirus Retreatment Trial. The Studies of Ocular Complications of AIDS Research Group in Collaboration with the AIDS Clinical Trials Group. The management of cytomegalovirus retinitis in AIDS. *Arch Ophthalmol* 1996;114:23–33.

Zegans ME, Walton RC, Holland GN, et al. Transient vitreous inflammatory reactions associated with combination antiretroviral therapy in patients with AIDS and cytomegalovirus retinitis. *Am J Ophthalmol* 1998;125:292–300.

Microsporidia

Summary

Microsporidia is a rare parasitic cause of chronic conjunctivitis and keratitis in patients with AIDS.

Etiology

Infection with microsporidia (Encephalitozoon or Nosema species most commonly).

Signs and Symptoms

Chronic irritation.
Photophobia.
Mild decrease in vision.

Demographics

Patients with AIDS, almost exclusively.

Ophthalmic Findings

- Diffuse, fine punctate epithelial keratitis (Figure 4.21A).
- Conjunctiva appears relatively unaffected.

Systemic Findings

Extraocular microsporidial infections:

Sinusitis.
Gastroenteritis.

Special Tests

Conjunctival scraping for Giemsa stain or electron microscopy.

Pathology

- Giemsa stain: multiple ovoid intraepithelial organisms (Figure 4.21B).
- Electron microscopy required for speciation.

Disease Course

Chronic fluctuating course.

Treatment and Management

- Fumagillin drops.
- Oral albendazole: systemic treatment may be necessary to destroy other mucosal reservoirs.

Differential Diagnosis

Toxic/medicamentosa.
Keratoconjunctivitis sicca.
Epidemic keratoconjunctivitis.

A
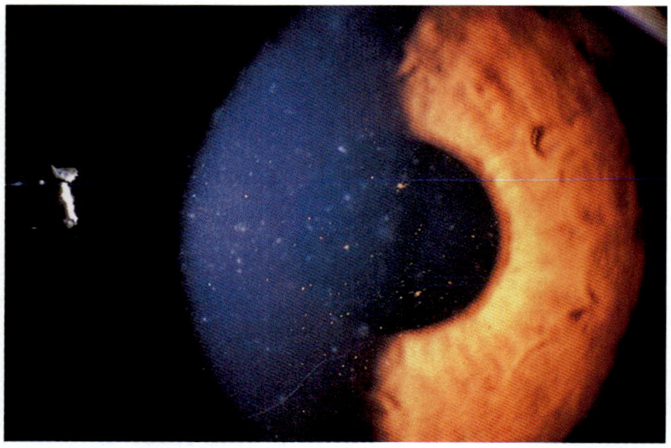
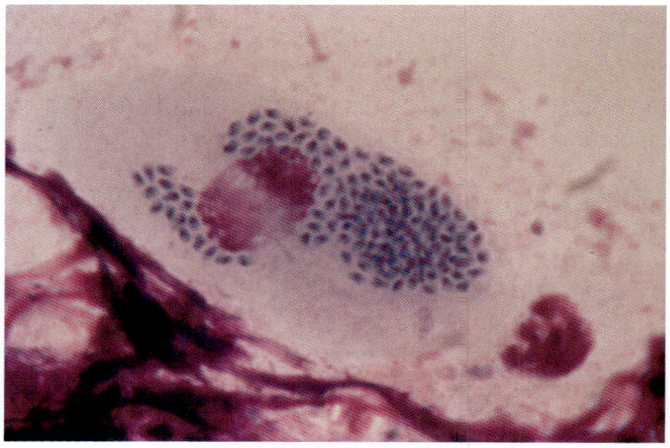
B

FIGURE 4.21. A: Diffuse punctate epithelial keratopathy found bilaterally in AIDS patients with microsporidial infection. **B:** Intraepithelial microsporidial organisms as seen on Giemsa stain.

References

Lowder CY. Ocular microsporidiosis. *Int Ophthalmol Clin* 1993; 33:145–151.

Shuler JD, Engstrom RE Jr, Holland GN. External ocular disease and anterior segment disorders associated with AIDS. *Int Ophthalmol Clin* 1989;29:98–104.

Molluscum Contagiosum

Summary

Molluscum contagiosum results from a pox virus infection and produces multiple umbilicated skin nodules, which, when found near the eye, can cause a chronic toxic follicular conjunctivitis.

Etiology

- Infection with the molluscum contagiosum virus, a member of the poxvirus family.
- Spread by hand-eye contact.

Signs and Symptoms

Chronic red, irritated eyes.

Demographics

Young, immunocompetent children.
Immunocompromised patients with AIDS.

Ophthalmic Findings

- Elevated skin nodules with a pearly border and central umbilication filled with white, cheesy-appearing material (Figure 4.22A)
- Chronic follicular conjunctivitis (Figure 4.22B).
- Punctate epithelial keratopathy.

Systemic Findings

- Molluscum lesions on skin of fingers and genital areas.
- Disseminated molluscum lesions in patients with AIDS.

Special Tests

Biopsy of nodule.

Pathology

Central cavity with degenerated epithelial cells surrounded by large, rounded epithelial cells containing cytoplasmic molluscum inclusions (molluscum bodies).

Disease Course

- In immunocompetent patients: spontaneous resolution.
- In immunosuppressed patients: chronic persistence or reinfection.

Treatment and Management

Excision.
Cautery.
Cryotherapy.
Application of caustic agents.
Incision with a needle.

Differential Diagnosis

Basal cell carcinoma.
Sebaceous cyst.
Keratoacanthoma.

Reference

Shuler JD, Engstrom RE Jr, Holland GN. External ocular disease and anterior segment disorders associated with AIDS. *Int Ophthalmol Clin* 1989;29:98–104.

Kaposi Sarcoma

Summary

Kaposi sarcoma is a vascular tumor caused by HSV-8 that produces red, fleshy tumors on the skin and mucosal surfaces of patients with AIDS.

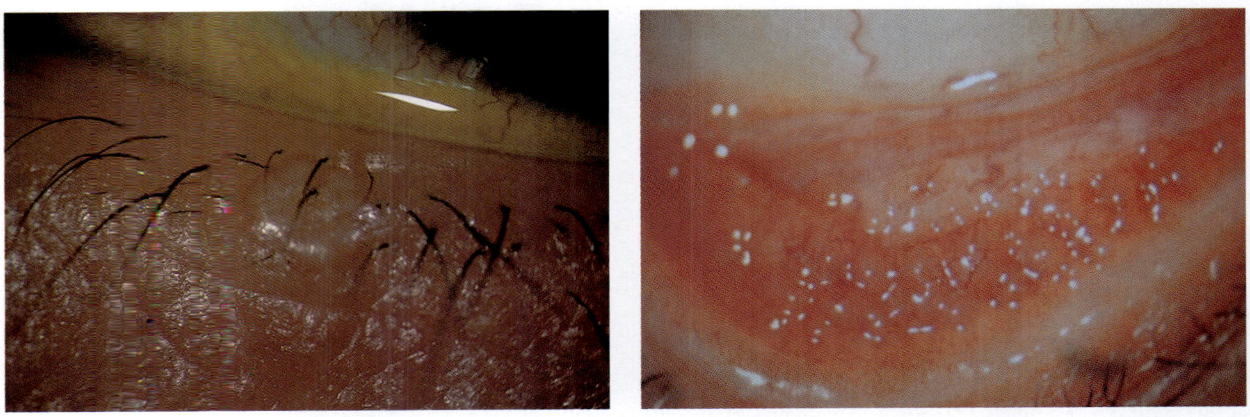

A B

FIGURE 4.22. **A:** Typical umbilicated molluscum lesion with cheesy-appearing necrotic central cavity. **B:** Toxic follicular conjunctivitis caused by viral particles shed by a molluscum lesion on the eyelid margin.

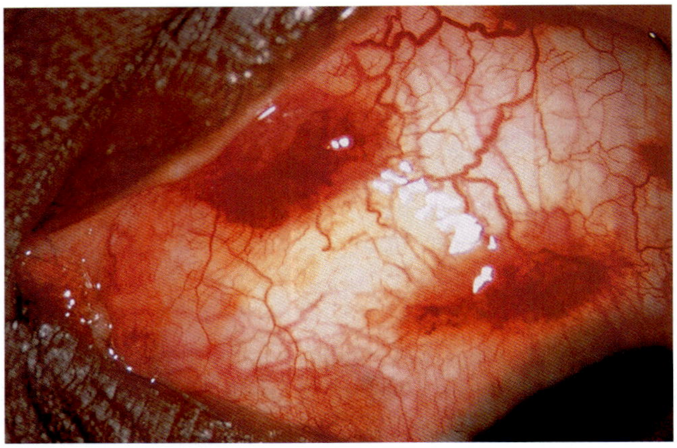

FIGURE 4.23. Fleshy vascular lesions on the conjunctiva in an AIDS patient with Kaposi sarcoma.

Etiology

Infection with human herpesvirus 8.

Signs and Symptoms

None.

Demographics

Patients with AIDS.

Ophthalmic Findings

Single or multiple raised, red, fleshy conjunctival or periocular masses (Figure 4.23).

Systemic Findings

May have Kaposi sarcoma elsewhere.

Pathology

Multiple dilated vascular channels.

Disease Course

May spontaneously disappear with immune reconstitution.

Treatment and Management

Antiviral medications with activity against herpes viruses may play a role.
Observation, since asymptomatic.
Surgical excision.
Chemotherapy, radiation therapy.
Immunoreconstitution with antiviral therapy.

References

Dugel PU, Gill PS, Frangieh GT, et al. Treatment of ocular adnexal Kaposi sarcoma in acquired immune deficiency syndrome. *Ophthalmology* 1992;99:1127–1132.

Shuler JD, Engstrom RE Jr, Holland GN. External ocular disease and anterior segment disorders associated with AIDS. *Int Ophthalmol Clin* 1989;29:98–104.

Herpes Zoster Ophthalmicus

Summary

Herpes zoster ophthalmicus can present as dermatitis, keratitis, or uveitis due to reactivation of VZV.

Etiology

Recurrence or reactivation of VZV infection.

Signs and Symptoms

Sharp stabbing or burning pain on forehead.

Demographics

Patients with AIDS.

Ophthalmic Findings

- Vesicular rash in V1 dermatome distribution (Figure 4.24).
- Epithelial keratitis.
- Iridocyclitis.
- Conjunctivitis, scleritis, episcleritis.
- Retinitis.
- Optic neuritis.

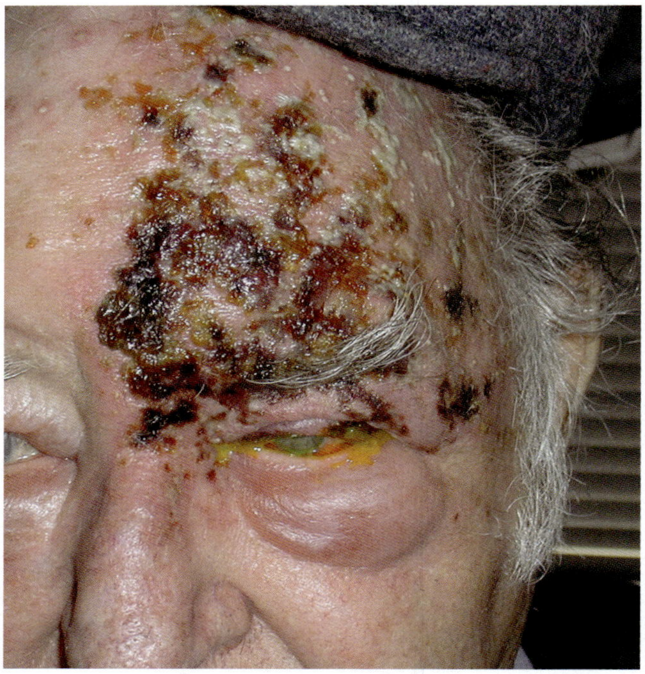

FIGURE 4.24. In a young or middle-aged patient, herpes zoster ophthalmicus affecting the V1 distribution may be indicative of an underlying immunodeficient state.

Disease Course

Rarely may become disseminated.

Treatment and Management

- Intravenous acyclovir.
- Maintenance therapy with acyclovir may be needed to prevent recurrences.

References

Sandor EV, Millman A, Croxson TS, et al. Herpes zoster ophthalmicus in patients at risk for the acquired immune deficiency syndrome (AIDS). *Am J Ophthalmol* 1986;101:153–155.

Seiff SR, Margolis T, Graham SH, et al. Use of intravenous acyclovir for treatment of herpes zoster ophthalmicus in patients at risk for AIDS. *Ann Ophthalmol* 1988;20:480–482.

Varicella-Zoster Retinitis and progressive Outer Retinal Necrosis

Summary

PORN is a necrotizing retinitis occurring in patients with AIDS that is attributed to VZV infection.

Signs and Symptoms

Decreased vision.
Peripheral scotoma.

Demographics

Patients with AIDS, CD4 cell counts usually less than 100 cells/mm³ (mean 20 cells/mm³).

Ophthalmic Findings

- Minimal vitreous inflammation.
- Multifocal deep retinal whitish lesions, usually found in periphery (Figure 4.25).
- Rapid coalescence of lesions (within days).

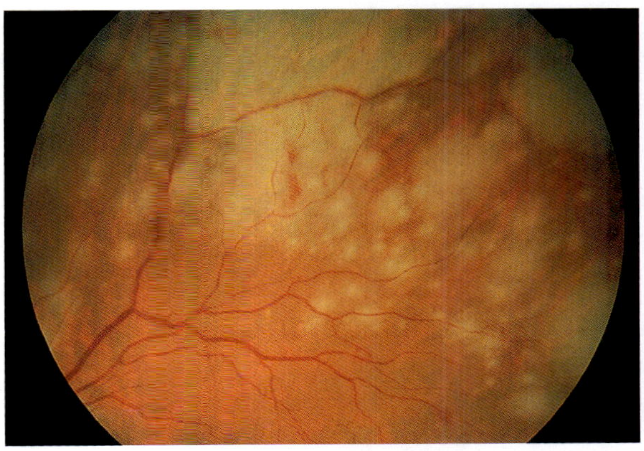

FIGURE 4.25. Outer retinal opacification with minimal vitritis as seen in a case of progressive outer retinal necrosis.

Systemic Findings

History of cutaneous zoster in 67% of patients.

Disease Course

Rapid, relentless progression of retinitis resulting in total destruction of retina and acuity of no light perception.

Treatment and Management

- High-dose i.v. acyclovir effective in some cases.
- Foscarnet (i.v. or intravitreal).

Differential Diagnosis

ARN.
CMV retinitis.
Lymphoma.
Syphilis.

References

Engstrom RE Jr, Holland GN, Margolis TP, et al. The progressive outer retinal necrosis syndrome: a variant of necrotizing herpetic retinopathy in patients with AIDS. *Ophthalmology* 1994;101:1488–1502.

Forster DJ, Dugel PU, Frangieh GT, et al. Rapidly progressive outer retinal necrosis in the acquired immunodeficiency syndrome. *Am J Ophthalmol* 1990;110:341–348.

Margolis TP, Lowder CY, Holland GN, et al. Varicella-zoster virus retinitis in patients with the acquired immunodeficiency syndrome. *Am J Ophthalmol* 1991;112:119–131.

Atypical Mycobacterial Infection

Summary

Atypical mycobacteria can cause a multifocal choroiditis, often in conjunction with systemic mycobacterial infection.

Etiology

Disseminated infection with atypical mycobacteria (*Mycobacterium avium* complex).

Signs and Symptoms

Decreased vision, photophobia, symptoms related to systemic mycobacterial infection.

Demographics

Patients with AIDS.

Ophthalmic Findings

- Multifocal choroiditis.
- May occur in conjunction with other AIDS-related ocular infections.

Systemic Findings

Disseminated systemic atypical mycobacterial infection (bone marrow).

Treatment and Management

Systemic antimicrobial therapy (rifabutin).

Differential Diagnosis

Pneumocystic choroiditis.

References

Morinelli EN, Dugel PU, Riffenburgh R, et al. Infectious multifocal choroiditis in patients with acquired immune deficiency syndrome. *Ophthalmology* 1993;100:1014–1021.

Whitcup SM, Fenton RM, Pluda JM, et al. *Pneumocystis carinii* and *Mycobacterium avium-intracellulare* infection of the choroid. *Retina* 1992;12:331–335.

Pneumocystic Carinii Choroiditis

Summary

An asymptomatic multifocal choroiditis caused by *Pneumocystic carinii*. More common in patients not receiving systemic prophylaxis for pneumocystitis.

Demographics

Patients with AIDS, CD4 cell counts less than 200 cells/mm^3.

Etiology

P. carinii (protozoa).

Signs and Symptoms

Asymptomatic.

Ophthalmic Findings

- Bilateral, multifocal, discrete, yellow, cream-colored, slightly elevated round or oval choroidal lesions 300 to 3,000 μm in diameter scattered in the posterior pole (Figure 4.26).
- No vitritis.

Systemic Findings

- *P. carinii* pneumonia.
- Fever, cough, shortness of breath (from pulmonary involvement).

Differential Diagnosis

Intraocular lymphoma, cryptococcus, atypical mycobacteria, metastatic infection, syphilis, sarcoid, VKH syndrome, sympathetic ophthalmia.

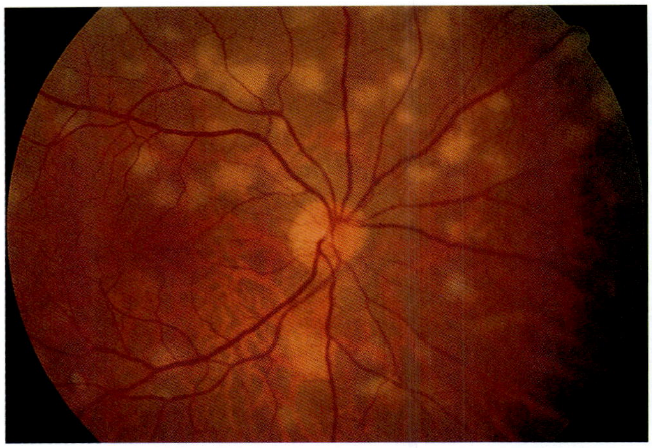

FIGURE 4.26. Multifocal choroidal lesions in an AIDS patient with *Pneumocystis carinii* pneumonia.

Special Tests

Chest x-ray, sputum analysis.

Pathology

Cysts in the choroid.

Treatment

Trimethoprim/sulfamethoxazole (Bactrim) or i.v. pentamidine.

Disease Course

- Slow growth of lesions, lesions may coalesce.
- Responds to treatment.

References

Rao NA, Zimmerman PL, Boyer D, et al. A clinical, histopathologic, and electron microscopic study of *Pneumocystis carinii* choroiditis. *Am J Ophthalmol* 1989;107:218–228.

Shami MJ, Freeman W, Friedberg D, et al. A multicenter study of *Pneumocystis* choroidopathy. *Am J Ophthalmol* 1991;112:15–22.

Whitcup SM, Fenton RM, Pluda JM, et al. *Pneumocystis carinii* and *Mycobacterium avium-intracellulare* infection of the choroid. *Retina* 1992;12:331–335.

Toxoplasmosis

See p. 248.

Fungal Retinitis, Choroiditis, and endophthalmitis

Summary

Hematogenous spread of fungi to ocular tissues usually causing a choroiditis or endophthalmitis.

Etiology

Hematogenous spread of fungal infection: Candida, Histoplasma, Sporothrix species.

Signs and Symptoms

Decreased vision.
Photophobia.

Demographics

Patients with AIDS.
History of i.v. drug abuse or indwelling catheters, hyperalimentation.

Ophthalmic Findings

Multifocal chorioretinitis.
Vitritis.
Perivasculitis.

Systemic Findings

Mucocutaneous candidiasis.
Systemic fungal infection.

Special Tests

Vitreous biopsy for culture and smear.

Treatment and Management

Vitrectomy and intravitreal antifungal agents.
Systemic antifungal therapy.
Voriconazole has broad spectrum and excellent oral bioavailability.

Differential Diagnosis

Toxoplasmosis.

Reference

Morinelli EN, Dugel PU, Riffenburgh R, et al. Infectious multifocal choroiditis in patients with acquired immune deficiency syndrome. *Ophthalmology* 1993;100:1014–1021.

Cryptococcus

Summary

Ocular involvement with cryptococcus may be manifest as papilledema, multifocal choroiditis, or endophthalmitis.

Etiology

Cryptococcal infection spread from the CNS to the eye.

Signs and Symptoms

Can be asymptomatic.
Decreased vision.

Demographics

Patients with AIDS.

Ophthalmic Findings

Cryptococcal papillitis.
Endophthalmitis.
Multifocal choroiditis or multiple retinal microabscesses.

Systemic Findings

Almost invariably have CNS cryptococcal meningitis.

Special Tests

Lumbar puncture for cryptococcal studies.

Disease Course

May resemble optic neuritis.

Treatment and Management

Vitrectomy and intravitreal amphotericin B in cases of endophthalmitis.

Medications

Intravenous amphotericin.
Itraconazole.

Differential Diagnosis

Pneumocystis choroiditis.
Fungal choroiditis.
CMV papillitis.

Reference

Winward KE, Hamed LM, Glaser JS. The spectrum of optic nerve disease in human immunodeficiency virus infection. *Am J Ophthalmol* 1989;107:373–380.

Drug-Related Inflammation

Rifabutin

Summary

Anterior uveitis in a patient with AIDS who is receiving prophylaxis for Mycobacteria may be due to rifabutin.

Etiology

Unknown.
Hypersensitivity to medication.

Signs and Symptoms

Decreased vision.
Light sensitivity.

Demographics

Patients with AIDS.

Ophthalmic Findings

Bilateral severe anterior uveitis.

Treatment and Management

Responds rapidly to topical corticosteroids.
Decrease or discontinue rifabutin.

References

Jacobs DS, Piliero PJ, Kuperwaser MG, et al. Acute uveitis associated with rifabutin use in patients with human immunodeficiency virus infection. *Am J Ophthalmol* 1994;118:716–722.

Saran BR, Maguire AM, Nichols C, et al. Hypopyon uveitis in patients with acquired immunodeficiency syndrome treated for systemic *Mycobacterium avium* complex infection with rifabutin. *Arch Ophthalmol* 1994;112:1159–1165.

Cidofovir

Summary

Among the ocular side effects of cidofovir are severe anterior uveitis and profound irreversible hypotony.

Signs and Symptoms

Decreased vision.

Demographics

Patients with AIDS.

Ophthalmic Findings

Severe anterior uveitis with fibrin.
Posterior synechiae.
Profound hypotony.

Disease Course

- Side effects can occur with both intravitreal and i.v. use.
- With discontinuation or reduction of dose of the cidofovir, the uveitis may resolve.
- Hypotony may be permanent and irreversible.

Treatment and Management

- Discontinuation or reduction of dose of cidofovir.
- Topical corticosteroids.

Reference

Chavez-de la Paz E, Arevalo JF, Kirsch LS, et al. Anterior nongranulomatous uveitis after intravitreal HPMPC (cidofovir) for the treatment of cytomegalovirus retinitis: analysis and prevention. *Ophthalmology* 1997;104:539–544.

CHAPTER 5

Glaucoma

Rohit Krishna • Ryan D. Vincent • Andrew Sorenson

INTRAOCULAR PRESSURE AND AQUEOUS HUMOR DYNAMICS

Glaucoma is a group of diseases resulting in an optic neuropathy that has characteristic changes in the optic nerve head (cupping) and progressive visual field loss. Elevated intraocular pressure is one of the primary associated risk factors but does not define the disorder.

- Intraocular pressure (IOP) is determined by the balance of aqueous humor production, outflow facility, and episcleral venous pressure.
- Quantified by the Goldmann equation:

$$P_o = F/C + P_v$$

where P_o = IOP (millimeters of mercury).
F = Formation of aqueous (microliters per minute) = 2 to 3 μL/min in normal patients (0.5% to 1%/min).
C = Facility of outflow (microliters per minute per millimeter of mercury) = 0.28 μL/min/mm of mercury in normal patients.
P_v = Episcleral venous pressure (millimeters of mercury) = 8 to 9 mm Hg.

Composition of Aqueous Humor

- Aqueous humor is a clear medium that is slightly hypertonic compared to plasma. It maintains IOP and nourishes the lens, cornea, etc.
- No blood cells in normal aqueous humor
- Inorganic ions:
  - Na^+, K^+, and Mg^{2+} concentration similar to plasma.
  - Ca^{2+} half of plasma level.
  - Cl^- and HCO_3^- are major anions.
- Organic anions:
  - Lactate most abundant organic ion.
  - Ascorbic acid at very elevated levels (15 to 50 times plasma levels).
- Carbohydrates:
  - Glucose about 70% plasma concentration, from facilitated transport into aqueous.
  - Higher levels in diabetics.
- Glutathione: important role in oxidative state of aqueous humor.
- Urea:
  - Approximately 85% of plasma concentration.
  - Crosses blood–aqueous barrier easily.
- Proteins:
  - Aqueous almost devoid of protein (1/200 to 1/500 of the protein found in plasma).
  - Enzymes with possible roles in the anterior chamber:
    - Hyaluronidase: may increase outflow facility of aqueous humor.
    - Carbonic anhydrase: regulation of bicarbonate levels in aqueous humor.
    - Lysozyme: antimicrobial role.
- Growth factors: higher levels in aqueous than plasma of TGF-β, acidic fibroblast growth factor (FGF) and basic FGF, insulin-like growth factor 1 (IGF-1), and transferrin.
- O_2 and CO_2.
  - O_2 at approximately 55 mm Hg: one third of atmosphereic concentration, corneal endothelium completely dependent on this source.
  - CO_2 present at 40 to 60 mm Hg.

Production of Aqueous Humor

- Produced by ciliary processes, each composed of a central core of capillaries and connective tissue surrounded by an inner nonpigmented and an outer pigmented layer of epithelium (Figure 5.1). The nonpigmented and pigmented layers are arranged so that they face apex to apex, and the basement membrane of the nonpigmented layer faces the posterior chamber (PC).
- Three basic mechanisms: simple diffusion (passive movement of solutes governed by charge and concentration gradient), ultrafiltration (movement of water and solutes down pressure gradient), and active secretion (pressure-independent movement of substances

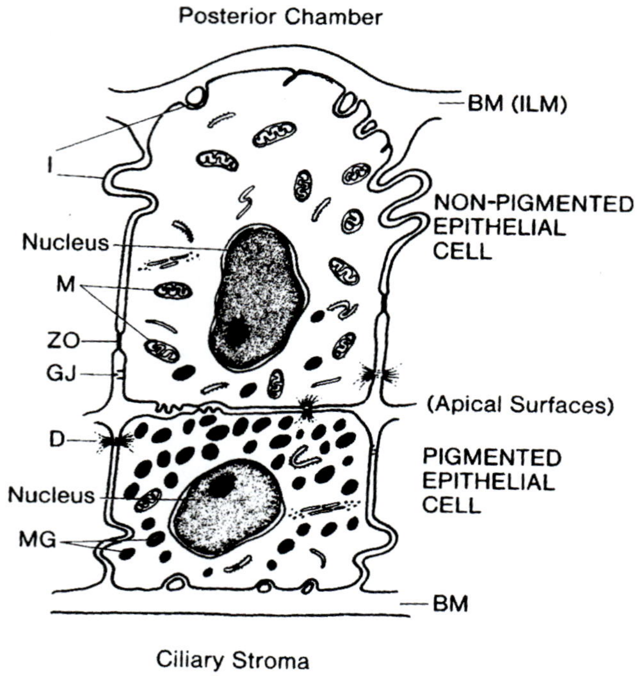

FIGURE 5.1. The ciliary body has two layers of epithelium aligned apex to apex. The pigmented epithelium is adjacent the stroma, whereas the nonpigmented epithelium is in contact with the posterior chamber. (From Shields MB. *Textbook of glaucoma*, 4th ed. Baltimore, MD: Lippincott Williams & Wilkins, 1998:10, with permission.)

against an electrochemical gradient by consumption of energy).

- Active transport is the major mechanism of aqueous formation; probably involves sodium pump at level of the nonpigmented epithelium.
- Inhibition by β-adrenergic antagonists (e.g., timolol), carbonic anhydrase inhibitors (CAIs) (e.g., acetazolamide and dorzolamide), and α_2-adrenergic agonists (e.g., brimonidine and apraclonidine).

Outflow

- Two pathways: trabecular (accounts for about 60% to 80% of outflow) and uveoscleral (remaining 20% to 40%).
- Trabecular meshwork (TM) is anatomically divided into uveal (most inner), corneoscleral, and juxtacanalicular (outermost) meshwork. Site of greatest resistance is the juxtacanalicular meshwork. Aqueous humor passes across meshwork into Schlemm's canal and ultimately drains into episcleral veins (Figure 5.2).
- Uveoscleral outflow from the anterior chamber through the ciliary muscle and into the suprachoroidal space and sclera, drained by emissarial channels of the sclera: increased by cycloplegia, adrenergic agonists (e.g., epinephrine), and prostaglandin analogues (e.g., latanoprost) in glaucoma therapy.

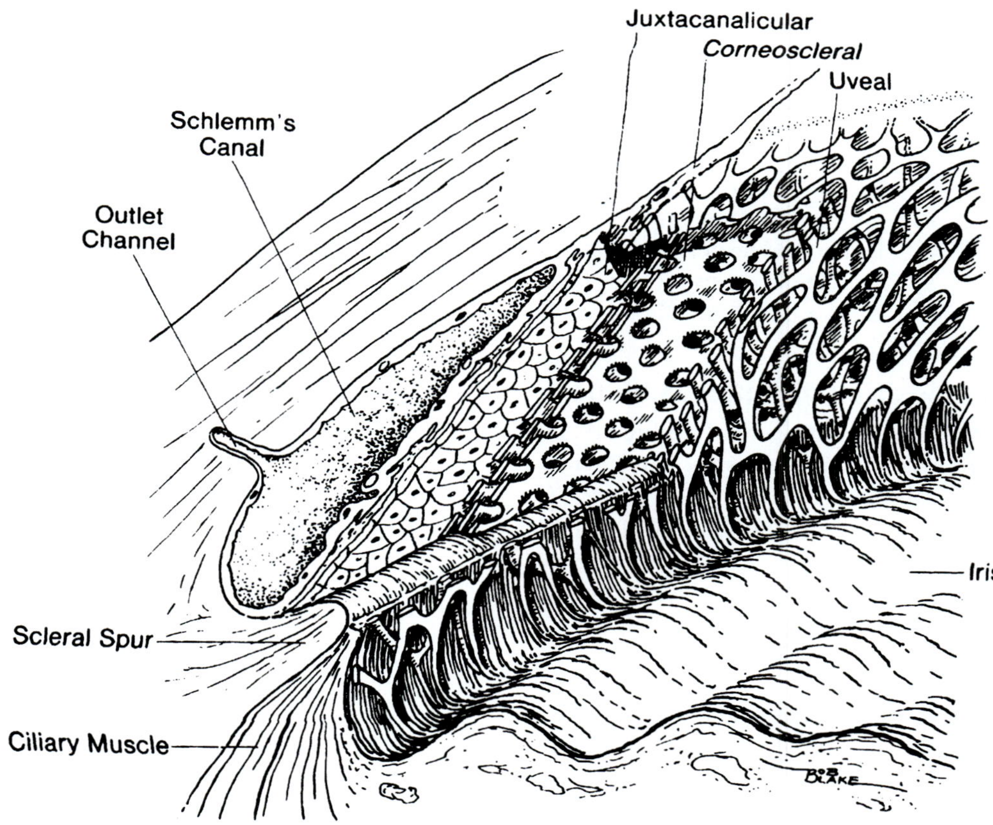

FIGURE 5.2. Diagram of the trabecular meshwork in cross section. (From Shields MB. *Textbook of glaucoma*, 4th ed. Baltimore, MD: Lippincott Williams & Wilkins, 1998:17, with permission.)

Intraocular Pressure Measurement Techniques

- Methods include indentation, applanation, rebound, noncontact, and pneumatic tonometry.
- Indentation tonometry exemplified by Schiotz tonometer:
    - Consists of concave footplate contiguous with plunger that slides within shaft. Shaft displaces a lever system and provides a reading that can be converted to millimeters of mercury. Performed in supine position.
    - Reading is strongly influenced by ocular rigidity: falsely high in rigid eyes (hyperopia) and falsely low in nonrigid eyes (high myopia, use of cholinesterase inhibitors, and prior ocular surgery).
- Applanation tonometry includes Goldmann tonometer, Perkins tonometer, and Tono-Pen:
    - Goldmann and Perkins tonometers function based on Imbert-Fick law:

$$P = F/A$$

    - where P = pressure, F = force, and A = area. IOP (P) is measured as the force (F) necessary to flatten the corneal apex a given area (A); diameter of 3.06 mm chosen because the surface tension of tears is counterbalanced by ocular rigidity at this diameter. In addition, multiplying the applied force by 10 gives IOP in millimeters of mercury. The area of flattening is assessed by placing fluorescein in the eye and using a split-field device to determine the flattened area (Figure 5.3)
    - Sources of error include excessive eyelid squeezing, Valsalva maneuver, pressure on the globe, extraocular muscle force applied to a restricted globe, corneal scarring or band keratopathy, corneal edema, excessive fluorescein (overestimates IOP), inadequate fluorescein (underestimates IOP), and astigmatism. Inaccuracy in cases of astigmatism can be minimized by rotating prism so that axis of least corneal curvature is opposite red mark on prism holder, or by taking average of two readings 90 degrees apart.
    - Tono-Pen uses constant area of applanation and determines force necessary to applanate this area. Several values are obtained and averaged to provide a digital readout. Less accurate at extreme values of IOP (overestimates low values and underestimates high values).
- Rebound tonometry (e.g., Icare tonometer):
    - A very light probe is used to make momentary contact with the cornea. Induction-based coil system measures probe deceleration, contact time, and other parameters during measurement. This information is used to calculate IOP.

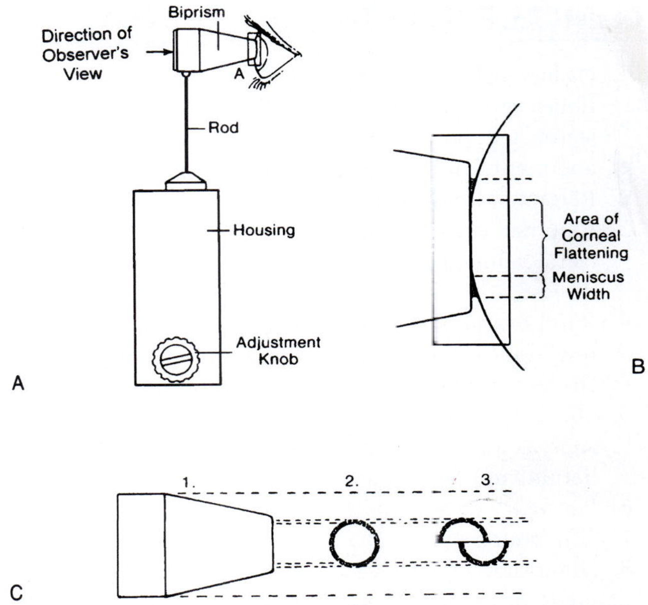

FIGURE 5.3. Diagram of the Goldmann applanation tonometer. The area of indentation is fixed, and the pressure can be derived. **A:** Diagrammatic representation of tonometer in apposition to the eye. **B:** Enlarged illustration of the corneal flattening created by the applanation by the tonometer tip. **C:** *1,* Appearance of the tonometer; *2,* tip cross section; *3,* view of meniscus when viewed through the slit lamp. (From Shields MB. *Textbook of glaucoma*. 4th ed. Baltimore, MD: Lippincott Williams & Wilkins, 1998:55, with permission.)

- Noncontact (air-puff) tonometry:
    - The force of the air stream increases linearly with time and stops when a given area of the central cornea is flattened. The duration of the air stream is converted to IOP.
    - Accurate in normal range but poor at extreme values, acceptable for mass screening.
- Pneumatic tonometry:
    - Composed in part of a probe with a floating pneumatic sensor and a rubber membrane that blocks the flow of air through the probe until the pressure buildup equals IOP.
    - Useful in cases of corneal scarring and edema.
- Central corneal thickness (CCT) effects on IOP measurement:
    - Thicker corneas overestimate IOP in a nonlinear fashion (~ 0.5 mm Hg difference for every 10 μm away from the population mean of 542 μm using Goldmann tonometry); conversely, thinner corneas underestimate IOP.
    - Hydration of the cornea (corneal edema) decreases its resistance to flattening and thus underestimates IOP (~ –2 mm Hg for every 70 μm change in corneal thickness, using Goldmann tonometry).
    - PRK/LASIK, which thin the cornea, cause underestimation of IOP.

CLINICAL EVALUATION OF GLAUCOMA

1. History including chief complaint, symptoms/onset/duration/severity, family history of glaucoma and vision loss, steroid use, previous IOP values, general medical history and medications, eye surgeries, and laser procedures.
2. Refraction for best acuity.
3. External examination to check for prominent episcleral veins or displacement of the globe from orbital disease.
4. Pupil examination to assess asymmetry of glaucomatous optic atrophy or possible corectopia or polycoria (iridocorneal endothelial [ICE] syndrome).
5. Slit-lamp examination to check for associated factors such as anterior chamber inflammation, pseudoexfoliation, and transillumination defects.
6. Perimetry to quantify visual field loss.
7. Tonometry.
8. Gonioscopy to assess angle width, presence of pigment, or peripheral anterior synechiae (PAS), etc.
9. Ophthalmoscopy to accurately assess optic disk contour and cup-to-disk ratio.
10. Special tests:
    - Tonography: assesses outflow facility by applying a known weight to the eye and measuring the change in IOP over time resulting from increased aqueous outflow.
    - Darkroom prone provocative test (DRPPT): compares IOP in supine position (not sitting) to IOP in prone position (in the dark and after 45 minutes). A rise of 9 mm Hg or more is considered a positive test result for occludable angle, and 4 to 8 mm Hg is equivocal.

Gonioscopy

Normal Angles

- Angle cannot be visualized without goniolens, since light reflected from angle undergoes total internal reflectivity at the air-cornea surface.
- Goniolens eliminates this interface with a surface of higher refractive index, allowing light from angle structures to leave at an angle greater than the angle of total internal reflectivity.
- Goniolenses are of two types, direct and indirect:
  - Direct includes Koeppe lens, which consists of 50-diopter (D) concave lens with a back surface that fits onto the anesthetized cornea. Other examples include the Layden, Swan-Jacobs, and Hoskins-Barkan lenses. The angle is visualized using a handheld binocular magnifier and a separate light source. Advantages of Koeppe gonioscopy include direct panoramic view of entire angle, ease of changing viewing angle into the angle of the eye (useful in cases of concave iris), and ability to rapidly compare the angle of both eyes.
  - Indirect includes Zeiss or Volk four-mirror and Goldmann mirror lenses. The Zeiss has an interface surface flatter than the corneal surface, eliminating the need for a coupling agent. The Goldmann lens is steeper than the cornea and requires a high-viscosity coupling agent; contact surface is actually on the sclera.
  - Advantages of the Zeiss lens include rapidity of application, no need for coupling interface solution (saline for Koeppe and high-viscosity agent for Goldmann), and ability to perform compression gonioscopy (the application of force on the cornea with the Zeiss lens to open the angle).
- Angle structures from anterior to posterior are cornea, Schwalbe's line, anterior TM, posterior TM, scleral spur, ciliary body band, and iris (Figure 5.4).
- Grading systems of angle depth include Shaffer, Spaeth, and van Herick systems.
  - Shaffer system is graded as follows:
    - Grade 0 = Closed angle.
    - Grade slit = 5 degrees or less.
    - Grade I = 10 degrees.
    - Grade II = 20 degrees.
    - Grade III = 30 degrees.
    - Grade IV = 40 degrees or greater.
    - Grades slit, I, and II are considered occludable angles.
  - Spaeth system includes Shaffer system but expands to include description of angle configuration and iris insertion.
    - R = Regular, no significant iris bowing.
    - S = Steep, iris arises from its root in steep convex curve.
    - Q = Quixotic, iris bows posteriorly (concave) from its root.
    - A = Above Schwalbe's line, closed angle.
    - B = Below Schwalbe's line, attachment to TM.
    - C = Scleral spur.
    - D = Deep, anterior ciliary body visible.
    - E = Extremely deep, unusually large portion of ciliary body band visible.
    - Current nomenclature for the description of an angle includes appearance of iris insertion in parentheses followed by anatomic insertion; for example, (C)D = anatomic insertion at the ciliary body but appears to be just below scleral spur without compression gonioscopy. Furthermore, an angle may be described with a number to indicate the angle of iris approach followed by letters to indicate iris insertion and angle configuration (e.g., 30CS).
  - van Herick technique grades angle depth based on slit-lamp examination, not gonioscopy. A thin beam is focused at an angle of 45 to 60 degrees on the cornea and anterior chamber (AC) at the temporal limbus.
    - I = AC depth < one fourth corneal thickness.

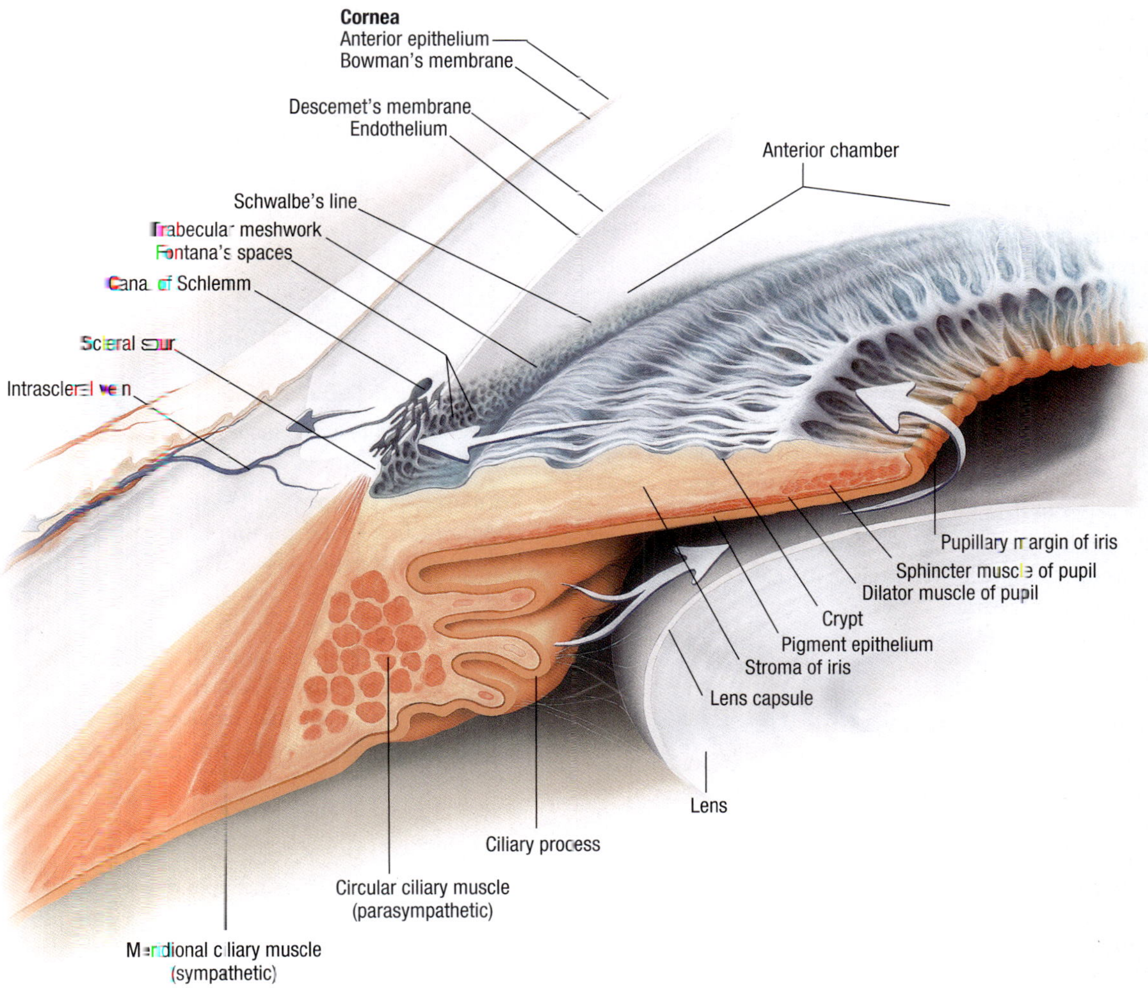

FIGURE 5.4. Gonioscopic view of the angle structures. (Asset provided by Anatomical Chart Co.)

II = One fourth corneal thickness.
III = One fourth to half corneal thickness.
IV = Up to full corneal thickness or greater.

Abnormal Angles

Abnormal angle vessels: Normal radial iris vessels may cross angle; neovascular vessels (Figure 5.5) typically arborize at the TM and can cause contraction and PAS.

Pigmentation: Increased meshwork pigmentation may be seen with aging and in pigmented individuals; however, heavy pigmentation or Sampaolesi line (accumulation of pigment along ridge where cornea transitions into the angle recess) suggests possible pseudoexfoliation, pigment dispersion syndrome, or trauma.

PAS: Adhesions between iris and TM; signify prior AC inflammation, appositional angle closure, angle neovascularization, corneal endothelial migration (ICE syndrome), or trauma. PAS tend to be sheetlike connections, whereas iris processes are fine, wispy extensions from the iris to the cornea.

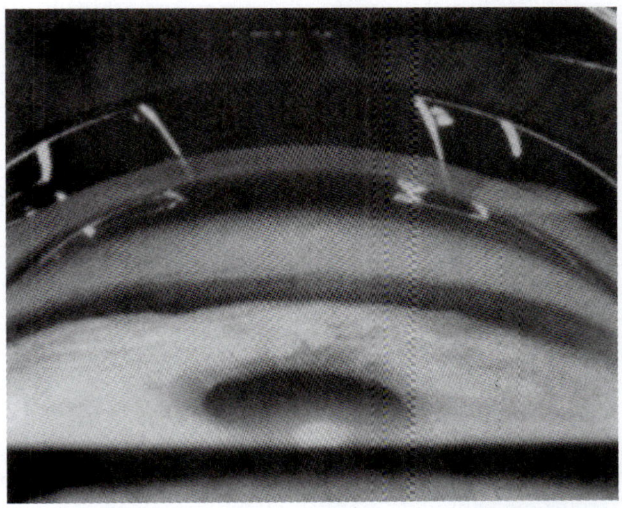

FIGURE 5.5. Neovascular vessels in the angle are evidence of severe posterior segment ischemia. (From Epstein DL. *Chandler and Grant's glaucoma*, 4th ed. Baltimore, MD: Lippincott Williams & Wilkins, 1997:72, with permission.)

Angle recession: seen months after blunt ocular trauma and characterized by abnormally deep angle allowing visualization of wide ciliary body band. Other clues to prior trauma may be present as well: torn iris processes, sphincter tears, phacodonesis, and/or iridodonesis. Histology typically reveals a tear between the longitudinal and circular muscle fibers in the ciliary body. These also can be associated with injury to the trabecular meshwork.

Cyclodialysis cleft: Typically after trauma, the ciliary body is separated from the ciliary sulcus and its attachment to the scleral spur, leaving a deep cleft. This can cause hyposecrection of aqueous humor and/or increased filtration of aqueous humor to the suprachoroidal space (uveoscleral outflow), leading to hypotony.

Iridodialysis: After blunt trauma, separation of the iris root from the ciliary body occurs. This can be seen along with or separate from a cyclodialysis cleft. Usually associated with hyphema, may not be recognized until anterior chamber blood has cleared. Can cause monocular diplopia and polycoria.

Optic Nerve

Assessment of Optic Nerve Changes

- Best method is use of slit lamp and a Hruby lens, a posterior pole contact lens, or a 60-, 78-, or 90-D lens.
- Cup-to-disk (c/d) ratio: Assess both horizontal and vertical dimensions. The physiologic c/d ratio is genetically determined. Two thirds of normal c/d ratios are less than 0.3, and only 6% of the normal population has c/d of 0.5 or greater. C/d ratios greater than 0.3 should be viewed with suspicion. The size of the disk correlates with the size of the cup. Smaller optic disks tend to have smaller physiologic cups and vice versa. Normal optic disk size is approximately 1.5 to 2.2 mm in diameter. For quantitative measurement of optic disk diameter, use the slit lamp and adjust the height of the slit beam to match the vertical diameter of the disk. The lens used must be taken into account for calculation: Multiply measurement by 1.1 for a 78-D lens and by 1.3 for a 90-D lens. Progressive enlargement of the cup is evidence of glaucoma, and c/d asymmetry of 0.2 or greater is very suspect for glaucoma. It should be noted that blacks have a higher physiologic c/d ratio in general.
- Rim contour: Focal neural rim damage may be detected as focal notching, thinning, or pallor and have corresponding visual field loss on perimetry. In normal individuals, neuroretinal rim thickness follows the ISNT rule: I = inferior rim is the thickest, followed by S = superior, N = nasal, and finally the T = temporal portion of the rim.
- Disk splinter hemorrhage: focal sign for glaucomatous damage; may signify progression of glaucoma and be recurrent. More commonly seen in normal tension glaucoma (Figure 5.6).
- Nerve fiber layer: best viewed with red-free illumination. Both wedge-shaped focal loss and diffuse atrophy can occur in glaucoma.

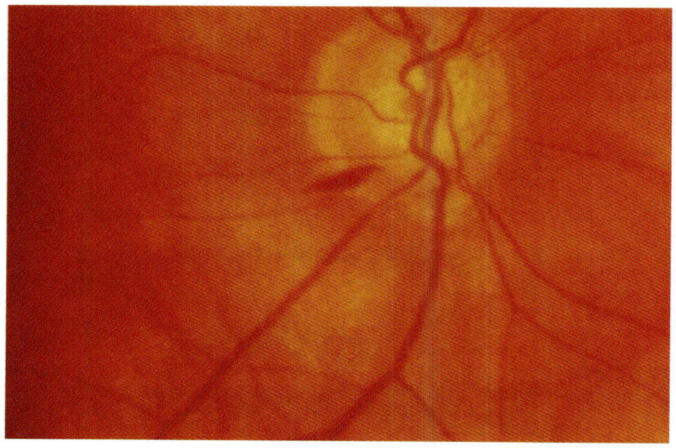

FIGURE 5.6. Splinter hemorrhage at the disk margin.

- Peripapillary atrophy (PPA) occurs as two types: alpha-zone and beta-zone peripapillary atrophy. It represents loss of choriocapillaris and RPE adjacent to the optic disk. Alpha-zone PPA is the outer or peripheral zone of PPA that can be seen in normal patients and other disease states (e.g., myopia). It has unknown impact on glaucoma. Beta-zone PPA is the central zone of atrophy adjacent to the disk that has been shown to be present with higher frequency and to a greater degree in patients with glaucoma.

Visual Fields

Defined as the entire visual space one can see at a given moment. For each eye, the visual field extends 90 degrees temporally, 70 degrees inferiorly, 60 degrees nasally, and 50 degrees superiorly.

- Hill of vision: refers to the three-dimensional representation of differential light sensitivity in the visual field (Figure 5.7). The best visual acuity is at the apex of the hill and descends from there, more steeply nasally than temporally.

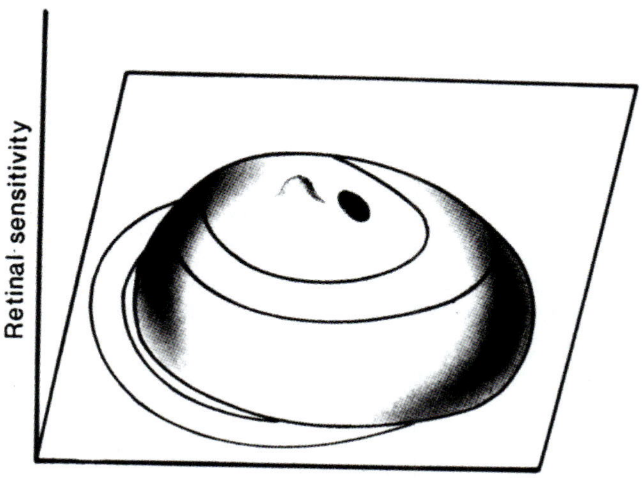

FIGURE 5.7. Hill of vision. The higher areas near the fovea represent greater light sensitivity.

- Perimetry refers to the testing of the visual field:
  - Threshold: dimmest spot able to be detected. The bracketing method is used to determine threshold in computerized static perimetry. Threshold testing is preferable in glaucoma patients and suspects.
  - Suprathreshold: light stimulus greater than threshold. Suprathreshold testing is useful for screening individuals not suspected of having glaucoma.
  - Kinetic testing: testing of sensitivity by moving a light stimulus from nonseeing to seeing portion of the visual field.
  - Static testing: testing of points in the visual field using fixed points.
  - Isopter: demarcation between visible and nonvisible parts of the visual field; represents edge of threshold.
  - Scotoma: area of depressed light sensitivity compared with surrounding visual field; may be relative or absolute.
  - Luminescence can be measured in apostilbs (asb) or decibels (dB). Apostilbs are nonlogarithmic units that increase with increasing intensity (decreasing light sensitivity). However, decibels are measured as 0.1 log units of light sensitivity and increase as the light stimulus becomes dimmer.
  - Isopter notations for the Goldmann perimeter are Roman numeral for spot size (area increases by fourfold per unit), Arabic numeral for light intensity (increases by 0.5 log unit or 3.15 per numeral), and lowercase letter for intermediate intensities (increases by 0.1 log unit per letter). Since spot size and intensity are related reciprocally, equivalent targets can be used by varying the two parameters (e.g., I4e = II3e = III2e = IV1e). Stimulus size, as stated above, increases fourfold per unit: 0 = 1/16 mm^2, I = 1/4 mm^2, II = 1 mm^2, III = 4 mm^2, IV = 16 mm^2, and V = 64 mm^2.

Static Versus Dynamic Perimetry

- Advantages of kinetic perimetry (e.g., Goldmann):
  - Rapid assessment of isopter contours and scotomas.
  - Familiarity among clinicians.
  - Goldmann perimeters are relatively inexpensive.
  - More dynamic interaction with patient.
- Disadvantages of kinetic testing:
  - Requires more skilled technical assistance.
  - Testing is usually suprathreshold and may not detect early changes.
  - Not as quantitative as computerized static perimetry.
- Advantages of computerized static perimetry (e.g., Humphrey, Octopus):
  - Quantifiable results that are reproducible.
  - Tests threshold with greater sensitivity.
  - Computer-programmed operation does not require highly skilled training.
- Disadvantages of computerized static perimetry:
  - More detailed data making interpretation more difficult.
  - Time-consuming and demanding on patient.
  - Equipment is more expensive.

Perimeter Defects and Errors

- Defects resulting from glaucomatous optic nerve damage:
  - Paracentral scotoma: round or ovoid defect within 10 degrees of fixation, an early defect seen in glaucoma; may be more common in low-tension glaucoma.
  - Arcuate Bjerrum scotoma: bowlike defect extending from blind spot to the horizontal raphe; occurs in the area 10 to 20 degrees from fixation (Figure 5.8).
  - Nasal step: defect in the nasal periphery respecting the horizontal raphe in which there is relative depression compared with the corresponding area of the opposite hemifield (Figure 5.9).
  - Temporal wedge: wedge-shaped defect extending from blind spot to the periphery.
  - Split fixation: central scotoma that respects the horizontal raphe; ominous sign.
  - Central island: both superior and inferior hemifield loss leaving only central island of tunnel vision; indicates very advanced glaucoma.

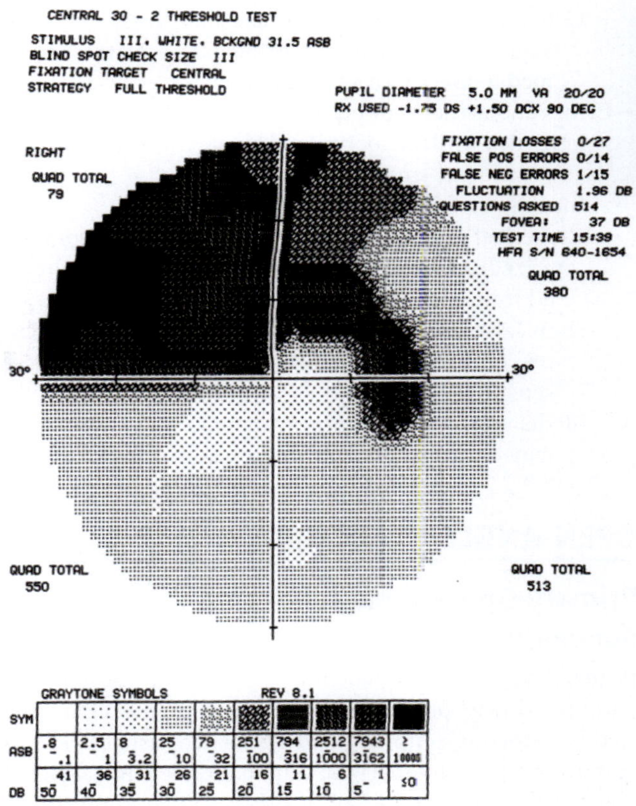

FIGURE 5.8. Bjerrum scotoma.

GLAUCOMA

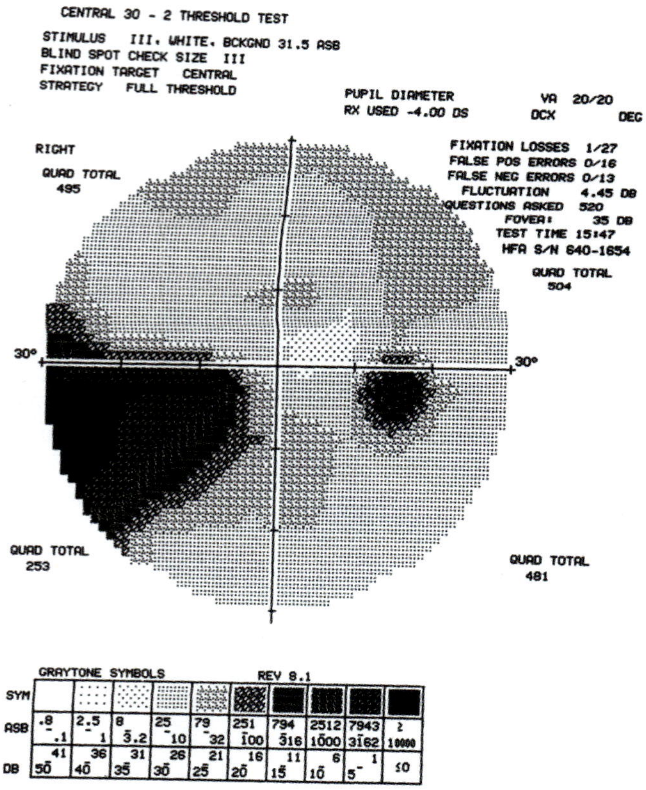

FIGURE 5.9. Nasal step.

Generalized depression: diffuse field loss; may be a sign of early field loss or artifact (cataract, other media opacity, or miotic pupil).

- Errors and artifacts in perimetry:

  Lens rim artifact: peripheral depression due to malpositioned lens.

  Incorrect refraction: generalized depression.

  Cloverleaf pattern: due to inattention late in computerized perimetry, since the program tests points in all four quadrants early on.

  High false-positive rate: results in "white scotomas" on computerized fields because of impossibly high sensitivities.

  Media opacity or miosis: cataracts and pilocarpine may cause generalized depressed fields.

OPEN-ANGLE GLAUCOMA

Primary Open-Angle Glaucoma

Summary

Primary open-angle glaucoma (POAG) is generally a chronic, slowly progressive optic neuropathy characterized by optic disk cupping and associated visual field loss patterns despite an otherwise unremarkable clinical examination; there is an absence of other known etiologies of open-angle glaucoma (OAG). Elevated IOP is a key modifiable risk factor.

Etiology

Not clearly established. Abnormalities of perfusion, ganglion cell metabolism, and/or mechanical factors are thought to play the central roles.

- Mechanical: Increased intraocular pressure directly compresses ganglion cell axons against the lamina cribrosa, interrupting axon function and leading to ganglion cell death.
- Ischemic: Abnormalities of the optic nerve head microvascular circulation, stressed by increased pressure or vessel compromise by lamina cribrosa plate distortion, leads to ganglion cell death.
- Neurotoxicity: Astrocytes or other CNS support cells may become dysfunctional resulting in disrupted axoplasmic transport, direct neurotoxicity from nitric oxide or TNF-α, and/or disruption of the neurotrophic extracellular matrix necessary to sustain ganglion cell function.
- A direct relationship between IOP and existing/subsequent optic nerve damage has been established.

Signs and Symptoms

Usually asymptomatic.

Loss of peripheral visual field early in disease; central visual field loss later in course.

Genetics

- Multifactorial inheritance with lack of penetrance and variable expressivity.
- First-degree relatives of glaucoma patients are at increased risk: 10% for siblings and 4% for offspring. Twenty-five percent of new cases of POAG have positive family history.
- Juvenile-onset glaucoma has been isolated to chromosome 1q. This form of juvenile-onset glaucoma is inherited as an atuosomal dominant trait. This gene has also been linked to some adult forms of open-angle glaucoma.
- Inherited form of glaucoma associated with aniridia: mutation in the *PAX6* gene located at 11p13. Sporadic form of aniridia associated with development of Wilms tumor.

Demographics

Occurs in 1.3% to 2.1% of general population over 40 years old.

Incidence increases with aging.

Estimates: 1 in 10 elderly blacks and 1 in 50 elderly whites (four to five times more prevalent in blacks).

Primary Risk Factors

- Family history
- Age
- Race
- Increased IOP
- Central Corneal Thickness (CCT)

Ophthalmic Findings

Bilateral (may be asymmetric).
Increased IOP (usually >22 mm Hg).
Gonioscopy: angle open, without visible pathologic features.
Optic disk:
Increased c/d ratio; asymmetry to fellow eye.
Asymmetry of the neuroretinal rim.
Focal thinning of the neuroretinal rim: "notching."
Optic disk splinter hemorrhage (Figure 5.6).
Vertical elongation of cup.
Retinal nerve fiber layer (NFL) loss.

Associated Ophthalmic Disorders

Increased incidence of central retinal vein occlusion in patients with glaucoma or OHTN.
Increased incidence of myopia (may be selection bias).

Systemic Findings

Increased prevalence of both elevated mean IOP and POAG in patients with diabetes mellitus. Diabetes as an independent risk factor for POAG remains controversial. Weak association exists between POAG and cardiovascular disease (hypertension, ischemic factors).

Special Tests

Gonioscopy: to rule out secondary causes, verify open angle.
Central corneal thickness (pachymetry): affects IOP measurements by all applanation methods.
Red-free illumination: to visualize NFL defects.
Diurnal IOP readings: to rule out spurious low IOP reading.
Automated visual field: to quantitatively evaluate visual field status.
Tonography: to measure relative outflow facility.
Blue-yellow perimetry (also known as short-wavelength automated perimetry, or SWAP): thought to detect visual field loss earlier. Projects a blue stimulus onto a yellow background, thereby isolating koniocellular, blue/yellow ganglion cells.
Frequency-doubling technology (FDT) perimetry: also thought to detect visual field loss earlier, it employs low spatial frequency sinusoidal grating undergoing rapid phase-reversal flicker. Isolates magnocellular cells.

Pathology

- Ganglion cell death (cells at inferior or superior aspect of disk appear to be more susceptible).
- Increased c/d ratio; loss of neuroretinal rim.
- Electron microscopy: decreased celluarity of TM and "extracellular plaques" in TM.

Disease Course

- Insidious, painless, slowly progressive.
- Nonreversible visual field loss; only rare instances of reversal of cupping.
- Optic disk changes may be observed before visual field changes.

Treatment and Management

- Lowering IOP is the only proven modifiable risk factor for preventing future disk damage and progressive visual field loss.
- Stereo photographs: to detect subtle changes in disk over time.
- Computerized imaging: provides a topographical map of disk for a more quantitative analysis.
- Periodic evaluation of visual fields: to assess treatment results.
- Correlate visual field changes with optic disk changes.
- "Target pressure" concept: Consistently achieve 25% to 66% of presenting IOP to limit further visual field loss (dependent on severity of glaucoma); continue to monitor visual field and disk changes even at target IOP for effectiveness of treatment, no matter how low the current IOP.
- "Glaucoma suspect" concept: patients who have high IOP or glaucomatous-appearing disks, but without corresponding visual field loss. There is no clear consensus on when or how to treat ocular hypertensives who do not have glaucomatous disks or visual field loss. A personalized assessment of risk factors and patient goals must guide treatment decisions. In general, initiate therapy if IOP is greater than 30 mm Hg, and lower than that if risk factors or evidence of glaucomatous optic nerve damage is present.
- There is no known "cure": The visual field loss is irreversible and the treatments have undesired effects. Therefore, the goal is to preserve visual field adequate for patient's lifetime and visual demands.

Medications

β-Blockers.
CAI inhibitors.
Prostaglandin analogues.
Adrenergic agonists.
Cholinergic agents.

Laser Surgery Indications

- Use laser trabeculoplasty in mild to moderate glaucoma.
- Effect may be temporary.

Filtration Surgery Indications (General Concepts)

- Progressive visual field loss or optic disk changes despite maximum tolerated medical therapy.
- Sustained highly elevated IOP (i.e., >40 mm Hg), even if without visual field loss or optic disk changes.
- Advanced visual field loss (small margin for tolerating further damage [i.e., loss progressing to fixation]).

Follow-Up

- Per specific case; at least every 6 months for IOP check.
- Recently diagnosed patients need repeated visual field tests in order to rule out learning artifact, and frequent visits to establish satisfactory IOP control.
- Up to 50% of patients with glaucoma (all types) have an initial screening IOP of less than 21 mm Hg.
- Establish consistency of visual field test-taking parameters.

Differential Diagnosis

Normal tension glaucoma: identical disease to POAG but patient never has documented IOP greater than 22 mm Hg.

Chronic/intermittent angle-closure glaucoma: peripheral anterior synechiae, occludable angles, symptoms, episodic IOP elevations.

Exfoliation glaucoma: anterior lens capsule changes, pupillary margin transillumination defects.

Pigmentary glaucoma: Krukenberg spindle, heavy deposition of pigment on TM, midperipheral iris transillumination defects, symptomatic with exercise or mydriasis.

Other optic neuropathies are generally nonprogressive and show no cupping of the optic disk.

Reference

Booth A, Churchill A, Anwar R, et al. The genetics of primary open angle glaucoma. *Br J Ophthalmol* 1997;81:409–414.

Normal Tension Glaucoma

Summary

Normal tension glaucoma (NTG) is a progressive optic neuropathy with typical glaucomatous optic disk damage and visual field loss with open angles as in POAG. However, the IOP is consistently less than 22 mm Hg. Also known as "low tension glaucoma" (LTG), it is probably a subset of POAG.

Etiology

Not well established. Thought to be due to relatively IOP-independent mechanisms such as microvascular damage; although not considered the main pathogenic factor, IOP has been established as a significant modifier of future disk damage and visual field loss.

Signs and Symptoms

Asymptomatic, visual field loss apparent later in natural history.

Demographics

Typically in elderly patients (over age 70 years).
No established racial predilection.

Ophthalmic Findings

Identical to POAG, except that IOP is normal.
When compared with POAG:
Visual field defects tend to be steeper, deeper, and closer to fixation.
Increased incidence of optic disk splinter hemorrhages.

Systemic Findings

Possible relationship to history of hypotensive shock, postural hypotension, migraines.

Special Tests

Diurnal IOP curve to rule out spurious low IOP reading.

Pathology

Obscure/undetermined but shares final common pathway of ganglion cell death.

Disease Course

Progressive nature is key characteristic. Some will have progressive damage despite very low IOPs.

Treatment and Management

- Progression of disease (further visual field loss or disk changes) should be documented before diagnosis and initiation of therapy.
- The only current therapeutic strategy is to lower IOP further.

Medications

Same as for POAG.

Follow-Up

Same as for POAG.

Differential Diagnosis

POAG with diurnal variation: on diurnal IOP curve testing has peaks in IOP greater than 22 mm Hg.

Angle-closure glaucoma (intermittent or chronic): has suggestive history, symptoms, features of occludable angle in both eyes, episodes of elevated IOP.

Previous glaucoma damage: burned-out pigmentary glaucoma, history (key feature of NTG diagnosis is progressive nature of visual field loss and disk changes despite "normal" IOP).

Nonglaucomatous optic neuropathy: nonprogressive (i.e., always inquire about a severe hypotensive episode such as massive blood loss during surgery that may explain a stable visual field loss).

Congenital optic nerve defect: nonprogressive.

Traumatic glaucoma: Previous eye trauma (usually blunt) may lead to dysfunction of TM and aqueous outflow compromise. The relative magnitude of the trauma may be implied by findings such as angle recession (though the angle recession itself may not be directly responsible for aqueous outflow compromise).

Reference

Grosskreutz C, Netland PA. Low-tension glaucoma. *Int Ophthalmol Clin* 1994;34:173–185.

Pigment Dispersion Syndrome and Pigmentary Glaucoma

Pigment dispersion syndrome (PDS) is characterized by spokelike midperipheral iris pigment epithelial thinning with pigment deposition on the corneal endothelium, TM, and lens periphery. If associated with consistently high IOP, visual field loss, and glaucomatous optic disk damage: "pigmentary glaucoma," a type of secondary open-angle glaucoma (SOAG).

Etiology

- Pigment dispersion is thought to be caused by direct mechanical contact between the anterior lens zonules and iris pigment epithelium.
- Blinking is theorized to create a stop-valve effect by increasing AC pressure relative to PC pressure (and thus the reverse pupillary block configuration of the iris).

Signs and Symptoms

Asymptomatic.

Episodic blurring, halos, and possible ocular pain (due to acute rises in IOP associated with exercise or mydriasis).

Demographics

Associated with moderate myopia.

Increased incidence in male patients.

Usually 20 to 50 years of age.

Whites (rare in blacks).

Approximately 25% to 50% of PDS patients progress to pigmentary glaucoma.

Ophthalmic Findings

- Krukenberg spindle: vertical pattern of pigment deposition on corneal endothelium.
- Open angle with dense, homogeneously pigmented TM (Figure 5.10).
- Sampaolesi line: pigment deposition anterior to Schwalbe's line.
- Iris transillumination defects: spokelike loss of pigment at iris midperiphery. In pseudophakes, the pattern follows the optic and haptic implant edges.
- Pigment "dusting" on iris surface.
- Pigmented cells in AC after dilation.
- Scheie stripe: pigment on lens capsule at zonule attachment site.

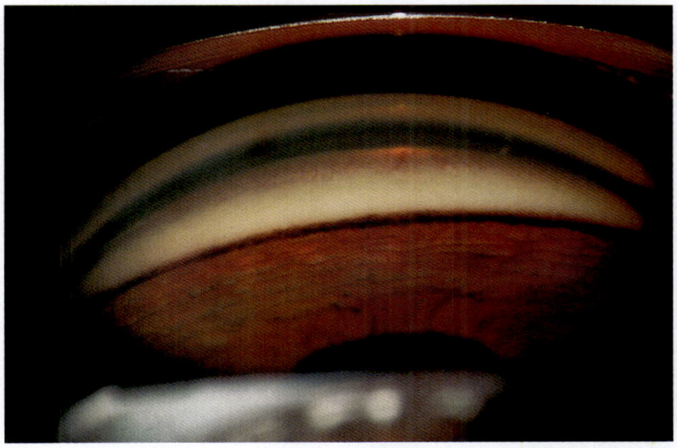

FIGURE 5.10. Pigment dispersion syndrome. The heavily pigmented meshwork band is evident.

- Large fluctuations in IOP (sudden large IOP elevation is observed following exercise or dilation).
- Iris contour concavity is frequently observed ("Q" configuration in the Spaeth classification).
- Nearly always bilateral.

Special Tests

Ultrasound biomicroscopy (UBM) confirms iris anatomic configuration of reverse pupillary block ("Q" shape).

Pathology

Direct dispersion of pigment into TM leads to degeneration of TM cells, trapping of cellular debris, and sclerosis of TM beams.

Disease Course

- In one study, 35% of patients with PDS and elevated IOP developed visual field loss or optic disk cupping (mean follow-up of 17 years).
- Signs and symptoms may decrease as patient ages.

Treatment and Management

- PDS with normal optic disks, visual fields, and IOP: Follow as a glaucoma suspect.
- If glaucomatous changes develop, treat medically as in POAG.
- Laser trabeculoplasty has good efficacy in these patients if medications are not effective.
- Laser iridotomy is indicated if reverse pupillary block component is observed (usually considered in young patients).

Medications

- Same as for POAG.
- Miotics have been shown to reduce iris transillumination defects and pigment dispersion.

Follow-Up

Patients with PDS are followed as glaucoma suspects.

Differential Diagnosis

Exfoliation syndrome/glaucoma: seen in older patients, pupillary margin iris defects, anterior lens capsule changes. Less dense pigment deposition, no symptoms.

POAG: no iris transillumination defects, less abundant pigment deposition, asymptomatic, older patients.

Inflammatory open-angle glaucoma: Nonpigmented cells and aqueous flare present, iris transillumination may be present.

Iris melanoma: has iris mass, very heavy pigment deposition.

Reference

Migliazzo CV, Shaffer RN, Nykin R, et al. Long-term analysis of pigmentary dispersion syndrome and pigmentary glaucoma. *Ophthalmology* 1986;93:1528–1536.

EXFOLIATION SYNDROME

Exfoliation syndrome or pseudoexfoliation (XS) is characterized by the deposition of a distinctive fibrillar material throughout the anterior segment, in particular, on the anterior lens surface. If associated with glaucoma, it is termed "exfoliative glaucoma" (XG), formerly called pseudoexfoliative glaucoma (PXG). This is in distinction to "true exfoliation" (i.e., that classically associated with glass blowing), which is now called "capsular exfoliation."

Etiology

A manifestation of a generalized basement disorder, the deposition of fibrillar material occludes the TM and thus compromises aqueous outflow.

Signs and Symptoms

Rarely symptomatic.

Patients may complain of foreign body sensation.

Demographics

- Varies considerably with population studied: XG accounts for greater than 50% of OAG cases in Scandanavian countries but for only 1.6% of OAG cases in the southeastern United States.
- Rarely seen in patients less than 50 years of age; most patients are more than 70 years old.

Ophthalmic Findings

- Corneal endothelium pigment deposition: usually diffuse, may rarely be in Krukenberg spindle pattern.
- Iris transillumination defects: "moth-eaten" iris appearance at pupillary margin (Figure 5.11); may be easier to observe with mydriasis.

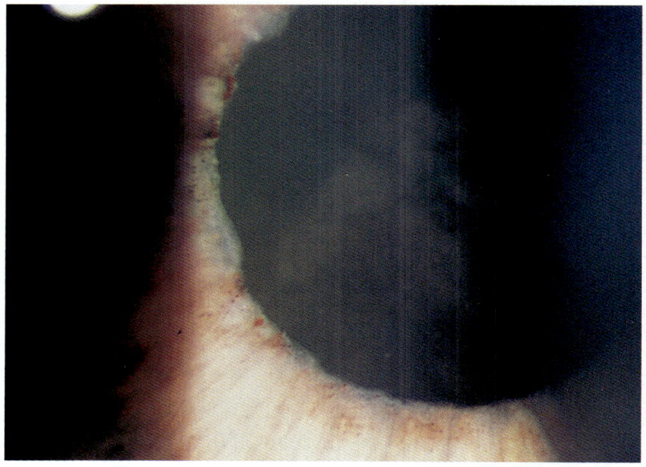

FIGURE 5.11. Exfoliation syndrome. The pupillary border of the iris may have a "moth-eaten" appearance.

- Pigment deposition on iris anterior surface.
- Diffuse spotty pigmentation throughout angle; pigmentation anterior to Schwalbe's line (Sampaolesi line) is frequently present.
- The anterior lens characteristically has a target pattern: A clear intervening area separates a central translucent zone from a peripheral area of granular deposition (best seen with mydriasis). The clear intervening zone is thought to be secondary to rubbing of the iris on the anterior lens capsule (Figure 5.12).
- Increased incidence of phacodonesis, lens subluxation, and increased risk of vitreous loss with cataract surgery attributable to weakened lens zonules.

Systemic Findings

Identical basement membrane findings throughout body: of no known consequence.

Pathology

- A primary basement membrane disorder.

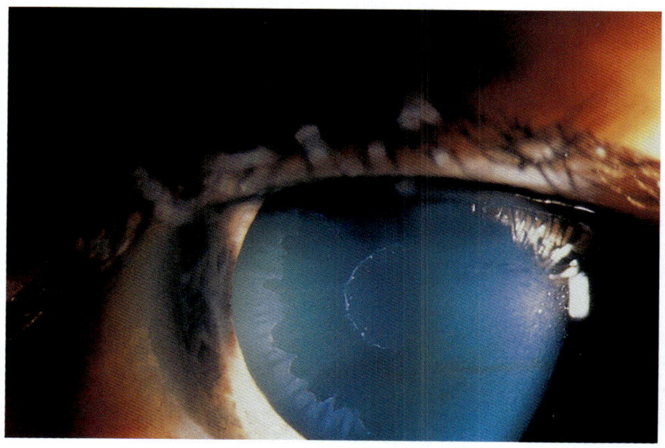

FIGURE 5.12. Target-shaped deposition of exfoliative material on the anterior lens capsule. The intervening clear zone is thought to be due to iridolenticular rubbing.

- Exfoliative material histochemically resembles elastic microfibrils and other extracellular matrix components.
- Obstruction of TM by pseudoexfoliative material and/or underlying TM dysfunction leads to compromised aqueous outflow.

Disease Course

- In an eye with XS and normal IOP, there is a 5.3% and a 15.4% chance of developing disk or field changes at 5 and 10 years, respectively.
- In an eye with XS and elevated IOP, there is a 35% chance of developing disk or field damage in 9 years (vs. 18% of ocular hypertensives).
- XG has a worse prognosis than POAG, frequently responding poorly to medical therapy and more likely to lead to development of visual field loss (48% vs. 19% for POAG).

Treatment and Management

- Approach is similar to POAG.
- Increased incidence of cataract extraction complications, since zonular weakness may lead to zonular dehiscence, tears in posterior capsule, vitreous loss, dropped nucleus.
- Lens extraction does not alleviate findings or alter disease course.
- Laser trabeculoplasty can be very effective with good uptake by pigmented TM, but there is shorter duration of response when compared to POAG.
- Trabeculectomy results are similar when compared to patients with POAG, but these patients have increased postoperative inflammation.

Medications

Same as for POAG, although generally less effective.

Follow-Up

XS patients are at increased likelihood of developing glaucomatous damage and therefore must be followed closely as glaucoma suspects.

Differential Diagnosis

PDS/pigmentary glaucoma: younger patients with midperipheral iris transillumination defects, more abundant pigmentary deposition on TM and cornea, lack of anterior lens capsule changes.

Capsular exfoliation (also known as capsular delamination, "true exfoliation"): history of glass blowing or welding.

Toxic exfoliation (uveitis and retained foreign body): symptoms, inflammation, and history of trauma.

References

Henry JC, Krupin T, Schmitt M, et al. Long-term follow-up of pseudoexfoliation and the development of elevated intraocular pressure. *Ophthalmology* 1987;94:545–552.

Kozart DM, Yanoff M. Intraocular pressure status in 100 consecutive patients with exfoliation syndrome. *Ophthalmology* 1982;89:214–218.

Naumann GO, Schlotzer-Schrehardt U, Kuchle M. Pseudoexfoliation syndrome for the comprehensive ophthalmologist: intraocular and systemic manifestations. *Ophthalmology* 1998;105:951–968.

Pohjanpelto P. Influence of exfoliation syndrome on prognosis in ocular hypertension >25 mm Hg: a long-term follow-up. *Acta Ophthalmol* 1986;64:39–44.

ANGLE-CLOSURE GLAUCOMA

Primary Angle-Closure Glaucoma

Primary angle-closure glaucoma (PACG) is acute, chronic, or intermittent elevation of IOP as a result of mechanical blockage of the TM by the iris root, without underlying secondary etiology (only anatomic predisposition). Identical glaucomatous optic neuropathy damage to POAG.

Etiology

PACG with pupillary block: Flow of aqueous humor from PC through pupil and into AC is limited anatomically; therefore aqueous humor accumulates in the PC. This creates a relative pressure gradient (high pressure in the PC and low in the AC), forcing the iris root to take a relatively anterior position and leading to angle narrowing or closure. Pupillary block may be absolute (i.e., posterior synechiae that totally obstruct aqueous flow into AC) or relative (i.e., anatomic factors create a pressure gradient). This is by far the most frequent etiology of PACG.

PACG without pupillary block ("plateau iris configuration"): an increasingly recognized anatomic variant, caused by relatively anteriorly positioned ciliary processes that create an anteriorly positioned iris root with planar configuration centrally. Plateau iris cannot be diagnosed with certainty until any possible pupillary block component is relieved with peripheral iridotomy.

Signs and Symptoms

- Acute angle closure (sudden, rapid increase in IOP):
  - Painful, red, congested, "steamy" eye.
  - Nausea and vomiting (has been misdiagnosed as an acute condition of the abdomen).
  - Blurred vision.
  - Rainbow-colored halos around lights.
- Intermittent (angle opens and closes spontaneously):
  - Transient blurry vision, halos, and/or headaches secondary to acute rises in IOP; IOP is normal between episodes.
  - Episodes occur over days or weeks.
- Chronic (progressive angle closure):
  - May be asymptomatic.
  - IOP may gradually rise over time.
  - Course may resemble POAG.

Demographics

- In a population over 40 years of age, PACG prevalence is 0.1% to 0.6% in whites, 0.1% to 0.2% in blacks, 2.1% to 5.0% in the Inuit, 0.4% to 1.4% in East Asians, 0.3% in Japanese, and 2.3% in a mixed ethnic group in South Africa.
- Highly prevalent in Eskimos and eastern Asians (studies have suggested that PACG accounts for 70% of all glaucoma cases in China).
- Two to four times more prevalent in female than in male patients, regardless of race.
- Small, hyperopic eyes are at increased risk.

Ophthalmic Findings

- Acute:
  - High IOP (40 to 80 mm Hg).
  - Middilated, sluggish, often irregular pupil.
  - Corneal edema.
  - Congested episcleral and conjunctival blood vessels.
  - Shallow AC.
  - AC cell and flare.
  - May have optic disk swelling.
- Intermittent:
  - Peripheral anterior synechiae.
  - During episodes, findings resemble acute ACG.
- Chronic:
  - PAS.
  - During episodes, findings resemble acute ACG.
  - The most frequent newly diagnosed ocular disease when glaucoma specialist enters region without prior glaucoma specialist care.
- "Glaukomflecken" are characteristic white anterior capsular opacities that represent focal necrotic lens epithelium remaining from prior angle-closure episodes.
- Gonioscopy of fellow eye shows a similar narrow, occludable angle.

Systemic Findings

Patients may present with abdominal pain, nausea, and vomiting in acute episodes.

Special Tests

- Compression gonioscopy to differentiate appositional from synechial angle closure (use Zeiss or Volk or Sussman four-mirror lens; Goldman three-mirror is inadequate for this test, since its large area of ocular contact suctions and distorts angle features).
- Provocative mydriatic test: compare predilation IOP with postdilation IOP. This is of controversial predictive value; an increase of 8 mm Hg is considered the upper limit of normal.
- DRPPT: Measure IOP in the maximum physiologic conditions that could precipitate angle closure (compare IOPs recorded at same body position).
- Anterior segment OCT and UBM may be useful in delineating the degree of angle closure in differing lighting conditions.

Pathology

Ganglion cell death similar to that seen in POAG.

Disease Course

- Depends on acute, intermittent, or chronic characteristics.
- In cases of acute angle closure, the untreated fellow eye has a 40% to 80% chance of developing acute angle closure over next 5 to 10 years. Prophylactic medical therapy with miotics does not significantly alter this course.
- "Mixed mechanism glaucoma": PACG leads to TM dysfunction and thus POAG-like disease course even after angle is anatomically reopened.

Treatment and Management

The definitive treatment is laser or surgical peripheral iridotomy (PI).

- Methods to facilitate laser PI:
  - Pretreat with argon laser, then Nd:YAG laser to open PI.
  - A sectoral pupilloplasty peaks the pupil or laser iridoplasty may relieve some pupillary block component (less congestion).
  - If attack broken medically, may wait until next day to perform PI, when less congestion is present.
- May need to reduce the IOP with other topical or systemic medications first, then use cholinergics.
- Globe compression (compression onto central portion of cornea only, since the goal is to force aqueous peripherally and open angle).
- Surgical paracentesis in extreme cases.
- Prophylactic laser iridotomy of contralateral eye (assuming similar anatomy) is highly recommended to decrease risk of future angle closure.
- Lensectomy/cataract extraction may need to be undertaken if the above treatments fail.

Medications

First, combination therapy with topical β-blockers, α_2-agonists, CAIs, prostaglandin analogues, and/or hyperosmotic systemic agents (e.g., mannitol). The goal is to relieve congestion until definitive therapy can be performed. Pilocarpine 1% may break mild attacks by inducing miosis which pulls peripheral iris away from the TM. However, it is often ineffective when pressure is high due to pupillary sphincter ischemia. Stronger miotics should be avoided and may, in fact, precipitate angle closure by advancing lens-iris diaphragm anteriorly. Nonselective adrenergic agonists (apraclonidine) should also be avoided due to vasoconstriction effects as this could worsen iris ischemia.

Follow-up

- Miotic therapy in fellow eye until prophylactic PI can be performed.
- There is a greater than 50% chance of developing angle closure in the fellow eye.

Differential Diagnosis

Always examine contralateral eye for narrow occludable angles, a key feature of PACG.

Secondary angle-closure glaucoma (SACG): Another ophthalmic disorder is identifiable as the etiology (see next section); the contralateral angle is nonoccludable.

Inflammatory open-angle glaucoma (glaucomatocyclitic crisis, Posner-Schlossman syndrome): has a more prominent component of aqueous inflammation; the contralateral eye has an open angle.

Traumatic glaucoma: history, angle recession, PAS.

POAG: no history or features of angle closure seen.

SOAG: angle is open; pigmentary or pseudoexfoliative features seen.

References

2007–2008 Basic and Clinical Science Course (BCSC), Section 10: Glaucoma. American Academy of Ophthalmology, San Francisco, 2007.

Erie JC, Hodge DO, Gray DT. The incidence of primary angle-closure glaucoma in Olmstead County, Minnesota. *Arch Ophthalmol* 1997;115:177–181.

Kim YY, Jung HR. Clarifying the nomenclature for primary angle-closure glaucoma. *Surv Ophthalmol* 1997;42:125–136.

Quigley HA, Broman AT. The number of people with glaucoma worldwide in 2010 and 2020. *Br J Ophthalmol* 2006;90:262–267.

Wilensky JT, Ritch R, Kolker AE. Should patients with anatomically narrow angles have prophylactic iridectomy? *Surv Ophthalmol* 1996;41:31–35.

Secondary Angle-Closure Glaucoma

A variety of ocular disorders may precipitate angle closure. Identifying and treating the underlying primary disorder is the definitive management. When both open-angle and closed-angle pathogenetic mechanisms are present (simultaneously or consecutively): "combined mechanism glaucoma."

There are two basic mechanisms of secondary angle closure:

- Iris root "pushed" anteriorly to close angle:
  - Lens-related.
  - Miotics.
  - Posterior segment masses or tumors.
  - Ciliary body swelling, choroidal effusion/hemorrhage, or ciliary-block glaucoma.
- Iris root "pulled" anteriorly to close angle:
  - Neovascularization of angle.
  - Inflammation.
  - ICE syndrome.

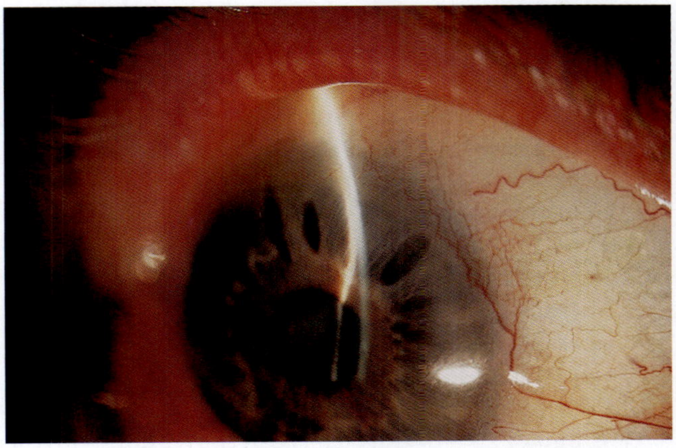

FIGURE 5.13. Iris bombe. Notice the anterior bowing of the iris and the apposition of the iris and cornea peripherally in the slit beam.

Etiology

- Anterior segment inflammation: may create posterior synechiae that adhere the iris pupillary margin to the lens, thus obstructing aqueous flow into the AC. The iris periphery then balloons outward in response to this increased pressure in the PC, creating an "iris bombe" configuration (Figure 5.13).
- Lens-induced glaucoma:
  - "Phacomorphic glaucoma": Enlargement of a hypermature lens may narrow the AC and precipitate angle closure.
  - Subluxed lens or microspherophakia may also cause angle closure.
  - AC intraocular lenses (IOLs) may occlude the pupil: Management is with PI and lens extraction as required.
- Postoperative flat AC: may lead to formation of PAS and permanent occlusion of angle.
- Drug-Induced: Topiramate (Topamax) is an oral antiepileptic, antidepressant, and headache therapy that can cause an acute syndrome of bilateral myopic shift, uniformly shallow AC, and elevated IOP from acute angle closure. Mechanism is choroidal effusion that causes profound rotation of the lens-iris diaphragm.
- Epithelial and fibrous downgrowth:
  - Occurs postoperatively when epithelium or other fibrovascular tissue migrates into the surgical wound and covers various anterior segment structures, including the TM.
  - Difficult to diagnose; flattened smooth-appearing iris surface that whitens with Argon laser treatment, but may need paracentesis specimen to confirm diagnosis (aqueous aspirate cytology).
- Miotics: may induce ACG by moving the lens-iris diaphragm anteriorly.
- Ocular trauma: may precipitate PAS formation and angle closure.
- Neovascular glaucoma.

- ICE syndrome.
- Posterior segment masses:
  - May mechanically force the lens-iris diaphragm anteriorly or stimulate angle neovascularization and thus close the angle (e.g., large ocular melanoma, large anterior uveal cysts).
  - Nonrhegmatogenous retinal detachments (RDs) may have an associated subretinal effusion or hemmorrhage that "pushes" the bullous RD anteriorly against the lens-iris diaphragm and thus narrows or closes the angle.
- Vitreoretinal disorders, other conditions:
  - Ciliary-block ("malignant") glaucoma: Aqueous humor is misdirected posteriorly into vitreous space.
  - Following panretinal photocoagulation, there may be ciliary body thickening and an anterior choroidal detachment that forces the lens-iris diaphragm anteriorly.
  - Severe central retinal vein occlusion (CRVO) may cause swelling of the choroid and ciliary body and thus shallow the AC.
  - Retinopathy of prematurity (ROP) is associated with cicatrization of retrolental tissue.
  - Persistent hyperplastic primary vitreous (PHPV) angle closure may be secondary to cataract and contracture of the primary vitreous.
- Nanophthalmos:
  - Has all the classic anatomic features (microphthalmia, hyperopia, small corneal diameter, thick sclera, narrow angles) that are susceptible to angle closure.
  - High incidence of angle closure.
  - High incidence of uveal effusions with intraocular surgery, which push lens-iris diaphragm forward. Avoid pilocarpine which can worsen pupillary block. Prophylactic sclerotomies can be used in select cases to prevent choroidal effusions.

Reference

Greenidge KC. Angle-closure glaucoma. *Int Ophthalmol Clin* 1990;30:177–186.

SECONDARY GLAUCOMA

Inflammatory Glaucoma

Uveitic Glaucoma

Summary

Ocular inflammation and uveitis can be associated with elevated IOP and glaucoma, which can involve an open or closed angle. Frequently, the cause of the inflammation is elusive (Table 5.1).

Table 5.1

Common causes of elevated intraocular pressure in acute uveitis
Herpes simplex virus
Varicella-zoster virus
Sarcoidosis
Posner-Schlossman syndrome
Fuchs heterochromic iridocyclitis

Etiology

- Open angle:
  - Trabecular obstruction with inflammatory cells, proteins, or other chemical mediators of the inflammatory process.
  - Trabeculitis.
- Closed angle (Figure 5.14):
  - Synechial angle closure.
  - Pupillary block from posterior synechiae.
- Steroid induced.

Signs and Symptoms

Pain.
Blurred vision.
Photophobia.

Demographics

Uveitis affects a wide variety of patients, depending on the specific disease entity.

Ophthalmic Findings

Anterior segment cells, aqueous flare, keratic precipitates.
Conjunctival hyperemia.
Keratitis.
Anterior and posterior synechiae.
Iris bombe.
Cataract.
Posterior segment inflammation (retinitis, vasculitis, choroiditis).
Macular edema.
Optic disk edema.
Sterile hypopyon.
Elevated IOP.

Systemic Findings

Arthritis (JRA, HLA-B27).
Skin lesions (herpes zoster, Behçet syndrome, Vogt-Koyanagi-Harada [VKH] syndrome, Lyme disease, sarcoid).
Pulmonary nodules (sarcoid).

Special Tests

HLA typing (HLA-B27).

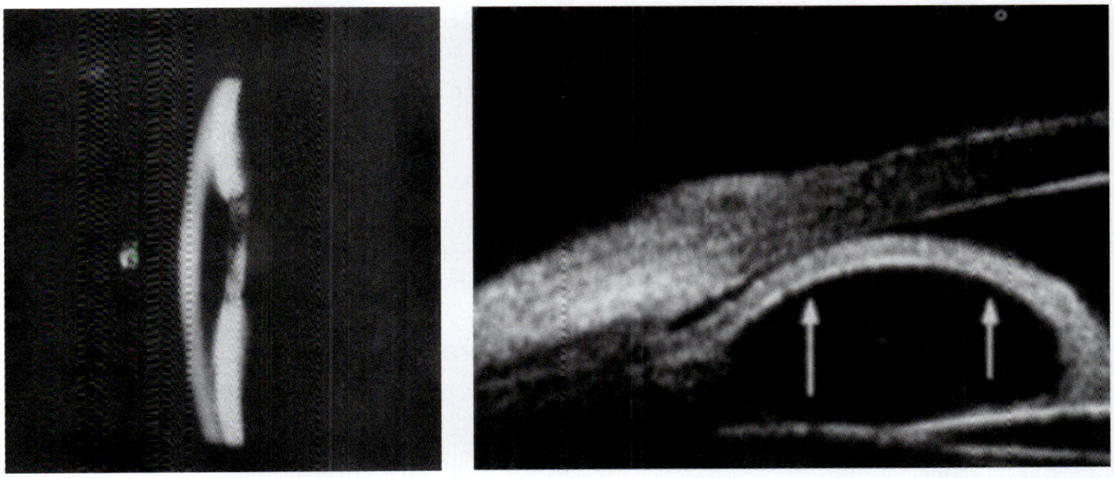

FIGURE 5.14 A, B Posterior synechiae at the pupillary margin prevent aqueous from entering the anterior chamber, resulting in iris bombe and angle closure. (Courtesy of Joel S. Schuman, MD.)

Chest x-ray.
Angiotensin-converting enzyme (ACE) and lysozyme.
Purified protein derivative (PPD) skin test.
Fluorescent treponemal antibody, absorbed (FTA-Abs) and Venereal Disease Research Laboratory (VDRL).
Antinuclear antibody (ANA).
Erythrocyte sedimentation rate (ESR).

Pathology

Tissues involved show signs of acute or chronic inflammation. Specific pathologic changes are highly dependent on disease entity.

Disease Course

- Acute process generally resolves within several months, but the glaucoma can linger if there are structural changes.
- Chronic uveitis and its sequelae can last several weeks to years and typically return after a quiescent period. The glaucoma can accompany acute exacerbations or remain as a result of chronic damage to outflow structures.

Treatment and Management

- Treat underlying cause of uveitis.
- Medical management of glaucoma.
- Surgical management of glaucoma (includes peripheral iridectomy, filtering procedures, ciliary body ablation, and aqueous shunt procedures).

Medications

1. Inflammation is treated with steroids (topical, subconjunctival, or systemic) and in severe cases with cytotoxic immunosuppressive agents.
2. Bacterial, viral, and parasitic causes are treated with appropriate antimicrobials.
3. Cycloplegic agents (atropine, scopolamine, phenylephrine) are used to break synechiae, treat ciliary pain, and stabilize the blood–aqueous barrier.
4. Glaucoma medications include β-blockers, α-agonists, and topical or oral CAIs. Miotics may cause breakdown of the blood–aqueous barrier and worsening of synechiae. Prostaglandins theoretically may worsen inflammation but are administered in very small concentrations. Prostaglandin analogues can also reactivate dendritic HSV keratitis or keratouveitis.

Follow-Up

Follow-up depends on the disease entity, but frequent visits are needed to assess IOP and inflammation.

Differential Diagnosis

Steroid-induced glaucoma: Elevated IOP can result from steroid treatment for ocular inflammation. The glaucoma usually remits following cessation of the steroids. Patients with POAG are more frequently steroid responders, and it may be difficult to separate the steroid effect from the primary glaucoma.

Reference

Moorthy RS, Mermoud A, Baerveldt G, et al. Glaucoma associated with uveitis. *Surv Ophthalmol* 1997;41:361–394.

Glaucomatocyclitic Crisis (Posner-Schlossman Syndrome)

Summary

This syndrome is an idiopathic open-angle inflammatory glaucoma occurring in young to middle-aged adults. It is typically unilateral and acute.

Etiology

- Actual pathogenesis is unknown but has been postulated to be due to an idiopathic trabeculitis. Herpesvirus infection has also been suggested.
- Prostaglandin-related vascular events may be related.
- Steroid-induced glaucoma.

Demographics

Ages 20 to 50 years.
Male and female patients equally affected.

Signs and Symptoms

Unilateral involvement.
Mild to moderate ocular pain.
Blurred vision.
Halos around lights.

Ophthalmic Findings

Keratic precipitates within 2 to 3 days of symptoms.
Little or no conjunctival hyperemia.
Corneal edema.
Elevated IOP, 40 to 70 mm Hg.
Few inflammatory cells.
Enlarged pupil in affected eye.

Systemic Findings

None.

Special Tests

- Tonography reveals decreased outflow facility in affected eye.
- Increase in aqueous humor production.

Pathology

Tissues involved show signs of acute or chronic inflammation. Specific pathological changes are highly dependent on disease entity.

Disease Course

Acute uveitis generally resolves within several months, but the glaucoma can linger if there are structural changes.

Treatment and Management

- Does not always necessitate long term or prophylactic treatment; in many cases the disease is self-limited.
- During the attack, IOP can be treated medically.

Medications

- Inflammation is treated with topical steroids and/or topical + systemic nonsteroidal anti-inflammatory drugs (NSAIDs).
- Glaucoma medications include β-blockers, α-agonists, and topical or oral CAIs. Prostaglandins theoretically may worsen inflammation but are administered in very small concentrations.

Follow-Up

The patient may be seen during attack recurrences and on a yearly basis to rule out development of open-angle glaucoma.

Differential Diagnosis

Uveitic glaucoma of other etiology.
Acute angle-closure glaucoma: The angle is closed in the involved eye and occludable in the fellow eye, pain is severe, no keratic precipitates.
Neovascular glaucoma: rubeosis iridis, pain is severe, synechial angle closure.
Pigmentary glaucoma: can also have an acute rise in IOP, especially after heavy exercise, accompanied by pigment release, heavily pigmented angle structures, radial iris transillumination defects.

References

Posner A, Schlossman A. Syndrome of unilateral recurrent attacks of glaucoma with cyclitic symptoms. *Arch Ophthalmol* 1953;39:517–535.

Raitta C, Vannas A. Glaucomatocyclitic crisis. *Arch Ophthalmol* 1977;95:608–612.

Fuchs Heterochromic Iridocyclitis

Summary

This syndrome is a chronic idiopathic inflammatory glaucoma associated with iris stromal atrophy and cataract. Presentation is often due to decreased vision secondary to cataract.

Etiology

Actual pathogenesis is unknown.

Demographics

- Usually unilateral, but can be bilateral in 13% of patients.
- Onset at ages 30 to 40 years.

Signs and Symptoms

Unilateral involvement.
No ocular pain.
Blurred vision.

Ophthalmic Findings

Stellate keratic precipitates diffusely scattered throughout cornea.

No conjunctival hyperemia.
Iris atrophy and heterochromia (involved eye is lighter, except in blue irides).
Elevated IOP, with 15% progressing to glaucoma.
Few inflammatory cells.
Cataract.
Fine blood vessels covering angle structures, which bleed when traumatized but do not cause synechial angle closure. Fine blood vessels can cause angle bleeding during intraocular surgery (Amsler's sign).

Systemic Findings

None.

Special Tests

Iris angiography reveals leakage from normal iris vessels.

Pathology

- Iris: reduction in the number of stromal melanocytes, degeneration of iris pigment epithelium, thickening of blood vessels.
- Inflammatory cells and membrane in the AC angle.

Disease Course

Chronic, smoldering iridocyclitis.
Gradual development of glaucoma and cataract.

Treatment and Management

- Do not treat iridocyclitis with long-term steroid therapy, since the inflammation is unresponsive to steroids.
- IOP can be treated medically but may eventually require surgery.
- Cataract extraction when necessary.

Medications

Glaucoma medications include β-blockers, α-agonists, and topical or oral CAIs. Prostaglandins theoretically may worsen inflammation but are administered in very small concentrations.

Follow-Up

The patient is followed up on a regular basis similar to follow-up for POAG.

Differential Diagnosis

Uveitic glaucoma of other origin.
JRA: occurs in younger patients and is often associated with joint disease.

Reference

Jones NP. Glaucoma in Fuchs heterochromic uveitis: etiology, management and outcome. *Eye* 1991;6:662–667.

Lens-Induced Glaucoma

Phacolytic Glaucoma

Summary

Phacolytic, or lens protein, glaucoma is caused by a blockage of the TM with lens proteins from an intact hypermature cataract.

Etiology

High molecular weight proteins leak through the intact lens capsule of a hypermature cataract. These proteins obstruct the aqueous outflow pathway, causing an elevated IOP. Macrophages ingesting the proteins and inflammatory debris may play a role in blocking the TM.

Demographics

Can be seen in any adult patient with a hypermature cataract.
Does not occur in children.

Signs and Symptoms

Decreased vision.
Moderate to severe ocular pain.
Halos around lights.

Ophthalmic Findings

See Figure 5.15.
Granulomatous keratic precipitates.
Significant conjunctival hyperemia.
Corneal edema.
Elevated IOP.
White cataract, may have white material on capsular surface or wrinkling of the anterior lens capsule.
AC flare.
The lens may be in place or dislocated into the vitreous.

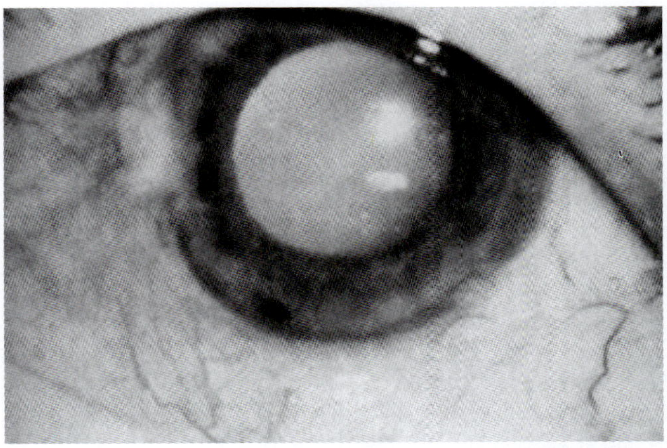

FIGURE 5.15. Phacolytic glaucoma. Hypermature cataract with leakage of lens proteins through the intact lens capsule. (From Epstein DL. Lens-induced open-angle glaucoma. In: Ritch R, Shields MB, eds. *The secondary glaucomas*. St. Louis, MO: Mosby, 1982:424, with permission.)

GLAUCOMA

Systemic Findings

None.

Special Tests

- Paracentesis shows engorged macrophages.
- High–molecular-weight proteins in aqueous humor.

Pathology

- Eosinophilic proteinlike material and engorged lipid-laden macrophages in the TM.
- The number of macrophages does not correspond to the severity of the glaucoma.

Disease Course

The glaucoma typically abates after cataract extraction.

Treatment and Management

- Reduce IOP by medical treatment.
- Reduce inflammation with topical steroids and cycloplegics.
- Cataract extraction following reduction in IOP and inflammation.

Follow-Up

The patient should be seen on the first postoperative day and regularly until the IOP normalizes.

Differential Diagnosis

Uveitic glaucoma.

Acute angle-closure glaucoma: The angle is closed in the involved eye and occludable in the fellow eye, pain is severe, no keratic precipitates.

Glaucomatocyclitic crisis: recurrent attacks of idiopathic inflammatory glaucoma without cataract.

Lens-particle glaucoma: history of lens trauma or surgery with retained lens particles and a violation of the capsule.

Reference

Flocks M, Littwin CS, Zimmerman LE. Phacolytic glaucoma: clinicopathologic study of 138 cases of glaucoma associated with hypermature cataract. *Arch Ophthalmol* 1955;54:37–47.

Lens-Particle Glaucoma

Summary

Lens-particle glaucoma is caused by retained lenticular material following trauma or surgery in which the lens capsule is violated.

Etiology

Liberated lens material obstructs the aqueous outflow pathway, causing an elevated IOP.

Demographics

Can be seen in any patient with lens material in the anterior or posterior chamber.

Signs and Symptoms

Decreased vision.
Moderate ocular pain.
Halos around lights.
Photophobia.
History of recent trauma, cataract surgery, or laser capsulotomy.

Ophthalmic Findings

See Figure 5.16.
Keratic precipitates.
Conjunctival hyperemia.

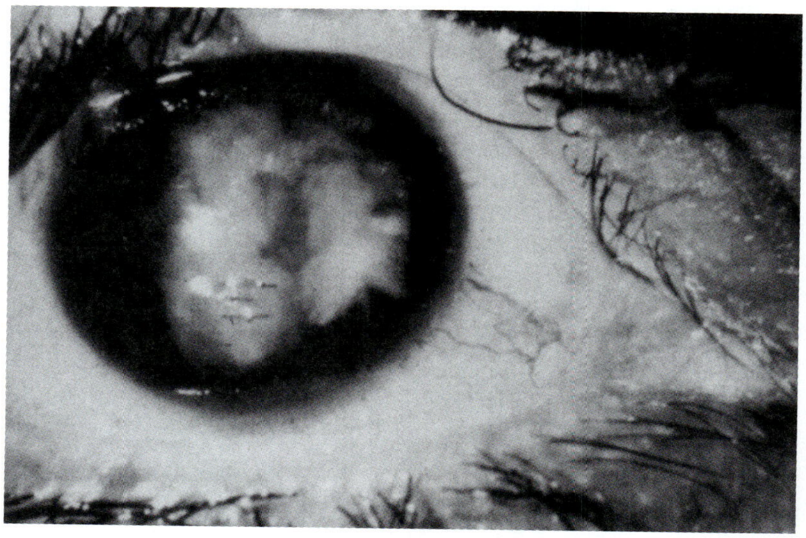

FIGURE 5.16. Lens-particle glaucoma. Retained lens fragments swell and occlude the outflow pathways. (From Epstein DL. Lens-induced open-angle glaucoma. In: Ritch R, Shields MB, eds. *The secondary glaucomas.* St. Louis, MO: Mosby, 1982:427, with permission. Courtesy of C. Davis Belcher III, MD.)

Corneal edema
Elevated IOP.
White fluffy lens material free in the anterior or posterior chamber.
AC flare.
Open AC angle by gonioscopy.

Systemic Findings

None.

Special Tests

None.

Pathology

Lens particles, inflammatory cells, and engorged macrophages are seen in the AC.

Disease Course

The glaucoma typically abates after removal of the lens particles.

Treatment and Management

- Reduce IOP by medical treatment.
- Reduce inflammation with topical steroids and cycloplegics.
- Remove lens particles via aspiration or vitrectomy for larger pieces of lens material.
- Examine optic nerve to assess damage and urgency of treatment.

Follow-Up

The patient should be seen frequently, especially during the first week.

Differential Diagnosis

Uveitic glaucoma.
Acute angle-closure glaucoma: The angle is closed in the involved eye and occludable in the fellow eye, pain is severe, no keratic precipitates.
Glaucomatocyclitic crisis: recurrent attacks of idiopathic inflammatory glaucoma without cataract.
Phacolytic glaucoma: mature or hypermature cataract with an intact lens capsule.
Infectious endophthalmitis: needs to be ruled out unless lens material is clearly visible.
Phacoanaphylactic glaucoma: absence of fluffy lens material, also follows trauma or surgery.

Reference

Epstein DL. Diagnosis and management of lens-induced glaucoma. *Ophthalmology* 1982;89:227–230.

Phacoantigenic Glaucoma

Summary

Phacoantigenic (phacoanaphylactic) glaucoma is a rare granulomatous inflammatory response to penetrating lens injury resulting from an immunologic response to lens protein.

Etiology

- Previously thought to be an immune rejection of previously sequestered lens material analogous to immune rejection of a foreign tissue transplant.
- Now hypothesized to be an immunologic disease resulting from a loss of normal immune tolerance to lens material.

Demographics

Can be seen in any patient after penetrating lens injury.

Signs and Symptoms

Decreased vision.
Moderate ocular pain.
Halos around lights.
Photophobia.
History of recent trauma, cataract surgery, or laser capsulotomy.

Ophthalmic Findings

Keratic precipitates (often granulomatous).
Conjunctival hyperemia.
Corneal edema.
Elevated IOP.
Synechiae formation.
AC flare.

Systemic Findings

None.

Special Tests

Aqueous aspiration shows polymorphonuclear neutrophils (PMNs).

Pathology

- Typical zonal granulomatous inflammation.
- The lens is surrounded by an inner layer of PMNs, a middle layer of multinucleated giant cells, and an outer layer of mixed mononuclear cells.

Disease Course

Without removal of the lens material, the glaucoma and inflammation worsen and may result in phthisis.

Treatment and Management

- Reduce IOP by medical treatment.
- Reduce inflammation with topical steroids and cycloplegics.
- Remove lens particles as soon as possible via aspiration or vitrectomy.

Follow-Up

The patient should be seen frequently, especially during the first week.

Differential Diagnosis

Toxic reactions to intraocular lens material or intracameral injections.
Lens particle glaucoma: fluffy white material in the AC.
Phacolytic glaucoma: mature or hypermature cataract with an intact lens capsule.
Infectious endophthalmitis: needs to be ruled out unless lens material is clearly visible.
Sympathetic ophthalmia: granulomatous panuveitis following ocular injury.

Reference

Marak GE. Phacoanaphylactic endophthalmitis. *Surv Ophthalmol* 1992;36:325–339.

Traumatic Glaucoma

Hyphema

Elevated IOP attributable to intraocular bleeding following eye trauma can be a result of hyphema, or later from ghost cell or hemolytic glaucoma. Spontaneous hyphema is managed differently and should alert one to coagulopathies, neovascularization, sickle cell disease, blood dyscrasias and, in children, juvenile xanthogranuloma.

Etiology

Hyphema: red blood cells in the AC obstruct the outflow pathway.

Demographics

Can be seen in any patient with blunt or penetrating ocular trauma, which is more common in young male patients.

Signs and Symptoms

Decreased vision.
Ocular pain.
Photophobia.
History of recent trauma.

Ophthalmic Findings

Hyphema: layered red blood cells (RBCs) or a blood clot in the AC.
Microhyphema: RBCs suspended in the aqueous humor.
Corneal blood staining.
Conjunctival hyperemia and edema.
Other signs of ocular trauma such as lens subluxation, ruptured globe, eyelid edema, and ecchymosis.

Systemic Findings

None.

Special Tests

- Hemoglobin electrophoresis in African American patients, especially those with spontaneous hyphema, mild ocular trauma, or IOP elevation that is out of proportion to hyphema or prolonged in nature.
- B-scan ultrasound if the posterior pole cannot be visualized.

Pathology

Blood and blood breakdown products are seen in the AC and outflow pathway tissues and in the corneal endothelium and stroma in corneal blood staining.

Disease Course

- The glaucoma typically resolves after spontaneous clearing of the blood.
- Rebleeding may occur and is most common at 3 to 7 days, when clot lysis and retraction occur. Rebleeding is estimated to occur in 5% to 10% of cases. This increases the risk of optic nerve damage, corneal blood staining, or vitreous hemorrhage. Risk factors for rebleeding include black race, patients using aspirin, those having systemic hypertension or ocular hypotony, or those presenting more than 24 hours after injury.
- Sickle cell disease may make the bleeding and the IOP elevation worse. The RBCs tend to become sickle shaped and rigid in the AC and are less able to be cleared through the outflow pathway.

Treatment and Management

- Medical management with aqueous suppressants, topical steroids, and cycloplegic agents to control inflammation and IOP. CAIs may worsen sickling of RBCs in patients with sickle cell disease by increasing aqueous ascorbic acid and thus changing the pH of the aqueous. Adrenergic agonists with α_1-agonist activity (epinephrine, dipivefrin, apraclonidine) should also be avoided in sickle cell patients because of their vasoconstriction effects which could cause anterior segment ischemia.
- Bed rest and elevation of the head of bed to promote layering of the blood. Bilateral patching may be indicated in severe cases (these are of unproven value).
- Surgical intervention is advised if there is a likelihood of optic nerve damage or corneal blood staining. Patients with sickle cell disease or prior glaucomatous optic atrophy should have a lower threshold for intervention.

AC washout without disturbing the clot is usually sufficient.

Surgical evacuation of the clot. This may increase the chance of rebleeding and should be approached with caution.

Trabeculectomy can afford temporary control of IOP and allow removal of RBCs or clot.

Medications

Glaucoma medications include β-blockers, α_2-agonists, hyperosmotics, and CAIs (avoid in sickle cell patients).

- Cycloplegia should be performed.
- Aminocaproic acid (50 mg/kg by mouth [p.o.] every 4 hours ×5 days) can be considered to prevent rebleeding but is usually unnecessary. It can cause postural hypotension and is contraindicated in patients with hepatic or renal disease, coagulopathies, cardiovascular or cerebrovascular disease, or pregnancy. Topical forms of this drug can be administered.
- Oral steroids can be used as an alternative to aminocaproic acid. A relatively high dose is needed: prednisone 1.5 to 2.0 mg/kg PO daily for clot stabilization.
- A topical form of aminocaproic acid (Caprogel) has been developed and studied for efficacy. Phase III, multicenter, placebo-controlled trial for use in traumatic hyphema provides evidence that Caprogel is safe and reduces rebleeding rates below that of placebo (authors do recommend a larger trial for more definitive conclusions).
- Tissue plasminogen activator (tPA) intracameral injection can accelerate the resolution of a hyphema, but may cause rebleeding.

Follow-Up

Follow-up examinations during the first week, 3 to 4 weeks after stabilization, and yearly. Examine the optic nerve for damage, the outflow structures for angle recession, and the rest of the eye for signs of traumatic damage.

Differential Diagnosis

1. Early:
   - Inflammatory cells and proteins causing increased IOP.
   - TM tears.
2. Late:
   - Traumatic angle recession: occurs later, characteristic gonioscopic appearance of widened ciliary body band.
   - Hemolytic glaucoma: Hemolytic debris and hemoglobin-filled macrophages block outflow.
   - Ghost cell glaucoma: Denatured RBCs from the vitreous block the outflow pathway when a break in the anterior hyaloid allows entrance into the AC.
   - Lens-induced glaucoma.
   - Epithelial or fibrous downgrowth: characteristic sheets of abnormal tissue covering and distorting structures.
   - Retinal detachment (Schwartz syndrome): Degenerated photoreceptor elements from an old RD block the outflow pathway.

References

Filipe JA, Barros H, Castro-Correia J. Sports-related ocular injuries: a three-year follow-up study. *Ophthalmology* 1997;104:313–318.

Pieramici DJ, Goldberg MF, Melia M, et al. A phase III, multicenter, placebo-controlled clinical trial of topical aminocaproic acid (Caprogel) in the management of traumatic hyphema. *Ophthalmology* 2003;110(11):2106–2112.

Sihota R, Sood NN, Agarwal HC. Traumatic glaucoma. *Acta Ophthalmol Scand* 1995;73:252–254.

Ghost Cell and Hemolytic Glaucoma

Summary

Ghost cell glaucoma occurs when degenerated RBCs from a vitreous hemorrhage gain access to the AC through a disrupted anterior hyaloid face and obstruct aqueous outflow. Hemolytic glaucoma usually follows a hyphema, and involves obstruction of the angle from blood breakdown products and hemosiderin-laden macrophages.

Etiology

Ghost cell: Ghost cells are RBCs that have lost their intracellular hemoglobin and are less pliable than normal RBCs. They gain entrance to the AC and obstruct the outflow pathway.

Hemolytic: Hemolytic debris from macrophages and the breakdown products of blood obstruct the TM.

Demographics

Can be seen in any patient with blunt or penetrating ocular trauma, which is more common in young male patients.

Signs and Symptoms

Decreased vision.
Ocular pain.
Photophobia.
History of trauma.

Ophthalmic Findings

Ghost cells (swollen, tan cells) or pigment-laden macrophages in the AC and angle (Figure 5.17).

Disrupted anterior hyaloid face.

Old hyphema.

Conjunctival hyperemia.

Other signs of ocular trauma such as angle recession, lens subluxation, ruptured globe, eyelid edema, and ecchymosis.

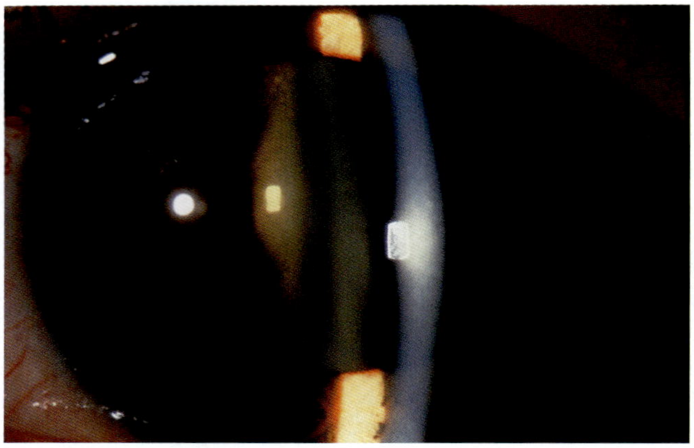

FIGURE 5.17. Ghost cell glaucoma. After a hyphema, degenerated red blood cells swell and do not traverse the trabecular meshwork as easily. Notice the layering of blood and khaki-colored cells. (From Tasman W, Jaeger E. *The Wills Eye Hospital atlas of clinical ophthalmology*, 2nd ed. Lippincott Williams & Wilkins, 2001.)

Systemic Findings

None.

Special Tests

- Cytologic examination of aqueous aspirate.
- Sickle preparation in African American patients.

Pathology

- Aqueous aspirate in hemolytic glaucoma shows pigment-laden macrophages.
- Aqueous aspirate in ghost cell glaucoma contains numerous degenerated "ghost cell" erythrocytes.

Disease Course

- Elevated IOP develops 3 to 4 weeks after a hemorrhage in the vitreous cavity.
- The severity of the glaucoma is related to the number of circulating ghost cells in the AC.
- Most cases can be treated with glaucoma medications.

Treatment and Management

- Medical management with topical β-blockers, α-agonists, CAIs (avoid in sickle cell patients), and prostaglandins.
- Topical steroids and cycloplegic agents to control inflammation.
- Surgical intervention is advised if the IOP cannot be controlled with medications. If the IOP is above 60 mm Hg (or 40 to 50 mm Hg for several weeks), surgery is probably needed to prevent corneal blood staining and to decrease IOP. Patients with prior optic nerve damage or corneal decompensation require surgical intervention earlier:

  AC washout of the ghost cells.

  Vitrectomy is sometimes necessary to remove the remaining ghost cells in the vitreous cavity.

Follow-Up

Frequent follow-up examinations during the first week, 3 to 4 weeks after stabilization, and yearly thereafter. Examine the optic nerve for damage, the outflow structures for angle recession, and the rest of the eye for signs of traumatic damage.

Differential Diagnosis

Inflammatory cells and proteins causing increased IOP.

Retinal detachment (Schwartz syndrome): Degenerated photoreceptor elements from an old RD block the outflow pathway.

Hemosiderotic glaucoma: results from a long-standing intraocular hemorrhage in which the hemosiderin from RBC breakdown is ingested by the trabecular endothelium and decreases their function by its toxic effects.

References

Montenegro MH, Simmons RJ. Ghost cell glaucoma. *Int Ophthalmol Clin* 1995;35:111–115.

Spraul CW, Grossniklaus HE. Vitreous hemorrhage. *Surv Ophthalmol* 1997;42:3–39.

Angle Recession

Summary

Ocular trauma results in a tear in the ciliary body which, if extensive enough, causes glaucoma by decreasing aqueous outflow.

Etiology

Damage to the TM from the traumatic angle recession results in decreased outflow of aqueous humor and glaucoma.

Demographics

- Can be seen in any patient with blunt or penetrating ocular trauma, which is more common in young male patients.
- Patients with a propensity to develop POAG may be more likely to develop glaucoma because of angle recession.

Signs and Symptoms

Unilateral glaucoma.

History of trauma.

Same signs and symptoms as open-angle glaucoma.

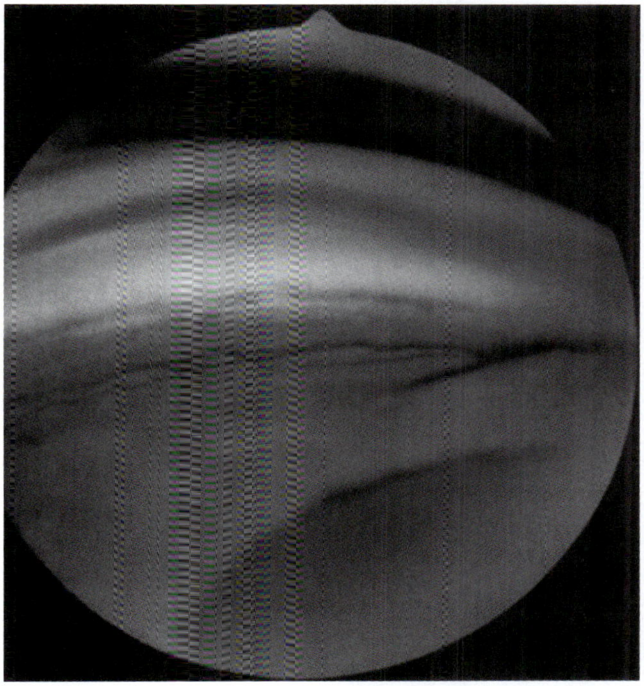

FIGURE 5.18. Angle recession following blunt trauma. The widened ciliary body band is apparent on gonioscopy. (From Epstein DL. *Chandler and Grant's glaucoma*, 4th ed. Baltimore, MD: Lippincott Williams & Wilkins, 1997:399 with permission.)

Ophthalmic Findings

- Deep chamber angle, asymmetric when compared with fellow eye.
- Widened gray ciliary body band on gonioscopy, sometimes intermittent (Figure 5.18).
- Torn iris processes.
- Other signs of ocular trauma such as angle recession, lens subluxation, ruptured globe, eyelid edema, and ecchymosis.

Systemic Findings

None.

Special Tests

None.

Pathology

- Recession occurs between the longitudinal and circular muscle layers of the ciliary body.
- A "glass membrane" may form over the angle as a late change of angle recession and may be an extension of Descemet membrane.

Disease Course

The risk of glaucoma is greater if 180 to 240 degrees or more of the angle is recessed.

Elevated IOP typically occurs late, even months to years following the injury.

Treatment and Management

- Medical management with topical β-blockers, α-agonists, CAIs, and prostaglandins.
- Laser trabeculoplasty is not helpful because of the nonfunctioning outflow structures and may make the glaucoma worse.
- Surgical intervention is advised if the IOP cannot be controlled with medications:
  - Trabeculectomy with antimetabolites because of the decreased success rate compared with filtering procedures in other glaucomas.
  - Aqueous shunt procedure.

Medications

Glaucoma medications include β-blockers, α-agonists, prostaglandins, and topical or oral CAIs. Miotics are not helpful because of the damage to the ciliary body and may make the glaucoma worse by decreasing uveoscleral outflow.

Follow-Up

Yearly visits with visual fields and optic nerve evaluation in patients with angle recession without glaucoma (treat as glaucoma suspects). If glaucoma develops, follow as a POAG patient. After the injury, examine the optic nerve for damage, the outflow structures for angle recession, and the rest of the eye for signs of traumatic damage.

Differential Diagnosis

Tears in TM: These can cause acute rises in IOP early after an injury.

Closure of a cyclodialysis cleft: A period of hypotony because of the cleft is followed by increased IOP after spontaneous or surgically induced closure.

Inflammatory cells and proteins causing increased IOP: occurs early after injury.

References

Salmon JF, Mermoud A, Ivey A, et al. The detection of post-traumatic angle recession by gonioscopy in a population-based glaucoma survey. *Ophthalmology* 1994;101:1844–1850.

Sihota R, Sood NN, Agarwal HC. Traumatic glaucoma. *Acta Ophthalmol Scand* 1995;73:252–254.

Neovascular Glaucoma

Summary

Growth of neovascular blood vessels over the angle leads to a fibrovascular membrane that contracts and closes the TM.

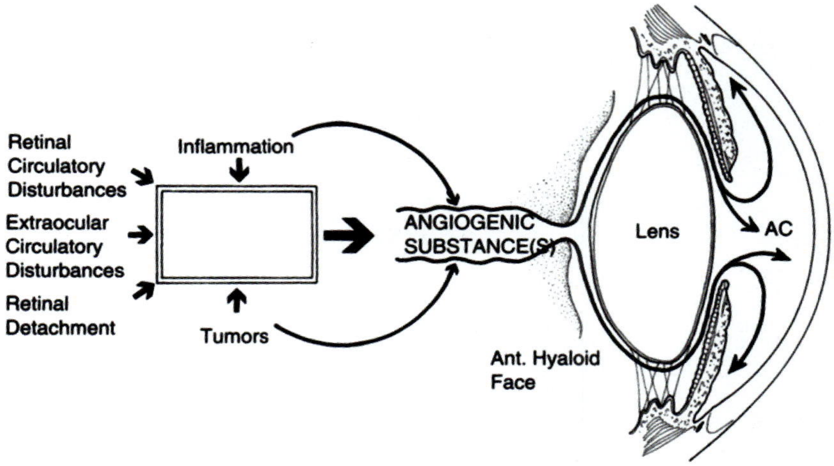

FIGURE 5.19. Diagram outlining causes of anterior segment neovascularization. (From Epstein DL. *Chandler and Grant's glaucoma*, 4th ed. Baltimore, MD: Lippincott Williams & Wilkins, 1997:311, with permission.)

Etiology

Neovascular glaucoma is classified as a secondary angle closure. Ocular tissue hypoxia (usually retinal ischemia) causes production of angiogenic factors (vascular endothelial growth factor, VEGF) that stimulate the formation of neovascular vessels in the iris and AC angle (Figure 5.19). Causes include:

- Central retinal vein occlusion.
- Proliferative diabetic retinopathy.
- Severe uveitis.
- Ocular ischemic syndrome (carotid artery insufficiency, after surgery on extraocular muscles, after irradiation).
- Central retinal artery occlusion.
- Intraocular tumors.
- Sickle cell disease.
- Retinal detachment.
- Eales disease.

Contraction of this fibrovascular membrane causes angle closure. With the formation of synechiae, angle closure becomes permanent and results in high elevations of IOP.

Demographics

Factors that cause ocular hypoxia:

- Retinal vascular occlusion: more common in patients with systemic hypertension.
- Proliferative diabetic retinopathy: more common in insulin-dependent diabetes, long-standing or poorly controlled diabetes.
- Anterior segment ischemia, patients who have undergone extraocular muscle surgery on more than two rectus muscles.
- Patients who have had irradiation for intraocular or head and neck tumors.

Smoking increases the risk of hypoxia in any disease.

Africans and African Americans are more likely to have a sickle cell hemoglobinopathy.

Cataract extraction, especially with unintentional or planned disruption of the posterior capsule, can increase the risk of anterior segment neovascularization by allowing the angiogenic factors access to the AC.

Signs and Symptoms

Decreased vision, halos around lights.
Severe ocular pain.
Photophobia.
Nausea and vomiting.
Can be asymptomatic.

Ophthalmic Findings

Neovascular blood vessels on the anterior iris surface and in the angle (Figures 5.20 and 5.21). Gonioscopy should be performed on all eyes at risk for neovascular glaucoma even without pupil/iris involvement, as 10% of CRVO patients develop NVA alone (without NVI).

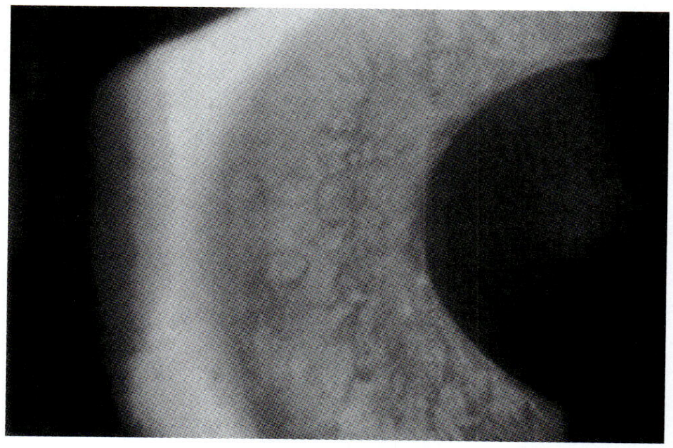

FIGURE 5.20. Iris neovascularization. (From Epstein DL. *Chandler and Grant's glaucoma*, 4th ed. Baltimore, MD: Lippincott Williams & Wilkins, 1997:313, with permission.)

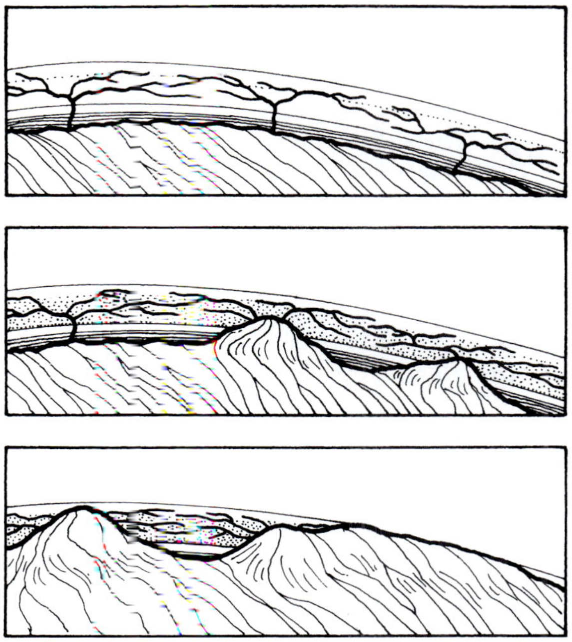

FIGURE 5.21. **A:** Early vessel growth in angle. **B:** Fibrovascular proliferation and synechiae. **C:** Extensive synechiae formation. Angle neovascularization. (From Epstein DL. *Chandler and Grant's glaucoma*, 4th ed. Baltimore, MD: Lippincott Williams & Wilkins, 1997:313, with permission.)

Synechial angle closure.
Hyphema.
Ectropion uveae.
AC inflammation.
Corneal edema.
Conjunctival hyperemia and edema.
Glaucomatous optic nerve atrophy and visual field loss.

Systemic Findings

Disease entities as listed above. Other signs of microvascular disease (transient ischemic attack [TIA], stroke, peripheral vascular disease, coronary artery disease, hypertension).

Special Tests

- Fluorescein angiogram (FA) to demonstrate retinal ischemia.
- Iris FA to demonstrate abnormal leaking iris neovascular vessels
- Carotid artery ultrasound to demonstrate insufficiency.
- Ophthalmic dynamometry to show ocular hypoperfusion.
- Hemoglobin electrophoresis if sickle cell disease is suspected
- B-scan ultrasound if the posterior pole cannot be visualized.

Pathology

1. Neovascular endothelial budding begins from iris capillaries and abnormal vessels with no muscularis layer, and little adventitia are seen in the iris and angle.
2. By electron microscopy, these vessels have gaps between and fenestrations in their endothelial cells.
3. Fibrovascular membrane consisting of myofibroblasts covers AC structures.
4. Contracture of membrane gives iris surface the characteristic flat configuration.
5. Further contraction results in ectropion uveae and obliteration of the angle by synechial closure.

Disease Course

If left untreated, the neovascularization progresses and causes total angle closure and intractable glaucoma. When adequate treatment is administered, the neovascularization may regress, but the damage to the angle and resultant glaucoma frequently remains. This is typically a very difficult disease to manage, and despite surgical treatment, many eyes continue to have glaucomatous damage. If the angle is open, greater chance exists to avoid surgery with early PRP and anti-VEGF therapy. Once the angle is closed, invariably surgical intervention becomes necessary.

Treatment and Management

1. Diagnosis and treatment of the underlying disease.
2. Panretinal photocoagulation (PRP) and anti-VEGF treatment (anterior chamber or intravitreal Avastin) to treat retinal ischemia and stop the production of angiogenic factor (VEGF). This is more successful if performed early when NVI develops and before permanent synechial closure has occurred. For CRVO, the Central Vein Occlusion Study showed that prophylactic PRP does not totally prevent iris and angle neovascularization and that prompt regression of the rubeosis is more likely to occur in response to PRP in eyes that were not previously treated. However, prophylactic PRP may still be considered before development of NVI/NVA in case of poor compliance/follow up.
3. Goniophotocoagulation is Argon laser treatment of NVA before the development of NVG. It is no longer done routinely but may be used in patients with high risk of developing NVG when PRP is not successful or is not possible.
4. Medical management with glaucoma medications, topical steroids, and cycloplegic agents to control inflammation and IOP.
5. Surgical intervention is often necessary:
   Trabeculectomy with antimetabolites has high failure rates but can be tried (71% success at 1 year, but only 28% successful at 5 years).
   Aqueous shunt procedure.

GLAUCOMA

Ciliary body ablation.
Retrobulbar alcohol injection to control pain in an eye with poor visual potential.
Enucleation for a blind, painful eye.

Follow-Up

Follow-up is usually daily until medical or surgical management has stabilized the disease.

Differential Diagnosis

Fuchs heterochromic iridocyclitis: Neovascularization can be seen in the iris and angle, but the eye is quiet, and synechial angle closure is not seen.
Exfoliation glaucoma: Neovascularization of the iris can be seen, but the eye is quiet and shows the deposition of fibrillar material characteristic of exfoliation syndrome.
Acute iridocyclitis: Inflammatory cells and debris can clog the TM, but neovascularization is generally not seen except in rare cases of chronic inflammation. Distinguish dilated radial iris vessels from superficial neovascular capillaries.
Angle-closure glaucoma: The presentation is identical, but there are no signs of neovascularization and the angle in the fellow eye is narrow and occludable.

References

The Central Vein Occlusion Study Group N report. A randomized clinical trial of early panretinal photocoagulation for ischemic central vein occlusion. *Ophthalmology* 1995;102:1434–1444.
Weber PA. Neovascular glaucoma: current management. *Surv Ophthalmol* 1981;26:149–153.

Steroid-Induced Glaucoma

Summary

Elevated IOP and glaucomatous optic nerve damage can occur as a result of the administration of topical, intravitreal, inhaled, systemic, or periocular (including skin) steroids.

Etiology

- A decrease in the outflow facility is seen with an open angle.
- Pathologic changes are seen in the endothelial cells of the trabecular meshwork and Schlemm's canal that leads to increased resistance to aqueous outflow.
- The underlying mechanism that causes steroid glaucoma is the subject of ongoing debate, but theories include the following:
  Increased deposition of glycosaminoglycans and proteoglycans in the TM that block aqueous flow (may be mediated through the TIGR/MYOC gene).
  Inhibition of phagocytosis by trabecular cells resulting in obstruction to aqueous flow.
  Steroids decrease the paracellular flow of aqueous through trabecular and Schlemm's canal cells by increasing the expression of cellular tight junction protein(s) and creating more intercellular junctions.
  Cytoskeletal rearrangement that increases trabecular resistance and may alter the function of trabecular cells.

Demographics

POAG: A high percentage of those with POAG (up to 80%) respond to corticosteroids with an increased IOP.
Age: Those under 10 years of age may be at increased risk.
Relatives of patients with POAG.
Diabetes.
High myopia.
Connective tissue diseases.

Signs and Symptoms

Similar to POAG, with asymptomatic visual field loss, optic nerve atrophy, and elevated IOP.

Ophthalmic Findings

Open angle.
Optic nerve atrophy.
Visual field loss.

Systemic Findings

The patient may have a systemic disease for which steroid treatment is necessary (asthma, organ transplantation) or even something as benign as a periocular dermatitis. All patients should be questioned regarding steroid use in any form.

Special Tests

Tonography reveals a decrease in outflow facility.

Pathology

- Accumulation of material in trabecular cells and Schlemm's canal cells.
- Changes in the cytoskeleton of trabecular cells from normal linear arrangement to stellate bundles.
- Increase in the number of tight junctions between Schlemm's canal endothelial and TM cells.

Disease Course

The glaucoma typically develops 2 to 6 weeks following steroid administration but can develop sooner. Once steroids are discontinued, the IOP elevation usually resolves in a time course that is similar to or slightly longer than the onset of elevation. If steroid use is continued, the glaucoma progresses and leads to optic nerve atrophy.

Treatment and Management

1. Discontinue the use of the corticosteroid, if possible.
2. Change to a less potent corticosteroid, or to a nonsteroidal anti-inflammatory agent. Preparations such as fluorometholone (FML), rimexolone (Vexol), or loteprednol (Lotemax) are less likely to raise IOP than prednisolone or dexamethasone or durezol.
3. Reduce the frequency of administration.
4. Glaucoma medications.
5. Surgical treatment with filtering procedures, aqueous shunts, or laser trabeculoplasty.
6. Prophylaxis: All patients should be questioned about steroid use of any kind; patients who need to use corticosteroids should have regular examinations (3 to 6 months) to detect glaucomatous changes.
7. A patient who develops steroid glaucoma after subconjunctival or sub-Tenon's injection of deposteroid may need to have the compound excised if the IOP remains elevated despite medical treatment.

Medications

- Glaucoma medications include β-blockers, α-agonists, prostaglandins, topical or oral CAIs, and miotics.
- Relative glaucoma risk of corticosteroids:
  Higher with a higher concentration of the same drug.
  Higher with an acetate or alcohol preparation (increased AC penetration with acetates).
  In general, the higher the anti-inflammatory effect of the steroid, the higher the risk of glaucoma (dexamethasone acetate > prednisolone acetate > dexamethasone alcohol > fluorometholone > prednisolone phosphate > rimexolone > medrysone).

Follow-Up

Follow-up is dictated by the severity of the disease. Once it has stabilized after discontinuation of the steroid, follow-up every 4 to 6 months is recommended. If steroid use is still needed, follow-up every 3 months is required if the IOP is stable.

Differential Diagnosis

POAG: does not have history of steroid use.

Uveitic glaucoma: This can be very difficult to distinguish from steroid glaucoma, and the two may also occur together. A patient with ocular inflammation treated with steroids may develop an elevated IOP as a result of the inflammation itself or the steroid. The IOP may be higher when inflammation is at its greatest, or may be low as a result of ciliary body inflammation and decreased aqueous production. Many of these patients require filtering surgery or aqueous shunts to enable adequate treatment of the inflammatory disease without exacerbation of steroid glaucoma.

Reference

Moorthy RS, Mermoud A, Baerveldt G, et al. Glaucoma associated with uveitis. *Surv Ophthalmol* 1997;41:361–394.

Malignant Glaucoma

Summary

Malignant glaucoma is a secondary angle-closure glaucoma that presents postoperatively with axial shallowing of the AC and forward displacement of the lens in the presence of a patent peripheral iridectomy.

Etiology

- Uniform flattening of the central and peripheral AC in contrast to pupillary block angle closure that narrows the peripheral angle.
- Angle narrowing causes elevated IOP.
- A patent iridectomy must be present to make the diagnosis and exclude pupillary block.
- The presence of suprachoroidal effusion or hemorrhage must be ruled out.
- The underlying mechanism that causes AC shallowing is unclear, but there are different theories:
  Aqueous misdirection: The aqueous is diverted posteriorly and pushes the vitreous forward, which shallows the AC by its mass effect.
  Anterior hyaloid: A decreased permeability of the anterior hyaloid results in the inability of fluid to perfuse into the AC and an increase in total vitreous volume, which shallows the AC.
  Ciliochoroidal effusion: Fluid in the ciliary body causes forward rotation of the ciliary processes and iris root, closing the angle. The effusion also causes a reduction in the diameter of the ciliary ring, leading to zonular laxity and forward movement of the lens, which shallows the AC and worsens the angle closure.
  Ciliary block: The lens equator comes into contact with the ciliary processes and blocks the flow of aqueous humor into the AC, forcing it into the vitreous cavity.

Demographics

Associated with small, hyperopic eyes.
History of chronic or acute angle closure.
History of recent ocular surgery.

Signs and Symptoms

Decreased vision, halos around lights.
Severe ocular pain.
Photophobia.
Nausea, vomiting.

Ophthalmic Findings

Shallow AC in the presence of a patent PI.
No choroidal effusion.
Highly elevated IOP: In the presence of a filtering bleb, the IOP may be normal or only mildly elevated but is higher than expected for an early postoperative trabeculectomy.
Conjunctival hyperemia.
AC inflammation.
Corneal edema.

Systemic Findings

None.

Special Tests

UBM of the anterior segment may show the vitreous face pushing the lens forward.

Pathology

Changes associated with high IOP and glaucomatous damage.

Disease Course

- If left untreated, the glaucoma progresses and leads to optic nerve atrophy.
- This condition mandates early medical and surgical intervention.

Treatment and Management

- Peripheral iridectomy, enlargement of existing PI, or creation of a more peripheral PI.
- Cycloplegia with short- and long-acting agents.
- Glaucoma medications and hyperosmotic agents.
- YAG laser disruption of the anterior hyaloid in aphakic or pseudophakic eyes. Argon laser photocoagulation of ciliary processes has been reportedly successful to treat this condition.
- Definitive treatment is vitrectomy with disruption of the anterior hyaloid and reformation of the AC. An iridozonulohyaloidectomy is useful in resolution of this condition.
- Long-term management with cycloplegic agents.
- Prophylactic PI in fellow eye.
- If fellow eye undergoes intraocular surgery, use viscoelastic material to prevent AC decompression when entering the eye.

Follow-Up

Follow-up is usually daily until medical or surgical management has stabilized the disease.

Differential Diagnosis

Angle-closure glaucoma secondary to pupillary block: The presence of a patent peripheral iridectomy rules this out, but verify that the PI is patent and peripheral enough so that it is not touching the lens.
Suprachoroidal hemorrhage: can be ruled out by B-scan ultrasound or UBM.
Suprachoroidal effusion: usually presents with hypotony, and can be ruled out by B-scan ultrasound or UBM.
Glaucoma following scleral buckle: Procedure may cause a suprachoroidal effusion and narrowing of the angle and AC.
"Loose lens" syndrome: In eyes with zonular laxity, when the diameter of the ciliary ring is decreased, as in a choroidal effusion or after administration of miotics, the zonular tension is released and the lens becomes mobile. Since it cannot be displaced posteriorly, because of the vitreous face, it moves anteriorly and causes pupillary block and axial shallowing of the AC.

References

Chandler PA, Simmons RJ, Grant WM. Malignant glaucoma: medical and surgical treatment. *Am J Ophthalmol* 1968;66:495–502.
Shaffer RN, Hoskins HD. Ciliary block (malignant) glaucoma. *Trans Am Acad Ophthalmol Otolaryngol* 1978;85:215–221.

Iridocorneal Endothelial Syndrome

Summary

ICE syndrome is a spectrum of diseases with three major clinical findings:
Essential iris atrophy: atrophic changes in the iris associated with glaucoma and resulting in heterochromia, corectopia, ectropion uveae, and hole formation.
Chandler syndrome: less extreme iris atrophy coupled with abnormalities of the angle and corneal endothelium likened to the appearance of beaten silver. Most common form of the three variants, accounting for 50% of ICE syndrome cases.
Cogan-Reese (iris nevus) syndrome: multiple iris nodules mimicking the appearance of iris nevi.

Etiology

Histopathologic, clinical, and molecular biological analyses point to an underlying corneal endothelial abnormality in the spectrum of diseases comprising the ICE syndrome. Normally, the endothelium remains confined to the posterior corneal surface seemingly held in place by contact inhibition. In the ICE syndrome, however, these cells migrate posteriorly over the AC angle and onto the iris surface and form multiple layers.

An alternative hypothesis is that the TM, iris, and corneal endothelium are all primarily involved. Trabecular cells normally exert contact inhibition on the corneal endothelium to prevent its migration. Derangement

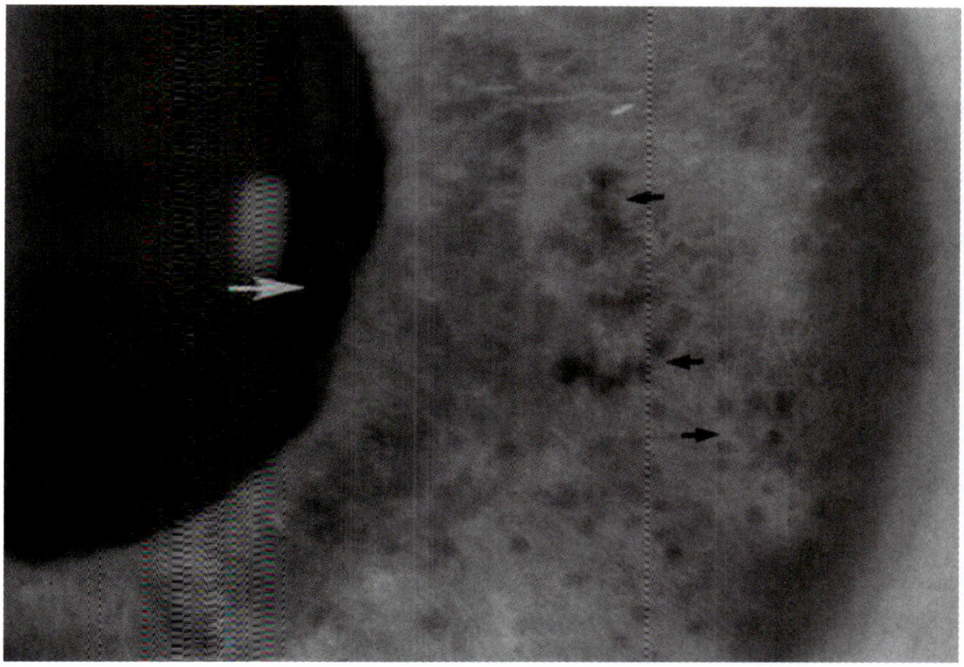

FIGURE 5.22. Pigmented iris nodules in the iridocorneal endothelial syndrome (*black arrows*) and ectropion uveae (*white arrow*). (From Shields MB. *Textbook of glaucoma*, 4th ed. Baltimore, MD: Lippincott Williams & Wilkins, 1998, with permission.)

of trabecular or iris cells may be the cause of endothelial migration in the ICE syndrome.

Studies of the chronology of Descemet membrane changes in ICE patients suggest that it may be an acquired disease. A viral origin with herpes simplex virus has been proposed.

Demographics

Unilateral.
Presents between 20 and 50 years of age.
More common in women.

Signs and Symptoms

Decreased vision.
Ocular pain.
Glare.

Ophthalmic Findings

- Corneal edema develops when cell migration results in a marked decrease in cell density and when dysfunctional endothelial cells are no longer able to maintain an optically clear deturgesced cornea.
- High peripheral anterior synechiae and membrane obstruction of the TM lead to the impediment of aqueous outflow, an elevation of IOP, and typical glaucomatous optic atrophy.
- Iris nevi are formed by contracture of the membrane around islands of normal iris stroma (Figure 5.22).
- Corectopia, polycoria, and ectropion uveae also result from contraction of the endothelial membrane and mechanical pulling of underlying tissues (Figure 5.23).

Systemic Findings

None.

Special Tests

- Polymerase chain reaction study of aqueous humor may show evidence of herpesvirus DNA.
- Specular microscopy can show changes in the corneal endothelium.

Pathology

- The corneal endothelium in patients with the ICE syndrome shows marked alteration of cell size, shape, and

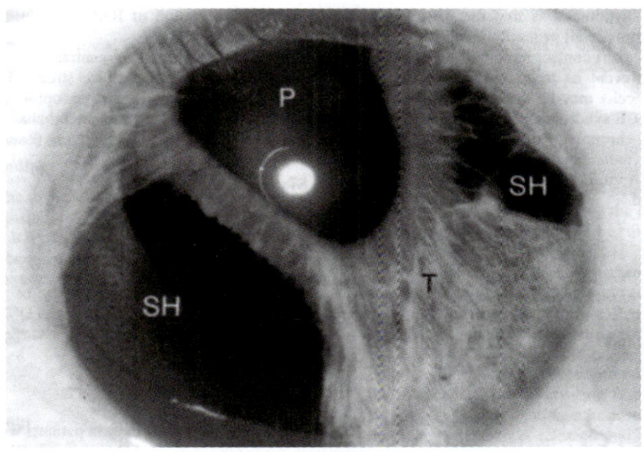

FIGURE 5.23. Eccentric pupil (*P*) and iris atrophy with stretch holes (*SH*) in the iridocorneal endothelial syndrome. (*T*, iris tissue) (From Shields MB. *Textbook of glaucoma*, 4th ed. Baltimore, MD: Lippincott Williams & Wilkins, 1998, with permission.)

GLAUCOMA

density. There is a great disparity in cell size with intermingling of large and small cells.

- Examination of the corneal endothelial apical cell surface demonstrates a variety of abnormalities. The normal intercellular border is rather narrow and formed by flat, undulating, and overlapping cell margins. In contrast, the cell borders in ICE syndrome are prominent as a result of the formation of numerous fingerlike interdigitating processes.
- Occasional lymphocytes provide evidence of a low-grade, chronic inflammation, and their presence is the source of a proposed viral cause for this disorder.
- The AC angle exhibits a cellular matrix composed of endothelial cells and a tissue resembling Descemet membrane that appears to extend posteriorly from the cornea.
- The iris nevi are composed of normal iris stroma and are also found with a surrounding endothelial membrane. These are presumably formed as the membrane surrounds a portion of normal iris stroma and contracts, creating a "pinched-off" elevated iris nodule.

Disease Course

The disease may be stable or slowly progress to glaucoma and corneal clouding. Glaucoma ultimately develops in 50% of patients with ICE syndrome and is more severe in the progressive iris atrophy and Cogan-Reese variants.

Treatment and Management

1. Glaucoma medications.
2. Filtering surgery or an aqueous shunt may be needed to treat the glaucoma, but trabeculectomy has a higher risk for failure attributable to migration of the endothelial membrane over the sclerostomy.
3. Hypertonic saline solution to treat corneal edema.
4. Corneal transplantation may be necessary for severe corneal clouding but should be undertaken only after the glaucoma is controlled.

Follow-Up

Follow-up when glaucoma is present depends on the severity of the disease but is usually every 1 to 3 months. If no glaucoma is present and the disease is stable, follow-up every 4 to 12 months is advised.

Differential Diagnosis

Fuchs endothelial dystrophy: lack of AC angle, iris, or synechiae findings.

Posterior polymorphous dystrophy (PPMD): similar corneal endothelial appearance; however, PPMD is bilateral and the endothelial abnormalities show a clear demarcation between zones of normal and epithelium-like cells.

The iris nevi can be mimicked by the Lisch nodules of neurofibromatosis, iris "tapioca" melanomas, melanosis of the iris, and even sarcoidosis.

Iris atrophy may be seen in anterior segment ischemia, herpetic keratouveitis, and other infectious and traumatic processes.

Axenfeld-Rieger syndrome: iris and angle abnormalities similar to ICE, but is bilateral, congenital, and often associated with systemic findings.

References

Chandler PA. Atrophy of the stroma of the iris: endothelial dystrophy, corneal edema, and glaucoma. *Am J Ophthalmol* 1956;41:607–615.

Cogan DG, Reese AB. A syndrome of iris nodules, ectopic Descemet's membrane, and unilateral glaucoma. *Doc Ophthalmol* 1969;26:424–432.

Eagle RC, Jr, Font RL, Yanoff M, et al. Proliferative endotheliopathy with iris abnormalities: the iridocorneal endothelial syndrome. *Arch Ophthalmol* 1979;97:2104–2111.

Congenital Glaucoma

Summary

Developmental abnormalities of the AC angle lead to obstruction of aqueous outflow and subsequent glaucoma that is present at birth or within the first few years of life.

Etiology

See Table 5.2.

- Classified as a developmental glaucoma.
- The common denominator in congenital glaucomas is a developmental abnormality of the outflow pathway, which physically obstructs the egress of aqueous in an open-appearing angle.

Demographics

Isolated congenital glaucoma is seen in approximately 1 per 10,000 live births.

Isolated trabeculodysgenesis is seen in 50% of patients with congenital glaucoma.

Cases are 90% sporadic, 10% autosomal recessive.

Bilateral in 75%.

Male patients, 65%; female patients, 35%.

Signs and Symptoms

Excessive tearing.

Blepharospasm.

Photophobia.

Ocular pain.

Irritability, crying (especially when exposed to light).

Decreased vision.

Ophthalmic Findings

Corneal edema.

Table 5.2

Hoskins' anatomic classification of developmental glaucomas

I. Isolated trabeculodysgenesis (malformation of trabecular meshwork in the absence of iris or corneal abnormalities)
  A. Flat iris insertion
    1. Anterior insertion
    2. Posterior insertion
    3. Mixed insertion
II. Iridotrabeculodysgenesis (trabeculodysgenesis with iris abnormalities)
  A. Anterior stromal defects
    1. Hypoplasia
    2. Hyperplasia
  B. Anomalous iris vessels
    1. Persistence of tunica vasculosa lentis
    2. Anomalous superficial vessels
  C. Structural anomalies
    1. Holes
    2. Colobomas
    3. Aniridia
III. Corneotrabeculodysgenesis (usually has associated iris anomalies)
  A. Peripheral
  B. Midperipheral
  C. Central
  D. Corneal size

Corneal stromal opacity and scarring attributable to Haab striae (horizontal breaks in Descemet membrane) (Figure 5.24)
Glaucomatous optic nerve atrophy and visual field loss.
Enlarged eye (buphthalmos).
Iris stromal hypoplasia.

Systemic Findings

Usually, no systemic abnormalities in isolated congenital glaucoma.

Special Tests

Diagnosis and evaluation of treatment usually require examination under anesthesia, paying special attention to the following:

Corneal diameters.
Gonioscopic appearance of the angle.
Optic nerve evaluation.
IOP.

Pathology

Flat iris insertion: The iris inserts into the TM anterior to the scleral spur.

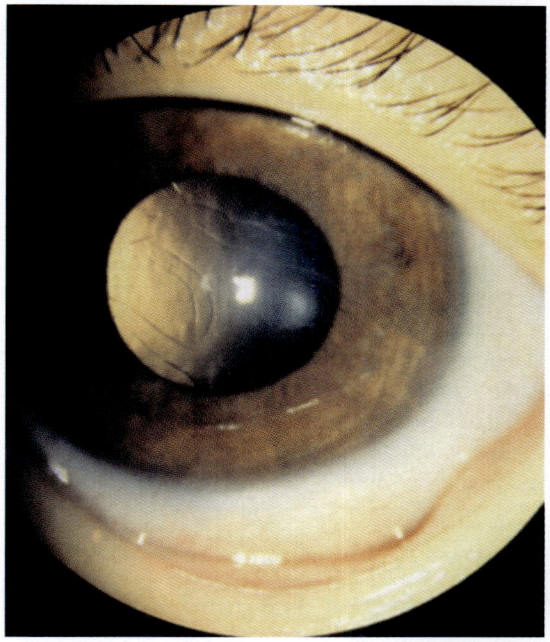

FIGURE 5.24. Breaks in Descemet membrane (Haab striae) as seen in congenital glaucoma. (From Epstein DL. *Chandler and Grant's glaucoma*, 4th ed. Baltimore, MD: Lippincott Williams & Wilkins, 1997:589, with permission.)

Wraparound iris: The iris is concave peripherally but sweeps up and over the TM with a "Barkan membrane."
TM: trabecular beam thickening, compression of trabecular spaces.

Disease Course

- If left untreated, the glaucoma progresses and the eye enlarges, causing buphthalmos and blindness.
- This is typically a very difficult disease to manage; despite surgical treatment, many eyes continue to have glaucomatous damage.
- Some patients have continued maturation of angle structures leading to a halt in the progression of the disease.
- Prognosis improves the later the disease presents in life.

Treatment and Management

See Figure 5.25.

1. Medical management with glaucoma medications, but definitive treatment is surgical.
2. Surgical intervention is usually necessary:
   Goniotomy if there is a clear view and obstructing membrane.
   Trabeculotomy.
   Trabeculectomy with antimetabolites.
   Aqueous shunt procedure.
   Ciliary body ablation as a last resort.
3. If monocular, aggressive treatment of axial myopia and resultant amblyopia is mandated.

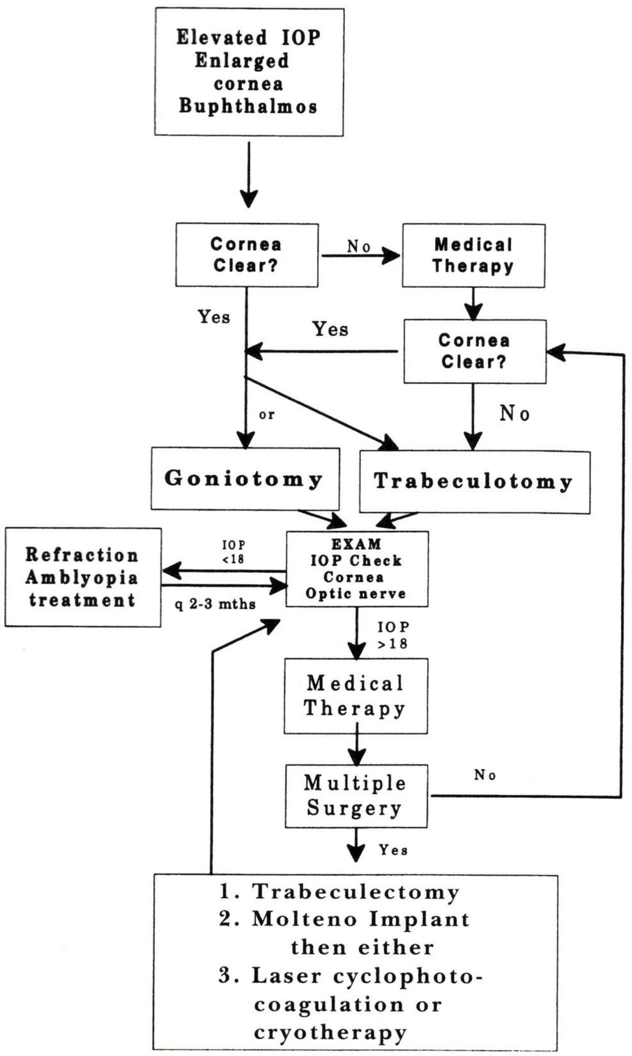

FIGURE 5.25. Treatment flow chart for congenital glaucoma. (From Epstein DL. *Chandler and Grant's glaucoma*, 4th ed. Baltimore, MD: Lippincott Williams & Wilkins, 1997:606, with permission.)

Follow-Up

- Follow-up is frequent until medical or surgical management has stabilized the disease.
- Examination under anesthesia should be performed every 3 to 6 months after stability is reached.
- Lifelong follow-up is needed, as many patients have recurrence.

Differential Diagnosis

- Nasolacrimal duct obstruction causes epiphora.
- Ocular or periocular infection or inflammation (dacryocystitis, canaliculitis, conjunctivitis) can cause redness and epiphora.
- Megalocornea is an X-linked condition with corneal enlargement in the absence of elevated IOP, Haab striae, and optic atrophy.
- Heritable corneal dystrophies and metabolic diseases can cause corneal clouding.
- Forceps trauma during birth can cause corneal tears (usually vertical).

Reference

Wagner RS. Glaucoma in children. *Pediatr Clin North Am* 1993;40:855–867.

Glaucoma and Elevated Episcleral Venous Pressure

Summary

Conditions that cause increased episcleral venous pressure (EVP) secondarily elevate the IOP and cause glaucomatous changes. Signs of elevated EVP can be obvious, as in a carotid-cavernous sinus fistula, or very subtle, as in dural shunts or Sturge-Weber syndrome.

Etiology

See Table 5.3.

Any condition causing elevated EVP (from venous obstruction, arteriovenous anomalies, or an idiopathic variant) can cause this type of glaucoma.

Demographics

Can be seen in any patient with the predisposing conditions, including trauma as a cause of arteriovenous anomalous shunts.

Table 5.3

Classification of elevated EVP

1. Venous obstruction
   a. Retrobulbar tumor
   b. Thyroid ophthalmopathy
   c. Superior vena cava syndrome (mediastinal tumor)
   d. Congestive heart failure
   e. Thrombosis of cavernous sinus or orbital vein
   f. Vasculitis involving episcleral or orbital vein
   g. Jugular vein obstruction
2. Arteriovenous anomalies
   a. Carotid-cavernous sinus fistula
   b. Orbital varix
   c. Sturge-Weber syndrome
   d. Orbital meningeal shunts
   e. Carotid jugular venous shunts
   f. Intraocular vascular shunts
3. Idiopathic
   a. Sporadic
   b. Familial

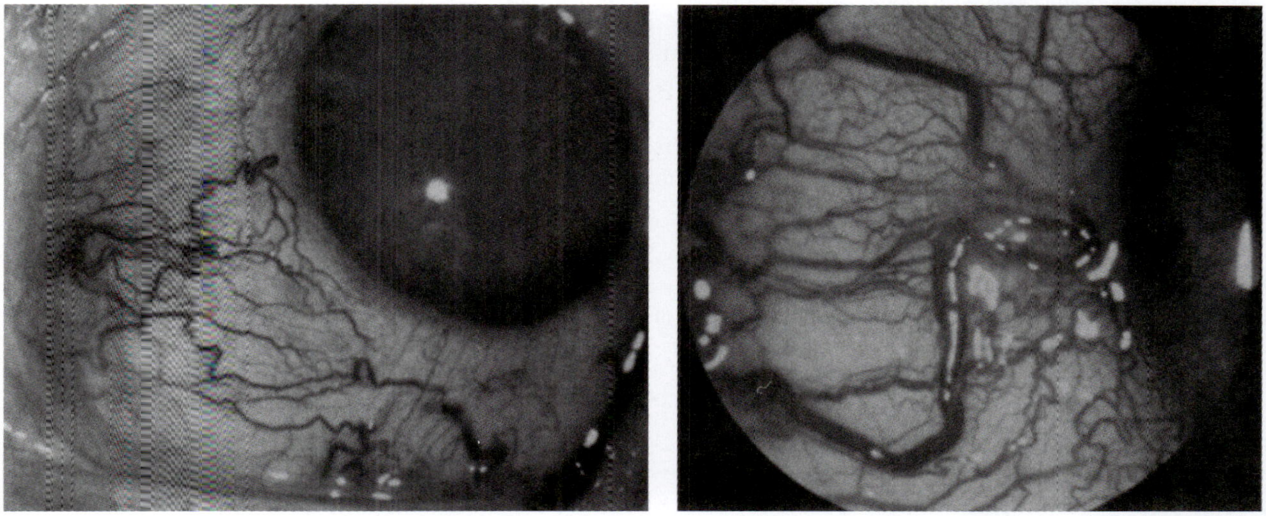

A B

FIGURE 5.26. A, B: Dilated episcleral vessels in Sturge-Weber syndrome. (From Epstein DL. *Chandler and Grant's glaucoma*, 4th ed. Baltimore, MD: Lippincott Williams & Wilkins, 1997:417, with permission.)

Signs and Symptoms

Head pain.
Ocular pain.
Red eye.
History of recent trauma.
Pulsating sensation and "whooshing" sound in the ears.

Ophthalmic Findings

- Dilated episcleral vessels and arterialization of conjunctival vessels (Figure 5.26).
- Exophthalmos with or without pulsations.
- Elevated IOP.
- Facial hemangioma of Sturge-Weber syndrome.
- Angle closure is possible.
- Signs of thyroid ophthalmopathy.
- Signs of arterial insufficiency such as AC cell and flare, extraocular muscle palsy, or neovascularization.
- Blood in Schlemm's canal on gonioscopy.

Systemic Findings

Sturge-Weber syndrome (encephalotrigeminal angiomatosis): typically unilateral facial cutaneous hemangioma (port-wine stain), cavernous hemangioma of the choroid, or leptomeningeal angiomas with ipsilateral seizures. Glaucoma in 30% to 70% of children with this syndrome. Increased risk of glaucoma with upper eyelid involvement.
Thyroid disease.
Pulmonary venous obstruction.
Superior vena cava obstruction.

Special Tests

- EVP can be measured with a device that applies pressure to flatten an episcleral vein.
- Outflow facility should be normal, except late in the disease.
- Arteriovenous anomalies can be demonstrated by magnetic resonance angiography (MRA) or cerebral angiography.

Pathology

The typical changes associated with glaucoma are seen in the eye.

Disease Course

The glaucoma progresses unless the primary condition is resolved or until the IOP can be brought under control medically or surgically if the underlying cause is not amenable to treatment.

Treatment and Management

1. Treatment of underlying causative condition.
2. Medical management of the elevated IOP.
3. Surgical intervention is advised if IOP cannot be managed medically and the underlying condition cannot be treated directly. Filtering surgery or tube shunt procedures are recommended over laser trabeculoplasty. However, these patients are at greater risk for choroidal hemorrhage or detachment and may require prophylactic posterior sclerostomies before the AC is entered.

Follow-Up

Follow up examinations frequently, until the cause is addressed or until the IOP is adequately managed. Follow up when stable is the same as for any stable glaucoma.

Differential Diagnosis

Inflammatory glaucomas: present not only with conjunctival and episcleral hyperemia but also with signs of anterior segment inflammation.

Angle-closure glaucoma: painful, red eye but angle is closed, in contrast to the open angle usually seen in glaucoma with elevated EVP.

Reference

Iwach AG, Hoskins HD, Jr, Hetherington J, Jr, et al. Analysis of surgical and medical management of glaucoma in Sturge-Weber syndrome. *Ophthalmology* 1990;97:904–909.

MEDICAL MANAGEMENT OF GLAUCOMA

See Table 5.4.

Adrenergic Agonists

Nonselective α-Adrenergic and β-Adrenergic Agonist

Epinephrine.
Dipivefrin (Propine).

Mechanism of Action

- IOP-lowering effect is a result of the balance between α-adrenergic and β-adrenergic stimulation.
- α-Adrenergic stimulation: Vasoconstriction in ciliary processes decreases ultrafiltration pressure and indirectly decreases aqueous humor formation.
- β-Adrenergic stimulation: increases aqueous production in ciliary epithelium, and stimulation of ciliary muscles increases uveoscleral outflow and trabecular outflow.

Common Side Effects

Systemic: hypertension, tachycardia, arrhythmia, headaches, nervousness.

Ocular: rebound conjunctival hyperemia, allergic blepharoconjunctivitis (20%).

Mydriasis: precipitates or aggravates angle closure.

Adrenochrome deposits from oxidized metabolites in the conjunctiva, cornea, and lacrimal system; also stains contact lenses.

Madarosis.

Cystoid macular edema in aphakics (10% to 20%), cause unknown.

Clinical Indications

- Good as a primary agent in asthmatic patients.
- Preferred over miotics in patients with cataracts; dilation improves the view.
- Preferred for young patients over pilocarpine, since it does not induce myopia.
- Used to sustain dilation during surgery.

Table 5.4

Common glaucoma medications

Class and drug name	Dosing	Mechanism of action	Common side effects
Adrenergic agonists (nonselective)			
Epinephrine 0.5%, 1%, 2%	b.i.d.	Decrease aqueous production, increase uveoscleral and trabecular outflow	Adrenochrome deposits, allergy, cystoid macular edema
Dipivefrin 0.1%	b.i.d.		
Adrenergic agonists (α-2 selective)			
Apraclonidine 0.5%, 1%	t.i.d.	Decrease aqueous production	Allergy, tachyphylaxis
Brimonidine 0.2%	t.i.d.		
β-Blockers (nonselective)			
Timolol 0.25%, 0.5%	q.d., b.i.d.	Decrease aqueous production	Hypotension, bradycardia, exacerbation of asthma, altered response to hypoglycemia in diabetics
Levobunolol 0.25%, 0.5%	b.i.d.		
Carteolol 1.0%	b.i.d.		
Metipranolol 0.3%	b.i.d.		
β-Blockers (β-1 selective)			
Betaxolol 0.25%, 0.5%	b.i.d.	Decrease aqueous production	Less effect on pulmonary system

(Continued)

Table 5.4

Common glaucoma medications (*Continued*)

Class and drug name	Dosing	Mechanism of action	Common side effects
Carbonic anhydrase inhibitors			
Acetazolamide Methazolamide	250 mg q.i.d. or 500 mg b.i.d. 50–100 mg b.i.d./t.i.d.	Decrease aqueous production	Sulfa allergy, systemic metabolic acidosis, tingling in extremities, aplastic anemia (rare)
Dorzolamide 2% Brinzolamide 1%	t.i.d. t.i.d.		Metallic taste
Cholinergics (direct acting)			
Pilocarpine 0.5%–10%	q.i.d.	Increase trabecular outflow	Brow ache, iris cyst formation, cataract formation, retinal detachment
Cholinergics (indirect acting)			
Echothiophate 0.03%–0.25% Demecarium 0.25%–0.5% Physostigmine ointment 0.25%–0.5%	q.d. q.d.–b.i.d.	Increase trabecular outflow	Brow ache, iris cyst formation, cataract formation, retinal detachment
Cholinergics (direct and indirect acting)			
Carbachol 0.75%–3%	t.i.d.	Increase trabecular outflow	Brow ache, iris cyst formation, cataract formation, retinal detachment
Hyperosmotic agents			
Mannitol Glycerin Isosorbide Urea	0.5–2.0 g/kg i.v. 1–1.5 g/kg p.o. 1.5 g/kg of 50% solution p.o. 0.5–2 g/kg i.v.	Dehydration and decrease of vitreous volume	Aggravation of CHF Hyperglycemia
Prostoglandin analogues			
Latanoprost 0.005%	q.d.	Increase uveoscleral outflow	Bitter taste, change in iris color, conjunctival hyperemia
Bimatoprost 0.01%, 0.03%	q.d.	Increase uveoscleral outflow	Bitter taste, change in iris color, conjunctival hyperemia
Travoprost 0.004%	q.d.	Increase uveoscleral outflow	Bitter taste, change in iris color, conjunctival hyperemia

CHF, congestive heart failure.

Pharmacologic Considerations

Epinephrine

- IOP is noted to decrease at 0.12% to 0.5% concentrations; to increase outflow, a 1% solution is needed.
- Onset of action is at 1 hour; peak effect is at 4 hours and lasts up to 12 hours.
- May produce irreversible corneal edema at higher concentrations when injected into the AC.
- Toxicity can produce drug-induced pemphigoid.
- Use with caution in patients using monoamine oxidase (MAO) inhibitors, tricyclic antidepressants, and antihistamines, since it can potentiate a systemic hypertensive crisis.
- Use with caution in patients with known cardiac disease or hyperthyroidism.

Dipivefrin

- Prodrug: converted into epinephrine by corneal esterases.
- Better penetration than epinephrine.

GLAUCOMA

- Twenty to forty percent decrease in IOP.
- Onset of action is in 30 minutes; maximum effect is at 1 hour.
- Dipivefrin 0.1% is equal to epinephrine 1% to 2%.
- Fewer systemic and topical side effects than epinephrine.
- Study found that dipivefrin is equivalent to betaxolol when used as a single agent.
- Long-term epinephrine therapy has the same degree of IOP control as timolol, although timolol is more effective in the initial year of therapy.

Concomitant Therapy

- Additive effect with pilocarpine and CAIs.
- Epinephrine with acetazolamide has greater reduction of aqueous formation than with either agent alone.
- Has a 10% to 15% additive effect when used with betaxolol.

Selective α-Adrenergic Agonist

Apraclonidine (Iopidine).
Brimonidine (Alphagan).

Apraclonidine

Mechanism of Action

- Lowers IOP by reducing aqueous humor production without altering outflow facility.
- Predominantly an α_2-agonist, but at higher concentrations can stimulate α_1-adrenoceptor, causing vasoconstriction and reducing blood flow to the ciliary body and aqueous production.
- May also decrease IOP by reducing episcleral venous pressure, which may be linked to reduced blood flow to the limbal area.

Pharmacologic Considerations

- Route of delivery to the ciliary body is through the sclera and conjunctiva.
- Does not cross the blood–brain barrier like clonidine.
- Thirty-five percent reduction in aqueous flow in 4 hours.
- One percent solution decreases IOP by 20% in 1 hour and by 30% to 40% at peak effect.
- Maximum effect is at 3 to 5 hours.
- Some studies noted that the 0.5% solution lowers IOP to a similar extent as the 1% solution.
- Dosage: 1% solution: one drop 1 hour before laser treatment and immediately postlaser; 0.5% solution: twice a day (b.i.d.) to three times a day (t.i.d.) for chronic use.
- Tachyphylaxis or lack of effect is observed in 20% of patients.

Clinical Indications

- One percent solution effective in preventing pressure rise following laser treatment and cataract extraction.
- One percent solution for treating acute angle closure.
- Adjunctive medication with other topical antiglaucoma medications.
- U.S. Food and Drug Administration (FDA)-approved as a short-term medication, but clinically used for long term.

Side Effects

- Allergic conjunctivitis and dermatitis (20% to 50%); increases with duration of use.
- Dry mouth/dry nose: Absorption in the lacrimal system causes vasoconstriction of the nasal and oral mucosa (20% of patients using 0.5% solution).
- Minimal cardiovascular side effects.
- Eyelid retraction (50%): probably due to stimulation of Müller muscle.
- Conjunctival blanching (85%): due to decreased blood flow in the perilimbal vessels.

Concomitant Therapy

- Timolol with apraclonidine lowers IOP better than timolol with dipivefrin.
- Apraclonidine has an additive effect with nonselective β-blockers.
- Significantly lowers IOP when used in combination with maximally tolerated medical therapy.

Brimonidine

Mechanism of Action

Reduces aqueous production without altering outflow facility (increases uveoscleral outflow). Much more highly selective for the α_2 receptor than apraclonidine.

Pharmacologic Considerations

- Sixty-seven percent decrease in aqueous humor production.
- Maximal IOP decrease of 20% to 30%.
- Efficacy and safety similar to apraclonidine.
- Unlike apraclonidine, it is a lipophilic drug, so absorption is through the cornea.
- Can pass through the blood–brain barrier and cause central nervous system (CNS) side effects.
- Some reports show fewer allergic reactions (e.g., follicular conjunctivitis) than with apraclonidine. Allergic reaction reported up to 40% with apraclonidine, less than 15% with brimonidine 0.2%, and less than 10% for Brimonidine-Purite 0.15%).
- Contraindicated in children under 7 to 8 years old, as can cause CNS depression.

Side Effects

Ocular: conjunctival blanching.
Systemic: dry mouth, hypotension.
CNS: drowsiness, fatigue.

β-Adrenergic Antagonists

Nonselective β_1-blockers (cardiac) and β_2-blockers (pulmonary):

Timolol.
Levobunolol.
Carteolol.
Metipranolol
Selective β_1-blocker (cardiac):
Betaxolol.

Mechanism of Action

- Reduces aqueous humor secretion by inhibiting cyclic adenosine monophosphate (camp) production in the ciliary epithelium.
- Site of action is on active secretion at the level of the nonpigmented ciliary epithelium.

Common Side Effects

Ocular: conjunctival hyperemia, superficial punctate keratitis, corneal anesthesia.
Cardiovascular bradycardia, hypotension, arrhythmia.
Pulmonary: bronchospasm, pulmonary failure.
Miscellaneous: depression, impotence, altered response to hypoglycemia.

Pharmacologic Considerations

Timolol

- One of the most commonly used drug in treatment of glaucoma.
- IOP decreases in 30 to 60 minutes.
- Forty-seven percent decrease in aqueous production at 1 week.
- Short-term escape partial loss of initial effect, due to drug-induced up-regulation of β receptors.
- Long-term drift: The response of β receptors is affected by continued exposure to an agonist. Reduction of aqueous flow is less pronounced in 1 year (25%) compared with 1 week (47%).
- More effective in lowering IOP than is epinephrine or pilocarpine.
- Binds to melanin.
- Secreted in breast milk.
- Exacerbates myasthenia gravis (depressive effect of β-blockers on neuromuscular fibers).
- Altered response to hypoglycemic episodes (pancreatic islet cell stimulation).
- Adversely affects lipid profiles: decreases high-density lipoprotein (HDL) values, increases triglyceride values.

Levobunolol

Analogue of propranolol.
Maximum effect: between 2 and 6 hours.
Previous studies: mean IOP reduction of 27% in 2 years.
Similar to timolol in efficacy: greater IOP-lowering effect than betaxolol.

Carteolol

- IOP reduction similar to other nonselective β-blockers (conflicting reports).
- Less ocular irritation.
- Less effect on serum lipid levels compared to timolol.
- Only β-blocker with intrinsic sympathomimetic activity (ISA); theoretically results in less bradycardia and vasoconstriction.
- No evidence shown of ISA when given topically.

Metipranolol

- Metipranolol 0.3% shown to be at least as effective as timolol 0.25%.
- Solution at 0.3% reduces IOP by 21%; 0.6% solution reduces IOP by 31%.
- Studies have shown more bradycardia, bronchospasm, and vasoconstriction than with timolol.
- Reports of granulomatous uveitis with use, cause of which is unknown.

Betaxolol

- Thirty-two to forty seven percent decrease in aqueous production.
- Lowers mean IOP by 14% to 17%.
- Onset of action, 30 minutes; maximum effect at 2 hours.
- Less effective in lowering IOP compared with timolol or levobunolol.
- Absorbed into systemic circulation four times less efficiently than timolol.
- Less pronounced systemic effects; better than other β-blockers for patients with pulmonary disease.

Concomitant Therapy

- β-Blockers in combination with miotics lower IOP more effectively than either drug alone.
- β-Blockers and CAIs reduce IOP slightly less than the additive percentage of each drug used alone.
- Betaxolol is the only β-blocker that preserves an outflow facility effect when used in combination with epinephrine, 10% to 15% additive effect.

α-Adrenergic Antagonists

Currently not used for glaucoma therapy.
Selective α-adrenergic antagonists:
Prazosin.
Thymoxamine.
Nonselective α-adrenergic antagonist: dapiprazole.

Prazosin

- Well tolerated, effective ocular hypotensive in animal studies.
- Reduced aqueous humor formation in rabbits by 27%.

- Ocular hypotensive effect lasts 6 to 8 hours; peak effect at 2 hours.
- No ocular toxicity noted in rabbits for 6 to 12 months.

Thymoxamine

- Inhibits iris dilator muscles.
- Topical 0.5% produces miosis without AC shallowing or accommodation.
- No changes in aqueous formation or outflow facility noted.
- Rabbit studies show an ocular hypotensive effect, which has not yet been seen in humans.
- Binds to melanin; therefore ineffective in darkly pigmented eyes.
- Side effects: hyperemia, burning, miosis, ptosis.
- Minimal systemic side effects.
- Potential uses:
  - May be used to break pupillary block in acute angle-closure glaucoma.
  - Reduces iris-zonular contact in pigmentary glaucoma.
  - Reversal of phenylephrine-induced mydriasis.
  - Treatment for lid retraction from thyroid disease.
  - Maintains position of IOLs.
  - As an adjunct to gonioscopy in distinguishing between a narrow and close angle.

Dapiprazole

- Inhibits iris smooth muscle dilators.
- Produces miosis without accommodation.
- Similar potential uses as thymoxamine.
- Also works poorly in darkly pigmented eyes.
- Can be used for pretreatment for Nd:YAG laser iridotomy; produces miosis with less iris vascular congestion than pilocarpine.
- Burning on installation noted.
- May produce conjunctival injection, which lasts 20 minutes.

Cholinergic Agonists (Parasympathomimetics)

- Direct acting (affects the motor endplates in the same way as acetylcholine): pilocarpine.
- Indirect acting: inhibits the enzyme acetylcholinesterase, thereby prolonging the action of naturally secreted acetylcholine:
  - Echothiophate.
  - Demecarium bromide.
- Direct and indirect acting: carbachol.

Mechanism of Action

- Ciliary muscle contraction pulls on the scleral spur and TM, thereby widening the trabecular spaces and increasing the outflow of aqueous humor.
- Pupillary sphincter contraction pulls the iris away from the TM.
- Decreases uveoscleral outflow.

Side Effects

- Induced myopia.
- Brow ache as a result of ciliary spasm.
- Visual disturbances, especially in dim light, because of the miosis.
- Increases pupillary block as a result of the forward movement of the lens-iris diaphragm, increase in anterioposterior diameter of the lens and miosis.
- Stronger indirect-acting miotics are cataractogenic.
- Can cause significant bleeding and severe fibrinous iridocyclitis postoperatively.
- Vasodilatory effect increases permeability of blood–aqueous barrier, intensifying inflammation.
- Reports of iris pigment epithelial cysts and retinal detachment.
- Malignant glaucoma is worsened with miotics.
- Induced ocular pseudopemphigoid.
- Corneal haze: carbachol > pilocarpine > phospholine.

Systemic Side Effects

Epiphora, diarrhea, abdominal cramps, increased salivation, nausea, vomiting, decreased pulmonary surfactant, worsening of Parkinson disease symptoms.

Pharmacologic Considerations

Pilocarpine

- Maximum effect occurs in 2 hours and lasts 6 to 8 hours.
- IOP decreases by 20% at 8 hours.
- Higher concentrations are needed in pigmented irides.
- Extremely high IOPs cause ischemia of the sphincter muscles to a degree that they are unresponsive to pilocarpine.
- Available in various concentrations from 0.25% to 4%, and as a prolonged-release (7 days) Ocusert system.

Carbachol

- Resistant to hydrolysis by cholinesterases, which makes it more potent with longer duration of action than pilocarpine.
- Intracameral carbachol (Miostat): used for intraoperative miosis; significantly reduces postoperative IOP after cataract surgery.
- Intracameral use can cause corneal clouding, bullous keratopathy, and increased postoperative iritis.
- Side effects are more severe and more common than with pilocarpine.

Echothiophate (Phospholine Iodide)

- Irreversible cholinesterase inhibitor.

- Susceptible to degradation, fresh solution should be kept cool.
- Extreme miosis occurs in 30 minutes.
- Maximum IOP reduction occurs in 24 hours.
- More marked systemic and ocular side effects than pilocarpine.
- May cause pigmented epithelial cysts at the pupillary border, especially in young phakic patients.
- More effective than pilocarpine in aphakics.

Demecarium Bromide

- Reversible cholinesterase inhibitor.
- Stable, insensitive to heat and hydrolysis.
- Action and effects are the same as echothiophate.

Concomitant Therapy

Miotics show an additive hypotensive effect when used in conjunction with other agents in the therapy of open-angle glaucoma.

Carbonic Anhydrase Inhibitors

- Systemic drugs:
  - Acetazolamide (Diamox).
  - Methazolamide (Neptazane).
- Topical drugs:
  - Dorzolamide (Trusopt).
  - Brinzolamide (Azopt).

Mechanism of Action

- Reduces aqueous humor formation (20% to 40%) by direct inhibition of carbonic anhydrase in the ciliary body without significantly affecting outflow mechanism.
- Reduces the flow of bicarbonate to the posterior chamber.
- A significant physiologic response requires greater than 99% inhibition of carbonic anhydrase in the target tissue.
- Systemic CAIs work to a lesser extent by production of generalized acidosis; systemic acidosis decreases aqueous production.

Side Effects

- Dose related.
- Paresthesias as a result of potassium loss.
- Metallic taste, gastrointestinal (GI) tract disturbances, loss of libido, drowsiness, loss of energy, depression.
- Increases formation of calcium oxalate and calcium phosphate renal stones: acetazolamide > methazolamide.
- Systemic metabolic acidosis: acetazolamide > methazolamide.
- As a sulfa derivative, similar allergic reactions and cross hyperreactivity.
- Idiosyncratic reaction (extremely rare, may not be causally related): aplastic anemia, thrombocytopenia, agranulocytosis.
- Can induce myopia: shallowing of the AC with no lens thickening suggests ciliary body swelling.
- Teratogenic effect in animals.

Pharmacologic Considerations

Acetazolamide

- Onset of action within 1 hour and peaks at 2 to 4 hours; effect lasts 12 hours.
- Hypotensive effect that is not due to diuretic action.
- Shown to increase rate of subretinal fluid absorption between retina and retinal pigment epithelium (RPE): used to treat chronic macular edema.
- Small amount can be excreted in breast milk.
- Also used to treat pseudotumor cerebri.
- Dose: 250 mg four times a day (q.i.d.) or 500 mg sequel b.i.d.

Methazolamide

- Longer duration of action and is less bound to serum proteins than acetazolamide.
- Less acidosis.
- Not as effective as acetazolamide.
- Dose: 25 to 50 mg b.i.d. to t.i.d.

Dorzolamide

- Access to ciliary body directly; also absorbed systemically.
- Ninety eight percent decrease in ciliary body carbonic anhydrase activity.
- Systemic side effects rare.
- IOP lowered 29% over 8 hours; IOP decreases 3 to 5 mm Hg through the day.
- Peak reduction of IOP at 2 hours after dose.
- Does not cause acid-base disturbances.
- Efficacy of dorzolamide 2% t.i.d. is comparable to betaxolol 0.5% b.i.d.
- Less effective than timolol.
- Additive when used with timolol (13% to 21% reduction in IOP).
- Formulated in an acidic pH of 5.6 for better absorption, this likely results in the common patient complaint of burning immediately after instillation.

Brinzolamide

- Absorbed through the cornea to the ciliary body.
- Highly lipophilic to promote corneal penetration.
- IOP reduction equivalent to dorzalamide in a high percentage of patients.
- Dissolved in a viscous ophthalmic suspension to increase ocular contact time (aids absorption).
- Viscous suspension allows for formulation at close to physiologic pH (7.5), but can cause patient complaints of blurred vision immediately after instillation.

Contraindications to Use

Primarily of concern in systemic CAI use.
Adrenal insufficiency.
Renal and hepatic disease.
Addison disease.
Severe pulmonary obstruction.
Caution in taking with salicylates: may lead to acid-base imbalance, salicylate intoxication.
Sulfa allergies.
Stevens-Johnson syndrome has been reported with systemic CAIs.

Osmotic Agents

Oral agents:
Glycerin.
Isosorbide.
Intravenous agent: mannitol.

Mechanism of Action

- Rapid increase in serum osmolality creates an osmotic gradient between the blood and the vitreous humor, thus drawing water from the vitreous cavity through the retinal and uveal vessels.
- IOP reduction is primarily caused by dehydration and reduction in vitreous volume.
- The reduction of vitreous volume allows posterior movement of the iris-lens plane, thereby deepening the AC.
- Factors that influence the osmotic gradient:
  The larger the dose and the faster the administration, the greater the osmotic gradient and the more pronounced reduction in IOP.
  The faster the metabolism of the drug, the shorter its duration of action.
  Drugs that remain extracellular (glycerin, mannitol) produce a greater osmotic effect than those distributed in total body water (isosorbide).
  The blood-ocular osmotic gradient decreases as the drug enters the eye. Drugs with poor ocular penetration (glycerin, mannitol) are more effective.
- IOP reduction may also be secondary to central effects on the hypothalamus.

Side Effects

- Headaches, nausea, vomiting, diarrhea.
- Mental confusion, cerebral dehydration, subdural and subarachnoid hemorrhages.
- Aggravation of congestive heart failure.
- Rebound elevation of IOP when agent penetrates the eye and the osmotic gradient reverses.
- Glycerin can cause hyperglycemia and ketoacidosis in diabetics.
- Electrolyte imbalances.

Pharmacologic Considerations

Glycerin

- Hypotensive effect starts in 10 to 30 minutes, maximal effect after 45 minutes to 2 hours.
- Duration of action is 4 to 5 hours.
- Metabolized by the liver, produces less diuresis than other agents.
- Metabolized into sugar and ketone bodies, so may be a serious problem in diabetics.
- Oral agents are slightly less effective and have a slower onset of action than intravenous (i.v.) drugs because of GI tract absorption.
- Dose: 1 to 1.5 g/kg body weight.

Isosorbide

- Well tolerated, can be used in diabetics, since it is not metabolized into sugar.
- Fewer side effects than glycerin.
- Chemically similar to mannitol.
- Peak hypotensive effect in 1 to 3 hours and lasts 3 to 5 hours.
- Dose: 1.5 g/kg body weight of a 50% solution.

Mannitol

- Greater and faster effect than oral hyperosmotics.
- Onset of action in 10 to 30 minutes, peaks in 30 to 60 minutes and lasts for 6 hours.
- No ocular penetration.
- Vitreous dehydration.
- Caution for patients with compromised cardiac and renal functions.
- Excreted unmetabolized in the urine.
- Dose: 1 to 1.5 g/kg body weight.

Prostaglandin Analogues

Latanoprost (Xalatan 0.005%)

Mechanism of Action

Increases uveoscleral outflow.

Side Effects

- Seven to 16% of hazel irides turn brown (increased melanogenesis with no increase in the number of melanocytes).
- Bitter taste, conjunctival hyperemia, burning, stinging, itching.
- Anterior uveitis—can cause recurrences, expecially of herpetic keratitis.
- Hypertrichosis—increased number, length, and thickness of lashes.
- Development of CME.
- Epithelial toxicity.

Pharmacologic Considerations

- Prodrug that penetrates the cornea and becomes active upon being hydrolyzed by corneal esterase.
- Dose: 1 drop in the evening, less effective when used twice daily. Peak effect 10 to 14 hours after administration.
- Lowers IOP by 25% to 32% (7 to 8 mm Hg).
- More effective in decreasing IOP than timolol (US and Scandinavian studies) or at least as effective as timolol (British studies).
- Hypotensive effect is maintained without drift from 2 weeks to 6 months of treatment.
- Less subjective ocular side effects than timolol.
- Does not alter heart rate.
- Reduces IOP equally well at night and during the day.

Concomitant Therapy

- Latanoprost 0.005% given once or twice a day decreased IOP by 15% to 25% (30% to 35% in another study) when added to timolol 0.5% b.i.d.
- Addition of latanoprost in patients on a regimen of pilocarpine resulted in an additional 14% to 18% drop in IOP.

Bimatoprost (Lumigan 0.01%, 0.03%)

Mechanism of Action

Increases uveoscleral outflow.

Side Effects

- Similar changes in iris pigmentation to latanoprost, hazel irides turn brown (increased melanogenesis with no increase in the number of melanocytes).
- Bitter taste, conjunctival hyperemia, burning, stinging, itching.
- Higher rates of conjunctival hyperemia than latanoprost.
- Anterior uveitis—can cause recurrences, expecially of herpetic keratitis.
- Hypertrichosis—increased number, length, and thickness of lashes.
- Development of CME.
- Epithelial toxicity.

Pharmacologic Considerations

- IOP-lowering effect similar to or perhaps slightly better than latanoprost, with studies showing additional IOP lowering upon switching from latanoprost to bimatoprost.
- Prostamide, which purportedly may have some alternative pathway effects.
- Dose: 1 drop in the evening, less effective when used twice daily. Peak effect 10 to 14 hours after administration.
- Lowers IOP by 27% to 33%.
- Hypotensive effect is maintained without drift from 2 weeks to 6 months of treatment.
- Reduces IOP equally well at night and during the day.

Concomitant Therapy

- Additive to other topical agents.

Travoprost (Travatan 0.004%)

Mechanism of Action

Increases uveoscleral outflow.

Side Effects

- Prodrug that penetrates the cornea and becomes active upon being hydrolyzed by corneal esterase.
- Similar changes in iris pigmentation to latanoprost, hazel irides turn brown (increased melanogenesis with no increase in the number of melanocytes).
- Bitter taste, conjunctival hyperemia, burning, stinging, itching.
- Anterior uveitis—can cause recurrences, expecially of herpetic keratitis.
- Hypertrichosis—increased number, length, and thickness of lashes.
- Development of CME.
- Epithelial toxicity.

Pharmacologic Considerations

- IOP-lowering effect similar to latanoprost.
- Dose: 1 drop in the evening, less effective when used twice daily. Peak effect 10 to 14 hours after administration.
- Lowers IOP by 25% to 32%.
- Hypotensive effect is maintained without drift from 2 weeks to 6 months of treatment.
- Reduces IOP equally well at night and during the day.
- Travatan Z—replaces benzalkonium chloride (BAK) preservative with sofZia, which is purportedly gentler to the ocular surface for patients with ocular surface disease.

Concomitant Therapy

- Additive to other topical agents.

New Medications on the Horizon

Rho Kinase Inhibitors

Mechanism of Action

Increases aqueous humor outflow facility. Rho Kinase is a downstream effector of Rho GTPase and its activity has effects on the formation of actin stress fibers, focal adhesions, and cellular contraction. It is currently under investigation for efficacy in human patients.

References

Butler P, Mannschreck M, Lin S, et al. Clinical experience with the long-term use of 1% apraclonidine. *Arch Ophthalmol* 1995;113:293–296.

Camras CB, Alm A, Watson P, et al. Latanoprost: a prostaglandin analog for glaucoma therapy. *Ophthalmology* 1996:103: 1916–1924.

Camras CB, the United States Latanoprost Study Group. Comparison of latanoprost and timolol in patients with ocular hypertension and glaucoma. *Ophthalmology* 1996;103:138–147.

DeSantis L. Preclinical overview of brinzolamide. *Surv Ophthalmol* 2000; 44 Suppl 2:S119–129.

Higginbotham EJ, Schuman JS, Goldberg I, et al. One-year, randomized study comparing bimatoprost and timolol in glaucoma and ocular hypertension. *Arch Ophthalmol* 2002; 120:1286–1293.

Netland PA, Landry T, Sullivan EK, et al. Travoprost compared with latanoprost and timolol in patients with open-angle glaucoma or ocular hypertension. *Am J Ophthalmol* 2001;132: 472–484.

Robin AL, Ritch R, Shin DH, et al. Short term efficacy of apraclonidine hydrochloride added to maximum-tolerated medical therapy for glaucoma. *Am J Ophthalmol* 1995;120:423–432.

Sugrue MF. Pharmacological and ocular hypotensive properties of topical carbonic anhydrase inhibitors. *Prog Retin Eye Res* 2000; 19:87–112.

SURGICAL MANAGEMENT OF GLAUCOMA

Peripheral Iridotomy

Indications

1. Acute angle-closure glaucoma with pupillary block: Patients presenting with acute angle closure should first be treated medically to break the acute attack, lowering IOP and decreasing corneal edema. However, laser PI may be performed if medical treatment is unsuccessful and can itself break the acute attack. The successful PI should be accompanied by a rush of aqueous from the posterior to AC and an opening of the peripheral angle with deepening of the AC.
2. Prophylaxis in contralateral eye of acute angle closure: The fellow eye of a patient with an episode of acute angle closure attributable to primary narrow-angle glaucoma should be treated prophylactically.
3. Narrow, occludable angle with pupillary block: An angle that is judged by gonioscopy to be narrow and occludable should undergo a PI. Positive darkroom prone and mydriatic provocative test results (IOP rise > 4 mm Hg) suggest that an angle is occludable.
4. Chronic angle-closure glaucoma with pupillary block: Chronic angle closure can cause intermittent angle closure or permanent trabecular damage and dysfunction. A PI reduces apposition of the iris to the outflow structures and further compromise.
5. Mixed mechanism glaucoma: This situation can rarely occur where there is true POAG and narrow-angle glaucoma with pupillary block. More commonly, the narrow angle is not diagnosed and chronic angle closure results in trabecular damage such that even when the angle is opened with a PI, the outflow is inadequate and a secondary open-angle glaucoma develops.
6. Malignant glaucoma: True malignant glaucoma persists despite a successful PI, but the procedure must be performed, to remove the pupillary block component and make the diagnosis.
7. Premalignant glaucoma: This situation describes an eye that has zonular laxity or a large lens, which may predispose to forward displacement of the lens and one type of malignant glaucoma.
8. Aphakic pupillary block: The anterior vitreous face may cause pupillary block in aphakic patients, and the initial treatment is a PI.
9. Pseudophakic pupillary block: The IOL or anterior capsule may become adherent to the iris, causing pupillary block and necessitating a PI.
10. Nanophthalmos: A short axial length causes narrow angles secondary to crowding of the AC and angle structures. The narrow angle commonly persists after PI, unless there is a large component of pupillary block.
11. Iris bombe: The iris becomes adherent to the lens (crystalline lens or IOL) or the vitreous face as a result of posterior synechiae, causing the typical bowing forward of the iris. A PI should be followed by a forward rush of aqueous, deepening of the angle, and release of the bombe configuration.
12. Pigment dispersion syndrome/pigmentary glaucoma: A PI in this situation remains controversial. The theoretical advantage is that the iridotomy relieves the reverse pupillary block and allows the iris to assume a flatter configuration, rather than the typical posterior concavity. It should be performed only when this posterior concavity can be demonstrated by gonioscopy or UBM. Treatment with miotics may be equally or more effective.
13. Plateau iris: The definition of plateau iris syndrome is the plateau iris configuration in the presence of a patent PI. Therefore, it is needed to make the diagnosis and to relieve any pupillary block that may coexist.
14. Nonpatent iridotomy/iridectomy: A laser PI should be used to complete an imperforate or secondarily closed laser or surgical iridectomy.
15. After glaucoma surgery: The iris may block the sclerostomy after trabeculectomy or the tube ostium after a tube shunt procedure and can be removed with the laser.

Contraindications

- There are no absolute contraindications, only relative ones:
  - Corneal edema.
  - Apposition of iris to cornea.
  - Angle closure without pupillary block.
- The synechial angle closures such as neovascular glaucoma, uveitic glaucoma, the ICE syndrome, or epithelial or fibrous downgrowth may not benefit from a PI because pupillary block is not the cause of angle closure.

Technique

1. Lens: Abraham, Wise, fundus contact lens. A contact lens is very helpful since it focuses laser energy, controls eye movement and lid closure, reduces reflection, and acts as a heat absorber. Goniosol is used as a contact medium.
2. Preoperative management may include any of the following:
   Pilocarpine 1% to 4% for pupillary constriction.
   Apraclonidine or brimonidine to prevent postoperative IOP spikes.
   CAI if significant visual field loss is present.
3. Aim laser (Argon, Nd:YAG, or combination of both) in peripheral iris crypt.
   Argon laser: more useful in thick brown or very vascular irides, less bleeding.
   Nd:YAG: penetrates iris tissue more quickly and effectively; bleeding if blood vessel encountered.
   Combined argon/Nd:YAG: thinning and coagulation of iris with argon, then completed with Nd:YAG.
4. Surgical peripheral iridectomy in patients with corneal edema in whom laser cannot be performed:
   Paracentesis.
   Deepen and reform AC.
   Prolapse iris through paracentesis.
   Cut iris with scissors.
   Replace iris in AC.
5. Postoperative management:
   Check IOP after 1 hour, 1 day, 1 week as needed (p.r.n.).
   Topical steroids p.r.n.
   Apraclonidine or brimonidine after procedure.
   Gonioscopic evaluation to assess effect.

Complications

Hemorrhage: This is more common with the Nd:YAG and can usually be controlled with moderate pressure from the contact lens.

Elevated IOP: This usually occurs within the first hour and lasts less than 24 hours, but may necessitate medical and even surgical treatment. It is caused by inflammation and dispersion of pigment by the laser. Its incidence is decreased by topical apraclonidine before or after surgery.

Uveitis: Postoperative inflammation is common and treated with topical steroids.

Corneal burns: The corneal endothelium can be damaged by both argon and Nd:YAG lasers, but are self-limited and rarely have long-term sequelae. These can be avoided by focusing the beam slightly posterior to the iris surface, especially when the iris is apposed to the cornea.

Diplopia or perceived white line in vision: This is more common with a large PI that is not covered by the upper lid. Treatment can consist of a colored contact lens or corneal tattoo to cover the defect. The subjective sensation of a white line in the vision often resolves without intervention.

Lens trauma: Anterior capsular opacities can occur, but are usually nonprogressive.

Pigment dispersion: This is commonly seen and can result in a transient increase in IOP and pigmentation of the TM.

Synechiae formation: This can be reduced by topical steroids or broken by dilation.

Corectopia: The pupil may become peaked toward the PI, but condition is usually transient and not visually significant.

Argon Laser Peripheral Iridotomy

- Long-pulse technique (light irides):
  Time: 0.2 seconds.
  Power: 1,000 mW.
  Spot size: 50 µm.
  Number: 1 to 30.
- Short-pulse technique (dark irides):
  Time: 0.02 to 0.05 seconds.
  Power: 1,000 to 1,500 mW.
  Spot size: 50 µm.
  Number: 25 to 100.

Nd:YAG Laser Peripheral Iridotomy

Power: 4 to 6 mJ.
Number: 1 to 10.
Shots/burst: 1 to 3.

Reference

Beckman H, Barraco R, Suger S, et al. Laser iridectomies. *Am J Ophthalmol Soc* 1971;77:674–706.

Laser Trabeculoplasty (LTP)

Indications

POAG.
Exfoliation glaucoma.
Pigmentary glaucoma.
Other SOAGs.

Contraindications

Poor visualization: may be due to corneal opacity, narrow or closed angles, or poor patient cooperation.

Angle closure: Primary or secondary angle-closure glaucomas rarely respond well to LTP.

Uveitic glaucoma: Uveitis is often exacerbated by LTP. Laser is generally not effective.

Congenital glaucoma: The abnormal angle of congenital or juvenile glaucoma is poorly responsive to LTP.

Angle recession glaucoma: traumatic glaucoma with torn, damaged, or poorly functioning TM responds poorly to LTP.

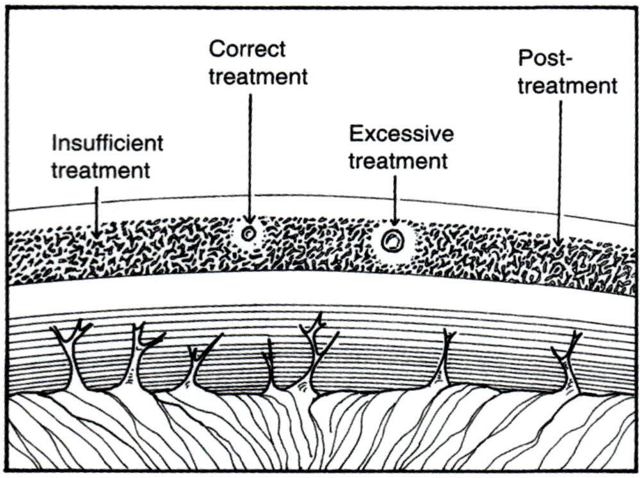

FIGURE 5.27. Argon laser trabeculoplasty. (From Epstein DL. *Chandler and Grant's glaucoma*, 4th ed. Baltimore, MD: Lippincott Williams & Wilkins, 1997:461, with permission.)

Technique

Lens: Goldmann three-mirror or Ritch trabeculoplasty lens. This procedure cannot be performed without a mirrored contact lens.

Preoperative management: apraclonidine or brimonidine.

Location: junction between nonpigmented and pigmented TM. Too anterior a position is not effective, too posterior a postion causes peripheral anterior synechiae.

Desired end point: mild blanching of the pigmented TM or a small cavitation bubble formation (Figure 5.27).

Postoperative management:

Check IOP after 1 hour, 1 day, and 4 weeks p.r.n.

Topical steroids p.r.n.

Apraclonidine or brimonidine.

Argon Laser Trabeculoplasty (ALT)

- Argon green laser.
- Spot size: 50 μm.
- Duration: 0.1 second.
- Power: Start at 500 to 800 mW (lower in pigmented angles), and titrate upward for effect.
- Number: 40 to 50 (180 degrees), 80 to 100 (360 degrees).

Selective Laser Trabeculoplasty (SLT)

- Q-switched, frequency-doubled (532-nm) Nd:YAG laser.
- Spot size: 400 μm.
- Duration: 0.3 nanosecond.
- Power: Start 0.4 to 1.0 mJ (lower in pigmented angles), and titrate upward for effect. Delivers only 1% of the energy of ALT.
- Number: 40 to 50 (180 degrees), 80 to 100 (360 degrees).

Complications

Hemorrhage: This is not common and can usually be controlled with moderate pressure from the contact lens or photocoagulation of the bleeding vessel.

Elevated IOP: This is fairly common but is usually transient and less than 10 mm Hg. Its incidence is decreased by topical apraclonidine/brimonidine before or after surgery.

Uveitis: Inflammation is common and is treated with topical steroids.

Corneal burns: The corneal endothelium can be damaged, but damage is self-limited and rarely has long-term sequelae.

Synechiae formation: This is more common with posterior treatment and can be reduced by topical steroids.

Progression of glaucoma: A reported 3% of patients may have worsening of their glaucoma following LTP. This may be related to postoperative IOP spikes or to trabecular damage. This should be considered when performing the procedure on patients with extensive visual field loss or split fixation.

Results

Studies comparing ALT to SLT showed they are both safe and effective, with similar reductions in IOP. On average, LTP is successful in 80% of eyes for 1 year, 50% for 5 years, and 30% for 10 years. SLT delivers less energy and causes less coagulative damage with fewer structural changes in the TM compared with ALT. SLT has the advantage of being repeatable.

Type of glaucoma: This is the main predictor of success, with exfoliation > pigmentary > POAG > low tension > aphakia.

Pigmentation: The more pigmentation there is in the angle, the higher the success rate is.

Age: Patients over 40 respond much better, and good response increases with age.

Mechanism

- LTP causes an increase in outflow facility.
- Mechanical theory: Laser treatment causes a shrinkage of the trabecular tissue, thereby separating the adjacent trabecular sheets and facilitating outflow.
- Cellular theory: Thermal injury causes a change in the metabolism and turnover of trabecular cells, resulting in a different cell population and a fluctuation in glycosaminoglycan deposition.

References

The Glaucoma Laser Trial Research Group. The Glaucoma Laser Trial, I: acute effects of argon laser trabeculoplasty on intraocular pressure. *Arch Ophthalmol* 1989;107:1135–1142.

The Glaucoma Laser Trial Research Group. The Glaucoma Laser Trial, II: results of argon laser trabeculoplasty versus topical medicines. *Ophthalmology* 1990;97:1403–1413.

Iridoplasty (Gonioplasty)

Indications

Acute angle-closure glaucoma: When medical therapy is unsuccessful in breaking an acute angle-closure attack and a PI cannot be performed, an iridoplasty may help to open the angle.

Plateau iris syndrome: The angle closure in plateau iris syndrome in the presence of a patent PI can be opened with iridoplasty, either primarily or after treatment with miotics has failed.

Nanophthalmos: A short axial length causes narrow angles secondary to crowding of the AC and angle structures. If the narrow angle persists after PI, an iridoplasty may be performed.

Phacomorphic glaucoma: A large or intumescent lens can push forward and cause angle closure, which may not respond to a PI and may be improved by iridoplasty.

Contraindications

Corneal edema.

Apposition of iris to cornea.

Synechial angle closure: The synechial angle closures such as neovascular glaucoma, uveitic glaucoma, the ICE syndrome, or epithelial or fibrous downgrowth do not benefit from an iridoplasty because the angle is scarred shut.

Technique

- Lens: Abraham. Goniosol is used as a contact medium.
- Preoperative management:
  - Pilocarpine 1% to 4%.
  - Apraclonidine or brimonidine.
- The contraction burns are placed circumferentially in the far periphery for 360 degrees (Figure 5.28).
- Postoperative management:
  - Check IOP after 1 hour, 1 day, and 1 week p.r.n.
  - Topical steroids p.r.n.
  - Apraclonidine or brimonidine.
  - Gonioscopic evaluation to assess effect.

Argon Laser Iridoplasty

Time: 0.5 seconds.

Power: 200 to 400 mW.

Spot size: 500 μm.

Number: 20 to 30.

Complications

Elevated IOP: This incidence is decreased by topical apraclonidine or brimonidine preoperatively or postoperatively.

Uveitis: Inflammation is common and is treated with topical steroids.

Corneal burns: The corneal endothelium may show diffuse burns, but these are self-limited and rarely have long-term sequelae.

Synechiae formation: These can be reduced with topical steroid use.

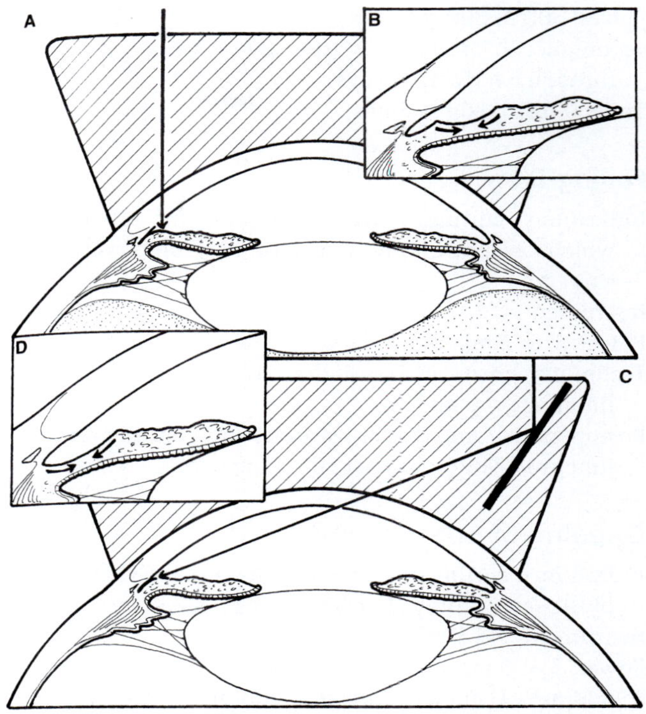

FIGURE 5.28. Laser irodoplasty technique. Direct laser application to the peripheral iris (**A**) shrinks the tissue, pulling the iris from the angle (**B**). As an alternative, the goniomirror (**C**) allows more peripheral application of the laser energy (**D**). (From Epstein DL. *Chandler and Grant's glaucoma*, 4th ed. Baltimore, MD: Lippincott Williams & Wilkins, 1997:505, with permission.)

Reference

Lim AS, Tan A, Chew P, et al. Laser iridoplasty in the treatment of severe acute angle closure glaucoma. *Int Ophthalmol* 1993;17:33–36.

Other Glaucoma Laser Procedures

Pupilloplasty

Indications: enlargement of miotic pupil, breaking of posterior synechiae, breaking of acute angle-closure pupillary block.

Instrument: argon laser.

Power: 150 to 600 mW.

Technique: 200 μm spots near pupillary border, 500-μm spots peripheral to first row.

Time: 0.2 to 0.5 seconds.

Laser Suture Lysis

Indications: for selective cutting of scleral sutures after filtration surgery to enhance egress of aqueous. The timing is very important, and cutting should be approached conservatively to prevent hypotony and a flat AC. Avoid cutting sutures on the first postoperative day, and do not cut more than one at a time.

Instrument: argon laser with Hoskins lens.

Power: 300 to 800 mW.
Technique: 1 or more 50-µm spots directly to suture through overlying tissues.
Time: 0.02 to 0.05 seconds.

Failing Bleb

Indications: cutting of tissue overlying the scleral flap, which is preventing aqueous flow after filtration surgery.
Instrument: Nd:YAG laser.
Power: 1 to 2 mJ.
Technique: Focus on tissues deep to the conjunctiva, outlining the scleral flap.
Postoperative care: digital massage, and consider subconjunctival 5-fluorouracil (5-FU) injections.

Opening of Sclerostomy

Indications: cutting of tissue blocking the internal aspects of the sclerostomy after filtration surgery.
Instrument: Nd:YAG laser.
Power: 3 to 8 mJ depending on the tissue.
Technique: Using a mirrored goniolens, use laser at the internal site of the sclerostomy and any tissues blocking it.
Postoperative care: digital massage, and consider 5-FU.

Goniophotocoagulation

Indications: adjunctive treatment in neovascularization of the angle. This is rarely performed, since the primary treatment is PRP and anti-VEGF injection.
Instrument: argon laser.
Power: 1,000 mW.
Technique: Using a mirrored goniolens and 50 µm spot size, apply laser to the trunk of the neovascular vessels as they branch over the angle structures.
Time: 0.1 seconds.
Postoperative care: topical steroids.

Cyclodestructive Surgery

Indications: decreased IOP (reduced aqueous humor formation) by ciliary process destruction, usually in patients who are poor surgical candidates or have poor visual potential.
Instrument: cyclocryotherapy or thermal lasers (Nd:YAG, argon, or diode). Cyclocryotherapy and Nd:YAG laser cyclophotocoagulation (CPC) are now rarely performed. Transscleral diode laser CPC is better tolerated with less pain and postoperative inflammation.
Power: 1.5 to 2.5 W for 1 to 2 seconds. Newer models have lower power/longer duration: 1,250 to 1,500 mW for 4 seconds.
Technique: Diode laser handpiece probe is applied directly to the limbus for transscleral delivery of energy to the ciliary processes. Typically treat 270 degrees around the limbus with 27 applications, sparing the superotemporal quadrant in initial treatment. Can be repeated with treatment of 180 degrees and 18 spots.

Endoscopic Cyclophotocoagulation (ECP)

Indications: decreased IOP (reduced aqueous humor formation) by ciliary process destruction. Better option for patients with visual potential, as it incites less inflammation with less risk for loss of vision compared to CPC. Anterior chamber approach with direct visualization, so can be done as a combined procedure with cataract surgery or used in pediatric pseudophakic, or aphakic eyes.
Instrument: Probe is 20 g in size and has a combined endoscope, laser, and light source. Diode laser is 810 nm wavelength.
Power: Start at 250 to 600 mW, titrating up to get shrinkage of the ciliary process with treatment.

Closure of Cyclodialysis Cleft

Indications: to close a cyclodialysis cleft that is causing hypotony.
Instrument: argon laser.
Power: 300 to 1,500 mW.
Technique: Using a mirrored goniolens, apply 50 to 200 µm spots to the cleft. Successful closure is often accompanied by rebound ocular hypertension. If unsuccessful, the treatment can be repeated or cryotherapy attempted or direct suturing can be performed surgically.
Time: 0.1 to 0.2 seconds.

References

Schultz JS. Additional uses of laser therapy in glaucoma. In: Ritch R, Shields MB, Krupin T, eds. *The glaucomas*, 2nd ed. St. Louis, MO: Mosby, 1996:1621–1630.

Schuman JS. Miscellaneous laser procedures. In: Epstein DL, Allingham RR, Schuman JS, eds. *Chandler and Grant's glaucoma*, 4th ed. Baltimore, MD: Lippincott Williams & Wilkins, 1997:504–508.

Goniotomy and Trabeculotomy

Indications

Goniotomy: This is most successful in primary congenital or juvenile glaucoma, especially in types with a membrane covering the chamber angle. It is much less effective in other types of pediatric glaucomas. It requires corneal clarity for gonioscopic visualization of the angle:

- Primary congenital glaucoma.
- Juvenile open-angle glaucoma.
- Sturge-Weber syndrome.
- Neurofibromatosis.
- Lowe's syndrome.

Uveitic glaucoma
Aniridia

Trabeculotomy: This is used in the same cases as goniotomy, but can be performed with a cloudy cornea and, occasionally, in combination with trabeculectomy. It can also be performed after goniotomy has failed. It causes much more scarring than goniotomy.

Goniotomy

This procedure is designed to incise the tissue overlying the TM and increase outflow.

Lens: Worst, Barkan, Lister, Swan-Jacob. All are direct goniolenses that permit insertion of a goniotomy blade into the AC through the peripheral cornea.

Goniotomy knife:
- Swan knife.
- Worst knife allows for irrigation.
- Barraquer knife.
- Needle (23 or 25 gauge) connected to viscoelastic cannula.
- Preoperative management: pilocarpine 1% to 2%.

Procedure:
- Corneal clarity can be enhanced by removal of the edematous epithelium.
- Operating loupes or the operating microscope must be used for magnification.
- The lens is placed on the cornea, and the angle is visualized.
- Viscoelastic or saline irrigation is used to maintain the AC.
- The knife is inserted 1 mm anterior to the limbus in peripheral cornea, parallel to the iris plane.
- Under direct visualization, incise the tissue overlying the TM, taking care to not cut too deeply. The tissue may be observed to fall away from the angle (Figure 5.29).
- The procedure is repeated at a site 180 degrees opposite.
- The AC is filled with saline, and the entrance closed with 10-0 nylon sutures.

Postoperative management:
- Topical steroids and antibiotics.
- Gonioscopic evaluation to assess effect.

Complications:
- Hemorrhage: A small amount of bleeding is common and resolves without treatment. A large hyphema with elevated IOP may cause corneal blood staining and requires an AC washout.
- Lens trauma can occur, but the likelihood is decreased by the use of miotics.
- Cyclodialysis is caused by an incision that is too posterior and disinserts the ciliary body from the sclera. If hypotony results, it can be treated with laser or cryotherapy.

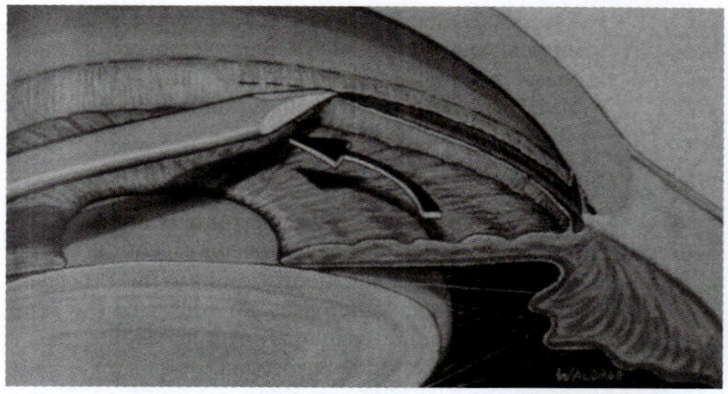

FIGURE 5.29. Goniotomy technique. The goniotomy knife is passed through a paracentesis to the trabecular meshwork opposite, and as it sweeps across the trabecular meshwork, the tissue can be seen to fall away. (From Buckley EG, Freedman SF, Shields MB. *Atlas of ophthalmic surgery*, vol 3. *Strabismus and glaucoma surgery*. St. Louis, MO: Mosby-Yearbook, 1995:612, with permission.)

Trabeculotomy

This procedure creates a direct communication from the AC to Schlemm's canal by cannulating the canal via an external approach and tearing the trabecular and other angle tissues.

- Preoperative management: pilocarpine 1% to 2%.
- Procedure:
  - A conjunctival flap is made, and a scleral flap is created as in a standard trabeculectomy.
  - A paracentesis is made, and viscoelastic is injected.
  - A radial scratch incision is made at the limbus and posteriorly in the scleral bed until Schlemm's canal is visualized.
  - To verify the canal, a 6-0 nylon suture is threaded in both directions and should meet no resistance. Threading with the suture 360 degrees and pulling through can be used as an alternative technique to a trabeculotome.
  - The internal arm of the trabeculotome is inserted into the canal and then rotated into the AC, using the external arm as a guide (Figure 5.30).
  - An opposite-handed trabeculotome is inserted in the other direction and again rotated into the AC.
  - The AC is filled with saline, and the scleral flap closed with 10-0 nylon.
- Postoperative management:
  - Topical steroids and antibiotics.
  - Gonioscopic evaluation to assess effect.
- Complications include all those for goniotomy, and the following:
  - Bleb formation from communication from the AC to the subconjunctival space.
  - Conjunctival scarring.
  - Scleral staphyloma from dissection.

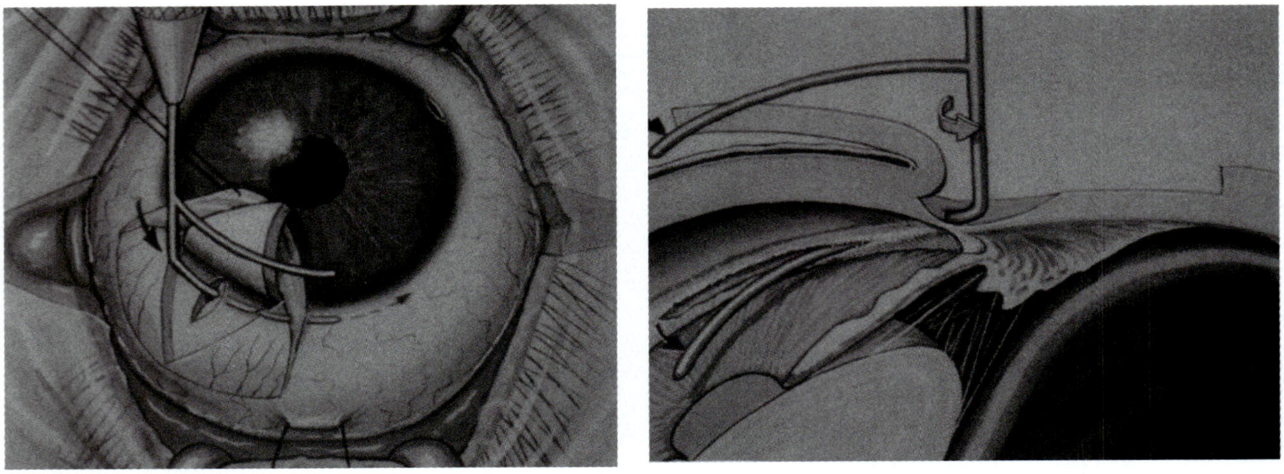

A B

FIGURE 5.30. Trabeculotomy technique. Under a partial-thickness scleral flap, the sclera is cut down to find Schlemm's canal. The trabeculotome is threaded along the canal (**A**). The trabeculotome is rotated to enter the anterior chamber (**B**). (From Buckley EG, Freedman SF, Shields MB. *Atlas of ophthalmic surgery*, vol 3. *Strabismus and glaucoma surgery.* St. Louis, MO: Mosby-Yearbook, 1995:615, with permission.)

References

Barkan O. Goniotomy. *Trans Am Acad Ophthalmol Otolaryngol* 1955;59:322.

Freedman SF. Medical and surgical treatments for childhood glaucomas. In: Epstein DL, Allingham RR, Schuman JS, eds. *Chandler and Grant's glaucoma*, 4th ed. Baltimore, MD: Lippincott Williams & Wilkins, 1997;472–483.

Hoskins HD, Shaffer RN, Hetherington J. Goniotomy vs. trabeculotomy. *J Pediatr Ophthalmol Strabismus* 1984;21:153.

Filtering Procedures

Trabeculectomy

Indications

- Consistently elevated IOP greater than 40 mm Hg.
- Progression of visual field loss on maximally tolerated medical therapy and laser trabeculoplasty.
- Progression of optic nerve cupping despite maximal therapy.
- Patients with progression of glaucoma as a result of noncompliance with medical therapy.
- These indications must be assessed in the light of the history of progression of the fellow eye, life expectancy of the patient, and the family history.

Contraindications

- Inability to undergo a surgical procedure.
- Certain glaucomas have a poor success rate with filtering surgery, and alternative treatment may be needed.
  - Neovascular glaucoma.
  - Congenital glaucoma.
  - Inflammatory glaucoma.
  - Previously failed filtration surgery.

Preoperative Preparation

- Glaucoma medications should be continued, with the following exceptions:
  - Miotics: may increase postoperative inflammation.
  - Epinephrine or dipivefrin: may cause conjunctival congestion, which increases surgical bleeding.
  - Some authors advocate stopping all medications to increase aqueous flow through the sclerostomy, to maintain patency.
- Aspirin and anticoagulants should be discontinued, if this does not jeopardize the patient's general medical condition.
- Assess the mobility of the conjunctiva, and plan the surgical approach.
- Minimize inflammation with steroid treatment.

Surgical Technique

The partial-thickness trabeculectomy is discussed. For information on full-thickness procedures, consult the references. There are many modifications to this procedure, and only the major differences are addressed (i.e., conjunctival flap, suture technique). Antimetabolite therapy is discussed in the following section.

- Retraction suture: This can be placed under the superior rectus muscle or within the superior corneal stroma to infraduct the globe. The corneal suture causes less bleeding and is more often used.
- Conjunctival flap:
  - Fornix-based (Figure 5.31):
    - Conjunctiva and Tenon's capsule incision made at the limbus.
    - Dissect bluntly posteriorly and to the sides.

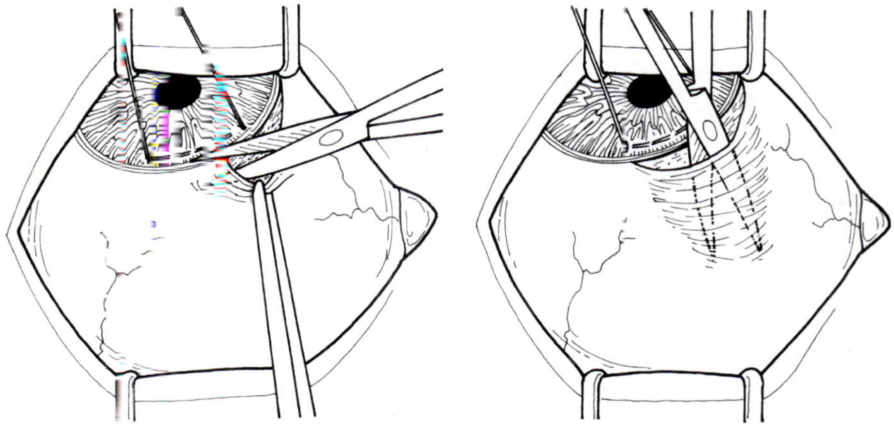

A B

FIGURE 5.31. A fornix-based flap for trabeculectomy is made by creating a peritomy (**A**) and extending the conjunctival flap posteriorly by spreading of the blades of the scissors (**B**). (From Epstein DL. *Chandler and Grant's glaucoma*, 4th ed. Baltimore, MD: Lippincott Williams & Wilkins, 1997:521, with permission.)

Advantages: more easily performed, better exposure, less manipulation of tissues, better posterior filtration.

Limbus based (Figure 5.32):

Conjunctival and Tenon incision made 8 to 10 mm posterior to the limbus.

Blunt dissection anteriorly to limbus.

Advantages: less likely to leak postoperatively.

- Scleral flap (Figure 5.33):
  - Outline the flap with cautery.
  - Incise the sclera to 50% depth with the blade.
  - Lift the posterior edge of the flap with forceps, and dissect underneath the flap toward the limbus.
  - Dissection is carried anteriorly until the surgical limbus is exposed (to peripheral cornea).
- Paracentesis and injection of viscoelastic (elective).
- Sclerectomy: This can be performed with a sclerectomy punch (e.g., Kelly or by removing a scleral block with a knife blade or the angled Vannas scissors. Avoid posterior removal since this may cause bleeding from the ciliary body and cyclodialysis.
- Iridectomy: Grasp the peripheral iris with forceps and retract outside the sclerectomy. The retracted iris is cut with scissors, and the remaining iris is reposited into the AC (facilitated by saline or viscoelastic, or with intracameral miotic).
- Scleral flap closure: The scleral flap is closed with 10-0 nylon sutures such that it does not leak but allows flow of aqueous humor with pressure or irrigation of saline into the AC:
  - Releasable sutures can be used, in addition to the permanent sutures, if Nd:YAG laser is not available or the sutures may not be visible postoperatively because of bleeding or Tenon's. They may exit through the cornea or conjunctiva.
  - Corneal: These are easier to perform and release.
  - Conjunctival: less foreign body sensation and theoretically less chance of endophthalmitis.
- Conjunctival closure:
  - Fornix-based: The conjunctiva and Tenon's capsule are attached to the peripheral cornea or lip of conjunctiva using overlapping interrupted or horizontal mattress sutures of 10-0 nylon or 8-0 or 9-0 vicryl on a vascular needle.
  - Limbus-based: The conjunctiva and Tenon's capsule (if remaining) can be closed together or in separate

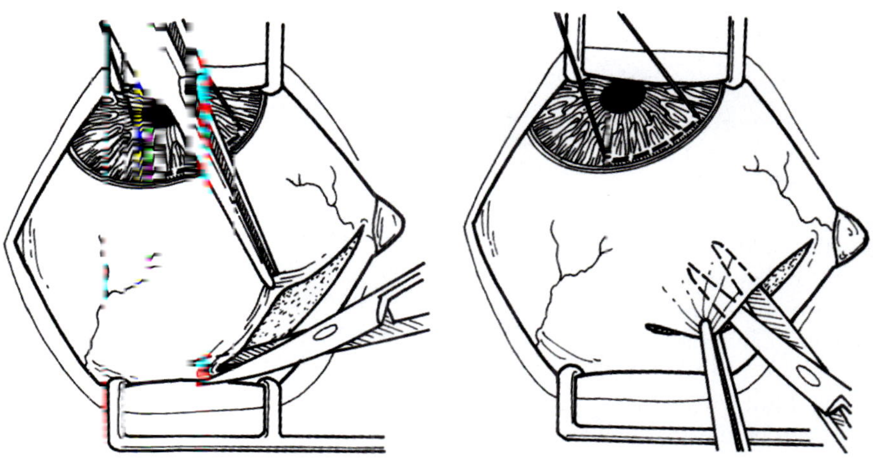

A B

FIGURE 5.32. Creation of a limbus-based flap for trabeculectomy by making a conjunctival and Tenon capsule incision in the superior fornix (**A**). The blunt dissection is carried anteriorly toward the limbus, taking care not to make conjunctival "buttonholes" (**B**). (From Epstein DL. *Chandler and Grant's glaucoma*, 4th ed. Baltimore, MD: Lippincott Williams & Wilkins, 1997:520, with permission.)

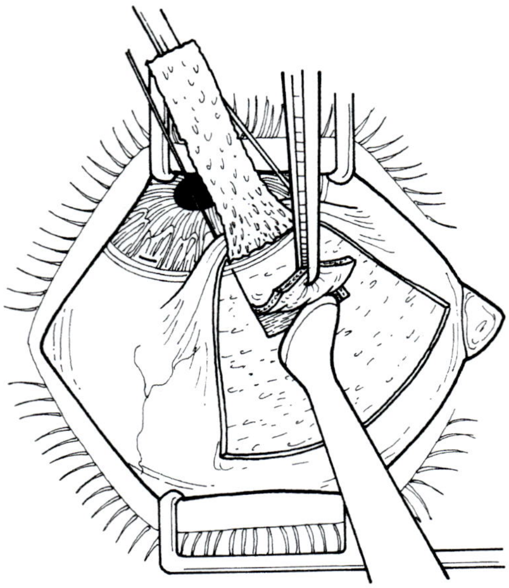

FIGURE 5.33. Creation of the partial-thickness scleral flap can be facilitated by lifting the flap with a small amount of tension and using a very sharp blade. (From Epstein DL. *Chandler and Grant's glaucoma*, 4th ed. Baltimore, MD: Lippincott Williams & Wilkins, 1997:521, with permission.)

layers with running 8-0, 9-0, or 10-0 sutures of permanent or absorbable material.

Conjunctival "buttonholes" are best closed with horizontal mattress sutures.

- Conclusion: The conjunctival closure is dried and checked for leaks by injecting saline into the AC via the paracentesis, which should form a bleb. Remaining viscoelastic should be removed.
- Recent Modifications to Classic Method of Trabeculectomy:

  Peng Khaw trabeculectomy technique: A British surgeon, Peng Khaw, developed a new technique for trabeculectomy that increases chance for success and reduces postoperative complications. His technique involves a very broad and posterior dissection under conjunctiva and tenons for creation of the bleb. Mitomycin C is similarly applied in a broad and posterior fashion to result in a more diffuse, shallow, and thicker-walled bleb. The scleral flap is constructed and sutured down to promote posterior flow of aqueous into the broad area of sub-Tenon space that was treated with MMC. This technique has been a significant contributor to improved trabeculectomy outcomes and avoids blebs that are localized, thin walled, and avascular. Newer blebs made with this technique have lower rates of bleb leak, hypoteny, blebitis, and bleb-related endophthalmitis.

  Express Mini Shunt: The Express Mini Shunt (Alcon) is a small stainless steel shunt that can be used in place of excising tissue with a traditional trabeculectomy. The surgery is similar to a trabeculectomy in creation of a bleb and partial-thickness scleral flap. However, instead of creating a sclerostomy under the flap with a Kelly punch, the anterior chamber is entered parallel to the iris plane with a 27-g needle or diamond knife at the limbus under the scleral flap. This passage is then used to place the 3-mm long, 400-μm wide Express Mini Shunt into the anterior chamber with the plate of the device flush against the sclera under the flap. The central bore of the shunt is 250 μm, and contains 50 μm openings for filtration of aqueous humor under the partial-thickness scleral flap. The design and pore size of this product is thought to produce less hypotony and other complications compared with traditional trabeculectomy. No iridectomy is required.

Postoperative Care

Frequent visits are needed to assess filtration function and wound healing.

- Medications:

  If possible, stop all aqueous suppressants, since these limit flow of aqueous humor through the filter and may lead to failure.

  Topical steroids.

  Topical antibiotics for 7 to 10 days, unless needed for prophylaxis of a very thin cystic bleb.

  Cycloplegics may help to maintain the AC and decrease the inflammatory response.
- The bleb should be elevated, especially after massage. If it is flat with a low IOP, check for wound leaks or evidence of hyposecretion (choroidals). If it is flat with a high IOP, check for blockage of the sclerostomy.
- If the AC is shallow with a low IOP, no intervention is necessary unless there is corneal-lenticular touch. In this case, the AC should be reformed with viscoelastic. If the IOP is high with a flat AC, a suprachoroidal hemorrhage or malignant glaucoma must be considered.
- Hyphema can be treated conservatively unless corneal blood staining is likely or a clot is blocking the sclerostomy, necessitating an AC washout or fibrinolytic treatment (i.e., tPA).
- Suture release can be performed with Nd:YAG laser of permanent sutures or by pulling releasable ones. If possible, avoid removing sutures during the first 2 postoperative days, and do not remove more than one at a time. The timing of release depends on the measured and target IOP and whether or not antimetabolites have been used. With antimetabolites, suture release up to 6 weeks after surgery may be effective.

Filtration Failure

The most common cause of failure is episcleral fibrosis and can be treated in several manners:

Bleb needling with or without 5-FU or MMC.

Internal revision of the sclerostomy. A paracentesis is made, and a blunt instrument such as a cyclodialysis spatula is used to push open the scleral flap and break adhesions from inside the AC.

External surgical bleb revision. The conjunctiva is reflected from a fornix-based approach, and the scar tissue over the flap is excised. The conjunctiva is closed in the same manner as a standard fornix-based trabeculectomy.

References

Allingham RR. Filtering surgery in the management of glaucoma. In: Epstein DL, Allingham RR, Schuman JS, eds. *Chandler and Grant's glaucoma*. 4th ed. Baltimore, MD: Lippincott Williams & Wilkins, 1997;516–537.

Sherwood MB, Migdal CS, Hitchings RA, et al: Initial treatment of glaucoma: surgery or medications. *Surv Ophthalmol* 1993;37:293–305.

Antimetabolite Therapy

Indications

Antimetabolites are used in patients who are at increased risk for filtration failure:

Young age.

Race: African Americans, Asians.

Previously failed filtration surgery.

Aphakic and pseudophakic glaucoma.

Congenital and juvenile glaucoma.

Neovascular glaucoma.

Other secondary angle-closure glaucomas.

Inflammatory glaucoma.

Contraindications

Antimetabolites should be used with caution in patients with very friable conjunctiva that may not heal well or an overfiltering bleb in the fellow eye after antimetabolite therapy, or if the AC has been entered prematurely during scleral flap dissection.

Mechanism

- Wound healing:
  - Coagulation and vasoconstriction.
  - Inflammation: white blood cells, cytokines, and enzymes.
  - Early repair: macrophages, fibroblasts, and epithelial cells
  - Granulation tissue: vascular buds by 3 to 4 days.
  - Scar formation: Fibroblasts secrete collagen and proteins over 2 to 3 weeks.
  - Remodeling: Scar tissue matures and healing is complete by 6 weeks.
- 5-FU: pyrimidine analog that inhibits thymidylate synthesis and DNA synthesis during the active phase (S phase) of the cell cycle.
- Mitomycin C: alkylating agent
  - Inhibits fibroblast proliferation by inhibiting DNA and RNA synthesis.
  - It is not cell-cycle specific and therefore has a lasting effect on a wide variety of tissues.
  - Much more potent than 5-FU (100 times).

Application

- 5-FU:
  - Intraoperative: applied to cellulose sponges over sclera and underneath conjunctiva and Tenon's capsule for 5 minutes before entering the AC. The sponge is then removed, and the area copiously irrigated with saline.
  - Postoperative: 0.1 mL (5 mg) injected into the subconjunctival space adjacent to or up to 180 degrees away from the bleb. This may be performed alone (5 to 10 injections) or following intraoperative application (up to 5 injections) for up to 4 weeks after surgery.
- Mitomycin C: 0.2 to 0.5 mg/mL applied intraoperatively for 2 to 5 minutes by the method described above. The concentration and time should be titrated to the tendency of the patient to scar.

Complications

Because of its potency, mitomycin C is accompanied by a higher rate of complications than is 5-FU:

Corneal epithelial defects: These are usually self-limited and should be treated conservatively with antibiotic ointment.

Corneal edema can occur, especially when the antimetabolite gains access to the AC during or after surgery, and is caused by corneal endothelial cell damage.

Conjunctival wound leaks: These should be repaired with a mattress suture. Scraping of the conjunctival epithelium or a small amount of bleeding may encourage healing.

Bleb overfiltration: The formation of thin, cystic, avascular blebs may lead to chronic hypotony from bleb overfiltration. Treatment includes:

Laser treatment of the bleb.

Autologous blood injection.

Scleral patch graft.

Bleb suturing.

Bleb rupture: A ruptured bleb can heal spontaneously or may require a conjunctival graft repair.

Scleral thinning and necrosis.

References

Palmer SS. Mitomycin as adjunct chemotherapy with trabeculectomy. *Ophthalmology* 1991;98:317–321.

The Fluorouracil Filtering Surgery Study Group. Three-year follow-up of the fluorouracil filtering surgery study. *Am J Ophthalmol* 1993;115:82–92.

GLAUCOMA

Aqueous Shunt Devices

Summary

The treatment of refractory glaucomas has evolved to include the use of drainage devices to facilitate the flow of aqueous humor through a tube implanted in the AC to the subconjunctival space.

Indications

Previously failed filtering surgery.
Neovascular glaucoma.
Uveitic glaucoma.
Congenital and juvenile glaucoma.
Aphakic and pseudophakic glaucoma.
Postpenetrating keratoplasty glaucoma.
ICE syndrome.
Keratoprosthesis.
Glaucomas with increased episcleral venous pressure.

Seton Devices

First, the device must be made of a material that is nonreactive and has poor fibroblast adhesion. It should establish a potential space in which aqueous humor can pool and be slowly absorbed. The bleb capsule must be posterior enough to minimize postoperative inflammation, thinning, and corneal dellen.

Most Commonly Used Devices

Molteno implant: The Molteno device consists of a silicone tube connected to a plate with a surface area of 270 mm^2. The double-plated device has a second plate attached to the first with another silicone tube. It relies on the formation of a capsule around the plates to limit the flow of aqueous humor.

Baerveldt implant: This device consists of a silicone tube connected to a plate with surface area of 250 or 350 mm^2. Like the Molteno device, it has no mechanism to impede aqueous flow and relies on capsule formation.

Krupin eye valve: The Krupin eye valve consists of a silicone tube for insertion into the AC and sidearms for support. The external portion of the tube has a slit where it is mounted onto the silicone plate. The valve function is a result of the slit providing unidirectional flow and resistance below a certain pressure, which is approximately 9 to 11 mm Hg.

Ahmed glaucoma valve: The Ahmed implant has a silicone tube connected to a plate via a protected sleeve valve. The aqueous humor flows through the tube and between two halves of a folded silicone elastomer membrane, which has been placed under tension perpendicular to the direction of flow. This configuration is designed to allow flow at a pressure of 8 to 10 mm Hg and requires that the valve be primed at the time of surgery.

Surgical Technique

All devices have in common the mounting of the implant on the sclera and the insertion of the tube into the AC. The nonresistive devices (Molteno, Baerveldt) also have several methods to help prevent postoperative hypotony, including the two-stage operation, internal suture occlusion, and tube ligature. A fenestration is typically made with suture needle tip to prevent high IOP in cases where tube ligature is required (e.g., Molteno and Baerveldt).

1. Conjunctival dissection: A fornix-based flap is made under conjunctiva and Tenon's capsule extending 90 degrees for a single-plate and 180 degrees for a double-plate implant. Relaxing incisions extending posteriorly aid in exposure.
2. The device should be primed with saline to ensure free flow of aqueous humor.
3. Mounting of device (Figure 5.34):
   - The implant is positioned between the superior rectus and horizontal rectus muscle with the anterior edge of the plate 8 to 10 mm posterior to the limbus.
   - The second plate of the double-plate Molteno device is passed under the superior rectus to the other superior quadrant.
   - The plate is secured to the sclera using a nonabsorbable suture.
   - The tube is cut to approximate length at an angle with the bevel up.
   - A paracentesis is made, and viscoelastic is injected to fill the AC.
   - A 23-gauge needle is inserted into the AC just anterior and parallel to the iris plane.

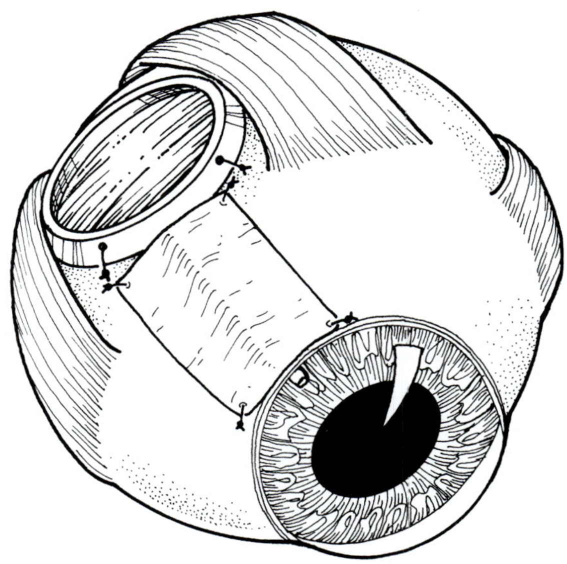

FIGURE 5.34. Placement of a seton. Notice the scleral patch covering the silicone tube that enters the anterior chamber. (From Epstein DL. *Chandler and Grant's glaucoma*, 4th ed. Baltimore, MD: Lippincott Williams & Wilkins, 1997:566, with permission.)

The tube is inserted through this tract.
The tube should be covered by a scleral flap or with a scleral patch graft (donor cornea or pericardium can alternatively be used), both of which are secured with nonabsorbable sutures.
The conjunctiva and Tenon's capsule are closed.
The AC is filled with saline, and the viscoelastic flushed out.

Complications

- Hypotony and related complications (flat AC, choroidal effusion [Figure 5.35], cataracts, hypotony maculopathy, retinal edema or folds, and corneal decompensation):
  - If there is corneal-lenticular touch, reform the AC with viscoelastic.
  - Repair conjunctival leaks.
- High IOP:
  - Early: Look for fibrin, viscoelastic, or blood blocking the tube. Digital massage often pushes the blockage through, or Nd:YAG laser or AC washout may be necessary. If there is a stent or ligature, loosen or remove it (this may cause hypotony).
  - Late: most likely a result of capsule formation limiting the flow of aqueous humor. Intraoperative mitomycin has not been shown to be beneficial.
- Tube erosion. This must be repaired with a scleral patch graft to prevent the risk of endophthalmitis.
- Corneal edema and corneal transplant rejection. These can be minimized by avoiding anterior entry of the tube and ensuring that the tip does not touch the endothelium. In corneal transplant patients, the violation of the anterior chamber autoimmune deviation (ACAID) response may increase rejection rates. In some cases, the tube can be placed into the sulcus in pseudophakic eyes or through the pars plana and into the vitreous cavity if the eye has been vitrectomized.

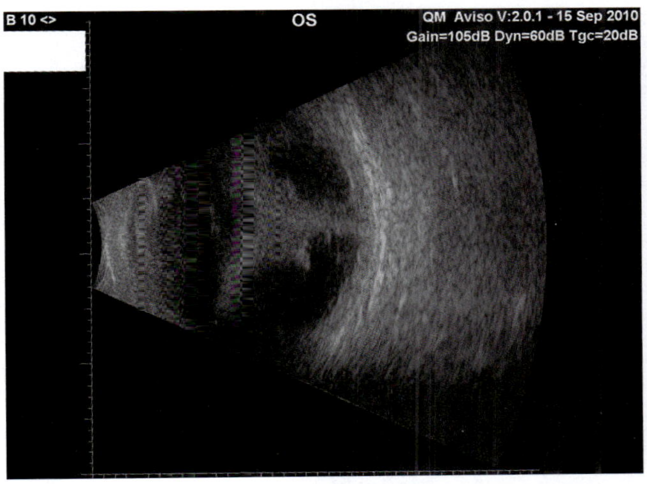

FIGURE 5.35. Ultrasound of choroidal effusions in a hypotonous eye following seton placement. (Courtesy of Thomas Patrianakos, MD.)

- Corneal dellen. This complication is a result of an elevation of conjunctiva at the limbus because of a thick scleral patch. It usually responds to aggressive therapy with lubricating ointment, but replacement of the scleral patch may be required.
- Diplopia. Diplopia can occur because of damage to the rectus muscle or, more commonly, a restriction attributable to the mass effect of the implant. Initial treatment is conservative, later treatment is with prism, and refractory cases may require reoperation on the muscles or removal of the shunt.

References

Lieberman MF, Ewing RH. Drainage implant surgery for refractory glaucoma. *Int Ophthalmol Clin* 1990;30:198–208.

Molteno ACB. The use of draining implants in resistant cases of glaucoma. *Trans Ophthalmol Soc N Z* 1983;35:94–97.

Nairne JEAH, Sherwood D, Jacob JSH, et al. Single stage insertion of the Molteno tube for glaucoma and modifications to reduce postoperative hypotony. *Br J Ophthalmol* 1988;72:846–885.

Ab Interno Trabeculectomy (Trabectome)

Summary

The Trabectome is a recently developed surgical procedure aimed at increasing aqueous humor outflow. It involves surgical removal of a strip of trabecular meshwork and inner wall of Schlemm's canal under gonioscopic visualization with a microelectrosurgical device.

Indications

Primarily for use in adult, open-angle glaucoma patients.
Can be done as a combined procedure with cataract surgery.

Surgical Technique

1. Clear corneal incision for access into the anterior chamber is made near the limbus with a 1.6-mm keratome blade after preoperative instillation of 1% pilocarpine.
2. Viscoelastic is used to stabilize/prevent flattening of the anterior chamber during the procedure. Recent reports indicate this step is not universally necessary.
3. The 19-g tip of the device is introduced into the anterior chamber under gonioscopic visualization to engage the nasal trabecular meshwork. The tip has a triangular, ceramic-coated footplate that is directed through TM into Schlemm's canal.
4. The body of the footplate is designed to act as a guide within Schlemm's canal, with the proximal portion of the tip containing a microbipolar cautery that catches and ablates the portion of the TM that is fed into it.
5. As the TM tissue is ablated, continual infusion/aspiration at the tip cools the tissue to avoid heat damage and to remove tissue debris.

6. The tip is used to treat TM in both directions starting opposite the corneal incision. Approximately 60 to 90 degrees of TM can be treated through a single incision.
7. Irrigation with balanced salt solution or use of the irrigation/aspiration tip from a phaco machine is used to remove remaining viscoelastic.
8. Single 10-0 nylon suture or anterior chamber air bubble may be used to ensure an adequate watertight seal at the corneal incision.

Complications

- Hemorrhage from Schlemm's canal frequently occurs during ablation but is usually minor and self-limited.
- Peripheral anterior synechiae development at the ablation or corneal incision site.
- Postoperative hypotony.
- Postoperative IOP spike.
- Descemet detachment/injury.

Postoperative Management

- Topical 1% pilocarpine BID ×2 weeks.
- Topical antibiotics and corticosteroids.

References

Minckler D, Baerveldt G, Ramirez MA, et al. Clinical results with the Trabectome, a novel surgical device for treatment of open-angle glaucoma. *Trans Am Ophthalmol Soc* 2006;104:40–50.

Minckler D, Mosaed S, Dustin L, et al. Trabectome (trabeculectomy-internal approach): additional experience and extended follow-up. *Trans Am Ophthalmol Soc* 2008;106:149–159.

Canaloplasty

Summary

Canaloplasty is a recent nonpenetrating surgical development aimed at increasing TM outflow. It involves circumferentially dilating Schlemm's canal with viscoelastic followed by placement of a tensioning suture 360 degrees around that is tied down to maintain patency of Schlemm's canal. It is based on the theory that increased IOP in OAG patients can contribute to compression and collapse of Schlemm's canal, which causes worsening of trabecular outflow facility.

Indications

Primarily for use in adult, open-angle glaucoma patients. Can be done as a combined procedure with cataract surgery. May have use in patients where anterior chamber entry is not desired, like nanophthalmic eyes or in cases with elevated episcleral venous pressure like Sturge-Weber.

Surgical Technique

1. Conjunctival dissection: A peritomy is made under conjunctiva and Tenon's capsule at the limbus and extended posteriorly to adequately allow for scleral flap construction.
2. Scleral flap is created as in a standard trabeculectomy.
3. A radial scratch incision is made at the limbus and posteriorly in the scleral bed until Schlemm's canal is visualized.
4. Viscoelastic is injected into Schlemm's canal (viscodilation) to dilate and aid in ease of passage of the cannula.
5. Schlemm's canal is intubated with a cannula that has a lighted tip and passed 360 degrees around until it emerges from the opposite end of the canal within the radial incision. The lighted tip allows for identification of location as the cannula is passed along the entire circumferential length of Schlemm's canal. Alternatively, the 10-0 Prolene suture tip can be passed blindly around the canal. Care should be taken if resistance is encountered to prevent dissection into the suprachoroidal space.
6. A 10-0 Prolene suture is then secured to the tip of the cannula, and the cannula is withdrawn leaving the suture in place. The suture, which is now present circumferentially 360 degrees, is tied down at the radial incision to create tension within Schlemm's canal.
7. The scleral flap and conjunctiva are tightly sutured down over top of the radial incision.

Complications

- Hemorrhage of episcleral vessels, common in patients chronically on glaucoma medications, can be controlled with light cautery to the scleral bed prior to scleral flap creation.
- Dissection of cannula or suture out of Schlemm's canal and into the suprachoroidal space posteriorly. Use of the lighted tip aids in visualization of tip location.
- Bleb formation from communication from the AC to the subconjunctival space.
- Conjunctival scarring.
- Scleral staphyloma from dissection.

Postoperative Management

- Topical steroids and antibiotics.

References

Grieshaber MC, Pienaar A, Olivier J, et al. Clinical evaluation of the aqueous outflow system in primary open-angle glaucoma for canaloplasty. *Invest Ophthalmol Vis Sci* 2010;51(3):1498–1504.

Lewis RA, von Wolff K, Tetz M, et al. Canaloplasty: circumferential viscodilation of Schlemm canal using a flexible microcatheter for the treatment of open-angle glaucoma in adults: two-year interim clinical study results. *J Cataract Refract Surg* 2009;35(5):814–824.

Surgical Procedures Under Investigation

Several newer technologies for treatment of open-angle glaucomas are being evaluated including the Glaukos iStent, Excimer trabeculoplasty, and the Solx (suprachoroidal shunt). These procedures are under investigation, and information on their efficacy will be available in the near future.

Nonpenetrating Procedures

Cyclodestructive Procedures

Indications

1. Severe glaucoma poorly controlled by medical treatment or filtering surgery.
2. Eyes in which filtering surgery is contraindicated or impossible, such as those with corneal transplants, extensive conjunctival scarring, or intraocular tumors.
3. Poorly seeing eye with pain and corneal edema secondary to elevated IOP.
4. Patient is unable to undergo incisional surgery because of general medical problems.

Contraindications

There are no true contraindications to this procedure, but it is generally performed in selected cases as a last resort.

Mechanism

The effect of these procedures is a reduction of aqueous production by destroying or altering the ciliary epithelium. Eyes with more pigment are more sensitive to treatment, presumably as a result of increased absorption of laser energy and greater tissue destruction.

Complications

The frequency and type of complications are related to the type of procedure used and the resultant tissue destruction. The most complications are seen after cyclocryotherapy, followed by transscleral cyclophotocoagulation (noncontact > contact) and direct endoscopic cyclophotocoagulation:

Pain: Pain is common and can be reduced by cycloplegia and steroids.

Uveitis: Inflammation is common and is treated with topical steroids. Sympathetic ophthalmia is a rare complication.

Decreased vision: This is usually due to macular edema.

Hypotony with or without phthisis bulbi: This is an uncommon complication but does occur as a result of hyposecretion and extensive tissue destruction.

Miscellaneous: Suprachoroidal effusion or hemorrhage, vitreous hemorrhage, scleral thinning, cataract formation, sympathetic ophthalmia (very rare).

Technique (for All Methods)

- Preoperative retrobulbar anesthesia.
- Postoperative management consists of adequate pain control, subconjunctival steroids, and topical steroids and atropine.
- All glaucoma medications are continued preoperatively and postoperatively and can be discontinued as indicated.

Cyclocryotherapy

Instrument: nitrous oxide cryounit with 2.5-mm cryoprobe tip.

Power: –80°C.

Location: 1 to 1.5 mm from the limbus at each clock-hour position for 180 to 270 degrees.

Time: up to 60 seconds (until an iceball forms 2 mm into the cornea).

Noncontact Transscleral Cyclophotocoagulation

Instrument: Nd:YAG laser.

Power: 4 to 8 J.

Location: 1 to 1.5 mm from the limbus, eight spots per quadrant for 360 degrees.

Time: 20-ms exposure.

Contact Transscleral Cyclophotocoagulation

Instrument: Nd:YAG laser or diode laser.

Power:

Nd:YAG: 4 to 8 J (reduce by 0.5 J if pops are heard with three consecutive treatments).

Diode: 1.5 to 2.5 W for 1 to 2 seconds. Newer models have lower power/longer duration: 1,250 to 1,500 mW for 4 seconds.

Location:

Nd:YAG: 1 mm from the limbus, eight spots per quadrant for 360 degrees.

Diode: 1.2 mm from limbus, 16 to 19 spots for 270 degrees.

Time:

Nd:YAG: 0.7 seconds.

Diode: 2 to 4 seconds, depending on the power of the diode laser being used.

Endoscopic Cyclophotocoagulation (ECP)

Indications: decreased IOP (reduced aqueous humor formation) by ciliary process destruction. Better option for patients with visual potential, as it incites less inflammation with less risk for loss of vision compared to

CPC. Anterior chamber approach under direct visualization, so can be done as a combined procedure with cataract surgery or used in pediatric, pseudophakic, or aphakic eyes.

Instrument: 20-g endoscope with fiberoptic light source, helium-neon (He-Ne) aiming beam, and 810-nm diode laser.

Power: 250 to 600 mW, titrating up to get shrinkage of the ciliary process.

Location: Direct visualization is obtained via intraocular insertion of the probe into the ciliary sulcus, which is expanded with viscoelastic. Treatment is for 270 to 360 degrees.

Time: 0.5 to 2.0 seconds, controlled by a foot switch to reach the end point of shrinkage and whitening of the ciliary process.

References

Schuman JS, Puliafito CA. Laser cyclophotocoagulation. *Int Ophthalmol Clin* 1990;30:111–119.

Uram M. Endoscopic cyclophotocoagulation in glaucoma management. *Curr Opin Ophthalmol* 1995;6:19–29.

GLAUCOMA STUDIES

Advanced Glaucoma Intervention Study (AGIS)

Summary

Assess the long-term outcomes of sequences of interventions involving trabeculectomy and argon laser trabeculoplasty in eyes that have failed initial medical treatment of glaucoma.

Study Population

- 789 eyes of 591 patients with medically uncontrolled open-angle glaucoma recruited from 1988 to 1992.

Study Design

- Multicenter, randomized clinical trial comparing 2 different treatment sequences: argon laser trabeculoplasty-trabeculectomy-trabeculectomy (ATT) versus trabeculectomy-argon laser trabeculoplasty-trabeculectomy (TAT).

Results

- After 7 years of follow-up, results revealed that blacks and whites differed in the way they benefited from the two treatment programs. The vision in eyes of black patients with advanced glaucoma tended to be better preserved in the program that started with laser surgery.
- From initial treatment through 7 years of follow-up, the average percent of eyes in black patients with decrease of vision was 28% in the program starting with laser surgery (ATT), as compared with 37 percent in the program starting with trabeculectomy (TAT).
- Lower IOP was associated with less visual field loss. Participants with an average IOP of 12 mm Hg, and an IOP of 18 mm Hg or less at all visits had significantly less visual field loss.

Conclusions

- Based on these results, it is recommended that black patients with advanced glaucoma begin a treatment program that starts with laser surgery.
- In contrast, white patients with advanced glaucoma who have no life-threatening health problems that would preclude surgery should start with trabeculectomy.
- Lower IOP reduces visual field loss (goal of 12 mm Hg, <18 mm Hg for all visits).

References

Nouri-Mahdavi K, Hoffman D, Coleman AL, et al. Predictive factors for glaucomatous visual field progression in the Advanced Glaucoma Intervention Study. *Ophthalmology* 2004;111:1627–1635.

The AGIS Investigators. The Advanced Glaucoma Intervention Study (AGIS): 7. The relationship between control of intraocular pressure and visual field deterioration. *Am J Ophthalmol* 2000;130:429–440.

Ocular Hypertension Treatment Study (OHTS)

Summary

To determine whether medical reduction of IOP prevents or delays the onset of glaucomatous visual field loss and/or optic disk damage in ocular hypertensive (OHT) subjects judged to be at moderate risk for developing open-angle glaucoma.

Study Population

- 1,637 patients with ocular hypertension recruited between 1994 and 1996.

Study Design

- Multicenter, randomized clinical trial comparing observation alone with medical therapy for ocular hypertension.
- OHT subjects included had an IOP of 24 to 32 mm Hg in one eye, and 21 to 32 mm Hg in the fellow eye. All participants had normal visual fields and optic nerves upon enrollment.
- Primary outcome variable was visual field loss or optic nerve damage.
- The goal for IOP reduction in the treatment arm was 20% reduction from baseline and IOP less than 24 mm Hg.

Results

- At 5 years of follow-up, the observation group had a 9.5% rate of progression to open-angle glaucoma compared to 4.4% in the treatment group.
- IOP reduction averaged 22.5% in the treatment group versus 4.0% in controls, and topical medications were generally well tolerated.
- Risk factors identified for development of open-angle glaucoma included: increased age, increased cup-disk ratio, greater pattern standard deviation, baseline IOP, and decreased central corneal thickness (CCT).
- CCT was found to be a powerful predictor of open-angle glaucoma development in this population.
- OHTS subjects had thicker corneas than the general population, and black patients had thinner corneas than white patients in the study.

Conclusions

- The findings of this trial verified that topical ocular hypotensive medications are effective in delaying or preventing the onset of open-angle glaucoma in patients with elevated IOP.
- The majority of patients in the observation group (90.5%) did not develop visual field loss or optic disk changes at the 5-year mark, implying that not all patients with borderline or elevated IOP should receive treatment.
- Clinicians should consider initiating treatment for individuals with OHTN who are at moderate or high risk for developing open-angle glaucoma, based on the risk factors identified in this study.

References

Gordon MO, Beiser JA, Brandt JD, et al. The Ocular Hypertension Treatment Study: baseline factors that predict the onset of primary open-angle glaucoma. *Arch Ophthalmol* 2002;120:714–720.

Kass MA, Heuer DK, Higginbotham EJ, et al. The Ocular Hypertension Treatment Study: a randomized trial determines that topical ocular hypotensive medication delays or prevents the onset of primary open-angle glaucoma. *Arch Ophthalmol* 2002;120:701–713.

Collaborative Initial Glaucoma Treatment Study (CIGTS)

Summary

To compare the long-term effect of treating newly diagnosed open-angle glaucoma with standard medical treatment versus filtration surgery.

Study Population

- 607 patients with open-angle glaucoma recruited from 1993 to 1997.

Study Design

- Multicenter, randomized clinical trial comparing initial medical treatment with initial surgical therapy for open-angle glaucoma.
- Primary outcome variable was progression of visual field loss.
- Secondary outcomes were quality of life, visual acuity, and IOP.

Results

- Initial medical and surgical therapy resulted in similar outcomes upon visual field testing for the 2 groups after 5 years of follow-up. Early visual acuity loss was greater in the surgery group, but this difference diminished with time.
- IOP averaged about 2 to 3 points lower in the surgical group (14 to 15 mm Hg) compared to medical group (17 to 18 mm Hg).
- Quality of life impact scores were very similar for the 2 groups, with the most consistent finding being increased local eye sympoms reported by the surgical group.
- Overall rate of progression was lower than many clinical trials, thought to be due to more aggressive IOP goals.

Conclusions

- Based on this trial, initial treatment of open-angle glaucoma with medical therapy or surgery results in similar visual field outcome.
- Patients who get early surgery for glaucoma have temporary decreased visual acuity and higher rates of cataract extraction, but the difference in visual acuity converges over time with medical treatment.

Reference

Lichter PR, Musch DC, Gillespie BW, et al. Interim clinical outcomes in the Collaborative Initial Glaucoma Treatment Study comparing initial treatment randomized to medications or surgery. *Ophthalmology* 2001;108:1943–1953.

Collaborative Normal-Tension Glaucoma Study (CNTGS)

Summary

This study was designed to establish the rate of progression, and to determine the effect of IOP reduction on open-angle glaucoma patients who have IOP in the normal range.

Study Design

- In patients with open-angle glaucoma and IOP in the normal range, patients were randomized to observation versus treatment by lowering IOP by 30% or more.
- Primary outcome variable was progression of visual field loss.

Results

- Reducing IOP by greater than 30% in the treatment group reduced the rate of visual field progression from 35% to 12%.
- Some patients continued to progress despite reduction in IOP.
- When visual field loss did occur, it tended to be slow.

Conclusions

- The results of this trial helped to establish a clear role of IOP in the management of patients with normal-tension glaucoma.
- Some patients continued to progress despite what was considered therapeutic reduction in IOP, and not all untreated patients did progress during the study, suggesting that other factors likely play a role as well.
- Given the rate of progression, each treatment strategy must be individualized to a given patient.

References

Collaborative Normal-Tension Study Group: Comparison of glaucomatous progression between untreated patients with normal-tension glaucoma and patients with therapeutically reduced intraocular pressures. *Am J Ophthalmol* 1998;126:487–497.

Collaborative Normal-Tension Study Group: The effectiveness of intraocular pressure reduction in the treatment of normal-tension glaucoma. *Am J Ophthalmol* 1998;126:498–505.

Early Manifest Glaucoma Trial (EMGT)

Summary

To compare the effect of immediate therapy to lower the IOP versus late or no treatment on the progression of newly detected open-angle glaucoma.

Study Population

- Newly diagnosed patients aged 50 to 80 years old with early visual field defects who were identified from population screening of 44,000 residents in Sweden.
- Patients with advanced visual field loss, mean IOP greater than 30 mm Hg or any IOP greater than 35 mm Hg, or visual acuity less than 20/40 were excluded.
- 255 patients were randomized to each study arm.

Study Design

- Multicenter, randomized clinical trial comparing observation alone versus betaxolol plus laser trabeculoplasty.
- Primary outcome variable was progression of visual field loss and optic nerve head changes.

Results

- At 6 years, 62% of untreated patients had visual field loss progression compared with 45% in the treated group. In multivariate analyses, progression risk was cut in half by treatment.
- The above treatment with betaxolol and ALT reduced IOP by 25%.
- Risk factors identified for progression included no treatment, older age, higher baseline IOP, exfoliation, disk hemorrhages, and bilateral disease.
- Progression risk decreased by approximately 10% for each 1 mm Hg drop in IOP from baseline.

Conclusions

- Early treatment of glaucoma decreases the risk for progression by 50%.
- Risk factors for progression include no treatment, older age, higher baseline IOP, exfoliation, disk hemorrhages, and bilateral disease.

References

Heijl A, Leske MC, Bengtsson B, et al. Reduction of intraocular pressure and glaucoma progression: results from the Early Manifest Glaucoma Trial. *Arch Ophthalmol* 2002;120:1268–1279.

Leske MC, Heijl A, Hussein M, et al. Factors for glaucoma progression and the effect of treatment: the Early Manifest Glaucoma Trial. *Arch Ophthalmol* 2003;121:48–56.

Glaucoma Laser Trial Study

Summary

Compared the efficacy and safety of argon laser trabeculoplasty (ALT) versus topical medication as a starting treatment for POAG.

Study Population

- Age greater than 35 years.
- IOP equal to or greater than 22 mm Hg in both eyes and glaucomatous visual field defects in at least 1 eye *or*.
- IOP equal to or greater than 27 mm Hg in one eye, and IOP equal to or greater than 31 mm Hg in the other eye, and cup-disk (c/d) ratio disparity equal to or greater than 0.67 and equal to or less than 1.5.
- Best corrected visual acuity of 20/70 or better in both eyes.
- Mean duration of follow-up, 7 to 9 years since diagnosis.

Major Variables

Change in visual field.
Change in optic disk.
Change in IOP.

Study Design

- Multicenter, randomized controlled clinical trial.
- One eye of each patient was randomly assigned to ALT as initial treatment, and the fellow eye was assigned to 0.5% timolol. Subsequent retreatment if necessary was

performed in the same stepped-medication regimen for both eyes.
- ALT performed in two sessions, 45 to 50 burns in 180 degrees each, 4 weeks apart. Power: 600 to 1,200 mW.

Results

- IOP: ALT group IOP decreased by 7 to 10 mm Hg; medical group: IOP decreased by 6 to 9 mm Hg; analysis of differences, ALT had 1.2 mm more IOP reduction.
- Visual fields: ALT group, mean change in decibels per test location of the visual field ranged from 0.5 to 1.1 dB during the first 2 years of follow-up indicating improvement; medical group: improvement through 3 years of follow-up (0.5 to 0.6 dB) with no change in negative mean changes at subsequent follow-ups.
- In both groups, C/D ratios showed slight increase in mean ratio of cup area to disk area over follow-up.
- Visual acuity: decreasing for both groups.

Conclusions

- Medication use was less for eyes initially treated with ALT.
- Similar proportions for both groups advanced to filtering surgery: 8% (23) in ALT group, 11% (31) in medical group.
- Initial treatment with ALT was at least as efficacious as initial treatment with topical medication.

References

Glaucoma Laser Trial Research Group. The Glaucoma Laser Trial, III: design and methods. *Controlled Clin Trials* 1991;12: 504–524.

The Glaucoma Laser Trial (GLT) and Glaucoma Laser Trial Follow-up Study: VII: results. *Am J Ophthalmol* 1995;120: 718–731.

5-Fluorouracil Filtering Surgery Study

Summary

To determine the long-term efficacy and safety of postoperative, subconjunctivally injected 5-FU in eyes with uncontrolled glaucoma and poor prognosis for filtering surgery, specifically, in aphakic and pseudophakic eyes and phakic eyes after failed filtering surgery.

Study Population

Patients with uncontrolled glaucoma (IOP > 21 mm Hg) who were receiving maximal medical therapy and had undergone cataract extraction *or* had at least one unsuccessful filtering procedure in a phakic eye without having previously received 5-FU.

Study Design

- Multicenter, randomized clinical trial.
- One eye per patient randomly assigned to trabeculectomy with 5-FU (5-FU group) versus trabeculectomy without 5-FU (standard group).
- The 5-FU group received 5.0 mg (0.5 mL) 5-FU solution injections 180 degrees from the operative site two times per day on postoperative days 1 through 7, and once daily on days 8 to 14.
- Failure defined as reoperation for control of IOP (IOP >21 mm Hg) during the first 3 years after surgery.

Results

- Failures: 49 of 100 (49%) in the 5-FU group in 3 years' follow-up; 73 of 99 (74%) in the standard group.
- Late-onset leakage more common in the 5-FU group (7/105 [7%]) as compared with the standard group (0/108 [0%]).

Conclusions

- Subconjunctival 5-FU after trabeculectomy was recommended in eyes with previous cataract surgery or unsuccessful filtering surgery.
- The increased risk of late-onset filter bleb leaks cautioned against the routine use of 5-FU in patients with good prognosis.

Reference

The Fluorouracil Filtering Surgery Study Group. Three-year follow-up of the Fluorouracil Filtering Surgery Study. *Am J Ophthalmol* 1993;115:82–92.

The Tube Versus Trabeculectomy Study (TVT)

Summary

Compare the safety and efficacy of nonvalved tube shunt surgery to trabeculectomy with mitomycin C in patients with previous intraocular surgery.

Study Design

- Multicenter randomized clinical trial.
- Patients aged 18 to 85 years of age with prior trabeculectomy, cataract extraction with IOL, or both and inadequate IOP control (between 18 and 40 mm Hg) on medical therapy randomized to undergo 350-mm^2 Baerveldt glaucoma implant or trabeculectomy with MMC (0.4 mg/mL for 4 minutes).
- Primary Outcome Measures: IOP, complication rates, visual acuity, visual field, quality of life, reoperation rates, and need for supplemental medical therapy.

Study Conclusions

- Ongoing clinical trial. Results from the TVT Study should help to provide direction between these two commonly used procedures for management in this patient population.

- Preliminary results: nonvalved tube shunt surgery more likely to maintain IOP control, avoid hypotony, and avoid reoperation than trabeculectomy with MMC during the first year of follow-up. Both with similar IOP reduction at 1 year, but less need for supplemental medical therapy in the trabeculectomy with MMC group.
- At 3 years, tube shunt surgery had higher success rates compared to trabeculectomy with MMC. Both had similar IOP reduction and rates of supplemental topical therapy required. The incidence of postoperative complications was higher in the trabeculectomy with MMC group (60%) compared with the tube shunt group (39%).

References

Gedde SJ, Schiffman JC, Feuer WJ, et al. The tube versus trabeculectomy study: design and baseline characteristics of study patients. *Am J Ophthalmol* 2005;140(2):275–287.

Gedde SJ, Schiffman JC, Feuer WJ, et al. Treatment outcomes in the tube versus trabeculectomy study after one year of follow-up. *Am J Ophthalmol* 2007;143(1):9–22.

Gedde SJ, Schiffman JC, Feuer WJ, et al. Three-year follow-up of the tube versus trabeculectomy study. *Am J Ophthalmol* 2009;148(5):670–684.

The Ahmed Versus Baerveldt Comparison (ABC) Trial

Summary

Compare the long term outcomes of Ahmed and Baerveldt tube shunt implants in the treatment of refractory glaucoma.

Study Design

- Multicenter randomized clinical trial.
- Trial to compare head-to-head surgical outcomes of the Ahmed versus Baerveldt tube shunts.

Study Conclusions

- Ongoing clinical trial to decide; results likely in 1 to 2 years.
- At the time of writing this chapter, Tsai et al. has reported a non-randomized study comparing outcome results from a single surgeon.

Reference

Tsai JC, Johnson CC, Kammer JA, et al. The Ahmed shunt versus the Baerveldt shunt for refracgtory glaucoma II: longer-term outcomes from a single surgeon. *Ophthalmology* 2006;113(6):913–917.

Beaver Dam Eye Study

Summary

Investigated the relationships of a history of migraine headaches, smoking, alcohol drinking, and diabetes with open-angle glaucoma.

Study Population

- Private census of Beaver Dam, Wisconsin, from September 15, 1987, to May 4, 1988.
- Total population: 5,925 in target age of 43 to 84 years; n = 4,926.

Study Design

Epidemiologic study of age-related eye disease.

Conclusions

- No evidence of relationship between open-angle glaucoma and migraine headache.
- No difference in frequency of glaucoma by drinking/cigarette-smoking status.
- Presence of open-angle glaucoma was increased in people with older-onset diabetes (7.8% of patients with diabetes compared with 3.9% of patients without diabetes).
- Prevalence of open-angle glaucoma, 2.1%; prevalence increased with age from 0.9% in individuals 43 to 54 years of age to 47% in individuals 74 years of age and older. No significant effect of patients' sex after adjusting for age. This prevalence is similar to that in other white populations.

References

Klein BE, Klein R, Meuer SM, et al. Migraine headache and its association with open angle glaucoma: the Beaver Dam Eye Study. *Invest Ophthal Vis Sci* 1993;34:3024–3027.

Klein BE, Klein R, Jensen SC. Open angle glaucoma and older onset diabetes: the Beaver Dam Eye Study. *Ophthalmology* 1994;101:1173–1177.

Klein BE, Klein R, Sponsel WE, et al. Prevalence of glaucoma: the Beaver Dam Eye Study. *Ophthalmology* 1992;99:1499–1504.

Klein BE, Klein R, Ritter LL. Relationship of drinking alcohol and smoking to prevalence of open angle glaucoma: the Beaver Dam Eye Study. *Ophthalmology* 1993;100:1609–1613.

United States Latanoprost Study Group

Summary

- Compared the ocular hypotensive efficacy and side effects of latanoprost with timolol.
- Determined the efficacy of latanoprost during 1 year of treatment.

Study Design and Population

- Multicenter, randomized, double-masked, parallel group study.
- Two hundred sixty-eight patients with ocular hypertension or early primary open-angle glaucoma received either latanoprost 0.005% once daily or timolol 0.5% twice daily for 6 months.
- Latanoprost 0.005% was applied topically once daily for 12 months in 272 patients.

Study Conclusions

- IOP reduction achieved with latanoprost (–6.7 ±3.4 mm Hg) was significantly greater than that produced with timolol (–4.9 ± [illegible] mm Hg) in 6 months.
- Pulse rate significantly reduced with timolol, but not with latanoprost.
- Slightly more conjunctival hyperemia was noted in the latanoprost-treated group than in the timolol-treated group.
- Fewer subjective side effects noted in the latanoprost group than the timolol group.
- Latanoprost significantly reduced diurnal IOP from 25.3 ±3.0 mm Hg at baseline to 17.4 ± 2.7 mm Hg (32% reduction) at [illegible] months in 198 patients.
- IOP reduction was maintained throughout the 12 months without evidence of drift and was not affected by sex, age, race and eye color.
- Possible or definite increase in iris pigmentation was noted in 1[illegible]% of 272 patients in 1 year.

References

Camras CB, the United States Latanoprost Study Group. Comparison of latanoprost and timolol in patients with ocular hypertension and glaucoma: a six-month, masked, multicenter trial in the United States. *Ophthalmology* 1996;103:138–147.

Camras CB, Alm A, Watson P, et al. Latanoprost: a prostaglandin analog for glaucoma therapy: efficacy and safety after 1 year of treatment in 19[illegible] patients. *Ophthalmology* 1996;103:1916–1924.

Apraclonidine Primary Therapy Study Group

Summary

Compared the long-term IOP-lowering efficacy of apraclonidine hydrochloride 0.25% and 0.5% with that of timolol maleate 0.5%.

Study Design

- Multicenter, randomized, double-masked clinical trial.
- Patients received apraclonidine 0.25% or 0.5% three times a day or 0.5% timolol twice a day for 90 days.

Study Conclusions

- Both apraclonidine 0.25% and 0.5% significantly reduced IOP when used as primary ocular hypotensive medication.
- Although apraclonidine 0.25% and 0.5% reduced IOP to a similar degree as timolol 0.5% 8 hours after morning dosing, neither concentration was as effective for reducing IOP after evening dosing.

Reference

Stewart WC, the Apraclonidine Primary Therapy Study Group. A 90-day study of the efficacy and side effects of 0.25% and 0.5% apraclonidine vs. 0.5% timolol. *Arch Ophthalmol* 1996;114:938–942.

CHAPTER

6

Neuro-Ophthalmology

Andrew G. Lee • Paul W. Brazis • Cynthia S. Chiu

NEURO-OPHTHALMOLOGIC HISTORY AND KEY TESTS

Three major categories of complaint in neuro-ophthalmology:

Afferent (e.g., visual loss, field or acuity, visual processing).
Efferent (e.g., diplopia, pupil abnormalities, eye lid abnormalities, jumping eyes).
Pain (e.g., headache, eye pain).

Questioning About Afferent System

Specifically define the following:

Onset (e.g., upon waking, following a headache).
Course (e.g., sudden, gradually progressive).
Duration (e.g., seconds, minutes, hours, days).
Severity of visual loss.
Q: "Could you see faces?"
Q: "Could you read?"
Q: "*Could you see motion?*"
Timing and onset of visual loss.
Laterality (and did the patient cover one eye to check?).
Monocular.
Binocular.
Progression.
Visual field defect versus acuity loss.
Associated pain (with eye movements?), headaches, nausea, or aura.
Associated motor or sensory dysfunction.
Associated scintillations or other visual phenomena.

Efferent Localization

Q: *"Where is the lesion?"*
Monocular or binocular (diplopia).
Vertical or horizontal diplopia.
Worse in fields of gaze (comitance) ?
Worse throughout day or fatigable?

Pain

Q: *"When, where, how much?"*
Palliative and precipitating factors.
Associated symptoms.

Motility Examination

- Head posture, head tilt, face position.
- Fixation preference (near and distance).
- Fixing with paretic eye or nonparetic eye.
- Dominance or better vision in fixing eye.
- Ductions (graded–4 [no movement] to 0 [normal]).
- Monocular movements.
- Cover fellow eye during testing.
- Movements (Table 6.1 and Figure 6.1):
  Supraduction or elevation: Eye moves up.
  Infraduction or depression: down.
  Abduction: away from midline.
  Adduction: toward midline
  Intorsion: inward rotation of the upper pole of the vertical meridian of each eye toward the midline of the face

Table 6.1

Muscle actions

Extraocular muscles	Primary	Secondary	Tertiary
Lateral rectus	Abduction	—	—
Medial rectus	Adduction	—	—
Superior rectus	Elevation	Adduction	Intorsion
Inferior rectus	Depression	Adduction	Extorsion
Superior oblique	Intorsion	Depression	Abduction
Inferior oblique	Extorsion	Elevation	Abduction

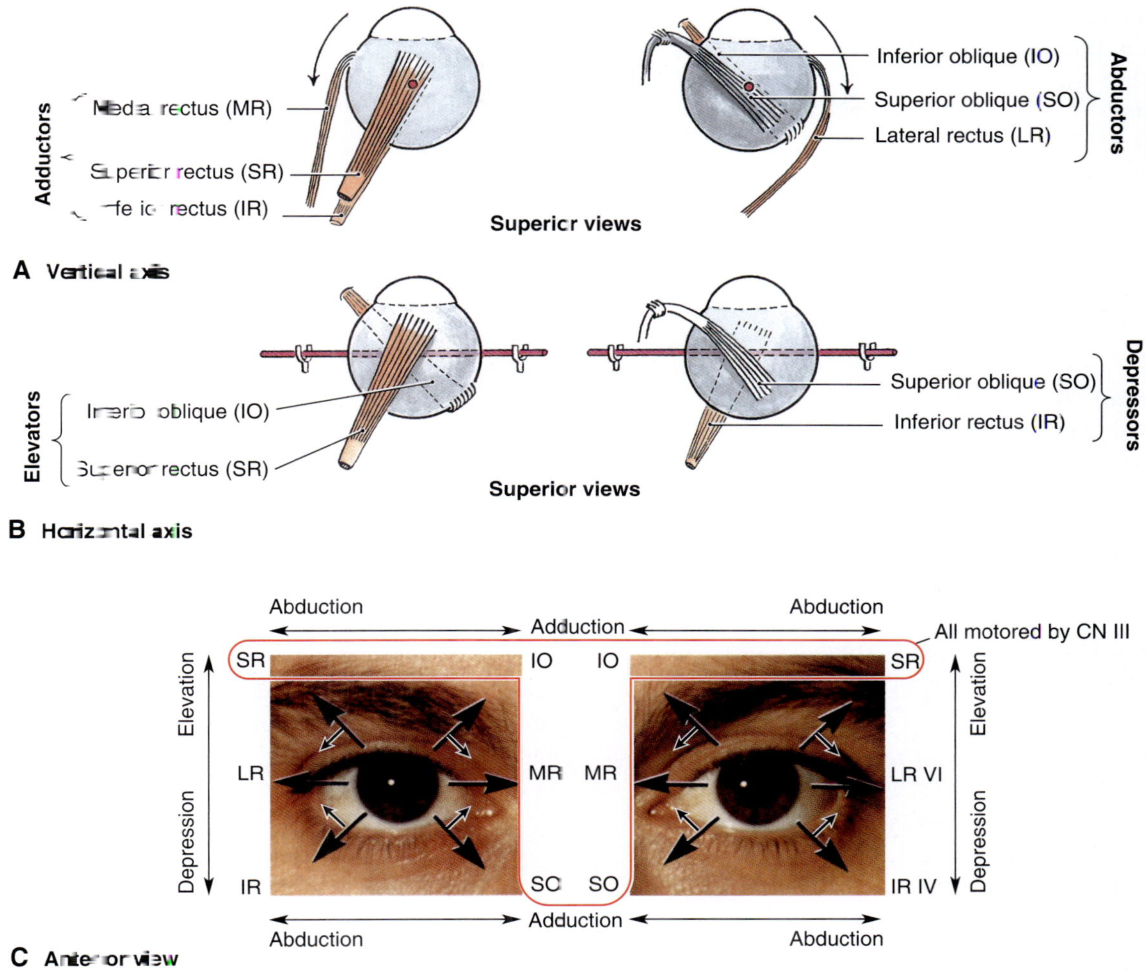

FIGURE 6.1. Basic eye movements. (CN, cranial nerve) (Adapted from Agur A, Dalley AF. *Grant's atlas of anatomy*, 11th ed. Baltimore, MD: Lippincott Williams & Wilkins, 2005:649, Figure 7.8.)

Extorsion: outward rotation of the upper pole of the vertical meridian of each eye away from the midline of the face

- Most elevation is due to superior rectus muscle (SRM) and most depression is due to inferior rectus muscle (IRM).
- Versions.
- Binocular movements.
- Ductions may be better than versions.

Accommodative Amplitude (Right Eye and Left Eye) Deviations

Distance with or without correction.
Near with or without correction.
Primary position and diagnostic positions.
Primary and secondary deviation.
Primary: fixing with nonparetic eye.
Secondary: fixing with paretic eye.
Secondary deviation greater than primary.
More innervational effort to keep paretic eye fixating on target.
Innervation drives fellow eye to greater deviation:
Esodeviation: turns in.
Exodeviation: turns out.
Hyperdeviation: eye turned up.
Hypodeviation: eye turned down.
Torsion (incyclotorsion or excyclotorsion).

Stereoacuity Testing

40 arc seconds: 20/20 acuity.
60 arc seconds: 20/40 acuity.
100 arc seconds: 20/200 acuity.
Titmus testing (i.e., fly, animals, circles).
Double Maddox rod testing for torsion.

Distance and Near Testing

Check primary and downgaze positions.
Especially useful for superior oblique palsy.

Can be compared to funduscopic torsion.
Saccades and pursuit (horizontal and vertical).
Latency.
Amplitude.
Accuracy.
Speed (velocity).

Motility: Special Tests

Cover-Uncover Test for Tropia or Manifest Deviation

Method

Have the patient fixate on target.
Cover one eye and look for shift in noncovered eye.
Uncover eyes.
Repeat test covering other eye.
Absence of shift: straight (orthotropia).
Shift of noncovered eye indicates tropia.
Requires vision good enough to fixate on target.

Alternate Cover Test for Phoria or Latent Deviation

Method

- Check cover-uncover test first; result must be negative (no tropia).
- Have the patient fixate on target.
- Cover one eye.
- Rapidly move cover to other eye and look for shift in eye as it is uncovered.
- Latent deviation kept in check by fusion.
- Cover-uncover test breaks down fusional control.
- Latent deviation revealed by eye movement when cover moved to other eye.

Hirschberg Test

For patients unable to fixate. See Figure 6.2.

Method

Hold fixation light at 33 cm.
Measure deviation of light reflex from pupil center, indicative of tropia.
Decentration of 1 mm = 7 degrees = 15 prism diopters.
Pupil edge margin = 15 degrees = 30 prism diopters.
Iris = 30 degrees = 60 prism diopters.
Limbus = 45 degrees = 90 prism diopters

Krimsky Method

For patients unable to fixate.

Hold fixation light at 33 cm.
Add prism in front of one eye until corneal light reflex is centered in both eyes.
Semiquantitative assessment of deviation.

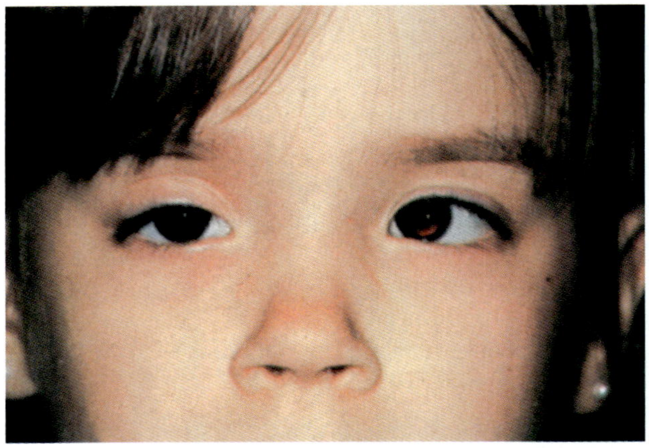

FIGURE 6.2. Left esotropia. Note lateral displacement of Hirschberg light reflex in the LE. Pupils are pharmacologically dilated. Photograph demonstrates right ptosis and asymmetry of the red reflex, which is caused by misalignment of the eyes.

Three-Step Test for Hypertropia (Bielschowsky/Parks Test)

Step 1: Which eye is higher? Right eye (RE) or left eye (LE)?
Step 2: Is the deviation worse in right or left gaze?
Step 3: Is the deviation worse in right head tilt (RHT) or left head tilt (LHT)?

Example

- RE higher = right hypertropia (RHT).
- Four possible paretic muscles.
  Right depressors (R-IR, right superior oblique muscle [R-SO]).
  Left elevators (L-SR, left inferior oblique muscle [L-IO]).
- If deviation is worse in left gaze:
  Only R-SO and L-SR act in gaze to the left (deviation worse in gaze toward paretic muscle).
- If deviation is worse in RHT:
  In tilt right, RE intorts and LE extorts to maintain position.
  Of the R-SO and L-SR, only the R-SO is an intorter of RE (L-SR is intorter of LE).
  Intorsion deficit is made up by the following: RE intorter = R-SR; therefore, secondary elevation by R-SR makes the RHT worse.
- Diagnosis: R-SO palsy.
  Step 4: Measure ocular torsion (if torsion mismatch consider alternative diagnosis of hyperdeviation such as skew/ocular tilt reaction).
  Mnemonic: SINRAD = Superiors INtort Recti ADduct.

FUNCTIONAL VISUAL LOSS

Summary

Nonorganic visual loss may manifest as loss of visual acuity or visual field. No organic lesion can be identified by examination, and nonphysiologic responses confirm the diagnosis.

Signs and Symptoms

May be unilateral or bilateral.
May be any form and severity of visual loss.

Evaluation of Nonorganic Visual Loss

Optokinetic Nystagmus Drum for Severe Loss (Not as Useful for Mild or Moderate Loss)

Horizontal jerk nystagmus.
One-inch-wide stripes indicate vision of at least 20/400.
If "loss" occurs in only one eye:
  Rotate drum before both eyes.
  Once good nystagmus elicited, cover unaffected eye.
  Nonorganic loss continues jerk.
Optokinetic nystagmus (OKN) may be suppressed by inattention.

Mirror Test for No Light Perception

Move mirror back and forth.
Rotate and twist mirror.
If acuity greater than LP, then nystagmoid movement.
Difficult to suppress response.

Proprioception Testing for Severe Visual Loss

Ask the patient to touch the left and right fingertips together.
A patient with organic disease performs the task easily; one with nonorganic disease cannot.
This is a test of proprioception, not vision.

Forced Acuity Testing

Start with smallest line (20/10).
Tell the patient that you are showing a line of "doubled" size.
Show next larger line (20/15).
Works best with computerized projections of multiple Snellen lines of same size.
Repeat until the patient is able to read line.
Express incredulously, *"You can't see these 'big' letters?"*

Near Vision Testing

A discrepancy of near versus distance vision, if not refractive error or media, is usually evidence of nonorganic loss.

Potential Acuity Meter

Measure best corrected acuity.
Dilate pupil.
Tell the patient that the test "bypasses" visual problem.
Improved PAM vision is evidence for ocular media opacity or nonorganic loss.

Red-Green Glasses

Method

Project red/green duochrome slide.
Red lens over abnormal eye.
If the patient is able to read the entire line, then nonorganic visual loss.
Red sees letters on both sides of the screen.
Green lens, only green side.
Mnemonic: "green over good eye."
May use Ishihara color plates.
Polarized lenses.
  American Optical polarizing test.
  Polarized glasses.
  Project-O-Chart slide.
Color testing.
Optic neuropathy often causes color defect.

Stereopsis

Test binocularly first.
RE 20/20 and LE 20/200 = stereo of 180 seconds of arc.
OU 20/20 has 40 seconds of arc.
Normal stereopsis = nonorganic acuity loss.

Pupil Responses

Eye with no light perception (NLP) should not react to light if from anterior visual pathway disease (patients will have normal pupil responses if cortical visual loss).

Evaluation of Nonorganic Visual Field Defects

Constricted Field

- Test with tangent screen.
  Test at two different distances (e.g., 1 and 2 m). Increasing the distance from the screen should increase the mapped field proportionately.
  Size of object varied (i.e., if double test distance, double test object).
  A field that fails to expand at any distance ("tunnel") is nonorganic.
- Monocular hemianopias or binasal or bitemporal hemianopia.
  Test monocular and binocular field.
- Overlapping field from other hemifield.
  If field loss persists under binocular conditions, then nonorganic.

Saccadic Testing

Saccades in supposedly blind peripheral field are a nonorganic finding.
Tell the patient that it is a test of eye movements.

Visual Field Defects Suggestive of Nonorganic Disease

Bilateral constriction without expansion at increasing distance (tunnel field).
Overlapping or inversion of isopters.
Spiraling of isopters.
Nasal hemianopias when tested monocularly that persist on binocular testing.

NEURO

VISUAL SENSORY SYSTEM

Types of Visual Field Defects

Etiology and evaluation based on pattern of visual field loss.

Unilateral Nerve Fiber Bundle Defect

Arcuate or altitudinal in shape.
Scotoma extends to blind spot.

Etiology

Ipsilateral optic nerve or retinal lesion.
Field defect size, density, and shape correspond to retinal or optic nerve lesion.
Central or paracentral scotomas suggest macular or optic nerve disease.
Bilateral nerve fiber layer or retinal defects may occur (e.g., glaucoma, retinal detachment).
Compressive lesions may cause nerve fiber defects (optic neuropathy).

Evaluation

Careful ophthalmoscopy.
Optic nerve head examination.
Exclude artifact of testing.
Exclude retinal disease.
Exclude glaucoma.
Exclude optic neuropathy.

Bilateral Cecocentral or Central Scotomas

May be bilateral optic neuropathy of any cause (e.g., compressive), but more common causes are listed below.

Etiology

Toxic or nutritional amblyopia.
Bilateral demyelinating (optic neuritis).
Syphilis.
Bilateral macula-involving occipital lesions.
Bilateral macular disease.
Leber hereditary optic neuropathy.

Evaluation

Exclude toxic optic neuropathies (e.g., heavy metals, ethambutol).
Consider nutritional amblyopia (vitamin B_{12}, folate, complete blood cell count [CBC]).
Neuroimaging.
Testing for Leber hereditary optic neuropathy.

Junctional Visual Field Defects

Etiology

- Usually, a mass lesion–compressing junction of optic nerve at chiasm (e.g., pituitary adenoma, craniopharyngioma, aneurysm).

Ophthalmic Findings

- Ipsilateral central or cecocentral visual field defect and superotemporal field defect in contralateral eye (junctional scotoma) (Figure 6.3).
- Monocular ipsilateral hemianopic (nasal or temporal) visual field defect (junctional scotoma of Traquair).

Although purported to be from contralateral crossing fibers extending into ipsilateral optic nerve (Willbrand knee), it is unlikely to exist anatomically, but the clinical localizing finding of the junctional scotoma to the junction of the optic nerve and chiasm remains valid.

Evaluation

Neuroimaging (preferably magnetic resonance imaging [MRI]) of junction of the optic nerve and chiasm.

Bitemporal Step or "Flavor" Visual Field Defect

See Figure 6.3.

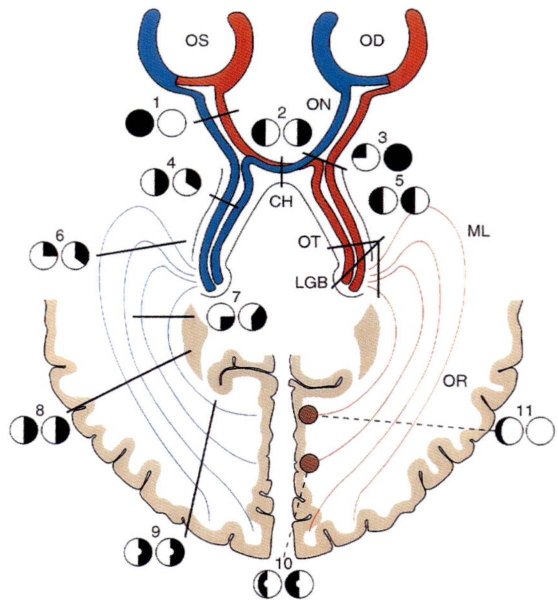

FIGURE 6.3. Schematic illustration of the visual pathway and visual field defects produced by lesions in various areas of the pathway. (ON, optic nerve; CH, chiasm; OT, optic tract; LGB, lateral geniculate body; ML, Meyer loop; OR, optic radiations) (Reproduced from Tasman W, Jaeger E. *The wills eye hospital atlas of clinical ophthalmology*, 2nd ed. Lippincott Williams & Wilkins, 2001, with permission.)

Etiology

Chiasmal lesion until proven otherwise.
Pseudochiasmal ones (not respecting midline).
Tilted disk.
Colobomas.
Bilateral nasal retinal disease (e.g., schisis).
Glaucoma.
Bilateral optic neuropathy.
Lesions affecting the chiasm:
- Pituitary adenoma.
- Meningioma.
- Craniopharyngioma.
- Internal carotid artery aneurysm.
- Other tumors.
- Demyelinating disease.
- Trauma.

Evaluation

Neuroimaging with attention to the chiasm.

Homonymous Hemianopsia

See Figure 6.3.

Etiology

- Retrochiasmal disease.
- Complete homonymous hemianopsia is not further localizing (i.e., localizes only to contralateral retrochiasmal pathway).
- More congruous (equal in appearance, size, shape of field) lesions are more posterior.
- Congruity does not apply to complete hemianopsia.

Signs and Symptoms

Signs and symptoms to help localize homonymous hemianopsia:

Optic tract:
- Contralateral APD.
- Band or bow-tie optic disk atrophy (contralateral).
- Generally incongruous homonymous hemianopsia.

Lateral geniculate body:
- Incongruous wedge defects "spears to fixation" (anterior choroidal branch of internal carotid artery).
- May spare or selectively involve horizontal strip of field (lateral choroidal branch).

Temporal lobe:
Defect denser superiorly (Meyer loop); "pie in the sky" scotoma (Figure 6.3).
Parietal lobe:
Incongruous defect denser inferiorly (Figure 6.3).
More likely congruous with macular splitting.
Other clinical signs:
- Right-sided lesions.
  - Constructional apraxias.
  - More severe neglect.
- Left-sided lesions.
  - Gerstmann syndrome:
  - Finger agnosia.
  - Right-left confusion.
  - Agraphia.
  - Acalculia.
- Aphasia.
- Neglect.

Occipital:
- Often isolated neurologically.
- Usually very congruous.
- May be paracentral.
- Macular sparing (central 5 degrees) due to dual circulation from middle and posterior cerebral arteries.
- May spare or selectively involve a temporal monocular crescent at anterior tip of calcarine cortex (Figure 6.3) supplied by anterior cerebral artery.

Optic Nerve Head Disorders

Coloboma

Summary

A coloboma is an excavated defect in the optic nerve that is due to incomplete closure of the embryonic fissure associated with a PAX6 mutation.

Etiology

Congenital: incomplete or abnormal closure of proximal end of embryonic fissure.

Signs and Symptoms

May be asymptomatic.
May have visual loss.

Ophthalmic Findings

- Abnormal appearance of optic nerve.
- Glistening white bowl-shaped excavation occupies an enlarged optic disk (Figure 6.4).
- Bare sclera visible because of absence of retina, retinal pigment epithelium (RPE), and choroid adjacent to and continuous with optic nerve.
- Usually inferonasal.
- Unilateral or bilateral.
- Absolute scotoma corresponding to coloboma.
- Associated findings:
  - May be isolated.
  - May be associated with iris, ciliary, or choroidal colobomas.
  - May be associated with other ocular abnormalities (microphthalmia, choroidal colobomas).
  - May be associated with other systemic abnormalities (e.g., Aicardi syndrome, Goldenhar syndrome, and CHARGE syndrome).

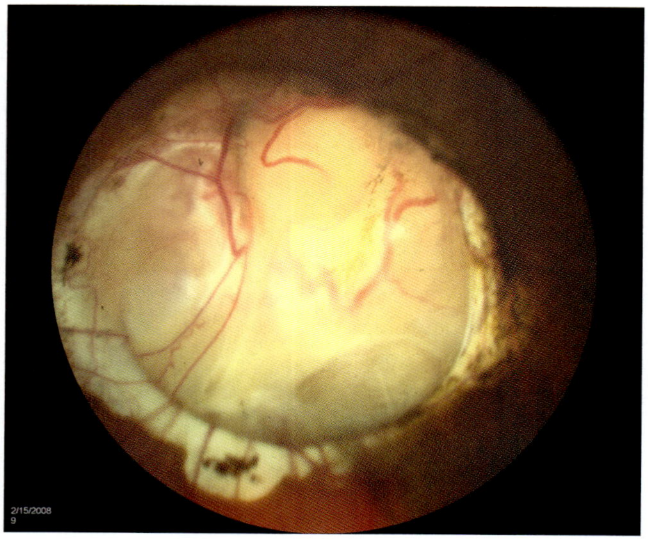

FIGURE 6.4. Optic nerve coloboma. Note the excavation of the sclera inferiorly. (Courtesy of Thomas Patrianakos, MD.)

Treatment

None.

Prognosis

Usually static.

Reference

Brodsky MC. Congenital optic disc anomalies. *Surv Ophthalmol* 1994;39:89–112.

Optic Pit

Summary

An optic pit is a congenital excavated defect or depression in the optic nerve due to a defect in the lamina cribrosa.

Etiology

Congenital.

Signs and Symptoms

May be asymptomatic.
May have visual loss.
May have metamorphopsia.

Ophthalmic Findings

Small excavated defect (pit) in optic nerve rim (Figure 6.5).
Usually temporal (may be nasal or central).
Bilateral in 15% of cases.
May be associated with serous retinal detachment.
Adjacent to optic pit.
May extend into macula.

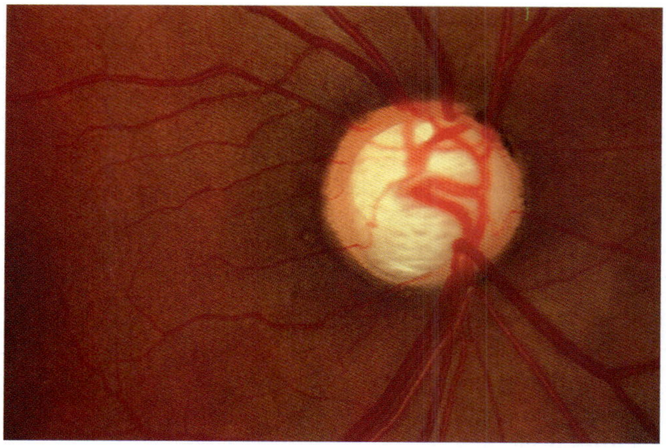

FIGURE 6.5. Optic pit temporally on the optic nerve. May have an associated serous retinal detachment. (Reproduced from Tasman W, Jaeger E. *The Wills eye hospital atlas of clinical ophthalmology*, 2nd ed. Lippincott Williams & Wilkins, 2001, with permission.)

Special Tests

Fluorescein angiography for serous detachment.

Treatment

No treatment unless serous detachment.
Laser treatment if serous detachment though often unsuccessful.
Vitrectomy in unresponsive cases.

Prognosis

Often, self-limited serous detachment.
May recur.

Reference

Brodsky MC. Congenital optic disc anomalies. *Surv Ophthalmol* 1994;39:89–112.

Optic Nerve Hypoplasia and Dysplasia

Summary

Optic nerve hypoplasia is a congenitally small optic nerve.

Etiology

Congenital.
Aplasia (rare).
Hypoplasia.
Dysplasia.

Signs and Symptoms

Sometimes asymptomatic.
May have decreased acuity.
Range: 20/20 to NLP.
Usually nonprogressive.

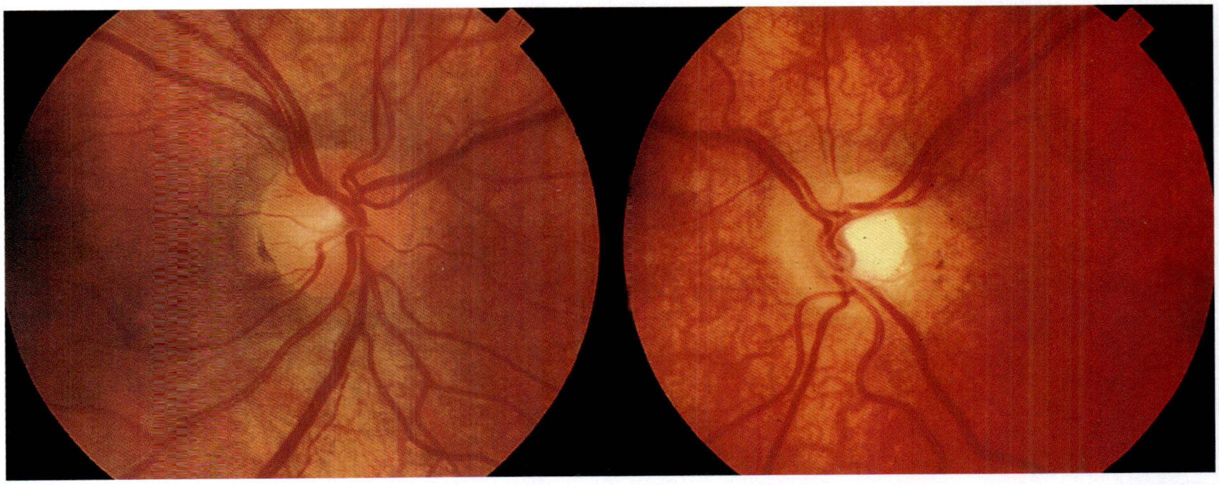

FIGURE 6.6. Hypoplasia of the optic nerve. The right optic disk is normal. A small amount of tissue is located nasally in the left disk. The rest of the disk is empty and a typical double ring sign is seen, particularly nasally. The nerve fiber layer is practically nonexistent. (Reproduced from Tasman W, Jaeger E. *The Wills eye hospital atlas of clinical ophthalmology*, 2 ed. Lippincott Williams & Wilkins, 2001, with permission.)

Cannot judge level of acuity from appearance of disk.
Visual field defects.

Ophthalmic Findings

Unilateral or bilateral.
Strabismus.
Nystagmus (including see-saw).
May have superimposed amblyopia.
Strong association with astigmatism.
Fundus signs.
Small optic disk.
One third to half the normal size.
With or without pallor.
Normal optic nerve dimension: horizontal, 1.38 mm; vertical, 1.46 mm.
"Double ring sign" (Figure 6.6).
May be confused with peripapillary atrophy.
Outer ring: junction of sclera and lamina cribrosa.
Inner ring: abnormal extension of retina and RPE.
Decreased nerve fiber layer thickness.
Normal-sized retinal vessels that may be tortuous.

Associated Signs

Developmental delay, most common.
Hypothalamic or pituitary dysfunction.
Endocrine dysfunction.
Facial abnormalities.
Skeletal abnormalities.
Ocular abnormalities (e.g., coloboma).

Risk Factors (Usually Idiopathic)

Young maternal age.
Use of medicines in pregnancy (e.g., alcohol, phenytoin).
Maternal diabetes (superior segmental hypoplasia).
Trisomies 13, 18, and 21.
Intrauterine cytomegalovirus and hepatitis.

Evaluation

Pediatric endocrinology consultation.
Hypothalamic hypopituitarism.
Neonatal hypoglycemia.
Diabetes insipidus.
Growth hormone deficiency.
Thyroid hormones.
Neuroimaging.

Special Tests

Stereo disk photos.
Formal visual field tests when the patient is old enough.

Treatment

Underlying endocrine disease.
Trial of patching for amblyopia.
Correct refractive errors (astigmatism).
Safety spectacles.

Developmental Abnormalities of Midline Brain Structures (De Morsier Syndrome—Septooptic Dysplasia)

Agenesis of anterior commissure.
Absent septum pellucidum and corpus callosum.
Central nervous system (CNS) basal encephalocele.
Testing for pituitary endocrine dysfunction is warranted.

Reference

Brodsky MC. Congenital optic disc anomalies. *Surv Ophthalmol* 1994;39:89–112.

Tilted Optic Disk

Other names:
Fuchs coloboma.
Inferior conus.
Inversion or dysversion of disk.

Summary

The optic disk may be congenitally tilted in one or both eyes, and this may result in a visual field defect.

Signs and Symptoms

Eighty percent of cases bilateral.

Ophthalmic Findings

See Figure 6.7.

Oval disk (with reduction in disk diameter).
Depression usually inferiorly.
Elevation usually superiorly.
Crescent, usually inferior (in direction of tilt).
Oblique direction of retinal vessels (emerging from superotemporal disk, sweep nasally before turning temporally).
Hypopigmentation (wedge-shaped area, opposite defective portion of the disc).
Visual field defects (usually superotemporal, may have bitemporal field defects simulating a chiasmal lesion, but defects do not respect vertical midline).

Evaluation

Optic disk photos.
Attention of field testing to vertical meridian.
Ectasia should match field defect location.
If vertical step in field, MRI scan.

Prognosis

Usually static.

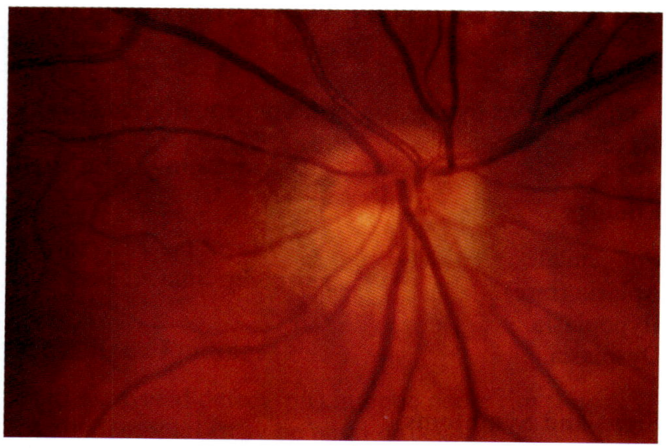

FIGURE 6.7. The congenital tilted optic disk is apparent as the oval of nerve tissue superiorly. There is no apparent optic cup.

Treatment

None.

Reference

Giuffe G. The spectrum of the visual field defects in the tilted disk syndrome: clinical study and review. *Neuroophthalmology* 1986;6:239–246.

Papilledema

Summary

Papilledema is a term that should be reserved for optic disk edema attributable to increased intracranial pressure. All other forms of optic disk swelling should be referred to as optic disk edema.

Etiology

Any cause of increased intracranial pressure:
Neoplastic (e.g., glioblastoma multiforme).
Infectious (e.g., abscess, meningitis).
Inflammatory (e.g., sarcoid).
Traumatic.
Infiltrative.
Vascular (e.g., arteriovenous malformation [AVM]).
Subarachnoid hemorrhage.
Venous sinus thrombosis.
Hydrocephalus.
Pseudotumor cerebri.

Signs and Symptoms

Usually bilateral but may be unilateral or asymmetric.
Usually preserved visual acuity and color discrimination early.
May have transient visual loss (TVL) lasting for a few seconds resulting in obscurations of vision.

Ophthalmic Findings

- Optic disk edema (Figure 6.8)
  Disk hyperemia: congestion of fine optic nerve capillaries.
  Opacification of nerve fiber layer.
  Peripapillary hemorrhages.
  Cotton-wool spots.
  Loss of the physiologic cup is a late sign.
  Venous dilation: elevation of optic nerve head.
  Retinal exudates.
  Circumferential retinal folds (Paton lines) in peripapillary region.
- Visual field defects (enlarged blind spot, generalized constriction).
  Glaucomalike defects.
- No afferent pupillary defect unless severe and asymmetric.
- Absent spontaneous venous pulsations.

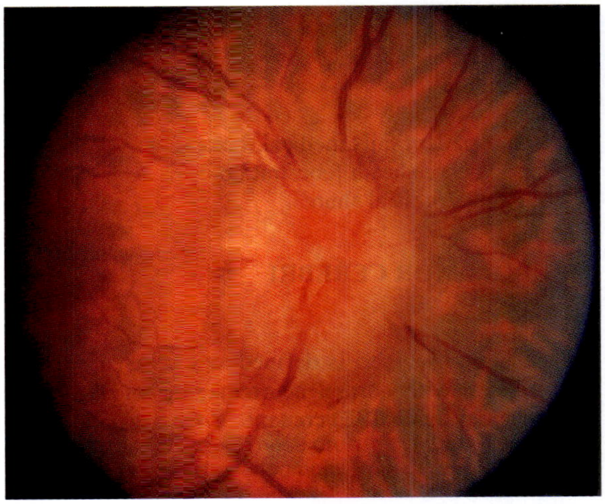

FIGURE 6.8. Florid papilledema. The swollen optic nerve fiber layer obscures the disk margins and fine disk capillaries and obliterates the optic cup nerve fiber layer hemorrhages and lipid exudates are seen.

Evaluation

Neuroimaging (to exclude mass lesion). Cranial MRI with contrast MR venogram (MRV) to exclude cerebral venous sinus thrombosis is recommended.
Lumbar puncture.
- Opening pressure.
- Cell count.
- Glucose, protein, cytologic testing, cultures.

Differential Diagnosis

Pseudopapilledema.
- Optic disk drusen.
- Hyperopic disks.

Other causes of bilateral optic disk edema.
- Anterior ischemic optic neuropathy (ION).
- Diabetic papillitis.
- Optic neuritis.
- Inflammatory or infiltrative optic disk edema.

Treatment

Treat underlying cause.
Acetazolamide.
Corticosteroids (but may worsen weight gain or pseudotumor cerebri).
Surgical, if the patient fails medical therapy.
- Optic nerve sheath fenestration.
- Ventriculoperitoneal or lumboperitoneal shunt.
- Bariatric surgery for weight loss in pseudotumor cerebri.

Pseudotumor Cerebri

Summary

Pseudotumor cerebri is defined as increased intracranial pressure with normal neuroimaging and normal cerebrospinal fluid (CSF) content.

Etiology

Usually idiopathic. Multiple associations:
- Venous outflow obstruction.
  - Sagittal sinus thrombosis.
  - Radical neck surgery.
- Endocrine, metabolic, or systemic diseases.
  - Hypoparathyroidism.
  - Addison disease.
  - Renal disease.
  - Systemic lupus erythematosus.
  - Behçet disease.
- Exogenous agents.
  - Vitamin A.
  - Tetracycline.
  - Steroid withdrawal.
  - Nalidixic acid.
  - Anabolic steroids.
  - Lithium.

Epidemiology

Usually young, obese women.
Beware of the diagnosis of pseudotumor cerebri in men, thin patients, or elderly individuals.

Signs and Symptoms

Papilledema (does not have to be present for diagnosis) (Figure 6.9).
Nonlocalizing sixth-nerve palsy, but no other cranial nerves involved or focal neurologic signs.
Headache.
Transient visual obscurations (seconds).
Pulsatile tinnitus.

Evaluation

Neuroimaging. Preferably MRI with contrast MRV.
Lumbar puncture, check opening pressure.

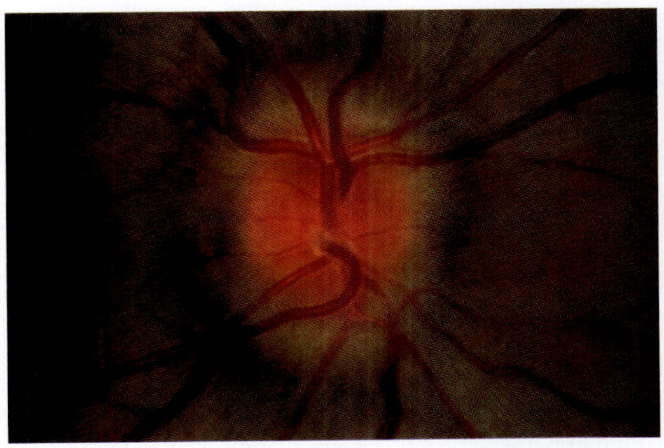

FIGURE 6.9. Papilledema secondary to pseudotumor cerebri. Both optic nerves had a similar appearance.

Treatment

Indications:
- Severe intractable headache unresponsive to headache medications.
- Progressive visual loss.

Treat underlying associated conditions.
Eliminate exogenous factors.
Weight loss.
Medications:
- Acetazolamide.
- Less commonly, other medicines (e.g., digoxin, furosemide, topiramate).
- Corticosteroids (see warning above).

Surgical therapy:
- Optic nerve sheath fenestration.
- Ventriculoperitoneal or lumboperitoneal shunt.

Special Testing

Visual field testing.
Optic disk photography.

References

Corbett JJ, Thompson HS. The rational management of idiopathic intracranial hypertension. *Arch Neurol* 1989;46:1049–1051.

Wall M, George D. Idiopathic intracranial hypertension (pseudotumor cerebri): a prospective study of 50 patients. *Brain* 1991;114:155–180.

Optic Nerve Head Drusen

Summary

Optic nerve head drusen are calcified hyaline bodies within the optic disk substance that may cause visual field loss.

Etiology

Congenital.
Autosomal dominant in some cases.

Histopathology

Hyaline bodies; may be calcified.
Acellular laminated concretions in optic nerve substance.

Demographics

Usually white patients.
Uncommon in black patients.

Signs and Symptoms

Usually asymptomatic.
May have visual field defects (slow progression).
(often arcuate, an enlarged blind spot, or visual field constriction).
Decreased visual acuity is rare, usually not due to drusen alone.
May have transient visual obscurations.

Differential Diagnosis

Arteritic ischemic optic neuropathy (AION).
Retinal artery or vein occlusion.
Subretinal neovascular membrane.
Subretinal exudation or heme.

Systemic Diseases

Associated conditions:
- Retinitis pigmentosa.
- Pseudoxanthoma elasticum.
- Angioid streaks.
- Retinal hemorrhages.
- Chorioretinal folds.
- Migraine.

Ophthalmic Findings

Usually bilateral (66%).
Discrete, amorphous deposits in optic nerve (Figure 6.10).
More often nasal than temporal.
Absent cup, small disk.
Anomalous disk vasculature.
No exudates or disk telangiectasias.
Tend to become more apparent with age.
Buried disk drusen in children.
Drusen transilluminate within disk head.
Subfoveal neovascularization.

Evaluation

A clinical diagnosis.
Examine family members.

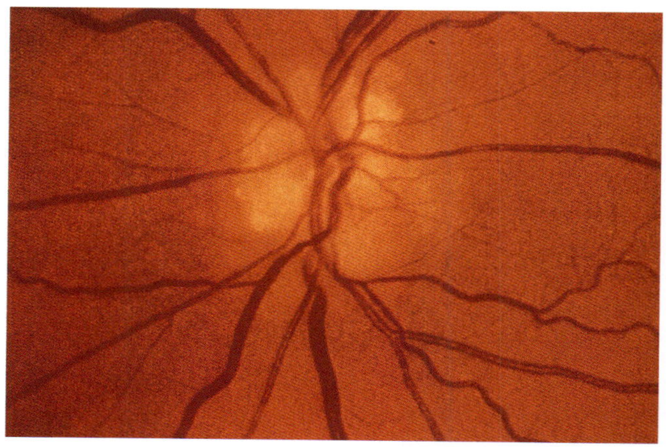

FIGURE 6.10. Optic nerve drusen cause the surface of the optic nerve to appear bumpy. These drusen can become calcified and are visible on ultrasonography.

Special Tests

Ultrasound of nerve head (for buried drusen).
Computed tomography (CT) scan (rarely needed) may show calcific drusen.
Preinjection fluorescein angiography.
- Autofluorescence.
- Probably not helpful in buried drusen.
- May show delay in filling of peripapillary choroid.

Stereo disk photos.

Reference

Rosenberg MA, Savino PJ, Glaser JS. A clinical analysis of pseudopapilledema. I. Population, laterality, acuity, refractive error, ophthalmoscopic characteristics, and co-incident disease. *Arch Ophthalmol* 1979;97:65–70.

Melanocytoma

Summary

A melanocytoma is a congenital pigmented abnormality of the optic disk head.

Etiology

Congenital.

Signs and Symptoms

Usually asymptomatic.

Ophthalmic Signs

Black optic nerve head lesion (Figure 6.11).
May be slightly elevated.

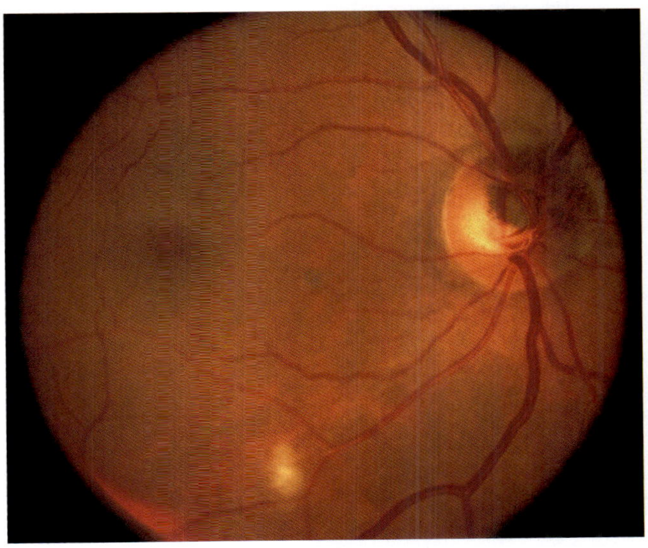

FIGURE 6.11. Melanocytomas are black lesions frequently found off the optic nerve. They represent benign melanocytic proliferation.

Special Tests

Usually, none needed.

Prognosis

May grow slowly.

Treatment

None.

Differential Diagnosis

Melanoma.
Combined hamartoma of the retina and RPE.

Reference

Joffe L, Shields JA, Osher RH, et al. Clinical and follow-up studies of melanocytomas of the optic disc. *Trans Am Acad Ophthalmol Otolaryngol* 1979;86:S1067–S1078.

Myelinated Nerve Fiber Layer

Summary

Myelination normally terminates at the lamina cribrosa but may occur in the nerve fiber layer of the retina.

Etiology

Congenital.

Signs and Symptoms

Usually asymptomatic.

Ophthalmic Findings

White myelin in distribution of nerve fiber layer, often radiating from the optic nerve, but may occur only in the peripheral retina (Figure 6.12).

Evaluation

Clinical diagnosis.

Prognosis

Static.

Treatment

None.

Differential Diagnosis

Cotton-wool patch.
Retinal infiltrate.
Arteriole occlusion.

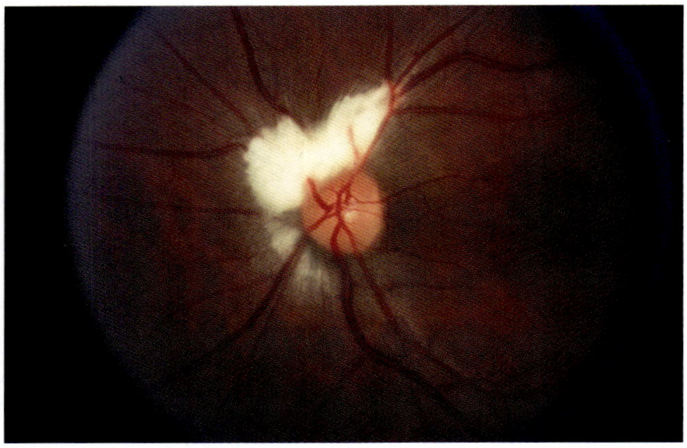

FIGURE 6.12. White feathery myelinated nerve fibers radiating from the optic disk.

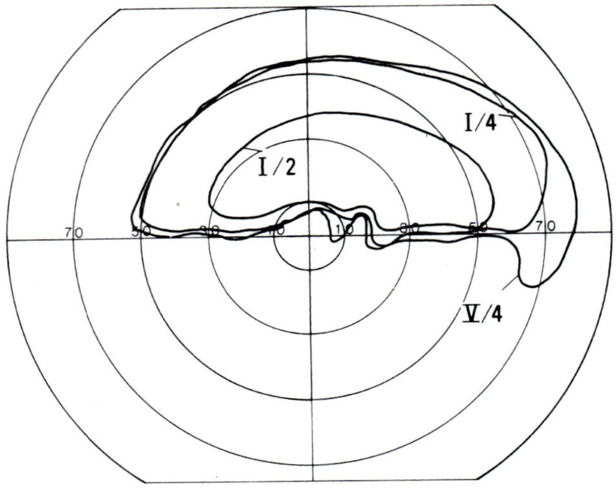

FIGURE 6.13. Inferior altitudinal defect in a patient with anterior ION. Notice that the defect respects the horizontal midline. (From Miller N, Newman N. *Walsh and Hoyt's clinical neuro-ophthalmology*, 4th ed., vol. 1. Baltimore, MD: Williams & Wilkins, 1995:213, with permission.)

Optic Nerve and Chiasm Disorders

Ischemic Optic Neuropathy

Summary

ION is a clinical syndrome characterized by acute loss of vision, evidence for an optic neuropathy, and usually a swollen optic nerve in an elderly patient.

Etiology

Arteritic ION: giant cell arteritis (GCA).
Nonarteritic ION: other vasculopathic risk factors (e.g., diabetes, atherosclerosis).

Signs and Symptoms

- Nonarteritic:
  Acute loss of visual acuity and/or visual field (usually altitudinal defect) (Figure 6.13).
  Dyschromatopsia.
  Usually unilateral.
  Usually painless.
- Arteritic:
  Usually more severe visual loss.
  May be bilateral.
  Constitutional symptoms and signs (headache, jaw claudication, scalp tenderness, malaise, fever, weight loss, anorexia, etc.).

Demographics

Usually occurs in older patients (>40 years).
Elderly patients evaluate for GCA (>50 years).
Patients often have vasculopathic risk factors.

Ophthalmic Findings

Usually swollen optic nerve (anterior ION).
Relative afferent pupillary defect in unilateral or bilateral asymmetric cases.
Absent anterior or posterior segment inflammation.

Systemic Findings

- Nonarteritic anterior ION:
  Diabetes.
  Hypertension (left ventricular hypertrophy).
  Smoking.
  Hypercholesterolemia.
  Hypotension (e.g., postsurgical, nocturnal, other) or anemia.
  Collagen-vascular disease.
- Arteritic:
  GCA.

Special Tests

Erythrocyte sedimentation rate (ESR) and/or C-reactive protein test for GCA.
Complete blood count with platelet count.
Temporal artery biopsy for GCA.

Pathology

Temporal artery inflammation with or without giant cells for GCA.
Disruption of internal elastic lamina.
Intimal hyperplasia.

Disease Course

- Nonarteritic:
  Often, static visual loss.

- May spontaneously improve.
- May have progressive visual loss.
- Small cup-to-disk ratio predisposing factor ("disk at risk").

- Arteritic:
  - Often, severe visual loss.
  - Untreated disease leads to bilateral severe visual loss.

Treatment

- Nonarteritic:
  - Treat underlying vasculopathic risk factors.
  - Aspirin (one per day) therapy may reduce risk in fellow eye (conflicting data).
  - No role for optic nerve sheath decompression (see Ischemic Optic Neuropathy Decompression Trial study).
- Arteritic:
  - Oral prednisone (1.0 to 1.5 mg/kg/day).
  - Consider intravenous (i.v.) steroids for monocular patients, bilateral, or severe visual loss.

Follow-Up

Nonarteritic: as needed.

Arteritic: 65% of patients develop arteric ION in fellow eye if untreated.

Follow ESR and clinical symptoms.

Taper steroids slowly.

Differential Diagnosis

Infectious optic neuropathy.

Inflammatory optic neuropathy.

Infiltrative optic neuropathy.

Compressive optic neuropathy.

Toxic optic neuropathy.

Hereditary optic neuropathy (Leber hereditary optic neuropathy).

References

Hayreh SS, Podhajsky PA, Raman R, et al. Giant cell arteritis: validity and reliability of various diagnostic criteria. *Am J Ophthalmol* 1997;123:285–296.

The Ischemic Optic Neuropathy Decompression Trial Research Group. Optic nerve decompression surgery for nonarteritic anterior ischemic optic neuropathy (NAION) is not effective and may be harmful. *JAMA* 1995;273:625–632.

The Ischemic Optic Neuropathy Decompression Trial Research Group. Characteristics of patients with nonarteritic anterior ischemic optic neuropathy eligible for the Ischemic Optic Neuropathy Decompression Trial. *Arch Ophthalmol* 1996;114:1355–1374.

Optic Neuritis

Summary

Optic neuritis is a general term that is used to describe idiopathic or demyelinating optic neuropathy.

Etiology

Idiopathic: most frequent.

Demyelinating diseases: multiple sclerosis (MS).

Infectious diseases: viral disease, syphilis, cat scratch disease, Lyme disease, etc.

Inflammatory diseases: collagen-vascular disease, sarcoid, etc.

Signs and Symptoms

- Typical optic neuritis is characterized by the following clinical features:
  - Unilateral, acute visual loss.
  - Pain worse with eye movement.
- Atypical features:
  - Bilateral simultaneous onset in adults.
  - Anterior or posterior segment inflammation.
  - Macular star figure.
  - Lack of pain.
  - Male.
  - NLP vision.
  - Significant retinal hemorrhages or cotton wool patches.
  - Lack of significant improvement.
  - History or examination findings suggestive of underlying inflammatory or infectious process.

Demographics

Usually young adults, but may occur in any age group.

Often female patients, but may be either gender.

Ophthalmic Findings

Decreased visual acuity and/or visual field.

Relative afferent pupillary defect in unilateral or bilateral but asymmetric cases.

Absence of anterior or posterior uveitis.

Normal (65%) or swollen (35%) optic nerve (most cases are retrobulbar).

Systemic Findings

Associated with MS.

Special Tests

MRI of the brain and orbits to look for demyelinating white matter disease (Figure 6.14).

Pathology

Optic nerve demyelination.

Disease Course

Ninety percent of cases improve to normal or near-normal vision with or without treatment.

Evaluation

Typical optic neuritis:
- MRI to evaluate for demyelinating disease.

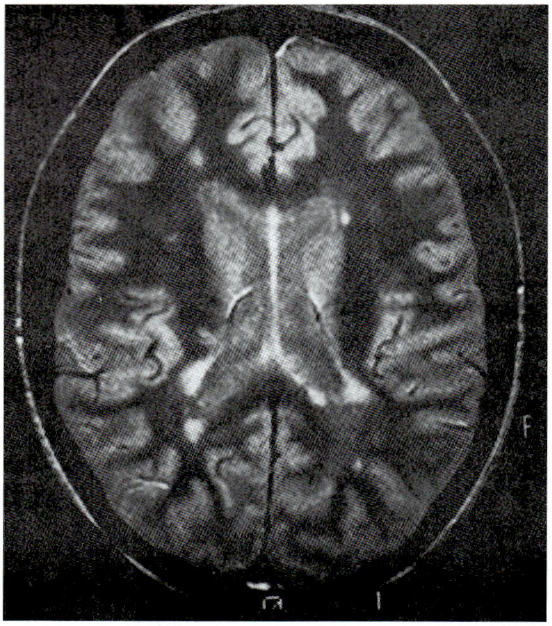

FIGURE 6.14. Multiple periventricular white matter lesions in a patient with MS on MRI. (From Miller N, Newman N. *Walsh and Hoyt's clinical neuro-ophthalmology,* 4th ed., vol. 1. Baltimore, MD: Williams & Wilkins, 1995:4339, with permission.)

No further laboratory evaluation necessary.

Atypical optic neuritis:

MRI head and orbit with fat suppression and contrast.

Laboratory evaluation directed by history and physical examination (e.g., syphilis serologic testing, antinuclear antibody testing, chest radiography, and lumbar puncture).

Treatment

- If normal MRI imaging and typical optic neuritis:
  Can observe for improvement.
  Consider i.v. steroids (methylprednisolone 1,000 mg/day for 3 days followed by oral steroid taper [See Optic Neuritis Treatment Trial study]). I.V. steroids hasten visual recovery but do not change ultimate visual outcome.
- If abnormal MRI consistent with MS:
  Consider i.v. steroids.
  Consider further evaluation for MS.
  Neurologic consultation for consideration of immunomodulatory treatments (interferon beta).

Follow-Up

Visual recovery over 4 to 6 weeks.

Risk of MS.

Differential Diagnosis

Infectious optic neuropathy.

Inflammatory optic neuropathy.

ION.

Infiltrative optic neuropathy.

Compressive optic neuropathy.

Toxic optic neuropathy.

Hereditary optic neuropathy (Leber hereditary optic neuropathy).

References

Beck RW, Cleary PA, Trobe JD, et al. The effect of corticosteroids for acute optic neuritis on the subsequent development of multiple sclerosis. *N Engl J Med* 1992;326:581–588.

Beck RW, Trobe JD, the Optic Neuritis Treatment Group. What we have learned from the Optic Neuritis Treatment Trial. *Ophthalmology* 1995:102;1504–1508.

Toxic or Nutritional Optic Neuropathy

Summary

Patients with toxic or nutritional optic neuropathies usually present with bilaterally symmetric, slowly progressive visual loss.

Signs and Symptoms

Visual field defect: typically central or cecocentral scotomas.

Visual acuity loss.

Bilateral and symmetric visual loss.

Slowly progressive.

Optic nerve may appear normal until late in course.

Optic atrophy usually develops eventually.

Etiology

- Nutritional deficiencies:
  Pernicious anemia.
  Dietary deficiency (e.g., veganism, alcoholism).
  Vitamin B_{12} deficiency.
  Folate.
- Toxins:
  Amantadine.
  Amiodarone.
  Amoproxan.
  Aniline dyes.
  Barbiturates.
  Cafergot.
  Cabromal.
  Carbon disulfide.
  Carbon tetrachloride.
  Cephaloridine.
  Chloramphenicol.
  Chlorodinitrobenzene.
  Clioquinol.
  Dichlorodiphenyltrichloroethane.
  Digitalis.
  Dinitrotoluene.
  Disulfiram (Antabuse).
  D-Penicillamine.

Diiodohydroxyquin.
Elcatonin.
Emetine.
Ethambutol.
Ethchlorvynol (Placidyl).
Ethylene glycol.
5-Fluorouracil.
Glue sniffing.
Halogenated hydroxyquinolone.
Heavy metals (e.g., arsenic, lead, mercury).
Hexachlorophene.
Iodoform.
Iodopyracet (Diodrast).
Isoniazid.
Lysol.
Methanol.
Methyl acetate.
Methyl bromide.
Octamoxin.
Organophosphate pesticides.
Penicillamine.
Phenazone (antipyren).
Pheniprazine (Catron).
Plasmocid.
Quinine.
Sodium fluoride.
Streptomycin.
Styrene (vinyl benzyl).
Sulfonamides.
Thallium.
Thioglycolate.
Tolbutamide (Orinase).
Trichloroethylene.
Vincristine.

Evaluation

MRI of the head.
Vitamin B_{12} level.
Folate level (serum and erythrocyte).
CBC.
Urine heavy metal screen (mercury, lead, arsenic) if history is suggestive.

Leber Hereditary Optic Neuropathy

Summary

Leber hereditary optic neuropathy is a rare inherited mitochondrial optic neuropathy that affects young male patients.

Etiology

Hereditary defect in mitochondrial DNA.

Demographics

Affects men, usually in their twenties.
Rarely affects women (10% to 20% of cases).
Mitochondrial inheritance.

Signs and Symptoms

- Visual acuity loss:
  Usually acute, rapid, unremitting, and painless.
  Usually 20/200 to hand motions but 20/20 to NLP range.
- Visual field loss (central or cecocentral scotomas).
- Bilateral involvement (second eye affected days to weeks to months later but 40% to 50% have simultaneous onset).
- Fundus findings at the time of visual loss.
- Triad of the "suspect fundus":
  1. Telangiectatic microangiopathy of optic neuropathy (Figure 6.15).
  2. Apparent swelling of nerve fiber layer around disk.
  3. Fluorescein angiogram often shows pseudoedema, but usually no leakage of dye at edge of disk.
- Fundus appearance after visual loss:
  Attenuated arterioles.
  Nerve fiber layer loss, especially, papillomacular bundle.
  Optic nerve pallor (temporally).
  May develop nonglaucomatous cupping.

Associations

Usually systemically normal but may have some associated findings.
Occasional cardiac conduction defects.
Dystonia and other minor neurologic deficits.

Evaluation

Exclude other causes for an optic neuropathy.
Primary mitochondrial DNA mutation (e.g., mtDNA 11778, 3460, 14484).

Treatment

Reducing metabolic stress on the optic nerve (e.g., smoking, known optic nerve toxins, and trauma).

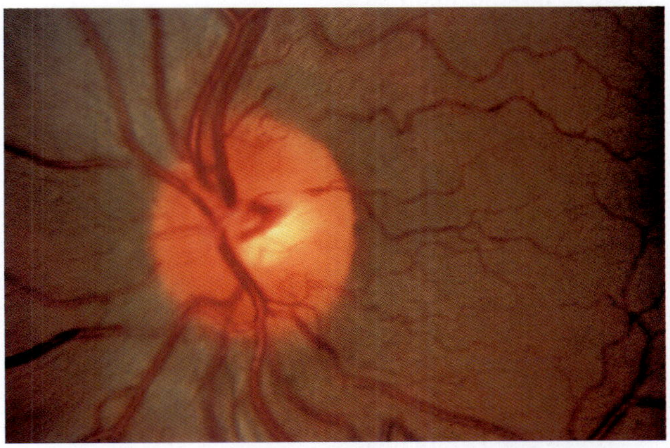

FIGURE 6.15. Hyperemic optic disk with telangiectatic vessels in a young male patient with Leber hereditary optic neuropathy.

NEURO

Medical therapy remains unproven.
- Multivitamins.
- Folate.
- Vitamin B_{12}.
- Thiamine.
- Idebenone and other coenzyme Q10 analogues.

Prognosis

Some patients experience spontaneous improvement.
Most remain unchanged.

References

Chalmers RM, Harding AE. A case-control study of Leber's hereditary optic neuropathy. *Brain* 1996;119:1481–1486.

Riordan-Eva P, Sanders MD, Govan GG, et al. The clinical features of Leber's hereditary optic neuropathy defined by the presence of a pathogenic mitochondrial DNA mutation. *Brain* 1995;118:319–337.

Infiltrative or Inflammatory Optic Neuropathy

Summary

Infiltration or inflammation of the optic nerve may mimic demyelinating or idiopathic optic neuritis.

Signs and Symptoms

Visual loss.
Decreased color vision.

Ophthalmic Findings

Unilateral or bilateral.
Afferent pupillary defect.
Optic disk pallor or swelling.
Optic disk may appear normal (retrobulbar).
Atypical features for optic neuritis:
- Bilateral simultaneous onset.
- Lack of pain.
- Lack of improvement.
- Anterior or posterior segment inflammation.
- Progressive or recurrent episodes.
- Steroid responsive or steroid dependent.

Etiology

- Neoplastic:
  - Plasmacytoma.
  - Carcinomatous meningitis.
  - Leukemia.
  - Lymphoma.
- Paraneoplastic disease.
- Infectious:
  - Cryptococcal meningitis.
  - Aspergillus.
  - Tuberculosis (TB).
  - Syphilis.
- Systemic inflammatory diseases:
  - Contiguous sinus disease.
  - Sarcoidosis.
  - Systemic lupus erythematosus.
  - Inflammatory bowel disease.

Evaluation

- MRI of the head (and orbit if orbital signs present).
- CBC.
- Syphilis serologic testing (e.g., fluorescent treponemal antibody, absorbed [FTA-Abs], rapid plasmin reagin [RPR]).
- Antinuclear antibody test.
- Chest radiograph.
- Angiotensin-converting enzyme, lysozyme.
- Lumbar puncture.
- Consider gallium or PET scan if suspect sarcoidosis.
- Purified protein derivative skin testing if TB suspected.
- Anti–double-stranded DNA, complement levels if systemic lupus erythematosus suspected.

Optic Pathway Tumors

Two common tumors of the optic pathway include optic nerve gliomas and meningiomas.

Optic Gliomas

Summary

Optic gliomas are glial tumors that may affect the optic nerve, chiasm, or tract and are found primarily in children and young adults.

Epidemiology

Age:
- Can occur at any age.
- Seventy percent of patients with gliomas are diagnosed by age 10.
- Ninety percent of gliomas are detected by age 20.
- Reported in adults.

No gender predilection.

Association

Neurofibromatosis (NF) type 1.

Incidence (Uncommon)

One to three percent of all orbital tumors.
One percent of intracranial neoplasms.
Three to six percent of intracranial tumors in childhood.

Location

One or both optic nerves.

Optic chiasm or tract.
In general, the more anterior, the better the prognosis.

Disease Course

Most gliomas are benign juvenile pilocytic astrocytomas.
Mortality: depends more on location than histologic appearance.
Optic nerve alone, 1[illegible]%.
Chiasm, 47% (variable).
- With hydrocephalus, 77%.
- Hypothalamic involvement, 91%.
- Malignant optic nerve gliomas occur rarely in adults, usually men.

Signs and Symptoms

Painless progressive visual loss (optic neuropathy).
- Overall vision loss 87%.
- Vision of 20/20 to 20/40, 26%.
- Vision of 20/50 to 20/200, 19%.
- Vision of 20/300 or worse, 55%.

Hypothalamic symptoms or endocrinologic.
- Diabetes insipidus.
- Diencephalic wasting.
- Precocious puberty.
- Somnolence.
- Growth failure.

Visual field defects (central or bitemporal).

Ophthalmic Findings

Proptosis (orbital, 9[illegible]%; chiasmal, 18%).
Disk swelling (3[illegible]%) or atrophy (60%).
- Rare optociliary shunt vessels.
- Fifty percent of intraorbital tumors have disk edema.
- Only 20% of chiasmal tumors have disk edema.

Strabismus (27%).
Nystagmus (spasmus nutans–like or see-saw nystagmus).

Evaluation

Consider glioma in any child with the following:
- Unexplained decreased visual acuity.
- Monocular or asymmetric nystagmus.
- Optic atrophy.
- Hypothalamic symptoms.
- Diencephalic syndrome.
- Spasmus nutans.
- See-saw nystagmus.
- Hydrocephalus.

Neuroimaging:
MRI scan head and orbit with fat suppression with gadolinium superior to CT scan (Figure 6.16).
Can appear as a fusiform enlargement of optic nerve and/or kinking of optic nerve.
Search for stigmata of NF.

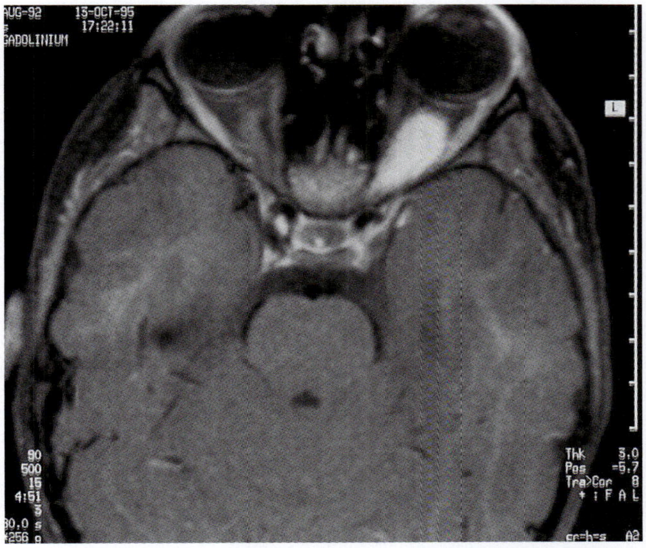

FIGURE 6.16. Magnetic resonance image with gadolinium enhancement of a fusiform, hyperintense lesion corresponding to an optic nerve glioma.

Assessment of growth and monitoring for precocious puberty.
Examine family members.
No biopsy usually indicated:
- If clearly intrinsic to nerve or chiasm.
- Intra-axial tumor.
- History of NF type 1.

Possible biopsy indications.
- Atypical features.
- Infiltration or compression of chiasm.

Differential Diagnosis

Parenchymal optic nerve enlargement.
- Sarcoid.
- TB.
- Syphilis.
- Optic neuritis.
- MS.
- Infiltration: leukemia, lymphoma.

Extraparenchymal.
- Sheath meningioma (Figure 6.17).
- Optic nerve sheath metastasis.

Treatment

- Controversial.
- Optic nerve glioma:
  Observation, since growth usually very slow.
  Excision is indicated for (a) severe vision loss in the setting of disfiguring proptosis or exposure keratopathy and (b) poor vision associated with intracranial extension or advancement threatening the chiasm.

NEURO

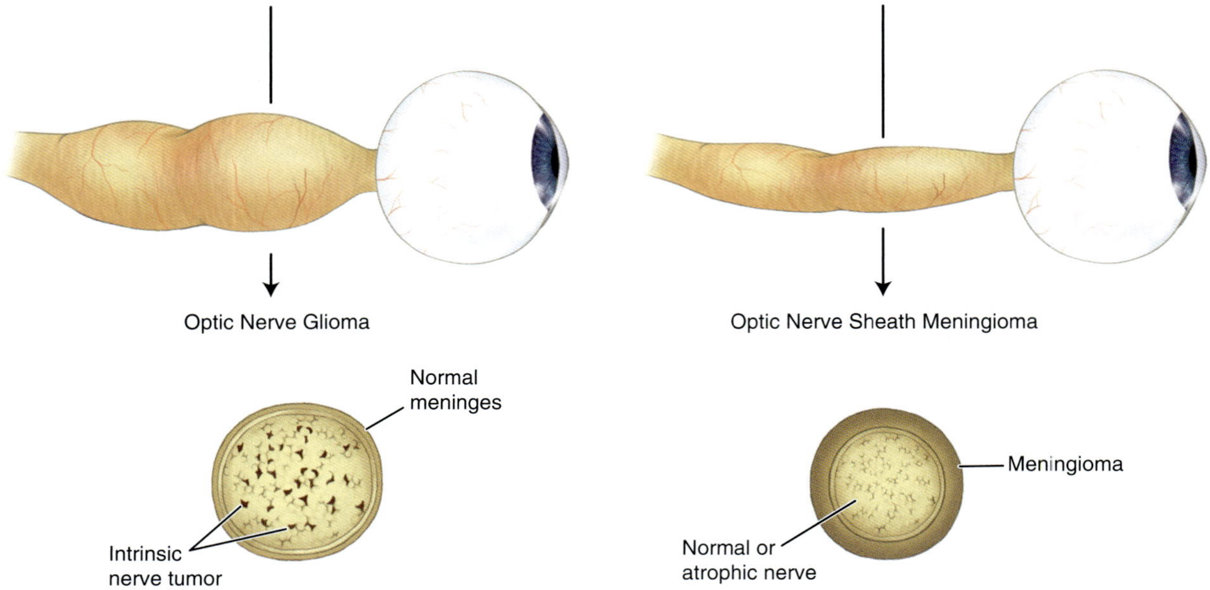

FIGURE 6.17. Optic nerve gliomas cause fusiform enlargement of the optic nerve, whereas optic nerve meningiomas cause a concentric enlargement of the nerve sheath.

- Chiasmal glioma:
  Observation.
  Possible treatment indications.
  Progressive visual loss.
  Hypothalamic symptoms.
  Hydrocephalus.
  Documented enlargement by MRI scan.
  Radiation therapy (usually reserved for progressive disease in older children).
  Chemotherapy (with or without radiation therapy).
  Actinomycin D/vincristine.
  Carboplatin.
  Vincristine and etoposide.
- There is no consensus on treatment.
  Natural history is variable and not well-defined.
  No randomized prospective clinical treatment trial.
  No clearly defined treatment protocols.
  Many studies have no tissue verification of diagnosis.

Possible Treatment Recommendations

- If visually and radiographically stable: observe.
- Large exophytic chiasmal lesion: debulk.
- Follow serially with MRI scans and clinical examinations.
- If progression (two successive eye visits or MRI), consider surgery.
- If the patient is not a surgical candidate, consider chemotherapy or radiotherapy.
- Shunt hydrocephalus.

Reference

Dutton JJ. Gliomas of the anterior visual pathway. *Surv Ophthalmol* 1994;38:427–452.

Meningiomas of the Anterior Visual Pathway

Summary

Optic nerve sheath meningiomas are benign proliferations of the meningeal sheath of the optic nerve causing compressive damage and interfering with pial blood supply to the optic nerve.

Epidemiology

Most commonly, middle aged (peak, fifth decade of life).
Female-to-male ratio, 3:1.
More often in white than in black patients.
Increased incidence in NF type 1

Signs and Symptoms

Painless.
Usually unilateral.
Gradually progressive loss of vision.
Proptosis.
Visual field defects.
Diplopia.
Intracranial meningomas, in particular those of the sphenoid wing, may cause compression of the optic nerve, cavernous sinus, and orbital structures.

Ophthalmic Findings

Disk edema and/or optic atrophy.
May see retinochoroidal venous collateral (also known as *optociliary shunt* vessel) (Figure 6.18).

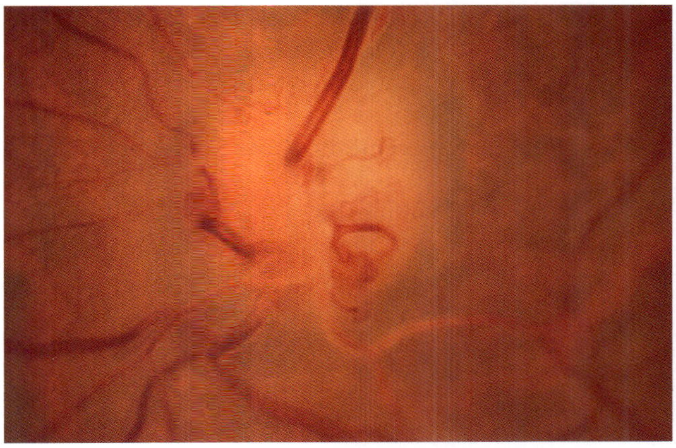

FIGURE 6.18. Opticiliary shunt vessels suggestive of an optic nerve sheath meningioma.

Evaluation

Neuroimaging (usually MRI) (Figure 6.19).
CT may show diffuse tubular enlargement of the optic nerve.
Calcification of the optic nerve sheath (train track sign).
Hyperostotis of adjacent bone.

Treatment

Optic nerve sheath meningiomas usually produce slow, progressive visual loss.
Cannot be surgically excised without sacrificing pial blood supply.
Radiation is first-line therapy.
Excision may be indicated for blind eyes with severe proptosis or to reduce risk of intracranial extension.

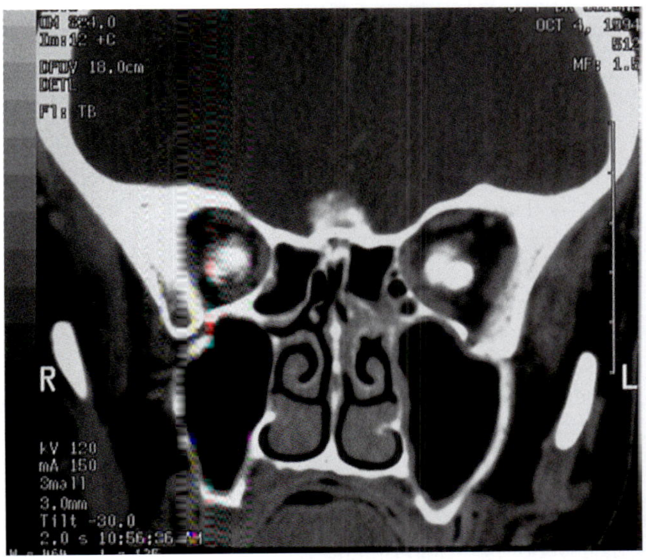

FIGURE 6.19. CT scan with contrast showing enhancement of an optic nerve sheath meningioma.

Traumatic Optic Neuropathy

Summary

Traumatic optic neuropathy is a clinical diagnosis that is characterized by a history of impact injury to the head, face, or orbit that is presumably transmitted directly or indirectly to the optic nerve and results in variable loss of vision.

Etiology

Trauma to the head, face, forehead, or orbit.
May be due to a number of mechanisms:
- Compressive.
- Direct mechanical injury.
- Retrobulbar hemorrhage.
- Increased intraorbital pressure.
- Subperiosteal or intrasheath hematoma or fluid.
- Optic nerve contusion, edema, or swelling.
- Vascular injury such as vasospasm or ischemia.
- Inflammation.

Signs and Symptoms

Loss of visual acuity ranging from 20/20 to NLP.
Loss of visual field.

Ophthalmic Features

Relative afferent pupillary defect in unilateral or bilateral but asymmetric cases.
Normal or, less commonly, swollen optic nerve.
Later develops optic atrophy.

Differential Diagnosis

Other causes of visual loss in the setting of trauma.
Open globe.
Traumatic cataract.
Vitreous hemorrhage.
Retinal detachment.

Evaluation

Neuroimaging: Incidence of visible canal fracture is variable. CT is the best test in the setting of trauma for detailed examination for bone fractures and bone fragments impinging on the optic nerve, and for the detection of acute hemorrhage.

Management

Medical Treatment

Megasode corticosteroids (numerous regimens, all unproven).
Dexamethasone, 3 to 5 mg/kg/day.
Dexamethasone, 1 mg/kg/day.
Methylprednisolone, 30 mg/kg load followed by 15 mg/kg every 6 hours i.v.
If vision improves on regimen of i.v. steroids after 48 hours, start rapid oral taper of prednisone.

If there is no clinical response after 48 hours or if the vision deteriorates during the steroid taper, surgical decompression of the optic canal is offered.

The International Optic Nerve Trauma Study did not find clear benefit for either corticosteroids or optic canal decompression.

Surgical Treatment (Reserved for Orbital or Sheath Hematoma, Bone Fragment Impinging Optic Nerve)

Perform canthotomy, cantholysis if the orbit is tense.

Drain subperiosteal hematoma if present.

Surgical decompression if medical therapy fails.

Surgery may be indicated to remove bone fragments impinging on the optic nerve.

Optic Tract and Occipital Lobe Disease

Visual Illusions and Hallucinations

Summary

Illusions are misperceptions of external environment attributable to disordered processing of visual stimuli (e.g., optical illusions) that disappear with eyes closed (unlike hallucinations). Hallucinations are subjective perceptions when no sensory stimulus is present.

Etiology of Illusions

- Optical aberrations.
  - Astigmatic lenses (distortions of shape).
  - Lenticular abnormalities (multiple images, altered color).
  - Brunescence (yellow-brown tint).
  - Cyanopsia (blue tint) after cataract removal.
  - Erythropsia.
  - Aphakia or pseudophakia.
  - After vitreous hemorrhage or hyphema.
  - Distortions in tear film or cornea.
  - Different indexes of refraction.
  - Retinal disease (micropsia, macropsia, metamorphopsia, xanthapsia).

Signs and Symptoms of Illusions

Disordered processing (visual and association cortex).

- Altered shape and size (acute occipital lesion).
  - Like "cubist" painting (coneheads or elongated fingers).
  - Cerebral metamorphopsia (overlap).
  - Illusory spread.
  - Often coexists with palinopsia.
- Altered position (occipital lobe).
  - Displace image into opposite hemifield.
  - Visual allesthesia.
  - Always have a homonymous hemianopsia.
  - Allesthetic image "seen" in hemianopic field.
  - Epileptic phenomenon.
    - May have associated tonic-clonic or focal electroencephalographic (EEG) discharge.
    - May cause perception of cerebral diplopia.
- Altered distance.
- Altered motion ("piecemealing" of motion, polyopia for moving objects).
- Multiple images (palinopsia).
  - Visual perseveration in time.
  - Images played back (may occur hours later).
  - Unilateral temporal parietal occipital lesions.
  - Right more often than left posterior hemisphere lesions.

Treatment of Illusions

Antiepileptic medications may be helpful.

Anticonvulsants may help.

Signs and Symptoms of Hallucinations

- Anterior visual pathway lesions with visual loss:
  - Vitreoretinal interface (tear, detachment).
  - Very brief flashes of white or colored lights.
  - Worse with eye movements.
  - Physical deformation of retinal receptors.
  - Often confined to one eye.
  - Silvery scintillations or dazzle.
  - Outer retinal disorders "snow or noise on television."
  - Sound-induced phosphenes in demyelinating optic nerve disease.
- Visual and temporal cortex lesions.
  - Animate figures typical of visual association cortex lesions.
  - Scenes with sense of familiarity: temporal lobe neural activity.
  - Vertebrobasilar insufficiency.
- Brainstem limbic circuits.
- Migraine.
  - Geometric scintillations (jagged lines, right angles).
  - Progression of scintillations across hemianopic field.
  - Over 20- to 30-minute period.
  - "Alice in Wonderland" syndrome.

Etiology of Hallucination

Partial seizure.

Imbalance in CNS neurotransmitters (drugs, toxins, diffuse CNS disease).

Disinhibition of "dreamlike" experiences.

- Altered consciousness.
- Visual deprivation.

May exist as isolated phenomenon (unlike auditory hallucinations).

Vestibulopathy (Wallenberg syndrome): "tilted" or "upside down."

Psychoactive agents.

Charles Bonnet phenomenon (associated with bilateral visual loss). These patients are aware that their hallucinations are not real.

Anton syndrome (associated with cortical blindness) occurs when patients hallucinate and confabulate about visual images despite no demonstrable visual perception. Occurs with damage to the visual cortex.

Evaluation

Reassure the patient if condition occurs in setting of blindness or visual loss.
Exclude medication-related side effects.
Distinguish between illusions and hallucinations.
Exclude migraine.
If atypical for migraine or other findings, MRI scan and EEG.

OCULAR MOTOR PARESIS

Third-Nerve Palsies

Anatomy

The third-nerve nucleus resides in the midbrain and is composed of several subnuclei that serve the IR, inferior oblique, and medial rectus muscles (MRMs) on the ipsilateral side; the levator (supplied by a single central nucleus) and the SR muscle on the contralateral side (Figure 6.20). The pupil fibers originate in the Edinger-Westphal nuclei. The fascicle of the third nerve passes by important structures in the midbrain (e.g., corticospinal tract) and enters the subarachnoid space. The third nerve then travels in the lateral wall of the cavernous sinus and enters the orbit via the superior orbital fissure, where it separates into a superior and inferior division (Figure 6.21A and Table 6.2).

Demographics

May occur at any age (may be congenital).
May occur in either gender.
Aneurysm uncommon but reported in children.

Ophthalmic Findings

Binocular vertical diplopia.
Ipsilateral hypotropia and exotropia.
May be partial or complete.
Pupil-sparing terminology only refers to a complete third-nerve palsy (ptosis, extraocular motility deficits) without involvement of pupil function.
The pupil may be spared initially in an evolving compressive third-nerve palsy.
Partial, complete, or no ptosis.
Partial, complete, or no pupil involvement (dilation, poor or no light reaction).

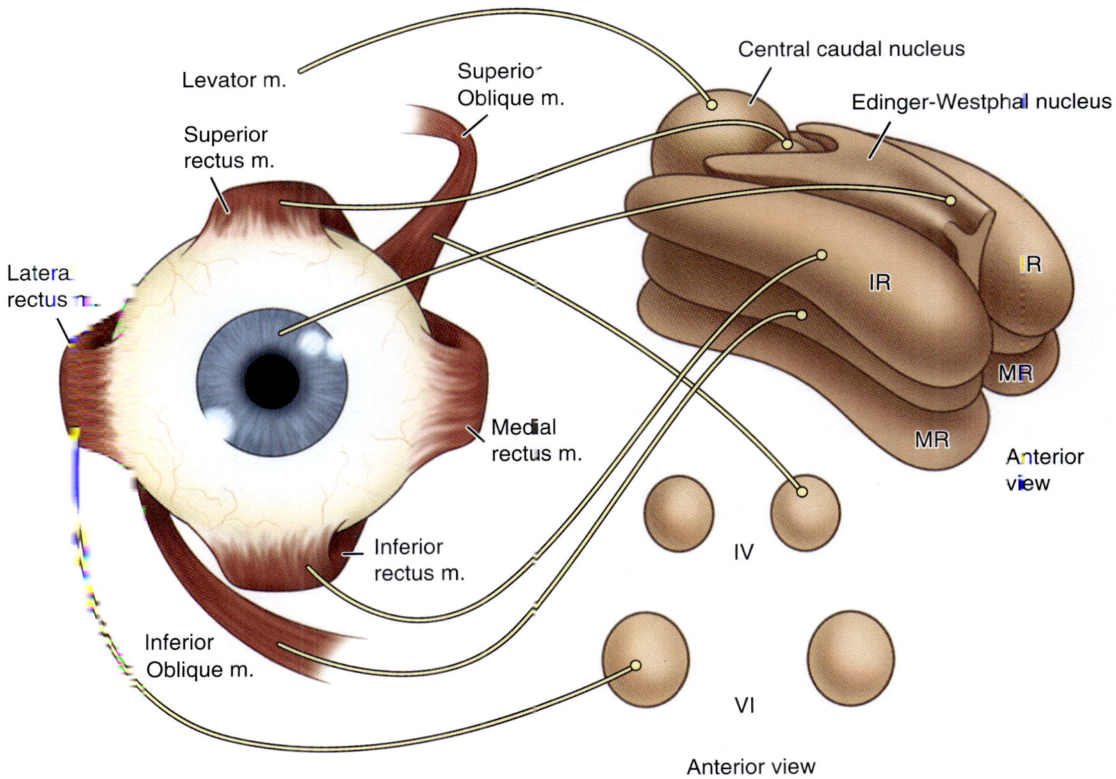

FIGURE 6.20 Innervation of the extraocular muscles. Note that the superior rectus and oblique muscles are innervated by contralateral nuclei and the levator by a fused central nucleus. (SR, superior rectus; SO, superior oblique; MR, medial rectus; IR, inferior rectus; IO, inferior oblique; LR, lateral rectus; EW, Edinger-Westphal nucleus; CCN, central caudal nucleus.)

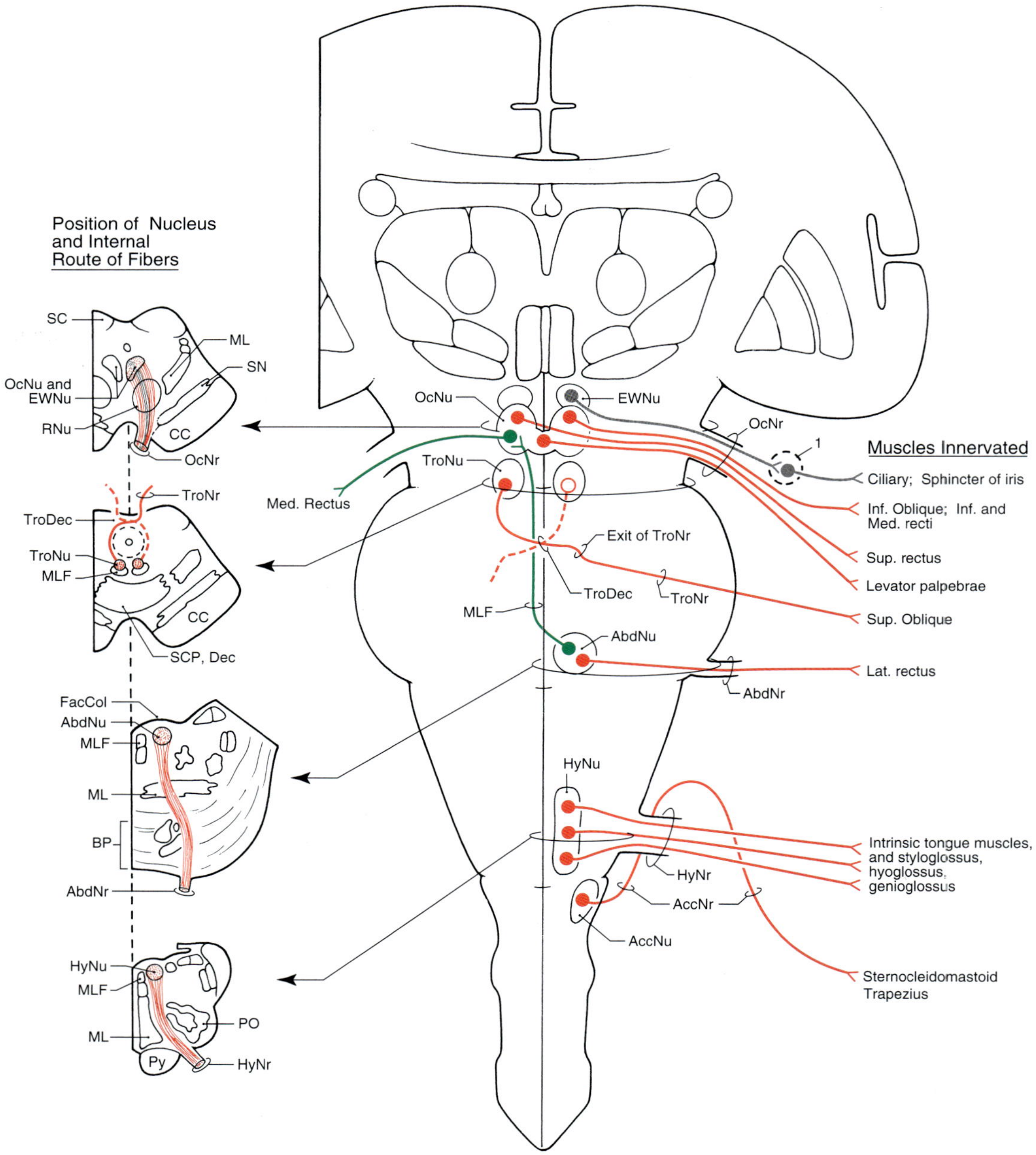

FIGURE 6.21. The origin and peripheral distribution of GSE fibers from the oculomotor, trochlear, abducens, spinal accessory, and hypoglossal nuclei. Also shown are GVE fibers arising from the Edinger-Westphal nucleus and the distribution of postganglionic fibers from the ciliary ganglion. Internuclear abducens neurons project, via the MLF, to contralateral oculomotor neurons that innervate the MRM (INO pathway). (Reproduced from Haines DE. *Neuroanatomy: an atlas of structures, sections, and systems*, 6th ed. Lippincott Williams & Wilkins, 2004, with permission.)

Differential Diagnosis

Aneurysm—usually at junction of posterior cerebral artery and posterior communicating artery.

Compressive lesion.
Ischemic.
Other (demyelinating, traumatic).
Myasthenia gravis.
Pseudotumor of orbit or orbital tumor.
Thyroid eye disease (TED).
Skew/ocular tilt reaction.

Evaluation

- Nonisolated (Figure 6.22):
  MRI of brain directed to topographic localization of associated signs.
  Lumbar puncture if negative imaging and meningeal signs.

Table 6.2

CN III lesions

Location	Etiology	Signs and symptoms	Other findings
Nuclear	Brainstem infarction/ischemia Neoplasm Trauma	Rare without other neurologic signs Unlikely to affect the pupil pathway alone	Obligatory nuclear lesions Unilateral third nerve and contralateral SR and bilateral partial ptosis Bilateral third nerve and spared levators
	Infection Demyelination Congenital hypoplasia	Usually associated with other midbrain signs (e.g., other cranial neuropathies, ataxia, or hemiparesis)	Possible nuclear lesions Bilateral total third nerve (e.g., basilar artery infarct) (Figure 6.23) Bilateral and symmetric ptosis (single midline nucleus) Isolated weakness of one muscle except levator and medial recti Cannot be nuclear lesions Complete III + normal contralateral SR (crossed innervation) Unilateral ptosis: levator (single caudal subnucleus bilateral innervation) Unilateral internal ophthalmoplegia (visceral nuclei are spread out) Isolated unilateral or bilateral medial rectus palsy (three separate subnuclei)
Fascicular	Infarct (most common) Hemorrhage Neoplasm Trauma Demyelination Inflammation (rare)	Red nucleus Contralateral ataxia Slow "rubral" tremor Claude syndrome Subthalamic region Contralateral hemichorea Hemitremor Benedikt syndrome Brachium conjunctivum below the decussation Cerebellar ataxia Vertical gaze palsy Nothnagel syndrome Cerebral peduncle Contralateral hemiparesis Face and tongue involvement Weber syndrome Other mesencephalic signs Disorders of gaze and convergence Somnolence Peduncular hallucinosis Paucity of speech (mutism) "Pseudoabducens palsy" "Midbrain corectopia"	

(Continued)

Table 6.2

CN III lesions (*Continued*)

Location	Etiology	Signs and symptoms	Other findings
Subarachnoid space third-nerve palsy	Aneurysm at junction of posterior communicating artery and posterior cerebral artery (most common) Basilar artery aneurysm Uncal herniation Basilar meningitis Neoplasm Ischemia/infarction (e.g., diabetic, hypertensive) Trauma Surgical Hydrocephalus	Pupil-involved third-nerve palsy should be considered to be a posterior communicating artery aneurysm until proven otherwise, especially if signs of subarachnoid hemorrhage are present.	CT scan (Figure 6.24), lumbar puncture if suspect subarachnoid hemorrhage or meningitis. Cerebral arteriography if suspect aneurysm.
Cavernous sinus/ superior orbital fissure, third-nerve palsy	Neoplasm Pituitary tumor Meningioma Metastasis Sphenoid sinus Lymphoma Craniopharyngioma Infections Mucormycosis *Aspergillus* sp. *Bipolaris hawaiiensis* Vascular Aneurysm of ICA Carotid-cavernous fistula Venous angioma Cavernous hemangioma Inflammatory lesions Trauma	Usually involves other cranial nerves (e.g., nerves IV, VI, and V1) (Figure 6.25) Proptosis indicates superior orbital fissure involvement	
Orbital third-nerve lesions	Inflammatory Ischemic Traumatic Neoplasm	Proptosis, chemosis, and conjunctival injection May have concomitant orbital optic neuropathy Progressive unilateral visual loss Disk swelling (followed by atrophy) Optociliary shunt vessels Occasionally enophthalmos	
Isolated nonlocalizing third-nerve palsy		Critical questions for TNP: Complete involvement or partial involvement? Pupil spared or pupil involved? Vasculopathic patient (e.g., hypertension, diabetes) or not?	

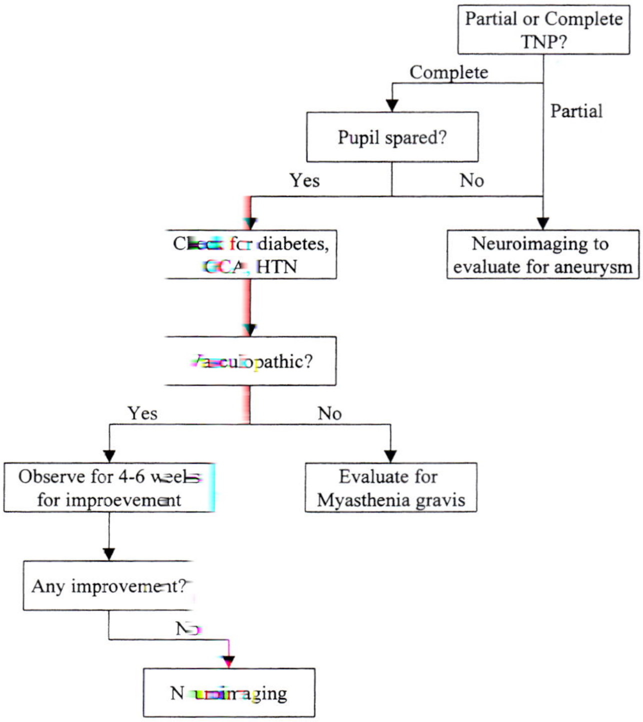

FIGURE 6.22. Evaluation of third-nerve palsy.

Consider GCA in elderly patients.
Consider myasthenia gravis if pupil spared.

- Isolated:
  Children:
  Consider congenital.
  Consider MRI
  Further evaluation based on history and examination.
- Congenital cases: no further evaluation.
- Traumatic cases: no further evaluation.
- Vasculopathic
  Typically complete, isolated, and pupil spared.
  Six to eight weeks.
  Observe for improvement.
  Evaluate and treat vasculopathic risk factors.
  Exclude GCA in elderly patients.
  If no better or progression, further evaluation including neuroimaging.
  Aberrant regeneration implies compressive lesion and warrants neuroimaging.
- Nonvasculopathic, bilateral, progressive, partial palsy, partial or complete pupil involvement (Figure 6.23):
  CT angiogram (CTA) usually first-line study.
  MRI and MRA or CTA negative.
  Catheter angiogram if aneurysm still suspected despite negative neuroimaging.
  Consider lumbar puncture if meningeal signs.
  Evaluate for vasculopathic risk factors.
  Consider myasthenia gravis if pupil spared.

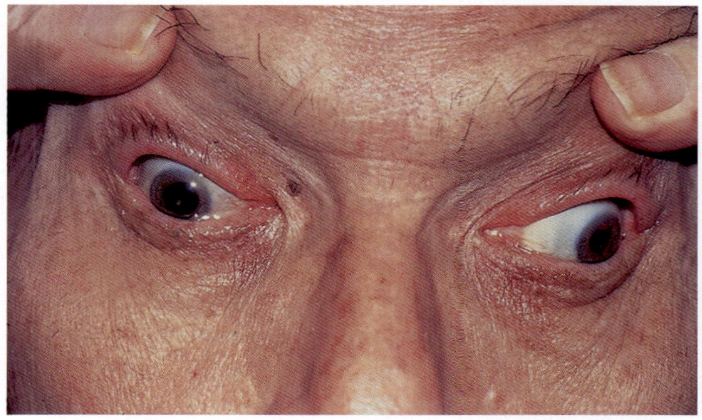

FIGURE 6.23. Bilateral complete oculomotor nerve palsy from damage to both oculomotor nuclei. Both eyes are deviated downward and outward with an accompanying bilateral ptosis.

Treatment

Patch.
Prism for comitant and relatively small deviations.
Strabismus surgery if stable deviation.

Reference

Brazis PW. Localization of lesions of the oculomotor nerve: recent concepts. *Mayo Clin Proc* 1991;66:1029–1035.

Fourth-Nerve Palsies

Anatomy

The trochlear nucleus lies caudal to the oculomotor nuclear complex at the level of the inferior colliculus and gives rise to the nerve fascicle, which courses posteroinferiorly around the aqueduct to decussate in the anterior medullary velum (the roof of the aqueduct) just caudal to the inferior colliculus. The trochlear nerve then emerges as one or more rootlets from the dorsal surface of the lower midbrain, immediately below the inferior colliculus and near the tentorium. The trochlear nerve axons leave the midbrain contralateral to their nucleus of origin. The cisternal segment then runs anteriorly over the lateral aspect of the brainstem; this cisternal portion of the nerve is closely related to the tentorium cerebelli. The nerve passes between the superior cerebellar and the posterior cerebral arteries and leaves the posterior fossa by piercing the dura at a point slightly below the point of entry of the oculomotor nerve into the cavernous sinus along the lateral aspect of the clivus, just below the petroclinoid ligament. Within the lateral wall of the cavernous sinus, the trochlear nerve lies below the oculomotor nerve and above the ophthalmic division of the trigeminal nerve, with which it shares a connective tissue sheath. It then crosses over the oculomotor nerve to enter the orbit through the superior orbital fissure, external to the tendinous ring that serves as an

Table 6.3

CN IV lesions

Location	Etiology	Signs and symptoms
Nucleus or fascicle	Infarct, ischemia, bleed, neoplasm, demyelination	Usually associated with other brainstem signs (e.g., third-nerve palsy, contralateral hemiplegia)
Subarachnoid space	Inflammatory or infectious meningitis, subarachnoid bleed, rarely aneurysm, trauma	Bilateral fourth-nerve palsies with trauma
Cavernous sinus	Sellar/parasellar tumors (e.g., pituitary, meningioma), ischemic, inflammatory (e.g., sarcoid), aneurysms, dissection of internal carotid artery, cavernous sinus thrombosis, fistula	Other cranial neuropathies of cranial nerves III, VI, or V or combination, or Horner syndrome
Orbit	Neoplastic inflammation, infectious, traumatic, etc.	Orbital signs (e.g., proptosis, chemosis)

attachment site for the extraocular muscles (the annulus of Zinn). The nerve supplies the SOM (Figure 6.21B and Table 6.3).

Signs and Symptoms

Binocular vertical diplopia.
Anomalous head position (e.g., typically head tilt contralateral to hypertropia).
Worse diplopia in downgaze toward the paretic SOM.
Subjective and objective torsion.
Congenital cases.
Large vertical fusional amplitudes.
Longstanding hypertropia.
Lack of subjective torsion.

Demographics

May occur at any age (may be congenital).
May occur in either gender.

Ophthalmic Findings

Binocular vertical diplopia worse in downgaze.
Ipsilateral hypertropia, worse in contralateral gaze, and worse in ipsilateral HT.
Decreased superior oblique function.
Subjective excyclotorsion on double Maddox rod testing.
Visible excyclotorsion on funduscopy.

Differential Diagnosis

Myasthenia gravis.
Pseudotumor of orbit or orbital tumor.
TED.
Skew/ocular tilt reaction.

Evaluation

- Nonisolated:
  MRI of brain directed to topographic localization of associated signs.
  Lumbar puncture if negative imaging and meningeal signs.
  Consider GCA in elderly patients.
  Consider myasthenia gravis.
- Isolated:
  Children:
    Consider congenital (e.g., review old photos for longstanding HT and subtle hemifacial hypertrophy).
    Consider MRI.
    Further evaluation based on history and examination.
- Congenital cases: no further evaluation.
- Traumatic cases: no further evaluation.
- Vasculopathic:
  Six to eight weeks.
  Observe for improvement.
  Evaluate and treat vasculopathic risk factors.
  Exclude GCA in elderly patients.
  If no better or progression, further evaluation including neuroimaging.
- Nonvasculopathic, bilateral, progressive:
  MRI along fourth nerve.
  Consider lumbar puncture if meningeal signs.
  Evaluate for vasculopathic risk factors.
  Consider myasthenia gravis.

Treatment

Patch.
Prism for comitant and relatively small deviations.
Strabismus surgery if stable deviation.

Reference

Brazis PW. Palsies of the trochlear nerve: diagnosis and localization—recent concepts. *Mayo Clin Proc* 1993;68:501–509.

Brown Syndrome

Summary

Brown syndrome is characterized by limitation of elevation in adduction of the involved eye attributable to presumed abnormalities in the superior oblique tendon sheath complex.

Etiology

Congenital.
Acquired.
Tenosynovitis (inflammation, rheumatoid arthritis).
Trauma.

Signs and Symptoms

Limited elevation in adduction.
May have a "clicking sound" or localized pain or tenderness in the area of the trochlea in attempted elevation in adduction.
Ipsilateral hypotropia.
May have an anomalous head position (chin up).

Evaluation

Forced ductions are positive.

Treatment

None if asymptomatic.

Superior Oblique Myokymia

Summary

Superior oblique myokymia is an intermittent firing of the SOM that results in transient diplopia or oscillopsia.

Etiology

Unknown.
May follow trauma.
May follow fourth-nerve palsy.
Usually not associated with intracranial disease (e.g., tumor or demyelination).

Signs and Symptoms

Intermittent vertical diplopia or oscillopsia.
Described as monocular "shimmering" or "quivering."
Paroxysms of vertical or torsional movements.

Evaluation

Observation at the slit lamp may reveal movements.
MRI if other signs suggesting intracranial disease (usually not necessary).

Treatment

Patching.
Medications (e.g., carbamazepine, propranolol).
Strabismus surgery (superior oblique tenectomy with inferior oblique myectomy).

Natural History

Exacerbations and remissions.

Reference

Brazis PW, Miller NR, Henderer JD, et al. The natural history and results of treatment of superior oblique myokymia. *Arch Ophthalmol* 1994;112:1063–1067.

Sixth-Nerve Palsies

Anatomy

The sixth-nerve nucleus is located in the caudal portion of the paramedian pontine tegmentum. The facial nerve fibers loop around the nucleus before exiting in the cerebellopontine angle. There are two populations of neurons with cell bodies in the abducens nucleus: one group forms the sixth nerve and the other group forms internuclear neurons that join the contralateral medial longitudinal fasciculus (MLF), which projects to the medial rectus subnucleus. The abducens nerve fibers pass ventrally to exit at the pontomedullary junction. The nerve then ascends the ventral surface of the pons, is crossed by the anteroinferior cerebellar artery, and pierces the dura of the clivus below the posterior clinoid. The nerve then runs beneath the petroclinoid ligament (Gruber canal) and enters the substance of the cavernous sinus. Some sympathetic fibers are briefly attached to the nerve in the cavernous sinus. From the cavernous sinus, the nerve passes through the annular segment of the superior orbital fissure and innervates the lateral rectus muscle (LRM) (Figure 6.21C and Table 6.4).

Signs and Symptoms

Binocular horizontal diplopia.
Worse diplopia in lateral gaze toward the paretic side.

Demographics

May occur in any age group.
May occur in either gender.

Ophthalmic Findings

Binocular horizontal diplopia worse ipsilateral gaze.
Uncrossed diplopia.
Abduction restricted or slowed.
May have an anomalous face turn for fusion.
May have an associated small vertical deviation.

Differential Diagnosis

Divergence insufficiency.
Duane syndrome, type I.
Myasthenia gravis.
Pseudotumor of orbit or orbital tumor.

Table 6.4

CN VI lesions

Location	Etiology	Signs and symptoms
Nucleus	Infarct, ischemia, bleed, neoplasm, demyelination	Horizontal gaze palsy not just an abduction deficit due to involvement of interneurons of MLF Usually associated with other brainstem signs (e.g., facial nerve palsy, contralateral hemiplegia)
Fascicle	Infarct/ischemia, bleed, neoplasm, demyelination	Adjacent structures involved (e.g., cranial nerves V, VII, and VIII, cerebellar ataxia, central Horner syndrome, contralateral hemiplegia)
Subarachnoid space	Any cause of increased intracranial pressure (e.g., pseudotumor cerebri, inflammatory or infectious meningitis, subarachnoid bleed, intracranial mass lesion)	Unilateral or bilateral
Petrous apex	Complicated otitis media, mastoiditis (Gradenigo syndrome) basilar skull fracture, or neoplasia (e.g., nasopharyngeal carcinoma)	Associated with cranial nerves VI, VII, and VIII and facial pain
Cavernous sinus	Sellar/parasellar tumors (e.g., pituitary, meningioma), ischemic, inflammatory (e.g., sarcoid), aneurysms or dissection of internal carotid artery, cavernous sinus thrombosis, fistula (Figure 6.27)	Other cranial neuropathies of nerves III, IV, VI, or V or combination, or Horner syndrome
Orbit	Multiple etiologies (e.g., neoplastic, inflammation, infectious, traumatic)	Orbital signs (e.g., proptosis, chemosis)

MLF, medial longitudinal fasciculus.

Spasm of the near reflex.
Thyroid eye disease.
Esophoria (decompensated).

Evaluation

- Nonisolated, progressive, or bilateral.
  - MRI of brain directed to topographic localization along sixth nerve.
  - Lumbar puncture (nonlocalizing sign of increased intracranial pressure) if negative result on imaging.
  - Consider GCA in elderly patients.
  - Consider myasthenia gravis.
- Isolated:
  - Children:
    - Consider postviral sixth-nerve paresis.
    - Consider MRI (rule out brainstem glioma or other structural lesion).
    - Further evaluation based on history and examination.
- Vasculopathic:
  - Observe for improvement in 6 to 8 weeks.
  - Could perform initial neuroimaging with MRI.
  - Evaluate and treat vasculopathic risk factors.
  - Exclude GCA in elderly patients.
  - If no better or progression, further evaluation including neuroimaging.
- Nonvasculopathic:
  - MRI.
  - Consider lumbar puncture.
  - Evaluate for vasculopathic risk factors.
  - Consider myasthenia gravis.

Treatment

Consider amblyopia treatment in children.
Patch.
Prism for comitant and relatively small deviations.
Strabismus surgery if stable deviation.

Localization of Lesion with Multiple Cranial Nerve Palsies

Etiology

- Brainstem:
  - Usually accompanied by other brainstem signs (e.g., hemiparesis, hemisensory loss).
- Subarachnoid space:
  - Often associated with other meningeal signs (e.g., headache, stiff neck).
- Cavernous sinus (Figures 6.24 and 6.25):
  - Any combination of cranial nerves (e.g., nerves III, IV, VI).

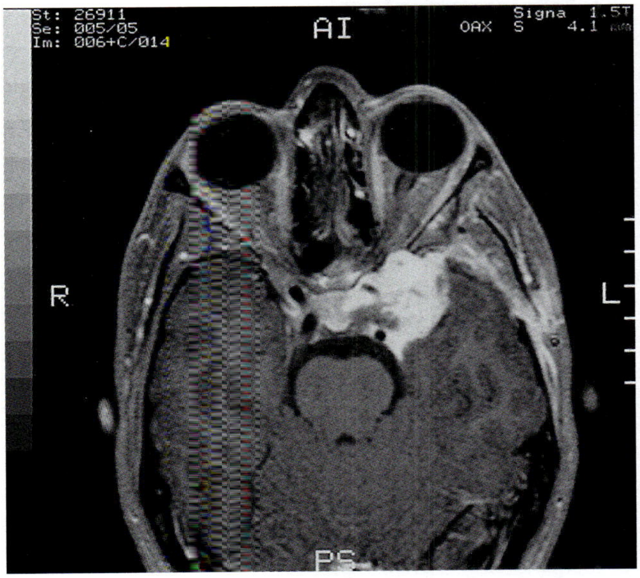

FIGURE 6.24. Contrast-enhanced CT scan of a cavernous sinus lesion.

May have Horner syndrome.
May have trigeminal dysfunction (V1 sensory loss or pain).

- Orbit:
  Usually accompanied by other orbital signs (e.g., proptosis, chemosis).
- Neuromuscular junction (NMJ) (e.g., myasthenia gravis).
- Multiple extraocular muscle involvement (e.g., thyroid).
- Multifocal disease (any combination of above).

Evaluation and Treatment

Neuroimaging and other appropriate evaluation should be directed to the underlying topographic localization and clinical signs.

Any patient with painless, pupil spared, nonproptotic ophthalmoplegia should be evaluated for myasthenia gravis.

Cavernous Sinus Syndrome and Tolosa-Hunt Syndrome

Summary

The cavernous sinus contains the ocular motor cranial nerves (III, IV, and VI), the first (anteriorly) and second (posteriorly) divisions of the trigeminal nerve, the internal carotid artery, and the ocular sympathetic nerves. Thus, lesions of the cavernous sinus may present with any combination of dysfunction of these nerves. Anterior extension of the lesion into the orbit through the superior orbital fissure may result in an optic neuropathy, proptosis, and other orbital signs. The Tolosa-Hunt syndrome (THS) describes an idiopathic, inflammatory, painful ophthalmoplegia syndrome that may be located within the cavernous sinus. THS, however, is a diagnosis of exclusion and

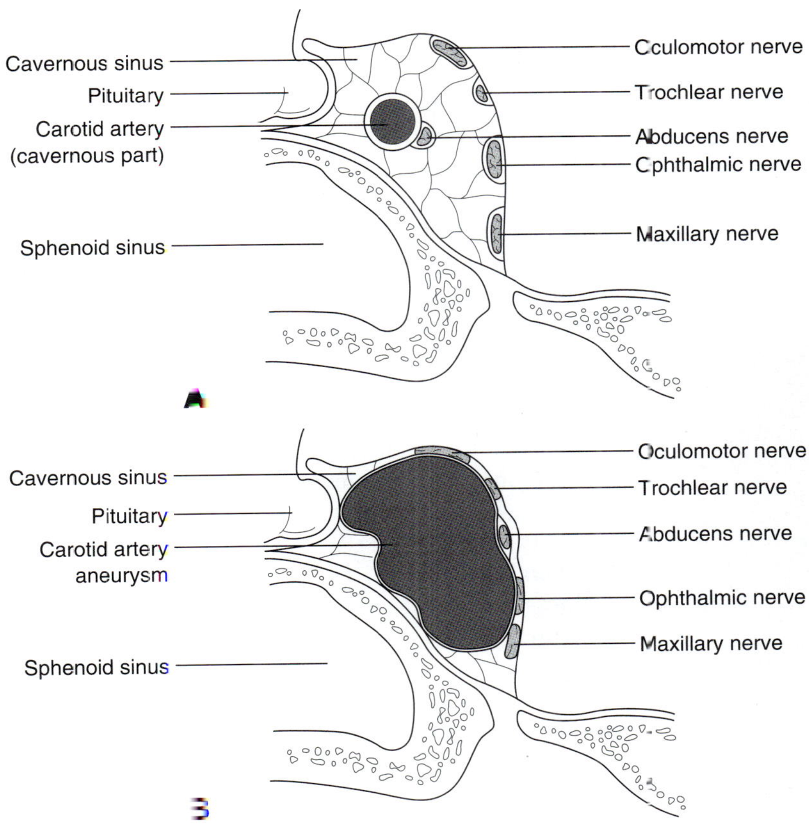

FIGURE 6.25. **A:** The cavernous sinus lies just lateral to the sella turcica. Within it lie the carotid artery and cranial nerves III, IV, and VI and branches of V. **B:** Pathological findings involving the cavernous sinus are not rare and can usually be recognized by the pattern of cranial nerve involvement.

requires a full evaluation of other causes of a cavernous sinus syndrome (Figure 6.25).

Epidemiology

Male and female patients equally affected.
Age: Fifth decade is most common age of onset (range, 35 to 75 years of age).

Signs and Symptoms

- Pain: steady, boring in and around eye, often in V_1 distribution, may precede ophthalmoplegia.
- Difficult to make this diagnosis without painful ophthalmoplegia: partial or total.
- Cranial neuropathy:
  Nerve III (86%).
  Nerve IV (29%).
  Nerve VI (70%).
  Any combination of above.
  V_1 distribution (30%), V2 (12%).
  Nerve VII (5%).
- With (22%) or without pupil involvement.
- May have (4%) Horner syndrome (pupil smaller) sensory defects (often, V_1 distribution; rarely in V_2 distribution).
- Optic neuropathy uncommon.
- Carotid cavernous fistulas may have additional findings related to high-pressure vascular flow (bruit, increased IOP).

Differential Diagnosis

Cavernous sinus syndrome with or without painful ophthalmoplegia:
Neoplastic (e.g., metastatic, lymphoma, multiple myeloma, carcinomatous meningitis, nasopharyngeal tumor, primary intracranial tumors).
Vascular (e.g., carotid-cavernous fistula) (Figure 6.26).
Infectious (e.g., fungal, syphilis, TB).
Inflammatory (e.g., sarcoid, Wegener granulomatosis, THS).
Ischemic (e.g., GCA).
Trauma.

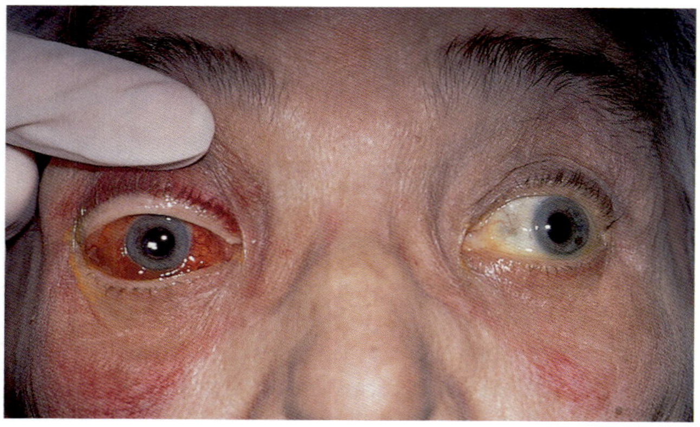

FIGURE 6.26. Complete right-sided ophthalmoplegia secondary to a carotid-cavernous sinus fistula. Ptosis and conjunctival chemosis are also evident.

Evaluation

Neuroimaging: preferably MRI scan.
Lumbar puncture if imaging result negative.
Laboratory studies (e.g., FTA-Abs or microhemagglutination–*Treponema pallidum* [MHA-TP], RPR, ANA, ESR, chest x-ray) based on the history and examination.

Treatment

Treatment of cavernous sinus lesions should be directed toward the underlying cause (e.g., tumor, infection).
THS.
Steroids (prednisone 1.0 to 1.5 mg/kg/day).
Consider i.v. steroids.
Exclude infectious causes before steroid therapy.

Primary Myopathies

Chronic Progressive External Ophthalmoplegia

Chronic progressive external ophthalmoplegia (CPEO) is an etiologically nonspecific term. Most generalized myopathies do not involve eye muscles, and specific syndromes causing CPEO have been identified.

Etiology (Types)

- Progressive ophthalmoplegia.
  Isolated CPEO.
  Kearns-Sayre syndrome.
  Oculopharyngeal muscular dystrophy.
  Myotonic dystrophy.
  Isolated oculopharyngeal myopathy.
- Distinguish from static ophthalmoplegias.
  Agenesis of extraocular muscles.
  Congenital fibrosis syndrome.
  Congenital myopathies.
- Other ocular myopathies.
  With proximal limb muscle involvement.
  With distal limb muscle involvement.
  Congenital myopathy.
- Associated with neurodegenerative disease.
- Presumed mitochondrial syndrome.
  Facial, bulbar, and limb myopathy.
  Ataxia.
  Spasticity.
  Peripheral neuropathy.
  Deafness.
  Dementia.
  Optic atrophy.
  Pigmentary degeneration of retina.
  Cardiac conduction abnormalities.
  Endocrine, skin, and skeletal abnormalities.
- Stephens syndrome (CPEO, ataxia, peripheral neuropathy).

Differential Diagnosis

Myasthenia gravis.
Inflammatory and infectious myopathies.
- TED.
- Idiopathic orbital myositis.
- Infectious myositis.
- Amyloidosis.

Progressive supranuclear palsy (PSP).
Myasthenialike syndromes.
- Eaton-Lambert syndrome.
- Organophosphate poisoning.
- Botulism.

Episodic ophthalmoplegia.
- Familial periodic paralysis.
- Muscle trauma and contusions.
- Ischemia and vasculitis.

Kearns-Sayre Syndrome

Epidemiology

- Onset: less than 20 years of age (childhood).
- May occur in infancy though usually normal at birth.
- Ophthalmoplegia after age 5 years.
- Usually isolated without family history.
- May be autosomal dominant.
- Most cases are sporadic (mitochondrial inheritance).

Ocular Findings

Usually develop in childhood.
Slowly progressive over years.
Bilateral and symmetric, affecting both horizontal and vertical muscles.
May initially spare downgaze.
No diplopia usually.
Ptosis initially (early childhood).
Cases reported with no ptosis.
May be total external ophthalmoplegia.
May involve orbicularis muscle.
Pupils normal.
Atypical pigmentary retinopathy ("salt and pepper").
- Rarely bone spicules (rare pigment migration).
- Usually posterior pole (widespread); mottled RPE changes.

Usually, vision normal; may have loss of central vision later in life.

Systemic Findings

- Cardiac:
  - Conduction block that can lead to sudden death (need sequential electrocardiogram [ECG]).
  - May require pacemaker.
- Neurologic symptoms and signs:
  - Deafness and vestibular dysfunction.
  - Cerebellar ataxia and corticospinal dysfunction.
  - EEG abnormalities.
  - CSF protein increased (>100 mg/dL).
  - Widespread muscular dystrophy.
  - Spongiform degeneration of CNS (cortex, basal ganglia, and brainstem).

Treatment

Coenzyme Q10.
Surgical repair of ptosis should proceed with caution because of the ophthalmoplegia and lack of Bell reflex.

Oculopharyngeal Muscular Dystrophy

Summary

Oculopharyngeal muscular dystrophy is an inherited ophthalmoplegia syndrome common in patients of French-Canadian ancestry.

Epidemiology

Usually, onset at age 40 years (older).
Most patients are of French-Canadian descent.
Autosomal dominant (100% penetrance).
Autosomal recessive and sporadic forms occur in other ethnic groups.

Signs and Symptoms

Difficulty swallowing.
Varying degrees of external ophthalmoplegia.
Weakness of orbicularis muscles common.
Temporalis wasting.

Evaluation

Clinical diagnosis.
Muscle biopsy specimen may show abnormalities.

Treatment

None.

Myotonic Dystrophy

Summary

Myotonic dystrophy is a generalized muscular disorder characterized by myotonia.

Ophthalmic Findings

Orbicularis weakness.
Myotonia on lid closure and ptosis.
Poor eccentric gaze holding, slow saccades.
Sluggish, miotic pupils.
Blepharitis.
Dry eye syndrome.
Hypotony.
Lens (may be seen even in "amyotonic forms").

- Polychromatic cataracts.
- Posterior cortex star.
- Posterior subcapsular.

Pigmentary changes in macula.
- May have "butterfly" pattern.
- RPE changes.
- Diminished response on electroretinogram (ERG).
- Increased dark adaptation threshold.

Visual field constriction.
May have tufts on iris that may bleed.
Intermittent lid lag (like thyroid).

Systemic Findings

Frontal baldness.
Testicular atrophy.
Cardiac abnormalities.
- Cardiomyopathy.
- Conduction defects.

Narrow hatchet facies due to temporalis and masseter atrophy.

Evaluation

Clinical diagnosis:

Exclude myasthenia gravis.
Consider systemic evaluation.
Lactate levels.
Muscle biopsy may provide definite diagnosis.
- Ragged red fibers.
- Cytochrome C oxidase.
- Mitochondrial DNA (mtDNA) studies in muscle.
- Electromyogram (distinguishes neuropathic and myopathic).
- Mitochondrial DNA mutations.

CSF.
- Increased protein.
- Not a requirement or diagnostic.

References

Daroff R. Chronic progressive external ophthalmoplegia: a critical review. *Arch Ophthalmol* 1969;82:845.

Kearnes TP. External ophthalmoplegia, pigmentary degeneration of the retina and cardiomyopathy: a newly recognized syndrome. *Trans Am Ophthalmol Soc* 1965;63:559.

Synkinesis

Marcus Gunn Jaw Wink

Summary

Abnormal elevation of the eyelid with jaw movement attributable to synkinesis of the levator (CN III) and jaw muscles (external and internal pterygoid muscles, CN V).

Etiology

Congenital aberrant neural connections.

Signs

Congenital ptosis.
Elevation of the eyelid with movement of the mandible to opposite side or forward, opening of the jaw, or clenching of the teeth.

Evaluation

Clinical diagnosis.

Treatment

Usually none.

Duane Syndrome

Summary

Abnormalities of abduction or adduction associated with cocontraction of the extraocular muscles with retraction of the globe and narrowing of the palpebral fissure.

Etiology

Congenital absence of the sixth-nerve nucleus with aberrant innervation of the lateral rectus from fibers of the third cranial nerve.

Signs

Three types:

1. Abduction deficit with retraction of the globe on attempted abduction.
2. Adduction deficit with retraction of the globe on attempted adduction (Figure 6.27).
3. Both abduction and adduction deficit.

All three forms are associated with narrowing of the palpebral fissure on attempted adduction.

May be bilateral.

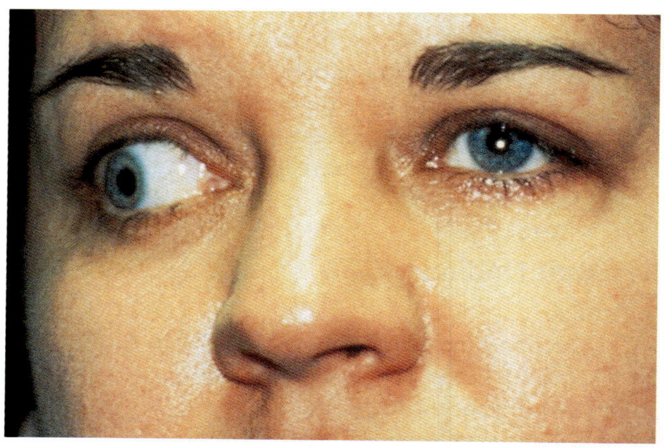

FIGURE 6.27. Duane syndrome type II. On right gaze, the LE is unable to adduct past the midline. The left palpebral fissure narrows secondary to retraction of the globe.

Evaluation

A clinical diagnosis.

Treatment

Usually none.

Aberrant Regeneration

Summary

Regeneration of the third nerve may result in abnormal innervation to any combination of the muscles innervated by the oculomotor nerve.

Etiology

Primary (no preceding third-nerve palsy) or secondary (following third-nerve palsy) phenomenon.
Does not occur with ischemic third-nerve palsies.

Signs and Symptoms

Elevation of the eyelid with eye elevation or adduction.
Pupil constriction on adduction, elevation, or depression.
Any combination of inappropriate third-nerve innervated extraocular muscle firing (e.g., adduction during attempted elevation).
Neuroimaging recommended for secondary aberrant regeneration of third nerve (MRI to rule out cavernous meningioma or intracavernous aneurysm).

Supranuclear Motility Disturbances

Saccades

Saccades are fast movements that allow corrective movements to maintain the object of regard on the fovea and bring the target rapidly onto the fovea. Saccades may be abnormally slow, inaccurate, or absent.

Signs and Symptoms

- Saccadic paresis (with intact infranuclear pathway).
  Bilateral lesion causes global saccadic palsy.
  Unilateral frontal lesions.
  Transient ipsilateral tonic deviation as a result of unopposed contralateral frontal lobe input.
  Decreased anticipatory saccades.
  Decreased saccades to remembered targets.
  Acute saccadic paresis.
- Inappropriate saccadic intrusions (ocular flutter and opsoclonus).
  Rapid, involuntary repetitive saccadic movements.
  Conjugate movements.
  Usually persist in sleep.
  Horizontal movements: flutter.
  Multivectorial: opsoclonus.
- Saccades may be abnormally slow or inaccurate (overshoot, undershoot).

Etiology

Slowed saccades:

- Any paretic process from muscle to brain.
  Peripheral nerve.
  Muscle.
  NMJ.
  Interneurons.
  Myopathy.
- Central lesions.
  Olivopontocerebellar atrophy and spinocerebellar degeneration.
  Huntington chorea.
  Wilson disease.
  Ataxia telangiectasia.
  PSP.
  Lipidoses.
  Parkinson disease (advanced cases).
  Alzheimer disease.
  Acquired immunodeficiency syndrome dementia.
  INO.
  Drugs (e.g., phenytoin [Dilantin], phenobarbital).
  Drowsy or inattentive state.
- Inaccurate saccades.
  Dysmetria (hypermetria or hypometria).
  Cerebellar or cerebral hemispheric disease.
  Wallenberg syndrome (PICA occlusion).
  After paretic adaptive phenomenon.
- Delayed saccades (increased latency).
  Congenital apraxia.
  Acquired apraxia.
  Huntington disease.
  Parkinson disease.
  Alzheimer disease.

Inappropriate saccades (saccadic intrusions):

- Square-wave jerks: eyes off target followed after 200 milliseconds by corrective saccade.
  Nonspecific (may be seen in normal individuals).
  Nonspecific dementias.
  Cerebellar atrophies.
  PSP.
  Huntington disease.
  Associated with strabismus.
  Nonspecific cerebral lesions.
  Nonspecific catechol depletion.
  Schizophrenia.
- Macrosquare-wave jerks.
  Brainstem or cerebellar disease.
  Friedreich ataxia.
  MS.
  Olivopontocerebellar atrophy.
- Ocular flutter (horizontal high-frequency, low-amplitude oscillations) and opsoclonus (conjugate, involuntary, large-amplitude saccades in all directions).
  Congenital myoclonic encephalopathy.
  Paraneoplastic (e.g., occult neuroblastoma).

Postinfectious or viral encephalitis.
Drugs (e.g., lithium, chlordecone, thallium).
Brainstem glioma.
Brainstem cerebrovascular accident (CVA).
Hydrocephalus.
Brainstem trauma.
Thalamic hemorrhage.

Smooth Pursuit

The smooth pursuit pathway allows tracking of an object in space. It may be abnormally slow or absent.

Signs and Symptoms in Smooth Pursuit Abnormality

Cogwheel "saccadic" pursuit: nonspecific.
Balint syndrome:
- Inability to look on command.
- Inability to find and group objects: "optic ataxia."
- Simultagnosia.
- Only see one object at a time.
- Cannot see the "big picture."
- Intact random and vestibular movements.

Etiology of Smooth Pursuit Defect

Drugs impairing pursuit:
- Benzodiazepines.
- Dilantin.
- Alcohol.
- Barbiturates.

Neurodegenerative diseases:
- PSP.
- Parkinson disease.
- Huntington chorea.
- Bilateral extensive parietooccipital disease.
- Dementia.
- Chiari malformation.
- Cerebellar degeneration.

Internuclear Ophthalmoplegia

Summary

The pons contains the final common pathway for horizontal saccades and pursuit. Lesions may disturb the parapontine reticular formation (PPRF) or the sixth-nerve nucleus and thus cause abnormalities in horizontal saccades and pursuit. Interneurons from the sixth-nerve nucleus travel to the contralateral MLF and may be damaged, resulting in an INO (Figure 6.28).

Clinical clues to PPRF lesions:
Causes unilateral horizontal gaze palsy.
If rostral lesion, can spare vestibuloocular reflex.
In acute lesions, eyes may deviate contralaterally.

Signs and Symptoms

Named for side of MLF lesion (side of adduction weakness).

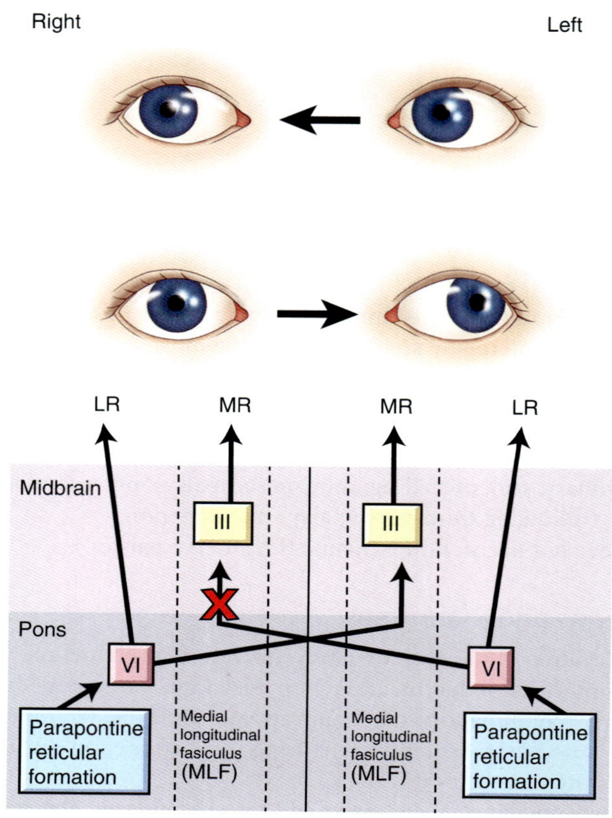

FIGURE 6.28. Internuclear ophthalmoplegia. A lesion in the right medial longitudinal fasciculus (MLF) interrupts the interneuron connection from the abducens nucleus (VI) to the oculomotor nucleus (III) resulting in the inability to adduct the RE on left gaze. (PPRF, parapontine reticular formation)

May have complete inability to adduct.
May have mild adduction lag.
May have abducting nystagmus in contralateral eye.
If midbrain lesion:
- More rostral disease.
- Called *Cogan's anterior INO.*
- Convergence involved (third-nerve nuclei).

If more caudal lesion may spare convergence.
May have an associated skew deviation.

Etiology

In a young adult, usually demyelinating disease.
In an older patient, usually a CVA.
Consider pseudo-INO of myasthenia.
Brainstem neoplasm.
Carcinomatous meningitis.
Paraneoplastic effect.
Chiari malformation.
Hydrocephalus.
Degenerative disease.
Drugs:
- Phenothiazines.
- Tricyclics.

Narcotics.
Lithium.
Barbiturates.
Propranolol.

Brainstem infarct.
Infectious (e.g., encephalitis, meningoencephalitis).
Metabolic:

Wernicke syndrome.
Pernicious anemia.
Hepatic encephalopathy.
Maple syrup urine disease.
Abetalipoproteinemia.
Fabry disease.

Postirradiation demyelination.
Brainstem or subdural hemorrhage.
Trauma.

Differential Diagnosis

Differential diagnosis of bilateral INO includes the following:

Intra-axial lesion.
Demyelination (MS).
Vascular.
Ischemic brainstem event.
Intraventricular extension of subarachnoid hemorrhage.
Brainstem AVM.
Basilar artery aneurysm.
Head trauma.
Neoplastic (e.g., brainstem glioma).
Infection (e.g., meningitis, syphilis, TB).
Metabolic or toxic (e.g., vitamin B_{12} deficiency, Wernicke syndrome).
Pseudo-INO of myasthenia gravis.
Extra-axial hematoma, aneurysm.
Obstructive hydrocephalus, Chiari malformation.
Spinocerebellar heredodegenerative disease.

Signs and Symptoms

Signs and symptoms of the "one and a half syndrome":

A combined lesion of PPRF or sixth-nerve nucleus and an INO (MLF lesion) on one side.
PPRF or sixth nerve nucleus lesion causes ipsilateral horizontal gaze palsy. Only contralateral CN VI is unaffected; therefore, only horizontal movement remaining is abduction of the contralateral eye.

Etiology

Brainstem ischemia.
MS.
Tumors (e.g., metastatic, malignant glioma).
Pontine hemorrhage.
Trauma.

Paralytic Pontine Exotropia

Unopposed drive from intact PPRF in a "one and a half syndrome" causes an exotropia, in addition to the findings for the "one and a half syndrome."

Bilateral Pontine Lesions

Signs and Symptoms

May abolish all horizontal movements.
Chronic lesions may spare reflexive movements.
Discrete lesions may cause selective saccadic loss.
May impair vertical movements.

Midbrain Lesions

Signs

Vertical gaze palsy (Figure 6.29).
Involvement of rostral interstitial nucleus of the MLF (riMLF) midbrain-thalamic junction.

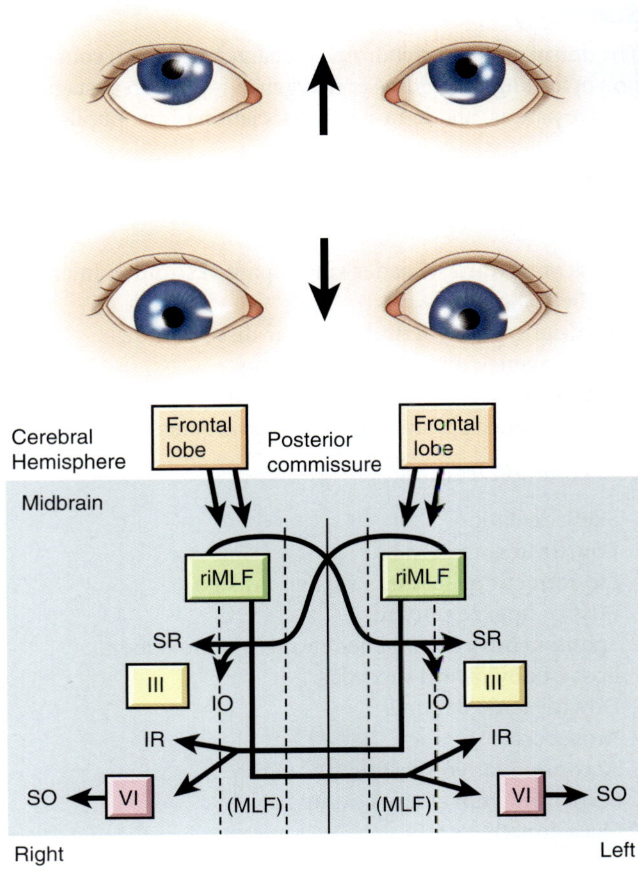

FIGURE 6.29. Control of vertical gaze is initiated by the frontal lobes through the rostral interstitial nucleus of the medial longitudinal fasciculus (riMLF).

Etiology

CVA.
Bilateral lesions of dorsomedial red nucleus.
Huntington disease.
PSP.
Thalamic bleed.
Diffuse degenerative processes.
PSP.
Infarct (basal ganglia, midbrain).
Cortical basal degeneration.
Whipple disease.
Parkinson disease (may limit upgaze).
Multiple sclerosis.
Fisher syndrome.
Syphilis.
Brucellosis.
Tetanus.
Encephalitis.
Neurofibromatosis.
Tuberculoma
Trauma (include neurosurgery).

Parinaud's Dorsal Midbrain Syndrome

Summary

The dorsal midbrain syndrome is characterized by a constellation of findings, including convergence-retraction nystagmus, upgaze paresis, and light-near dissociation of the pupils.

Signs and Symptoms

Common features:

- Loss of upward saccades (may spare vestibuloocular and Bell's).
- Mydriatic pupils with light-near dissociation.
- Convergence retraction nystagmus.
- Papilledema and/or obstructive hydrocephalus.
- Convergence spasm or paresis (divergence paralysis).

Less common features:

- Skew deviation.
- Fourth-nerve palsy.
- Lid retraction (Collier's tucked lid sign).
- Loss of upgaze pursuit.
- Spontaneous convergence retraction movements.
- Loss of downward saccades.
- Downbeat nystagmus.
- Anisocoria.
- Accommodative spasm with upgaze.
- Serpentine movements on upgaze.
- Occasionally, ptosis.

Infrequent features:

- Peduncular hallucinosis: vivid colored imagery.
- Precocious puberty.
- Pseudoabducens palsy.
- "Setting sun sign in infant" (hydrocephalus).
- "A" or "V" pattern exotropia.
- Square-wave jerks.

Etiology

Pineal gland tumors.
Germinoma (classically in adolescent boys).
Teratoma.
Glioma.
Metastasis.
Hydrocephalus (aqueductal stenosis usually).
May be only or presenting sign of shunt malfunction.
Infiltrating tumors of the third ventricle.
Pituitary apoplexy.
Metabolic.
- Niemann-Pick disease.
- Gaucher disease.
- Tay-Sachs disease.
- Maple syrup urine disease.
- Wilson disease.
- Kernicterus.

Neurosyphilis and other encephalitis.
Whipple disease.
TB.
Drugs.
- Barbiturates.
- Carbamazepine.
- Neuroleptics.

Demyelination.
Trauma (including neurosurgical).
Vascular (midbrain or thalamic).
- Stroke (infarct or bleed).
- AVM.
- Giant aneurysm.
- Hypoxia.

Degenerative (vertical gaze palsy).
- PSP.
- Huntington disease.
- Cortical basal degeneration.
- Diffuse Lewy body disease.
- After jejunal-ileal bypass for obesity.
- Shunt malfunction (early sign even with normal MRI).
- Benign transient form in childhood.

Evaluation

MRI of dorsal midbrain.
Exclude other causes for dorsal midbrain syndrome.

Facial Nerve Palsy

Anatomy

Bilateral innervation to the brow and orbicularis muscle and contralateral innervation to the lower two thirds of the face.

Etiology

Supranuclear syndrome:
- Frontal cortex lesion may result in upper extremity, hand, or tongue weakness on the contralateral side.

Nuclear or cerebellopontine angle syndrome: Causes include demyelination, neoplastic (e.g., acoustic neuroma), infarct, bleed.

Signs and Symptoms

- Nuclear or cerebellopontine angle.
  - Total ipsilateral facial weakness.
  - Decreased tearing (nervus intermedius).
  - Hyperacusis (nerve to stapedius).
  - Decreased taste to anterior two third of the tongue (chorda tympani).
  - Thus, nuclear syndromes are defined by the "company they keep": Foville syndrome (e.g., cranial neuropathies of nerves V, VI, and VIII; Horner syndrome); Millard-Gubler syndrome (nerve VI, gaze palsy, contralateral hemiparesis).
- Gradenigo syndrome (petrositis): due to mastoiditis or otitis media. Cranial neuropathy, nerves V (facial pain), VI, and VII.
- Geniculate ganglionitis: Ramsay Hunt syndrome (herpes zoster oticus).
- Greater superficial petrosal nerve: Causes include nasopharyngeal cancer, schwannoma, inflammation (e.g., herpes zoster, petrositis, sphenoid sinus disease).

Evaluation

Nonisolated:
- MRI of seventh nerve.
- Further evaluation based on history and physical examination.

Isolated:
- Most commonly idiopathic Bell palsy.
- Consider MRI.

Treatment

Ocular lubrication.
Lateral tarsorrhaphy if exposure keratopathy.
Gold weight placement in the upper eyelid.
Corticosteroids.

Nystagmus

Summary

Nystagmus is a rhythmic abnormal eye movement. It may be unilateral, bilateral, or asymmetric. It may be pendular (equal amplitude and frequency in each direction) or jerk (fast and slow phases). It may be present in primary gaze or appear in particular gaze positions, or present as a combination of these. It may be congenital or acquired.

Physiologic Forms

End point or end gaze.
OKN.
Caloric testing of vestibuloocular reflex.
Rotational.

Localizing Forms

INO

Clinical features:
- Abduction nystagmus (contralateral to lesion).
- Adduction weakness ipsilateral to lesion.

Localization to ipsilateral MLF.

Etiology

Young person: MS.
Older person: stroke.
Myasthenia can cause pseudo-INO.
Other lesions of brainstem (e.g., neoplasm).

Downbeat Nystagmus

Clinical Features

Fast phase down.
Worse in downgaze.

Etiology

Cervicomedullary junction lesions (e.g., spinocerebellar degeneration, hydrocephalus, Chiari malformation).
Alcohol related (e.g., cerebellar degeneration, thiamine deficiency, magnesium deficiency, vitamin B_{12} deficiency).
Brainstem or cerebellar stroke or encephalitis demyelinating disease.
Medicines and toxins (e.g., lithium, phenytoin, carbamazepine, toluene abuse).
Acquired and familial cerebellar disease.
Head trauma.
Paraneoplastic.
Lower motor neuron syndromes as described below as well as idiopathic "Bell's Palsy".

Congenital Downbeat Nystagmus

Transient finding in normal newborns.

Clinical Features

Usually better in upgaze and worse in downgaze.
Present in primary position.

Upbeat Nystagmus

Ophthalmic Findings

Fast phase up.

Etiology

Vermis of cerebellum.
Intrinsic brainstem.

- Pontomesencephalic or pontomedullary.
- Infiltrating tumors of fourth ventricle.
- Demyelination.
- Medulla (infarct or tumor).

See-Saw Nystagmus

Ophthalmic Findings

Elevation and intorsion in one eye (one half-cycle).
Synchronous depression and extorsion in other eye.

Etiology

Most suprasellar or parasellar mass:
- Rostral brainstem (midbrain/thalamic).
- Interstitial nucleus of Cajal lesion.
- Trauma.
- Neoplasia.
- Congenital (septooptic dysplasia).
- Brainstem CVA.
- Demyelination.
- Syringobulbia, syringomyelia (rare).
- Chiari malformation.

Convergence-Retraction Nystagmus

Ophthalmic Findings

Asynchronous (nystagmoid movement vs. nystagmus).
Disjunctive, convergent cocontraction saccades.
Usually horizontal.
Seen with dorsal midbrain syndrome findings.

Etiology

Dorsal midbrain at level of posterior commissure.

Age in years and cause:
- Age 0: infant aqueductal stenosis.
- Age 10: pinealoma.
- Age 20: trauma.
- Age 30: brainstem AVM.
- Age 40: MS.
- Age 50: basilar artery stroke.

Periodic Alternating Nystagmus

Ophthalmic Findings

Sixty- to ninety-second beats one way and then changes direction.
Present in primary position; therefore must observe all horizontal nystagmus for reversal of nystagmus.
Uniplanar (does not change horizontal nature in upgaze or downgaze).

Etiology

Medulla and craniocervical:
- Congenital.
- Brainstem stroke or trauma.
- MS.
- Cerebellar or spinocerebellar degeneration (Friedreich ataxia).
- Craniocervical disease (e.g., Chiari malformation).
- Vestibular nuclei or vestibulocerebellum.
- Neurosyphilis affecting the cerebellum.
- Cerebellar tumor, abscess, or cyst.

Torsional Nystagmus

Ophthalmic Findings

Rotary nystagmus.
May have horizontal or vertical component.

Etiology

Purely torsional suggests CNS disease.
- Lateral medulla syndrome.
- Mesodiencephalic junction.
  - Syringobulbia or syringomyelia.
  - Chiari malformation.
  - Vascular anomalies.
  - MS.
  - Possible paraneoplastic syndrome.
- Pons lesion.

Congenital Nystagmus (Less Than 3 Months Old)

Summary

Congenital nystagmus may be divided into *sensory* congenital nystagmus and *motor* nystagmus. Although this is a somewhat arbitrary distinction, we believe it is useful for clinical decision making.

Etiology

Sensory afferent disease is more common (10:1 vs. "motor" form), and all infants with congenital nystagmus should be evaluated for visual loss.
- Albinism.
- Aniridia.
- Achromatopsia.
- Atrophic or hypoplastic optic nerve.
- Anterior segment disease (cataract, cornea, coloboma).
- Leber congenital amaurosis.
- Retinal abnormalities (e.g., cone dystrophies [blue cone monochromat, congenital stationary night blindness], Norrie disease, familial exudative vitreoretinopathy, primary foveal hypoplasia).
- Systemic infections (e.g., syphilis).
- Motor nystagmus occurs when there is no sensory loss.

Signs and Symptoms

Does not usually develop before 10 weeks of age.
- Usually diagnosed in infancy.
- May not present until first few months of life.

Sensory nystagmus is not due to *cortical* visual loss.
In general, vision in the presence of sensory nystagmus is 20/200 or worse.

Ophthalmic Findings

Mnemonic: "CONGENITAL":
Convergence and eye closure dampens.
Oscillopsia absent.
Null zone that is present increases foveation time, which results in increased acuity.
Gaze position does not change *horizontal* direction of nystagmus (i.e., nystagmus remains uniplanar, horizontal in upgaze and downgaze).
Equal amplitude and frequency in each eye.
Near acuity is good (convergence dampens nystagmus).
Inversion of optokinetic response (OKN).
Turning of the head to achieve null point.
Abolished in sleep, usually.
Latent (occlusion) nystagmus occurs.

Evaluation

Evaluation of nystagmus and normal fundus in infants:
- Neuroimaging (e.g., MRI scan of head).
- ERG: scotopic and photopic if imaging is negative.
- Laboratory tests (if systemic indications).
  - Phytanic acid.
  - Very long chain fatty acids.
- Consider biopsy of conjunctiva (if systemic indications) for neuronal ceroid lipofuscinosis.

Bruns Nystagmus

Ophthalmic Findings

Large amplitude and low frequency, looking toward lesion.
High frequency and low amplitude, away from lesion.

Etiology

Cerebellopontine angle (tumors).
Most commonly acoustic neuroma.

Spasmus Nutans

Summary

Spasmus nutans is an acquired dissociated nystagmus of childhood that is usually benign but may be associated with optic glioma. The nystagmus usually spontaneously resolves by age 5 years.

Ophthalmic Findings

Asymmetric if bilateral (may be very variable).
May be strictly unilateral.
Fine "shimmering" horizontal movement.
May be rotary or vertical.
Dissociated.
Small amplitude and high frequency.
May precede head nodding.
Constant or intermittent.

Epidemiology

Age of onset: 4 to 14 months (first year of life).
Disappears by age 5 years usually.

Etiology

Usually self-limited and benign.
May be mimicked by glioma or third-ventricle tumor.

Evaluation

Consider MRI scan of head with attention to anterior visual pathway.

Acquired Binocular Pendular Nystagmus

Ophthalmic Findings

Equal amplitude in both directions (pendular).
Horizontal or vertical.

Etiology

Disorders of myelin.
Oculopalatal myoclonus.
Mitochondrial cytopathy.
Lesions of chiasm.
Brainstem or cerebellum stroke or tumor.
Whipple disease.

Evaluation

Evaluate congenital nystagmus for visual loss.
Exclude medicines and toxins as causes.
Neuroimaging for unexplained acquired nystagmus.
Direct imaging to selected sites based on specific form of nystagmus.

PUPIL ABNORMALITIES

Anatomy of Pupillomotor Pathway

Afferent Loop

See Figure 6.30.

Retinal nerve fiber layer and retinal ganglion cells.
Optic nerve axons.
Optic chiasm.
Optic tract.
Fibers to the brachium of superior colliculus.
Dorsal midbrain synapse in pretectal nuclei.
Edinger-Westphal nuclei.

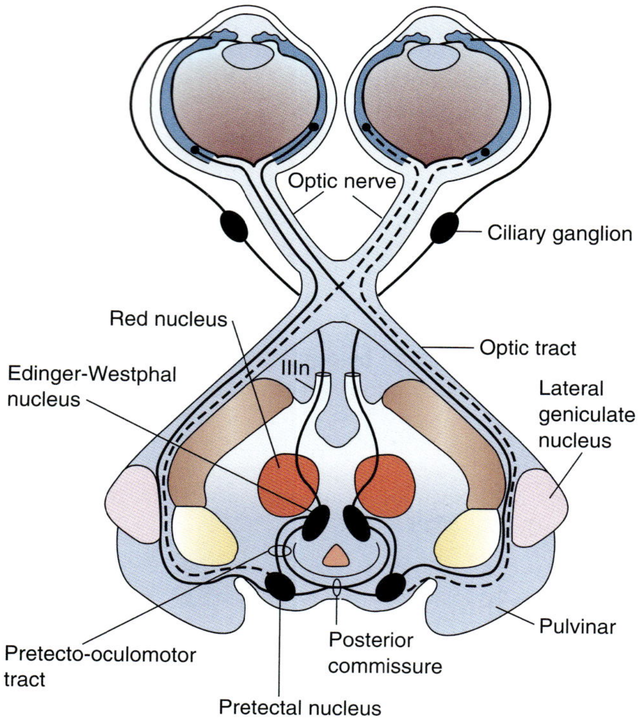

FIGURE 6.30. Diagram of the path of the pupillary light reflex. (Reproduced from Walsh FB, Hoyt WF. *Clinical neuro-ophthalmology*, 3rd ed., vol. 1. Baltimore, MD: Williams & Wilkins, 1969, with permission.)

Efferent Loop of Parasympathetic Pathway

See Figure 6.30.

Third cranial nerve.
Pupil fibers lie superior in subarachnoid space.

Efferent Loop of Sympathetic Pathway

See Figure 6.31.
Three neuron arc:

First-order neuron (central neuron): hypothalamus to level of C8 to T2 in the spinal cord (ciliospinal center of Budge).
Second-order neuron (preganglionic intermediate): travels up (without synapse) through paraspinal ganglia to synapse in the superior cervical ganglion (angle of the jaw).
Third-order neuron (postganglionic): travels with carotid artery to the cavernous sinus; within the substance of sinus some fibers join briefly with the sixth nerve and then proceed onto the V_1 (ophthalmic branch) nasociliary branch to the iris dilator via long posterior ciliary nerves.

Afferent Pupil Defect (or Marcus Gunn Pupil)

Testing (Swinging Flashlight Test)

- Low background illumination.
- A patient fixating distant target (relax accommodation).
- Use a bright light source (e.g., indirect head lamp or Fenhoff transilluminator).
- Look from below, and instruct the patient not to look directly at light source.
- Move light briskly and rhythmically from eye to eye for fast count of 3 seconds with equal time to each eye.
- Test multiple times.
- Observe and record pupil response to direct, consensual, and direct response after swinging flashlight from contralateral eye (swinging flashlight test).
- If strabismus is present, direct light on pupil axis.

Ophthalmic Findings

- Normal response: pupil constriction ipsilateral (direct) and contralateral (consensual).
- Abnormal response on swinging flashlight test:
  Type I: immediate pupil dilation, 4+ APD.
  Type II: slower but definite dilation, 3+ APD.
  Type III: initially no change, then dilation, 1 to 2+ APD.
  Type IV: initial constriction but then escapes to a larger size more rapidly than fellow eye, trace APD.
  Might be better to quantitate RAPD with neutral density filters.

Etiology

Optic nerve disease.
Large amount of retinal disease.
Optic tract lesion (contralateral APD to lesion).
Rarely amblyopia.
Rarely vitreous hemorrhage (?).
May occur contralateral to pretectal lesion without visual loss.

Evaluation

Look for optic neuropathy or retinal disease.
Unexplained APD is evidence for an optic neuropathy.
Evaluation should proceed for an optic neuropathy.

Anisocoria

See Figure 6.32.

Evaluation

Determine pupillary light reaction.

Differential Diagnosis

Differential diagnosis of normal light reaction:

Physiologic.
Horner syndrome.
Sympathetic overaction (e.g., pharmacologic).

Physiologic Anisocoria

Occurs in about 20% of normal individuals.
Lid position normal (no ptosis).

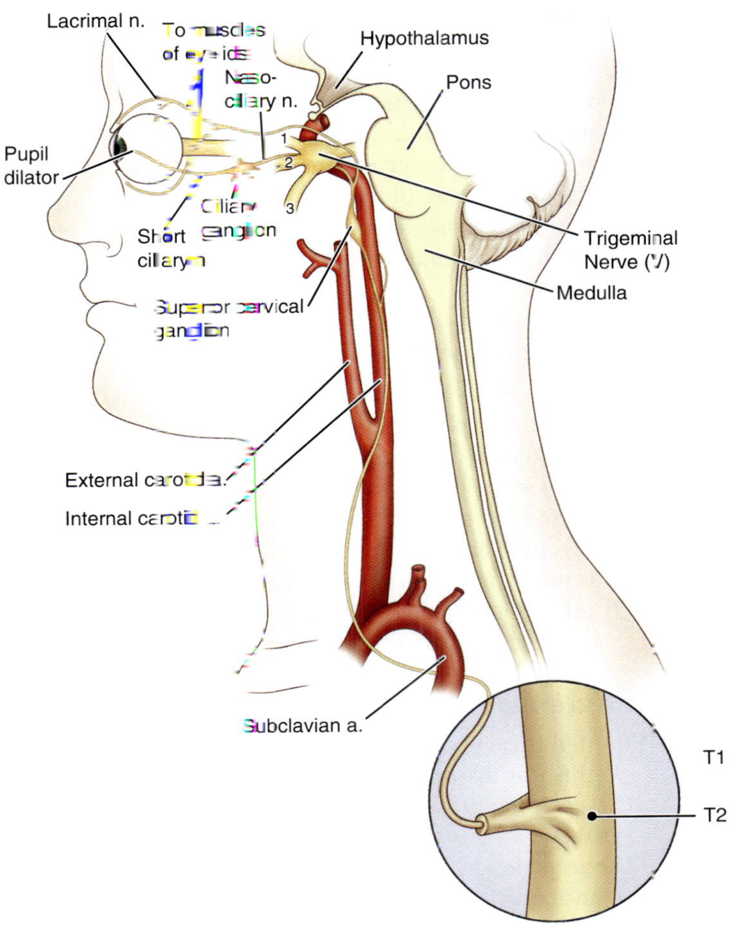

FIGURE 6.31. Sympathetic pathway. The first-order neuron travels from the hypothalamus to vertebrae C8 to T1, synapsing with the second-order neuron continuing to the superior cervical ganglion. The third-order neuron continues through the ciliary ganglion (without synapsing) to the pupillary dilator.

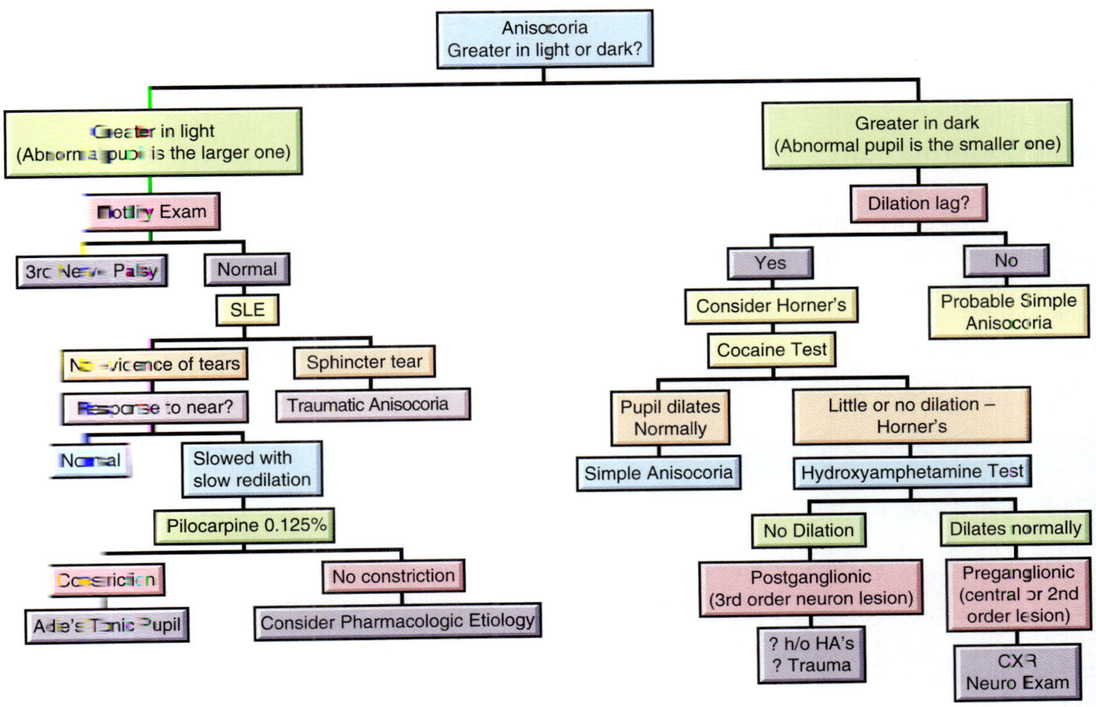

FIGURE 6.32. Evaluation of anisocoria.

Table 6.5

Etiology of Horner syndrome by location

Author	No. of cases	Central	Intermediate	Postganglionic
Grimson (1979)	120	Rare	50%	33%
Maloney (1980)	450	13%	43%	44%
Giles (1958)	216	10%	—	—
Keane (1979)	100	63%	25%	12%

No dilation lag.
Pupil size may vary from day to day.
Equal anisocoria in light and dark.
Usually less than 1 mm anisocoria.
Result of topical cocaine or apraclonidine testing negative.

Horner Syndrome

Signs and Symptoms

Normal light and near reaction.
Mild ptosis (usually <2 mm).
Moderate ipsilateral miosis.
Apparent enophthalmos.
Lower lid "upside-down ptosis" or "reverse ptosis."
Anhidrosis of face and neck.
Iris heterochromia (usually congenital Horner syndrome).

Etiology

See Table 6.5.

Pharmacologic Confirmation

- Topical cocaine:
  Inhibits reuptake of norepinephrine.
  Failure or diminished reaction of ipsilateral pupil to dilate: Horner syndrome.
- Topical apraclonidine.
  Alpha 1 and alpha 2 effects.
  Denervation supersensivity in Horner syndrome.
  Smaller pupil (Horner syndrome) dilates and larger normal pupil constricts.
  Reversal of anisocoria = end point (confirms but does not localize Horner syndrome).
  Pharmacologic localization of Horner syndrome.
  Hydroxyamphetamine (Paredrine 1%).
  Stimulates release of norepinephrine.
  Distinguishes preganglionic from postganglionic lesion.
  If no dilation, implies postganglionic lesion.
  See Table 6.6.

Evaluation and Management

- Central: MRI of central neuron (i.e., hypothalamus to C-8 to T-2 level of spinal cord).
- Preganglionic intermediate: imaging of T-2 level of spinal cord to superior cervical ganglion, including apex of the lung and the neck (exclude dissection of carotid artery).
- Postganglionic:
  If isolated, no further evaluation is usually needed.
  If other signs, imaging from superior cervical ganglion to orbit (consider internal carotid artery).

Differential Diagnosis

Poor light reaction and normal near reaction:
Light-near dissociation of the pupils.
Severe afferent pathway disease.
Diabetic autonomic neuropathy.
Pretectal lesion (Parinaud, sylvian aqueduct syndromes).
Chronic alcoholism.
Encephalitis.
Argyll-Robertson pupils (associated with syphilis).
MS.
Neurodegenerative disease.
Poor light and near reaction:
Tonic pupil.
Third-nerve palsy.
Iris sphincter damage.
Pharmacologic pupil.

Adie's Tonic Pupil

Summary

A tonic pupil has a poor light reaction and a tonic near reaction.

Table 6.6

Response to pharmacologic testing

Topical drop	Preganglionic Horner syndrome (first- or second-order Horner syndrome)	Postganglionic Horner syndrome (third-order Horner syndrome)	Normal pupil
Cocaine	No dilation	No dilation	Dilation
Hydroxyamphetamine	Dilation	No dilation	Dilation
Apraclonidine	Dilation	Dilation	Constriction

Epidemiology

Usually, young women (70%).
Age, 20 to 40 years; mean age, 32 years.
Incidence: 4.7 per 100,000 population.
Ten to twenty percent of cases are bilateral.

Signs and Symptoms

Twenty percent of cases are asymptomatic.
"Blurry vision" attributable to accommodative paresis.
Difficulty reading.
Photophobia and glare.
May have ciliary spasm or brow ache with near work.
Accommodative induced astigmatism.

Ophthalmic Findings

Slit-lamp findings:
- Sector paresis of sphincter (regional palsy) "tadpole pupil."
- Vermiform movements (hippus in uninvolved iris).

Pupil findings:
- Early in disease, pupil is dilated.
- Poor tonic constriction to light and near.
- Slow redilation after accommodation.
- Irregular dilated pupil.
- May become miotic over time ("little old Adie's").

Systemic Findings

Decreased deep tendon reflexes.
Finding of normal reflexes does not exclude the diagnosis.

Evaluation

A clinical diagnosis.
Pharmacologic testing with low-dose pilocarpine (1/8%).
- Cholinergic denervation supersensitivity (80%).
- Pilocarpine 1/8% constricts Adie's tonic pupil.
- Normal pupil does not constrict to low-dose pilocarpine.

Differential Diagnosis

Infectious (e.g., syphilis, zoster, measles, chickenpox).
Trauma (e.g., surgery, including cataract surgery).
Tumors (e.g., orbit, choroid, paraneoplastic).
Iatrogenic (e.g., retinal laser photocoagulation, retrobulbar alcohol, cryotherapy).
Diabetes and other neuropathies.
GCA (rare).
Migraine.
Inflammatory (e.g., sarcoid).
Amyloid.
Dysautonomias (e.g., Riley Day, Shy-Drager syndromes), chronic alcoholism.
Fisher variant of Guillain-Barré syndrome.
Hereditary motor sensory neuropathy types 1 and 2.
Pharmacologic blockade.

Management

- Consider ESR if indicated in elderly patients (rare).
- Perform syphilis serologic testing (e.g., MHA-TP and RPR) for the following unexplained pupil abnormalities:
  Any irregular bilateral miotic pupils.
  Light-near dissociation without explanation.
  Bilateral tonic pupil.

Treatment

Glare treatment: sunglasses, weak pilocarpine (0.05%).
Ciliary spasms: weak anticholinergic.
Accommodation paresis: bifocals (may be unequal adds).
Most require *no* treatment.

Disease Course

Pupil and light reaction usually do not recover.
Pupil may get smaller with time.
Most symptoms resolve spontaneously.
May remain hyporeflexic.
Up to 4% of cases per year become bilateral.

Third-Nerve Palsy

In the neurologic intensive care setting, an isolated dilated pupil is an ominous sign of third-nerve dysfunction (e.g., uncal herniation). In the outpatient setting, however, an isolated dilated pupil without ptosis or motility disturbance is almost never a third-nerve palsy. The evaluation of the dilated pupil in isolation should exclude more common causes of mydriasis, including the tonic pupil, pharmacologic dilation, and iris damage. Third-nerve palsy is discussed in more detail in a separate section.

Structural iris changes may also result in anisocoria; usually, a careful history and slit-lamp examination are all that is required for the diagnosis.

Etiology

Sphincter tear.
Old transillumination defects.
Evidence for old or new inflammation (e.g., keratic precipitates, anterior chamber cell and flare, iris nodules).
Posterior synechiae.
Previous intraocular surgery.
Iris ischemia (e.g., angle-closure glaucoma).
Iris atrophy.

Pharmacologic Dilation

Summary

Pharmacologic dilation can usually be diagnosed based on the history and examination. Pharmacologic confirmation with topical pilocarpine 1% can confirm the diagnosis.

Demographics

Be wary of patients with access to dilating drops (health care personnel, recent emergency room visits).

Ophthalmic Findings

Middilated to widely dilated, fixed pupil.
Unilateral conjunctival blanching (if using neosynephrine).

Evaluation

Pupils dilated with a pharmacologic agent do not constrict to pilocarpine 1%.

Etiology

Inadvertent exposure to topical mydriatics (e.g., tropicamide, Cyclogyl, atropine), scopolamine patches.
Pupil can also be pharmacologically constricted (e.g., pesticides, pilocarpine).
Factitious intentional use of mydriatics.
Plants (e.g., moonflower, jimsonweed).

SYSTEMIC DISEASES

Multiple Sclerosis

MS refers to a demyelinating disease causing multiple CNS lesions separated in time and space.

Epidemiology

- Northern latitudes: increased risk.
- Genetic: slight increase in first-degree relatives.
- Concordance rate of 25% for monozygotic twins.
- Any age; most patients are 20 to 40 years old.
- Male-to-female ratio, 2 to 1.
- White patients more often than black patients.

Neuro-ophthalmologic Features

- Afferent disease:
  Optic neuritis is most common.
  May affect chiasm, tract, and retrochiasmal pathways.
- Efferent disease:
  INO.
  Wall-eyed, bilateral INO (WEBINO).
  One-and-a-half syndrome.
  Skew deviation.
- Nystagmus:
  Upbeat.
  Downbeat.
  Acquired pendular.
  Elliptical or torsional.
  Rebound.
  Periodic alternating.
  Gaze evoked.
  Central vestibular.
- Cerebellar dysfunction (e.g., dysmetria).
- Saccadic abnormalities.
  Square-wave jerks.
  Flutter.
  Myoclonus.
  Opsoclonus.
  Prolonged latency.
  Inaccuracy and decreased velocity.
- Rarely cranial neuropathy.

Diagnostic Criteria

Attack: neurologic symptom lasting more than 24 hours.
Clinical evidence of lesion: signs on neurologic examination.
Paraclinical evidence of lesion: CNS lesion not producing neurologic signs (e.g., MRI, CT, electrophysiology, urologic testing).
Laboratory support (e.g., oligoclonal bands, increased immunoglobulin G in CSF).
Separate lesion (cannot be explained on a single lesion).

Types of MS:

- Clinically definite MS:
  Two attacks (separated by remission).
  Involving different parts of CNS separated by 1 month and one of the following:
  Evidence for two anatomic sites by examination.
  One clinical lesion and one historical.
  One clinical and paraclinical for another ("laboratory-supported [LS]") lesion.
- Clinically probable MS:
  History of one attack and two anatomic lesions.
  History of two attacks and one anatomic lesion.
  One attack and two clinical, separate lesions.
  One attack, one clinical lesion, and a second paraclinical lesion.
- Possible MS:
  Single attack from a single lesion.
  Multiple attacks with normal examination.
  Modifiers: LS definite or probable MS (paraclinical) CSF oligoclonal bands *plus*.
  Two attacks separated by remission.
  Or one attack and clinical evidence for two lesions.
  Or one attack and one clinical lesion and paraclinical.

Treatment

There is no definitive treatment for MS. The following are used:

- Steroids and other immunosuppression.
- Immunomodulatory therapy (e.g., interferon β_1, copolymer I [analog of myelin basic protein]).
- Other unproven therapies (e.g., calcium blockers, hyperbaric O_2, and plasmapheresis).

References

Beck RW, Trobe JD. What we have learned from the optic neuritis treatment trial. *Ophthalmology* 1995;102:1504–1508.

Wikstrom J, Poser S, Ritter G. Optic neuritis as an initial symptom in multiple sclerosis. *Acta Neurol Scand* 1980;61:178–185.

Thyroid Eye Disease

Epidemiology

Twenty to fifty percent of hyperthyroid patients develop TED.
Can occur with Hashimoto thyroiditis.
Can occur in any thyroid state.
Twenty to forty percent of patients have TED at systemic diagnosis.
Most patients develop TED within 18 months of systemic diagnosis.
Age, 30 to 40 years (any age).
Female-to-male ratio 4:1 to 7:1.

Signs and Symptoms

Systemic signs
- Nervous, irritability, weakness, weight loss.
- Palpitations, tremor, sweating, tachycardia.
- Dyspnea, diarrhea, heat intolerance.
- Emotional lability, insomnia.
- Increased appetite.
- Goiter, thyroid bruit, or thrill.

Skin changes
- Dermatopathy.
- Moist skin.
- Pretibial myxedema.
- Vitiligo.
- Hair loss, brittleness.

Ophthalmic Findings

Dysthyroid myopathy.
- Most common cause of diplopia in adults.
- Eyelid signs:
  - Lid retraction (stare).
  - Lid lag on downward gaze.
  - Inferior scleral show.
  - Decreased blink.
  - Lid edema ("jelly roll").

Conjunctival vessels over horizontal recti dilated.
Strabismus.
Proptosis.
- Most cases symmetric and bilateral (90%).
- If asymmetric by more than 7 mm, consider tumor.
- Most common cause of proptosis in adults.

Exposure keratopathy.
Optic neuropathy.

Evaluation

- Systemic thyroid control.
- Orbital imaging
  - CT findings.
    - Diffuse muscle enlargement.
    - Usually confined to muscle belly (tendon normal).
    - Muscle involvement: IRM > MRM > SRM > LRM.
- Possible indications for CT scan in TED:
  - Rule out tumor or pseudotumor or the orbit if diagnosis is unclear or atypical signs are present.
  - Preoperative decompression.
  - Before XRT for thyroid optic neuropathy or comfort.
  - Graves optic neuropathy (compression).
  - Probably not needed for routine cases.
  - Iodinated CT contrast might precipitate or worsen systemic thyroid disease.

Differential Diagnosis

Differential diagnosis of CT findings:
Arterialized orbital veins (e.g., cavernous sinus fistula).
Neoplastic (e.g., metastasis).
Secondary extension from paranasal sinuses.
Acute orbital myositis (e.g., pseudotumor).
Acromegaly.
Acute enlargement with systemic cardiac myositis.
Systemic inflammation (e.g., Wegener granulomatosis, systemic lupus erythematosus, vasculitis).
Trichinosis.

Treatment

Control thyroid status.
Observation.
Stop smoking (associated with worsening of TED).
Elevate head of bed.
Dark glasses.
Prednisone (1 mg/kg/day by mouth [PO] for 10 days with rapid taper).
- Tends to worsen edema (side effect of steroids).
- Not a good long-term therapy.
- Possible indications.
- Acute inflammatory TED.
- Optic neuropathy.
- Preoperatively.
- Before XRT.
- Recent (<3 months) soft tissue signs.
- Postoperative XRT or decompression.

Preradioactive Iodine Therapy

Short-course trial:
- Prednisone 80 mg/day.
- If no better after 1 week, stop.
- If stable for 1 month, taper 10 mg/month.
- Fifty percent of patients respond but then relapse with taper.
- Could use i.v. administration and higher doses.

Radiation Therapy

Conflicting evidence base
Probably not needed for mild disease
Low dose (differential effect of T cells?).

2,000 rads (well-tolerated dose).
Ten treatments over 2 weeks.
Low-dose steroids with XRT.
Day 7 through third posttherapy week.
Reduce inflammation.
Worst in second week of treatment.
Possible indications:
Optic neuropathy.
Primary therapy after failing steroid therapy.
Intolerable steroid side effects.
Patients who refuse steroid.
Poor surgical candidates.
"Comfort."
Short term.
Recent-onset soft tissue signs.
"Wet," "juicy" TED.

Exposure Keratopathy

Mild: topical drops, ointments; tape lids at bedtime.
Moderate: Consider tarsorrhaphy.
Beware of increased orbital volume.
May cause worse problems.
Severe: Consider decompression.

Lid Retraction

Sympatholytic drops (guanethidine).
Lid retraction.
Toxic to cornea.
Limited usefulness.
Consider lid surgery alone (reconstructive).
Only if stable.
May mask minimal proptosis (<22 mm).

Strabismus

Observe:
If single binocular vision.
In primary and reading position.
Patching.
Prisms if:
Less than 10 prism diopters.
Fairly comitant deviation.
Strabismus surgery (stable after 3 to 6 months).
Almost never resection.
Recession.
On adjustable suture.
Dissect adhesions.
Intraoperative forced ductions.
May require multiple surgeries.
Botulinum toxin not generally useful.

Orbital Decompression

Indications:
Optic neuropathy.
Unresponsive to steroids or XRT.
Emergent vision threatening.
Vision threatening corneal exposure.
Severe proptosis after conservative therapy fails.
Reconstructive (cosmetic).
May cause postoperative strabismus.
Multiple surgical approaches.
Preferred sequence of surgical procedures: orbital decompression, strabismus surgery, and then eyelid surgery.

Myasthenia Gravis

Summary

Myasthenia gravis is a disease of skeletal muscle acetylcholine (ACh) receptors that results in a neuromuscular transmission deficit and variable muscle weakness.

Etiology

Antibodies to ACh receptors (binding, blocking, modulating).
Rare medication-induced cases.
Uncommon congenital, neonatal, or childhood cases.
Seronegative muscle specific kinase positive cases.

Systemic Associations

Thymoma.
Thyroid disease.
Other autoimmune diseases (e.g., rheumatoid arthritis, systemic lupus erythematosus).

Demographics

Gender:
Ocular myasthenia (OM): ratio of men to women, 57:43.
Generalized myasthenia (GM): ratio of men to women, 41:59.
Both OM and GM: ratio of men to women, 43:57.
Age:
Mean age of onset for OM, 38 years; for GM, 33 years.
Usually less than 40 years of age but can occur in infancy and childhood.
No racial predilection.

Signs and Symptoms

OM: double vision and/or ptosis.
GM: systemic weakness (e.g., swallowing, extremity weakness).

Ophthalmic Findings

Ninety percent eventually have ocular signs.
Ptosis (75% initially, 90% eventually).
Fatigue on sustained upgaze.
Variable.
Enhanced ptosis ("see-saw ptosis" [i.e., increased ptosis if contralateral eyelid lifted, due to Hering's Law of Equal Innervation]).
Lid twitch (lid overshoot from downgaze to primary gaze) (Cogan sign).
Ophthalmoparesis (any nonpainful, pupil-spared diplopia).

Fatigues and is variable.

Any pattern (e.g., mimics sixth, fourth, or pupil-sparing third nerve, pseudo-INO, gaze palsy).

Evaluation

Ice test.

Rest or sleep test.

Tensilon test (edrophonium).

Neostigmine (Prostigmin).

Anti-ACh receptor antibodies.

Electromyography and repetitive nerve stimulation studies in selected cases.

Neurology consultation.

CT of chest (rule out thymoma).

Differential Diagnosis

Intracranial lesions can cause fatigue and positive Tensilon test.

Eaton-Lambert syndrome.

Midbrain lesion.

CPEO.

Myotonic dystrophy.

Oculopharyngeal dystrophy.

Medication-induced myasthenia syndrome.

Penicillamine.

Aminoglycosides.

Procainamide.

Vincristine/vinblastine.

Other antibiotics (e.g., tetracycline, clindamycin, ampicillin, polymyxin).

Furosemide, colchicine, gemfibrozil.

Topical beta-blockers.

Chloroquine.

Treatment

- Ocular:
  Patch eye.
  Ptosis crutch.
  Prism not usually helpful due to variability of deviation.
- Medications:
  Mestinon (pyridostigmine).
  Prednisone.
- Ptosis or strabismus surgery if stable.
- Plasmapheresis.
- Thymectomy (especially if thymoma).
- Immunosuppressives (e.g., azathioprine, cyclosporine, cyclophosphamide).

Carotid Disease and Carotid Surgery

Risk of Cerebrovascular Accident

After hemispheric transient ischemic attack (TIA):

Risk: 8% per year of CVA.

Twenty percent of these in first month and 50% in first year.

Twenty-three percent cumulative 3-year risk.

After TVL:

Risk: 2% per year.

No good data on untreated TVL.

After 4.5 years, about 6% rate of CVA and 11% rate of retinal infarct.

Cumulative risk for CVA at 2 years: 17% for TVL versus 44% for TIA.

After retinal emboli, risk of CVA: 3% to 5% per year.

Recommendations of Amaurosis Fugax Study Group (1990) for Considering Carotid Endarterectomy

High-grade stenosis (70% to 99%).

Clearly demonstrated benefit in multiple studies.

Symptomatic patients *only*.

Not a high risk surgically.

Perioperative CEA morbidity and mortality rate of less than 2%.

Index treatment to individual patient.

No significant cardiac or pulmonary disease.

Nonobese.

Age: less than 75 years.

Medical treatment alone for 0% to 29% stenosis.

Value for 30% to 69% is unknown.

Emerging role for carotid stenting and angioplasty.

TRANSIENT VISUAL LOSS

Summary

TVL may be monocular or binocular; may last seconds, minutes, or hours; and may be the result of intraocular, intraorbital, or intracranial processes.

Signs and Symptoms

Temporal profile of the transient loss of vision.

Acute versus gradual.

Seconds versus minutes versus hours.

One eye or both eyes.

Gaze-evoked visual loss looking to one side or the other is very suggestive of an intraorbital mass, which compresses or stretches the optic nerve with eye rotation.

Systemic Symptoms Suggestive of Carotid Ischemia

Unilateral weakness.

Unilateral sensory loss.

Dysarthria (not in isolation).

Transient monocular blindness.

Rarely homonymous hemianopsia.

Systemic Symptoms Suggestive of Migraine

- Area of visual loss gradually spreads: *"march."*
- Progressive increase over 15 to 20 minutes: *"buildup."*

- March and buildup: highly characteristic of migraine.
- Headache: need not be present to be ocular migraine.
- Visual loss typically scintillations around an area of scotoma. Area within the area of visual disturbance resembles "heat waves" or "water running down a glass."
- Absence of scintillations does not exclude migraine.
  Positive phenomenon more likely to be migraine.
- Atypical ocular migraine (retinal): usually no scintillations or headache.
- Attempt to see the patient during an attack.
  Retinal arteriolar and venous narrowing reported.
  Retinal edema, venous dilation, and delayed fluorescein filling.
  May have actual retinal infarction.
  Migraine can cause anterior ION.
  Migraine can cause central serous choroidopathy.
- May be stereotyped (carotid disease can be stereotyped).
- History of migraine.
  Family history.
  History of motion sickness, somnambulism, cyclic vomiting.
  Stereotyped phenomenon.
  Migraine accompaniments.

Ophthalmic Findings

Exclude ocular causes of TVL.
Tear film (blink clears debris).
Physiologic halos or monocular diplopia.
Retinal circulation (entoptic phenomenon).
Accommodative problems.
Vitreoretinal interface (e.g., floaters).
Glare or afterimages.
Recurrent hyphema.
Recurrent angle closure.
Posner-Schlossman syndrome.
Look at fundus carefully.
Papilledema.
Retinal emboli or ischemia.
Optic disk abnormalities.

Etiology and Differential Diagnosis

- Transient obscuration of vision lasting seconds at a time in one or both eyes (may be precipitated by Valsalva maneuver or standing up) suggests papilledema.
  Ocular etiologies.
  Optic disk drusen.
  Rarely thromboembolic disease.
- Transient monocular visual loss suggests thromboembolic disease (e.g., carotid disease) or migraine.
  Migrainelike visual phenomenon and headache may rarely occur in AVMs or meningioma. These usually do not have characteristic buildup, timing, or resolution and often have progressive symptoms (e.g., increase in frequency and duration).
- Transient binocular visual loss suggests migraine or vertebrobasilar disease. Other less common causes include seizures, AVMs, neoplasms, meningoencephalitis, and trauma.
- Posterior vertebrobasilar circulation disturbances are typically accompanied by other signs (e.g., dysequilibrium, diplopia, dysarthria, dysphagia, dizziness, "drop attacks," dysesthesias of perioral region or limbs).

Evaluation

- Exclude ocular causes.
- Exclude migraine.
- Exclude papilledema.
- Evaluate for inflammatory, thrombotic, and thromboembolic disease.
  Carotid disease (e.g., carotid Doppler, angiography).
  Cardiac embolic source (e.g., echocardiogram, ECG, Holter monitor).
  Vasculitis (e.g., systemic lupus erythematosus, rheumatoid arthritis).
  Exclude coagulopathy in younger patients (e.g., antiphospholipid antibodies, CBC, lipids, prothrombin time, partial thromboplastin time).
  Consider GCA in elderly patients.

Treatment

Depends on underlying cause or origin.
Papilledema.
Migraine therapy.
Carotid disease.
Control of stroke risk factors (e.g., blood pressure).
Antiplatelet drug (e.g., aspirin).
Encourage risk reduction (e.g., smoking cessation).
Consider carotid endarterectomy if significant stenosis is present.
Cardiac disease therapy.

MAJOR NEURO-OPHTHALMOLOGIC STUDIES

Optic Neuritis Treatment Trial

Summary

- I.V. methylprednisolone speeds the recovery of visual loss in optic neuritis but does not alter eventual visual outcome (compared with natural course of disease).
- Oral prednisone alone is contraindicated in patients with optic neuritis.
- I.V. methylprednisolone may delay the onset of demyelinating signs and symptoms, especially in patients with abnormal white matter changes on the MRI.

Study Population

Acute unilateral optic neuritis with visual symptoms of 8 days' duration or less.

Relative afferent pupillary defect and a visual field defect in the affected eye.

Study Design

Randomized controlled clinical trial.

Patients randomly assigned to one of three treatment groups:

1. Oral prednisone (1 mg/kg daily) for 14 days.
2. I.V. methylprednisolone (250 mg four times daily for 3 days) and then oral prednisone taper (1 mg/kg daily) for 11 days.
3. Oral placebo for 14 days.

Results

- More rapid visual recovery in i.v. methylprednisolone group, but final acuity at 30 days was similar among the three groups.
- Visual acuity was 20/40 or better in 93% of patients at 12 months
- Greater rate of recurrent optic neuritis in oral prednisone group (almost two times greater).
- Treatment with i.v. or oral steroids reduced the rate of clinically definite MS during the first 2 years. By 3 years, the effect was negligible.

References

Beck RW, Cleary PA. Optic Neuritis Treatment Trial: one year follow-up results. *Arch Ophthalmol* 1993;111:773–775.

Beck RW, Trobe JD. What we have learned from the Optic Neuritis Treatment Trial. *Ophthalmology* 1995;102:1504–1508.

Ischemic Optic Neuropathy Decompression Trial

Summary

Optic nerve decompression does not improve the visual outcome of nonarteritic anterior ION and may be harmful. The spontaneous improvement rate is better than previously reported.

Study Population

Patients with nonarteritic anterior ION:

Acute unilateral loss of vision.

Afferent pupillary defect.

Lack of underlying causes.

Study Design

- Single-masked, multicenter, randomized clinical trial.
- Twenty-five clinical centers.
- Two hundred and fifty-eight patients randomly assigned to optic nerve sheath decompression or observation.

Results

Of the surgery group, 32.6% improved compared with 42.7% of the group receiving careful follow-up. Patients receiving surgery had a significantly greater risk of losing three or more lines of vision at 6 months: 23.9% in the surgery group worsened compared with 12.4% in the group receiving careful follow-up. No difference in treatment effect was observed between patients with progressive nonarteritic anterior ION and all others.

References

Smith DB. Characteristics of patients with nonarteritic anterior ischemic optic neuropathy eligible for the Ischemic Optic Neuropathy Decompression Trial. *Arch Ophthalmol* 1996;114:1366–1374.

The Ischemic Optic Neuropathy Decompression Trial Research Group. Optic nerve decompression surgery for nonarteritic anterior ischemic optic neuropathy (NAION) is not effective and may be harmful. *JAMA* 1995;273:625–632.

Carotid Endarterectomy Studies

North American Symptomatic Carotid Endarterectomy Trial

Summary

Carotid endarterectomy is beneficial for patients with high-grade carotid stenosis (stenosis of 70% to 99%). The study is ongoing for patients with carotid stenosis of 30% to 69%.

Study Population

- Hemispheric TIA/CVA or amaurosis fugax *and* ipsilateral carotid stenosis.
- Two strata: 30% to 69% versus 70% to 99% carotid stenosis.

Study Design

- Randomized controlled clinical trial.
- Fifty centers nationwide, 659 patients enrolled.
- Patients randomly assigned to carotid endarterectomy and medical therapy to medical therapy alone. All patients optimized on medical therapy (aspirin).

Results

Life Table Analysis (Less Than 70% Stenosis)

- For the end point of any CVA risk at 2 years:
  Medication only: 26%.
  Medication plus CEA: 9%.
  Relative risk reduction: 65%.
  Ninety-five percent of CVAs were ipsilateral to stenosis.
- Major CVA:

Medication only: 13%.
Medication plus CEA: 2.5%.

- Subgroup analysis:
  Higher risk reduction if 90% to 99% stenosis was present.
  Annual risk with CVA medications alone: 15%.
  Surgical morbidity and mortality same, regardless of grade of stenosis.

References

North American Symptomatic Carotid Endarterectomy Trial. Beneficial effect of carotid endarterectomy in symptomatic patients with high-grade carotid stenosis. *N Engl J Med* 1991;325:445–453.

Mayo Asymptomatic Carotid Endarterectomy Study Group. Results of a randomized controlled trial of carotid endarterectomy for asymptomatic carotid stenosis. *Mayo Clin Proc* 1992;67:513–518.

CHAPTER

7

Oculoplastics and Orbital Disease

Susan Carter • H. Jane Kim

ORBIT

Anatomy

Orbital Dimensions

Volume: 30 mL.
Height: 35 mm.
Width: 40 mm.
Medial wall length: 45 mm.
Globe to optic canal: 18 mm.
Optic nerve: 5 cm.
 Intraocular: 1 mm.
 Intraorbital: 25 mm.
 Intracanalicular: 10 mm.
 Intracranial: 15 mm.

Orbital Bones

See Figure 7.1.

Orbital Apertures

See Figures 7.2 and 7.3, and Table 7.1.

Evaluation of Orbital Disorders

Axial displacement (Table 7.2).
Nonaxial displacement (Table 7.3).
Imaging (Table 7.4).
Destructive lesions of bone (Table 7.5).
Classification of orbital disorders (Tables 7.6 and 7.7).

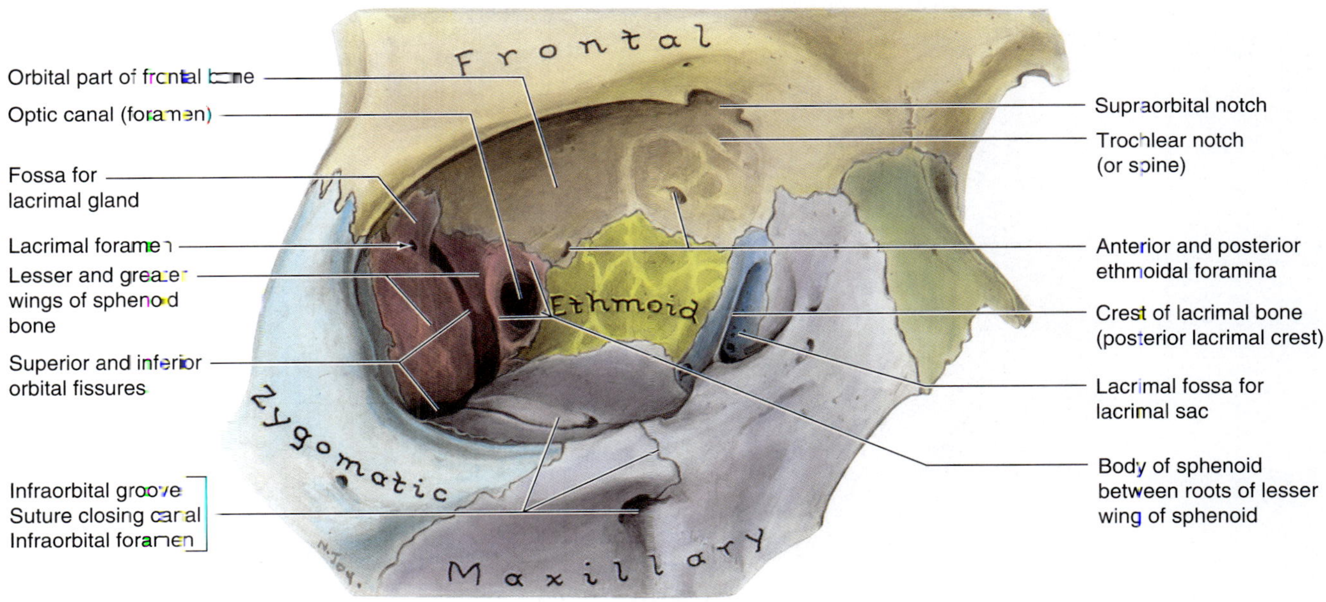

Anterior view

FIGURE 7.1. Seven orbital bones: sphenoid, ethmoid, zygomatic, maxillary, frontal, lacrimal, and palatine, with the ethmoid being the thinnest bone. Observe the optic canal situated within the lesser wing of the sphenoid bone, separated by optic strut from the superior orbital fissure. (From Moore KL, Dalley AF II. *Clinical oriented anatomy*, 4th ed. Baltimore, MD: Lippincott Williams & Wilkins, 1999, with permission.)

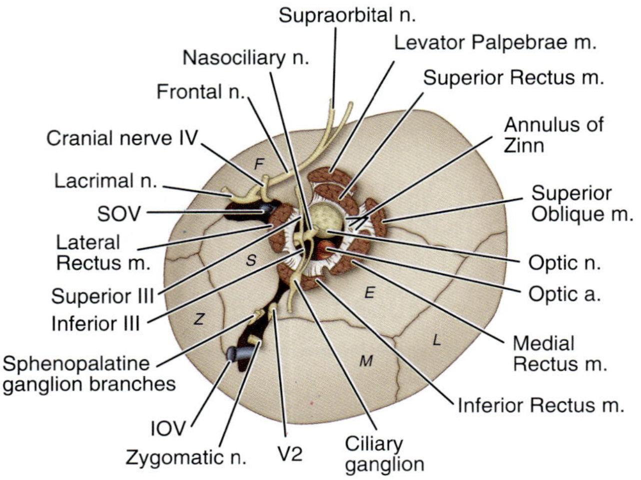

FIGURE 7.2. The orbital apex. (*E*, ethmoid bone; *F*, frontal bone; *IOV*, inferior orbital vein; *L*, lacrimal bone; *M*, maxillary bone; *S*, sphenoid bone; *SOV*, superior orbital vein; *Z*, zygomatic bone.)

ORBITAL INFLAMMATION

Orbital Cellulitis

Summary

Bacterial and fungal infections of the orbit may occur in children (usually monomicrobial) and adults (polymicrobial) with vision-threatening and life-threatening sequelae. Preseptal cellulitis occurs only in the periorbital structures anterior to the orbital septum, unlike orbital cellulitis, which involves more posterior structures. Orbital cellulitis most commonly occurs in the setting of active paranasal sinus disease or trauma with associated infected facial wounds.

Etiology

Periorbital structures: paranasal sinus, face and eyelid, lacrimal sac (dacryocystitis), or dental infections.
Intraorbital structures: endophthalmitis, dacryoadenitis.
Exogenous: trauma, surgery.
Endogenous: septic embolization.
Most common organisms: *Staphylococcus aureus*, *Streptococcus* sp., *Haemophilus influenzae* (in children), Gram-negative rods, *Mucor* (in diabetics), *Aspergillus*.

Signs and Symptoms

See Table 7.8 and Figure 7.4.

Special Tests

- Cultures and/or Gram stain: blood, conjunctiva, nasopharynx, external wounds, cerebrospinal fluid, as necessary.
- Complete blood cell count (CBC) with differential.

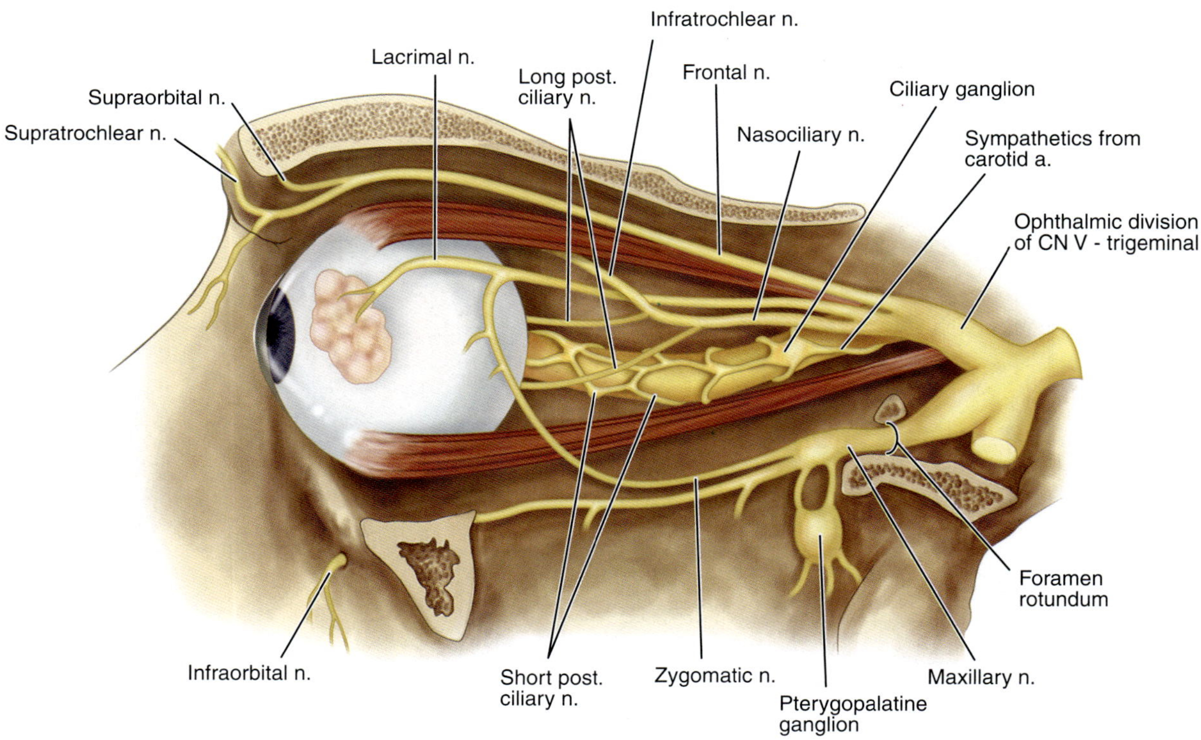

FIGURE 7.3. The nerves of the orbit. Observe the ciliary ganglion that receives sensory fibers from the nasociliary branches of CN V1, sympathetic fibers from the internal carotid plexus (traveling around the ophthalmic artery), and parasympathetic fibers (which synapse in the ganglion) from the inferior branch of the CN III.

Table 7.1

Orbital apertures

Aperture	Location	Contents
Optic canal	Lesser wing of sphenoid	Optic nerve, ophthalmic artery, sympathetic nerves
Superior orbital fissure	Greater and lesser wings of sphenoid	Divided by lateral rectus: outside muscle cone, lacrimal (V_1), frontal (V_1), trochlear (fourth) nerves; inside muscle cone, oculomotor (superior and inferior division of third cranial), nasociliary (V_1), abducens (V_1) nerves Sympathetic nerves Superior ophthalmic vein
Inferior orbital fissure	Sphenoid, maxillary, and palatine bones	Infraorbital and zygomatic nerves (V_2) Inferior ophthalmic vein
Anterior ethmoid canal	Frontal and ethmoid bones	Anterior ethmoid nerve (becomes dorsal nasal) and artery
Posterior ethmoid canal	Frontal and ethmoid bones	Posterior ethmoid nerve and artery
Nasolacrimal canal	Maxillary and lacrimal bones	Nasolacrimal duct
Zygomaticofacial and zygomaticotemporal canals	Zygoma	Branches of zygomatic nerves and arteries
Supraorbital notch/foramen	Frontal bone	Supraorbital nerve (V_1) and artery
Infraorbital foramen	Maxillary bone	Infraorbital nerve (V_2) and artery

Table 7.2

Axial displacement

Unilateral proptosis	Bilateral proptosis[a]	Enophthalmos
Thyroid orbitopathy: most common cause in adults	Thyroid orbitopathy: most common cause in adults	Structural: trauma, asymmetry
Cavernous hemangioma	Lymphoma and leukemia	Atrophy: trauma, x-ray therapy
Glioma	Vasculitis and Wegener granulomatosis	Cicatrization: metastatic breast carcinoma, sclerosing inflammation, after trauma
Meningioma	Idiopathic orbital inflammation	Asymmetric palpebral fissures
Orbital cellulitis: most common cause in children	Cavernous sinus thrombosis	
	Metastatic lesions	

[a]All causes listed below may cause unilateral proptosis as well.

Table 7.3

Nonaxial displacement

Superior	Inferomedial	Inferolateral	Pseudoproptosis
Maxillary sinus tumor	Lacrimal gland tumors Dermoids	Frontoethmoidal mucocele Sinus carcinoma	High-level myopia Contralateral enophthalmos Asymmetric orbits Asymmetric palpebral fissures

Table 7.4

Imaging

Modality	Description	Advantages/disadvantages
Plain film x-rays	Caldwell, Waters, facial series	*Advantages*: useful in trauma, especially with metallic foreign bodies *Disadvantages*: poor soft tissue visualization
Ultrasound	Reflected sound waves originate from tissue interfaces Good sound transmission: cystic or angiomatous tumors Poor sound transmission: solid or infiltrative tumors	*Advantages*: quick, inexpensive *Disadvantages*: poor anatomic detail of entire orbit
CT	Two-dimensional image obtained by x-rays	*Advantages*: useful in trauma setting, metal foreign body, bony lesion *Disadvantages*: more expensive than plain films
MRI	Magnetic field aligns nuclei of hydrogen atoms, radiofrequency pulse excites nuclei, nuclei emit radiomagnetic energy, which is detected, processed, and imaged: T_1-fat is bright; T_2-fat is dark	*Advantages*: excellent anatomic detail, magnetic resonance digital subtraction angiography possible *Disadvantages*: no bone anatomy, cannot be used in presence of metal foreign body, more expensive than CT, longer image acquisition time, often more difficult to schedule or obtain

CT, computed tomography; MRI, magnetic resonance imaging.

Table 7.5

Destructive lesions of bone

Solid lesions	Cystic lesions	Hyperostotic lesions
Histiocytosis X	Dermoid cyst	Meningioma
Bony metastases: lung, prostate cancers, neuroblastoma	Mucocele	Fibrous dysplasia
Sinusitis and sinus malignancies		Ossifying fibroma
Wegener granulomatosis		Osteoma
Osteogenic sarcoma		Osteogenic sarcoma

Table 7.6

Common orbital disorders

Pediatric patients	Adult patients
Orbital cellulitis (most common)	Thyroid orbitopathy (most common)
Capillary hemangioma	Cavernous hemangioma
Lymphangioma	Lymphangioma
Dermoid and epidermoid cysts	Orbital cellulitis
Rhabdomyosarcoma	Idiopathic orbital inflammation
Idiopathic orbital inflammation	Meningioma
Optic nerve glioma	Lacrimal gland tumors
Neurofibroma	Lymphoproliferative lesions
Metastatic tumors—neuroblastoma, leukemia	Metastatic tumors: breast, lung

Table 7.7

Craniofacial deformities

Disorder	Description	Examples
Craniofacial cleft syndrome	Failure of bony sutures to close	Treacher Collins syndrome (mandibulofacial dysostosis): lateral lid defects, malar hypoplasia, micrognathia Goldenhar (oculoauriculovertebral dysplasia): lid colobomas, preauricular skin tags, limbal dermoids, vertebral anomalies
Craniostenosis syndromes	Premature closure of bony sutures	Crouzon disease (craniofacial dysostosis): exophthalmos, exotropia, optic atrophy, superior rectus hypoplasia, parrot-beak nose Apert disease (arachnocephalodactyly): similar to Crouzon's, but with syndactyly

- Computed tomography (CT) scan: Order with contrast, evaluate preseptal versus postseptal location, look for paranasal sinus disease, subperiosteal abscess.
- Biopsy for microscopy.
- Fungus: *Mucor*—nonseptate hyphae, *Aspergillus*—septate branching hyphae.

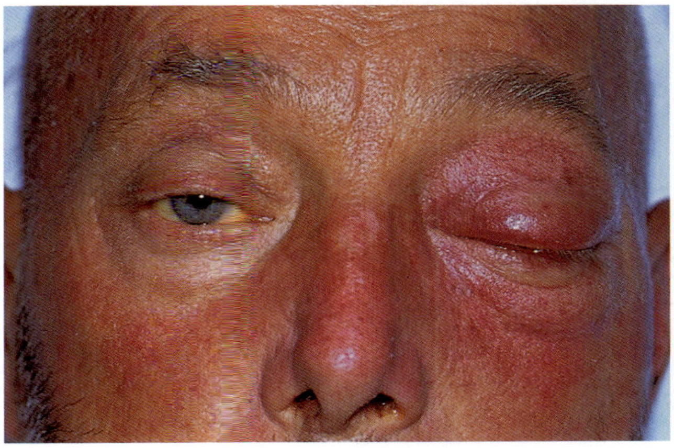

FIGURE 7.4. Left orbital cellulitis with marked periorbital edema, erythema, and proptosis.

Mucormycosis

- Severe infection with genera Rhizopus, Mucor, Absidia belonging to the family Mucoraceae, a subset of the class Phycomycetes.
- Blood vessel invasion, vascular occlusion, necrosis, black eschar (late finding) on roof of mouth or nose.
- Begins in sinus—invades orbit.
- Risk factors: diabetics in ketoacidosis or with antecedent bacterial infection, alcoholics, and immunocompromised patients.
- Histopathology: nonseptate, large branching filamentous hyphae seen on periodic acid-Schiff and Gomori methenamine-silver stains.
- Treatment: extensive debridement of necrotic tissues with irrigation with amphotericin B.
- Intravenous amphotericin B (nephrotoxic, aplastic anemia).

Disease Course

- May progress from preseptal to orbital cellulitis, orbital cellulitis to cavernous sinus thrombosis or intracranial abscess, without appropriate treatment. Must follow patients closely for development of deeper infection, decreased vision or ocular motility, or afferent pupillary defect.

Table 7.8

Signs and symptoms of orbital cellulitis

Feature	Preseptal cellulitis	Orbital cellulitis
Pain	Yes	Yes
Fever	Possible	Possible
Periorbital edema, warmth, tenderness	Yes	Yes
Proptosis	No	Yes
Restricted extraocular movement	No	Yes
Conjunctival chemosis	No	Yes
Decreased vision	No	Yes
Afferent pupillary defect	No	Yes
Optic nerve head swelling	No	Yes

Table 7.9

Chandler's classification of orbital infection

	Intravenous antibiotics	Surgical drainage	Other
I. Preseptal	Oral in mild cases with close follow-up, intravenous if severe or with progression	—	—
II. Orbital cellulitis	Yes	Yes (if no improvement despite 72 hours of intravenous antibiotics or progression of symptoms)	—
III. Subperiosteal Abscess	Yes	Yes if >9 years old. Expectant if <9	—
IV. Orbital abscess	Yes	Yes	—
V. Cavernous sinus thrombosis (diagnosis confirmed by MR venogram)	Yes	—	IV heparin

- Cavernous sinus thrombosis: bilateral orbital involvement, decreased skin sensation affecting ophthalmic (V_1) or maxillary (V_2) divisions of the trigeminal nerve, complete ophthalmoplegia, headache, nausea, vomiting, and fever.
- Subperiosteal abscess formation (commonly superomedial or inferomedial orbit) can result in sudden loss of vision with posterior extension of the abscess toward the orbital apex.

Treatment and Management

- After cultures and blood work are obtained, the patient should be immediately placed on a regimen of antibiotics. Infectious disease consultation may be obtained.
- Patients with preseptal cellulitis are occasionally treated as outpatients with oral antibiotics; otherwise, intravenous antibiotics are given.
- Patients with sinus disease should be evaluated by an otolaryngologist.
- Mucormycosis, a rare, rapidly progressive fungal orbital infection, should be suspected in all diabetics and immunosuppressed patients; definitive diagnosis and treatment should be performed immediately; treatment consists of orbital debridement, possible exenteration and local irrigation, and systemic treatment with amphotericin B.
- A lag time of 24 to 48 hours commonly occurs between initiation of antibiotics and clinical response.
- If there is no improvement or if new signs such as decreased vision or development of an afferent pupillary defect develop, repeat CT scan and suspect abscess formation or resistant organisms.
- Abscesses in adults should be surgically drained, particularly in the setting of visual compromise; abscesses in children may be followed closely if under the age of 9, with surgical drainage for any deterioration.
- Aspergillosis, a fungal infection that may be acute or chronic and local or disseminated, is treated with orbital debridement, possible exenteration and local irrigation, and systemic treatment with amphotericin.

Medications

Antibiotic choice depends on origin or cause of cellulitis.

- Trauma: third-generation cephalosporin and clindamycin for Gram negative organisms Gram-positive skin flora, and anaerobes, respectively.
- Sinus: second-generation cephalosporin for sinus bacteria.
- Children: single aerobe, second-generation cephalosporin for *H. influenzae*.
- Adults (>14 y/o): polymicrobial (average five species). Third-generation cephalosporin, nafcillin, or vancomycin (if methicillin-resistant *S. aureus* suspected), and metronidazole (crosses blood–brain barrier) or clindamycin for anaerobes.
- Fungus: amphotericin B (liposomal amphotericin B reserved for immunocompromised host with renal failure), voriconazole (more effective for invasive *Aspergillus*).

Follow-up

- Patients should be followed extremely closely until signs of improvement are evident, such as decreased lid edema and erythema, decreased chemosis, improved ocular motility, improved visual acuity, or decreased proptosis.
- Intravenous antibiotics should be continued for approximately 1 week before switching to oral antibiotics.

Differential Diagnosis

- Idiopathic orbital inflammation: no signs of infection.
- Carotid cavernous fistula: no signs of infection.
- Orbital vasculitis.

References

Bilyk J. Periocular infection. *Curr Opin Ophthalmol* 2007;18: 414–423.

Epstein VA, Kern RC. Invasive fungal sinusitis and complications of rhinosinusitis. *Otolaryngol Clin N Am* 2008;41(3):497–524.

Harris GJ. Subperiosteal abscess of the orbit. Age as a factor in the bacteriology and response to treatment. *Ophthalmology* 1994;101(3):585–595.

Necrotizing Fasciitis

Summary

- Periocular necrotizing fasciitis is a rapidly progressive infection that spreads along the subcutaneous soft tissue planes and that can eventually lead to shock and organ failure.

Etiology

- Idiopathic but has been associated with blunt or surgical trauma (blepharoplasty) in healthy patients.
- Group β-hemolytic *Streptococcus*.

Signs and Symptoms

- Mimics preseptal cellulitis initially but results in necrosis of adjacent tissue and cyanosis (subcutaneous hemorrhage and thrombosis).
- Painful, erythematous, and/or blue eyelids.
- Possible retinal artery occlusion due to thrombosis or ischemic necrosis of the deep orbit.

Treatment and Management

- Subcutaneous debridement, resection of necrotic skin, and β-lactam antibiotics (penicillin, ceftriaxone, or clindamycin)

Reference

Elner VM, Demirci H, Nerad JA, et al. Periocular necrotizing fasciitis with visual loss. *Ophthalmology* 2006;113:2338–2345.

Thyroid Orbitopathy

Summary

Thyroid orbitopathy, the most common cause of unilateral or bilateral proptosis in adults, occurs in 50% of patients with Graves disease. Patients with thyroid orbitopathy may be hyperthyroid, hypothyroid, or even euthyroid. Ocular complications attributable to thyroid orbitopathy include ocular exposure, strabismus, and optic nerve compression.

Etiology

- Autoimmune disorder with antibodies to orbital fibroblasts demonstrated in some patients.
- Fibroblasts can transform into adipocytes.
- Stimulation of glycosaminoglycans or collagen production.

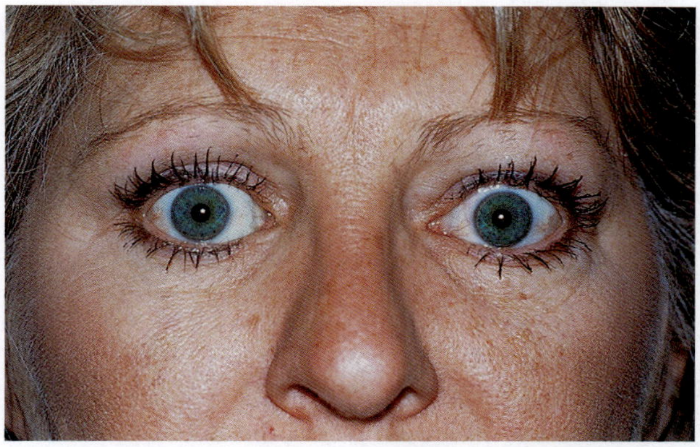

FIGURE 7.5. Bilateral thyroid orbitopathy with exophthalmos and lid retraction.

Signs and Symptoms

See Figure 7.5.

- Lid retraction (early sign).
- Lid lag on downgaze (early sign).
- Periorbital edema.
- Proptosis.
- Conjunctival chemosis.
- Enlarged vessels over rectus muscle insertions.
- Corneal exposure, ulceration.
- Extraocular motility restriction, with preferential extraocular muscle involvement (inferior > medial > superior > lateral rectus) sparing the tendons.
- Elevated intraocular pressure with upgaze.
- Compressive optic neuropathy with decreased visual acuity, decreased color vision, afferent pupillary defect, visual field defects.

Demographics

- Age: 25 to 50 years.
- Ratio of women to men: 6 to 1.

Ophthalmic Findings

Werner's "NOSPECS" (mnemonic) classification:
Class 0: No signs or symptoms.
Class 1: Only signs (eyelid retraction).
Class 2: Soft tissue periorbital swelling.
Class 3: Proptosis of eyes.
Class 4: Extraocular muscle involvement, diplopia.
Class 5: Corneal involvement, exposure.
Class 6: Sight loss by optic nerve compression.

Systemic Findings

- Pretibial dermopathy.
- Other features associated with a dysthyroid state: restlessness, tremor, weight loss with hyperthyroidism or lethargy, constipation, weight gain with hypothyroidism.
- Associated with myasthenia gravis, smoking, family history.

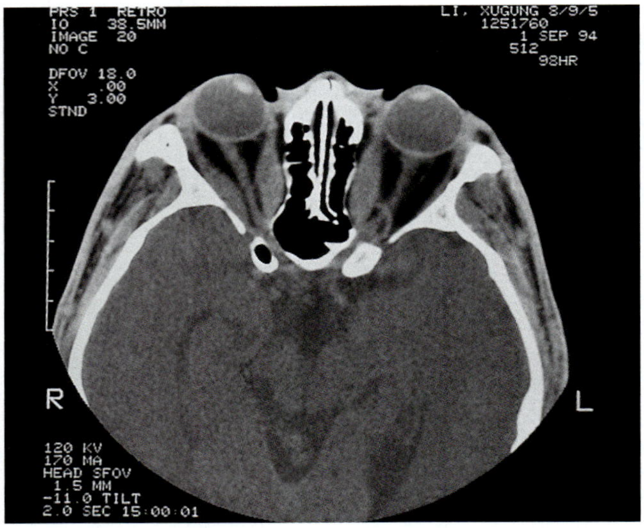

FIGURE 7.6. Computed tomography scan demonstrating enlarged extraocular muscles.

Special Tests

- Evaluate thyroid function: sensitive thyroid-stimulating hormone (TSH); T3 and T4 (thyrotropin receptor) antibodies; antithyroid antibodies; thyrotropin-releasing hormone (TRH) stimulation test; Werner or T3 suppression test.
- Orbital imaging (Figure 7.6).
    - Extraocular muscle enlargement sparing tendons:
        - Most commonly involved (in order): inferior rectus, medial rectus, and superior rectus muscles.
    - Least commonly involved: lateral rectus.
    - Increased fat volume.
    - Optic nerve compression by muscles in orbital apex.
    - Rule out other causes of proptosis.
    - Define anatomy of paranasal sinuses before orbital decompression with CT scan.

Pathology

Inflammation and enlargement of orbital tissues, specifically the nontendinous portions of the extraocular muscles:

- Early: lymphocyte and plasma cell infiltration of muscles, deposition of mucopolysaccharide by activated fibroblasts, and formation of collagen.
- Late: fibrosis and fatty infiltration of muscles.

Disease Course

- Acute inflammatory phase (6 to 18 months) evolves into chronic stable fibrotic phase.
- Spontaneous remissions and exacerbations can occur.
- Thyroid disease and orbital disease run independent courses; however, orbital disease may worsen after radioactive iodide thyroid gland treatment.
- Optic neuropathy may occur in patients without significant proptosis, because of posterior compression of the nerve.
- Fifty percent of patients with upper lid retraction may improve without intervention.
- Motility fluctuates during the acute phase.

Treatment and Management

- Local supportive measures: artificial teardrops, lubricating ointment, elevating head of bed.
- Corticosteroids: given with H_2 receptor antagonist, bisphosphonate, and calcium.
    - For acute inflammatory phase.
    - For compressive optic neuropathy.
    - Prednisone 60 to 100 mg for up to 1 week to assess steroid responsiveness.
    - Pulse IV methylprednisolone (10 mg/kg, max 1 g) repeat at 48-hour intervals × 3; may be repeated after 3 months if no response or recurs. Side effects of cardiac arrhythmia, liver toxicity, relapse.
    - Rebound effect may occur after cessation of steroids.
- Other immunomodulators are being studied in refractory cases with active inflammation.
    - Cyclosporin A: inhibits T-cell and IL-2 activity; start 2 mg/kg BID.
    - Tacrolimus: inhibits T-cell and IL-2 activity.
- Orbital radiation:
    - Traditionally recommended for acute inflammatory phase or compressive optic neuropathy; however, recent studies have failed to demonstrate significant benefits 12 months after radiotherapy, whether administered early or late in the course of Graves ophthalmopathy.
    - Risks include cataract formation and radiation retinopathy, especially in diabetics and patients receiving systemic chemotherapy.
    - For compressive optic neuropathy: dosage: 2,000 cGy in ten fractions over 2 weeks to posterior orbit.
- Surgical management: a staged approach must be taken to the surgical rehabilitation of the patient with thyroid orbitopathy so as to avoid unnecessary procedures.
    - Orbital decompression.
    - Extraocular muscle surgery.
    - Adjustment of eyelid margin position.
    - Blepharoplasty.
- Orbital decompression:
    - For optic neuropathy, corneal exposure, proptosis.
    - Remove bony walls of orbit to allow prolapse of orbital soft tissues and enlargement of orbital volume.
    - Medial wall, ethmoid sinus, orbital floor, maxillary sinus, lateral wall, temporalis fossa.
    - Good success rates in improving decreased vision attributable to optic neuropathy.
    - Complications: diplopia, hemorrhage, infection, cerebrospinal fluid leak, optic nerve injury.
- Extraocular muscle surgery:
    - Perform only after motility disturbance is stable for 6 months.
    - Steroids and radiation therapy have minimal effect.

Inferior and medial rectus muscles most often affected: recess with adjustable sutures.

- Lid margin position surgery.
    - Lid retraction due in part to fibrotic levator or Müller muscle, increase in sympathetic activity.
    - Recess either muscle to lower the lid, especially laterally, with or without spacer grafts such as sclera.
    - Raise the lower lid to help cover the cornea, with spacer grafts.
- Blepharoplasty: Remove excess skin and fat to improve cosmesis.

Differential Diagnosis

Idiopathic orbital inflammation (pseudotumor).
Orbital amyloidosis
Carotid cavernous fistula.
Orbital tumor.
Eyelid retraction: see p. 29 for differential.

References

Gorman CA, Garrity JA, Fatourechi V, et al. A prospective, randomized, double-blind, placebo-controlled study of orbital radiotherapy for Grave's ophthalmopathy. *Ophthalmology* 2001;108:1523–1534.

Krassas GE, Boboridis K. Recent developments in the medical treatment of thyroid eye disease. *Orbit* 2006;25:117–122.

Meyer PAR. Avoiding surgery for thyroid eye disease. *Eye* 2006;20:1171–1177.

Sergott RC, Glaser JS. Graves' ophthalmopathy: a clinical and immunologic review. *Surv Ophthalmol* 1981;26:1–21.

Shorr N, Seiff SR. The four stages of surgical rehabilitation of the patient with dysthyroid ophthalmopathy. *Ophthalmology* 1986;93:476–483.

Idiopathic Orbital Inflammation (Orbital Pseudotumor)

Summary

Acute idiopathic orbital inflammation typically presents with pain and may be diffuse or localized to a specific area of the orbit. Treatment is typically with oral steroids. Many systemic processes such as sarcoid, Wegener granulomatosis, or metastatic carcinomas may present in a similar fashion. These must be considered before the diagnosis of idiopathic orbital inflammation is made.

Etiology

Idiopathic.

Signs and Symptoms

- Anterior orbit inflammation/diffuse inflammation:
    - Pain.
    - Erythema and edema of lids.
    - Chemosis.
    - Decreased vision.
    - Decreased extraocular motility.
    - Uveitis.
- Apical inflammation:
    - Pain.
    - Decreased vision.
    - Decreased extraocular motility.
- Myositic inflammation:
    - Pain with eye movements.
    - Decreased extraocular motility.
    - Localized chemosis.
- Lacrimal inflammation:
    - Pain.
    - S-shaped eyelid deformity.
    - Localized chemosis.

Demographics

All ages, men and women.

Ophthalmic Findings

Children may develop papillitis.

Special Tests

CT scan:
- Anterior, diffuse, apical: enhancing infiltrative mass with irregular margins.
- Myositic: fusiform enlargement of extraocular muscle involving the tendon.
- Lacrimal: irregular swelling of lacrimal gland.

Pathology

Polymorphous infiltrate of inflammatory cells including lymphocytes, neutrophils, plasma cells, and macrophages.

Disease Course

Generally resolves with treatment but may recur.

Treatment and Management

- Obtain orbital scan.
- NSAIDS for myositis.
- Corticosteroids: first line in a typical case.
    - Start with 1.0 to 1.5 mg/kg/day × 1 to 2 weeks, with slow taper over 6 to 12 weeks.
    - Methylprednisolone 1 g/day × 1 to 3 days for vision loss
    - Rapid resolution usually occurs with steroids.
- Biopsy if no improvement with steroids or if recurrence occurs, or atypical presentation.
- Add immunosuppressants as steroid-sparing drugs.
- Orbital irradiation or immunobiologic agents (infliximab) can be used in refractory cases.

Differential Diagnosis

- Adults:
    - Orbital cellulitis.

Orbital inflammation secondary to the following:
Sarcoidosis:
Uveitis, dacryoadenitis, rare orbital lesions.
Tests: angiotensin-converting enzyme, lysozyme, chest x-ray (CXR): hilar adenopathy, positive gallium scan.
Pathology: noncaseating granulomas.
Wegener granulomatosis:
Upper and lower respiratory tract lesions, vasculitis, nephritis, orbital inflammation, uveitis.
Tests: antineutrophil cytoplasmic antibodies (ANCA), abnormal urinary sediment, abnormal CXR.
Pathology: necrotizing granulomatous inflammation and vasculitis
Sjögren syndrome:
Dry eyes, dry mouth, other associated autoimmune diseases, enlarged lacrimal glands.
Tests: Antinuclear antibodies (ANA, rheumatoid factor [RF], Sjögren antibodies).
Pathology: polymorphous nongranulomatous inflammatory infiltrate
Ruptured dermoid cyst.
Arteriovenous fistulas.
Orbital metastasis.

- Children:
  - Orbital cellulitis.
  - Ruptured dermoid cyst.
  - Rhabdomyosarcoma.
  - Metastatic neuroblastoma.
  - Leukemic orbital infiltrate.

References

Harris GJ. Idiopathic orbital inflammation: a pathogenetic construct and treatment strategy. *Ophthal Plast Reconstr Surg* 2006;22:79–86.

Mombaerts I, Glodschmeding R, Schlingemann RO, et al. What is orbital pseudotumor? *Surv Ophthalmol* 1996;41:66–78.

Rootman J, Nugent R. The classification and management of acute orbital pseudotumors. *Ophthalmology* 1982;89:1040–1048.

ORBITAL TUMORS

Congenital Orbital Tumors

Dermoid and Epidermoid Cysts

Clinical Features

- Onset: childhood.
- Smooth cystic mass in lateral or superolateral orbit.
- Differentiate superomedial lesion from encephalocele by CT scan.

Pathology

- Dermoid: cyst lined by keratinized epidermis with dermal appendages such as hair follicles and sebaceous glands.
- Epidermoid: cyst lined by keratinized epidermis without dermal structures.

Treatment

- Complete excision.
- Ruptured cyst results in severe inflammation.

Lipodermoid

Clinical Features

- Solid choristoma located lateral to lateral limbus with orbital extension.
- Associated with Goldenhar syndrome.

Pathology

Solid tumor with adipose tissue, hair follicles.

Treatment

- Excise anterior component only if hairs cause irritation.
- Extensive resection may result in motility problems and damage to lacrimal ductules.

Reference

Fry CL, Leone CR Jr. Safe management of dermolipomas. *Arch Ophthalmol* 1994;112:1114–1116.

Vascular Tumors

See Table 7.10.

References

Harris GJ. Orbital vascular malformations: a consensus statement on terminology and its clinical implications. *Am J Ophthalmol* 1999;127:453–455.

Rootman J. Vascular malformations of the orbit: hemodynamic concepts. *Orbit* 2003;22:103–120.

Capillary Hemangioma

Clinical Features

- Onset at few weeks of life, grows over first year, involutes over several years.
- Superficial strawberry surface lesion or deep bluish orbital lesion.
- Kasabach-Merritt syndrome: capillary hemangiomas associated with thrombocytopenia.

Pathology

Fine network of endothelially lined vascular channels.

Treatment

- Amblyopia, strabismus, anisometropia: treat; otherwise, may observe, since involution will occur.

Table 7.10

Vascular lesions

Type	Characteristics
Arteriovenous malformation	*Arterial flow lesion*: congenital lesion of anastamosing arteries and veins, without intervening capillaries; severe hemorrhage may occur with excision unless feeding branches are occluded before surgery
Arteriovenous fistula	*Arterial flow lesion*: traumatic or degenerative connection between arteries and veins *Carotid cavernous fistula*: high flow, pulsating proptosis, tortuous epibulbar vessels, bruit, CT with enlarged superior ophthalmic vein, motility disturbances; embolization by neurointerventional radiology *Dural cavernous fistula*: low flow, injected conjunctival vessels, elevated intraocular pressure, motility disturbances; may spontaneously close
Orbital varix	*Venous flow lesion*: large venous dilation, proptosis with Valsalva maneuver, conservative management

CT, computed tomography

- Steroids:
  - Intralesional (betamethasone and triamcinolone): risk of emboli of steroid particles through vessels that anastomose with the orbital circulation and cause central retinal artery occlusion.
  - Topical (clobetasol [Temovate] steroid cream): risk of atrophy and hypopigmentation of skin and subcutaneous tissues.
  - Systemic oral steroids.
  - Watch for adrenal suppression and growth retardation with steroids.
- Propranolol, systemic
  - Effective treatment for disfiguring infantile capillary hemangiomas.
  - Potential mechanisms of action: vasoconstriction, down-regulation of the RAF/mitogen-activated protein kinase pathway resulting in decreased expression of proangiogenic factors, and triggering apoptosis of capillary endothelial cells.
  - Risk of bradycardia, hypotension, hypoglycemia, bronchospasm.
- Surgery: useful only in well-circumscribed deep lesions.

References

Shorr N, Seiff SR. Central retinal artery occlusion associated with periocular corticosteroid injection for juvenile hemangioma. *Ophthalmic Surg* 1986;17:229–231.

O'Keefe M, Lanigan B, Byrne SA. Capillary haemangioma of the eyelids and orbit: a clinical review of the safety and efficacy of intralesional steroid. *Acta Ophthalmol Scand* 2003;81:294–298.

Leaute-Labreze C, Dumas de la Roque E, Hubiche T, et al. Propranolol for severe hemangiomas of infancy. *N Engl J Med* 2008;358:2649–2651.

Lymphangioma

Clinical Features

- Infiltrative nonencapsulated lesion of eyelid, orbit with onset in first decade
- Abrupt enlargement with hemorrhage into lymphangioma (chocolate cyst)
- May enlarge with upper respiratory tract infection.
- Fluid levels on MRI, but no flow on MRA or MRV.

Pathology

- Large serum-filled spaces lined by endothelial cells.
- Chocolate cysts: hemorrhage from interstitial capillaries.

Treatment

- Monitor and treat amblyopia, strabismus, and anisometropia, particularly after hemorrhage.
- Drain hemorrhage.
- Avoid surgical resection because of infiltrative nature.
- Debulk lesion anteriorly as needed.

Differential Diagnosis

- Orbital varices: weakened venous system that enlarges with increased venous pressure (e.g., **Valsalva maneuver) and enhances on CT.**

Reference

Harris GJ, Sakol PJ, Bonavolonta G, et al. An analysis of thirty cases of orbital lymphangioma: pathophysiologic considerations and management recommendations. *Ophthalmology* 1990;97:1583–1592.

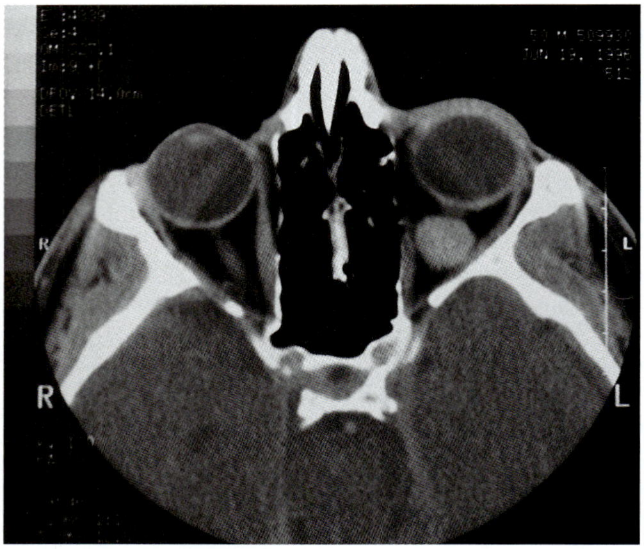

FIGURE 7.7. Computed tomography scan of well-circumscribed intraconal cavernous hemangioma.

Cavernous Hemangioma

Clinical Features

- Most common benign primary orbital tumor of adults, particularly middle-aged women.
- Gradual proptosis, decreased vision with optic nerve compression or induced hyperopia (Figure 7.7).
- CT: well-circumscribed mass with homogeneous enhancement.

Pathology

Encapsulated lesion consisting of large, dilated vascular spaces filled with red blood cells.

Treatment

Surgical excision for lesions compromising ocular function.

Hemangiopericytoma

Clinical Features

- Uncommon tumor of middle-aged adults.
- Similar presentation as cavernous hemangioma.
- May cause conjunctival engorgement and prolapse, motility restriction.
- CT: well-circumscribed lesion.

Pathology

Large pericytes surround a capillary network.

Treatment

- Complete surgical excision.
- May recur, undergo malignant transformation, metastasize.

Neural Tumors

Optic Nerve Glioma

See Figure 7.8.

Clinical Features

- Optic nerve glioma develops during the first decade.
- Twenty-five to fifty percent associated with neurofibromatosis type 1.
- Painless proptosis, vision loss, afferent pupillary defect.
- Chiasmal involvement may occur.

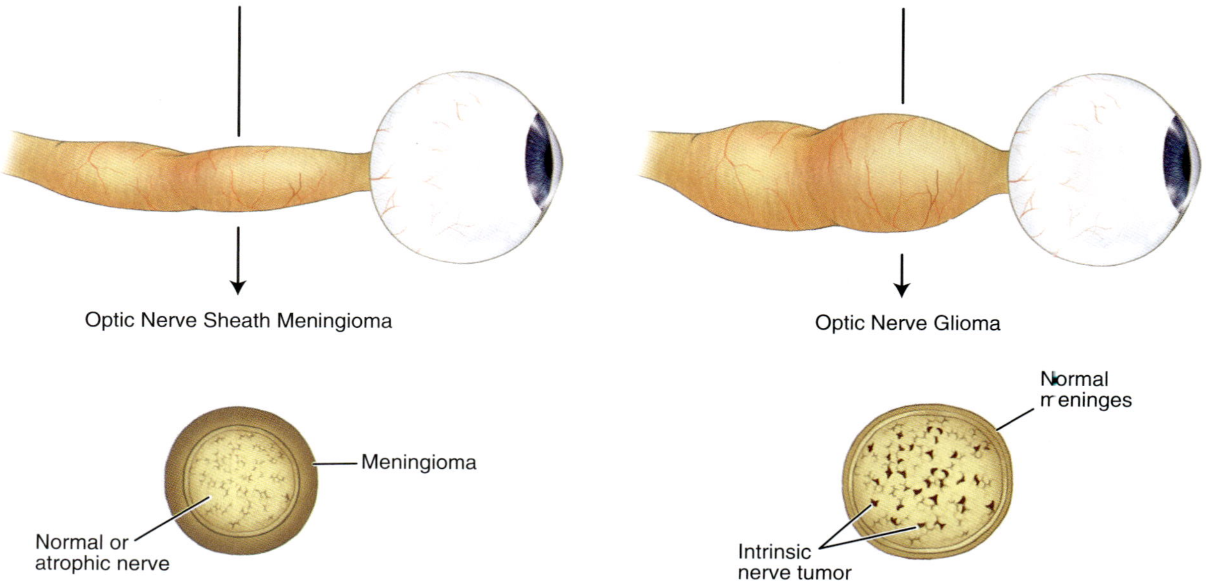

FIGURE 7.8. Comparison of optic nerve meningioma (**A**), optic nerve glioma (**B**), (**C**).

- Imaging:
  - Plain film: enlargement of optic canal greater than 6.5 mm in diameter.
  - CT: S-shaped fusiform enlargement of optic nerve.
  - Magnetic resonance imaging (MRI): better than CT for evaluation of posterior extension of tumor (more common in NF). Isointense or hypointense on T1 and hyperintense on T2.

Pathology

Pilocytic astrocytoma (hairlike elongated neoplastic glial cells) with Rosenthal fibers (eosinophilic cell processes).

Treatment

- Management of optic nerve gliomas is controversial because of the variability in natural history of these tumors; although most remain stable or progress slowly, others may grow rapidly.
- Treatment includes observation with serial MRI, chemotherapy (first line for progressive lesions), radiation (if chemotherapy fails), or surgical excision.
- Radiation therapy is given for nonresectable tumors with chiasmal invasion.
- Surgical excision involves optic nerve resection and therefore results in blindness; thus, tumor should be excised for growth toward the chiasm or for a blind proptotic eye.

References

Lee AG. Neuroophthalmological management of optic pathway gliomas. *Neurosurg Focus* 2007;23(5):E1.

Liu GT. Optic gliomas of the anterior visual pathway. *Curr Opin Ophthalmol* 2006;17:427–431.

Meningioma

Clinical Features

- Intracranial meningioma:
  - More common than primary optic nerve meningioma and can invade the orbit resulting in secondary optic nerve sheath meningioma.
  - Middle-aged adult women.
  - Sphenoid bone most commonly involved.
  - Proptosis, chemosis, lid edema, temporal fullness, late visual loss.
  - CT: bony change, hyperostosis.
- Optic nerve meningioma (Figure 7.8):
  - Middle-aged adult women; less commonly, children with neurofibromatosis.
  - Proptosis, decreased vision, papilledema or optic atrophy, optociliary shunt vessels (collaterals from retinal to choroidal venous circulation; seen in 25% to 30%), choroidal folds.
  - CT/MRI: diffuse thickening or fusiform enlargement of optic nerve, nodular surface, "train track" sign (central lucent zone), intralesional calcification.

Pathology

- Meningothelial cells in various patterns.
- Psammoma bodies (calcified whorls of degenerated cells).

Treatment

- Meningiomas are slow-growing tumors that may be observed while following the patient carefully for vision loss, motility disturbances, or ocular exposure that is due to proptosis.
- Intracranial meningioma:
  - Excise for vision loss, motility disturbance, or ocular exposure.
  - Combined approach with neurosurgery for surgical resection or debulking.
- Optic nerve meningioma:
  - More conservative treatment of optic nerve than intracranial meningioma, because of tumor location.
  - Tumor is resected with risk of intracranial tumor spread, progressive growth, or poor vision.
  - Complete surgical excision of optic nerve is performed with a blind eye and progressive tumor.
  - Stereotactic radiotherapy is considered an early treatment option to stabilize and even improve vision.

References

Dutton JJ. Optic nerve sheath meningioma. *Surv Ophthalmol* 1992;37:167–183.

Jeremic B, Pitz S. Primary optic nerve sheath meningioma. *Cancer* 2007;110:714–722.

Plexiform Neurofibromas

Clinical Features

- Infiltrative, well-vascularized tumor within eyelid, orbit.
- Upper lid lesion: "bag of worms," S-shaped eyelid.
- Associated with neurofibromatosis type 1.
- Higher incidence of glaucoma in the ipsilateral eye.

Pathology

Intertwining bundles of Schwann cells, axons, and endoneural fibroblasts

Treatment

Debulk lesions with caution.

Schwannoma

Clinical Features

- Painless proptosis in middle-aged individuals.
- Ten percent of schwannomas occur in patients with neurofibromatosis.
- Usually benign with slow progression, rare malignant transformation.
- CT: well-circumscribed ovoid tumor.

Pathology

- Encapsulated proliferation of Schwann cells.
- Antoni A: tightly packed Schwann cells; Verocay body (palisading nuclei).
- Antoni B: loosely arranged Schwann cells; degeneration within the tumor.

Treatment

Excision.

Neuroblastoma

Summary

- Most common metastatic orbital lesion in children.
- Primary malignancy located in the adrenal medulla and less commonly in the cervical ganglia that can result in ipsilateral Horner syndrome.
- Abrupt ecchymotic proptosis, bilateral in about 50%.

Mesenchymal Tumors

Rhabdomyosarcoma

Summary

Rhabdomyosarcoma, the most common primary orbital malignancy of childhood, should be suspected in any child with the rapid onset of an orbital process. Biopsy of a suspected lesion should be performed immediately. The survival rate of patients with rhabdomyosarcoma has improved significantly with the use of chemotherapy and radiation therapy.

Signs and Symptoms

- Sudden onset of unilateral proptosis.
- Eyelid swelling, injection, ecchymosis.
- Pain and decreased vision are uncommon.

Demographics

Onset: age 7 to 8 years.

Ophthalmic Findings

- Proptosis (80% to 100%), downward and lateral displacement of globe.
- Palpable mass: superonasal quadrant in 70%.
- Ptosis: may be the first sign.
- Conjunctival and lid edema and erythema.

Systemic Findings

Regional lymphadenopathy with metastatic spread to lung and bone.

Special Tests

- CT: Look for bony destruction; lesion may appear circumscribed or infiltrative.
- Immediate biopsy.
- Metastatic workup: CXR, bone marrow biopsy, lumbar puncture.

Pathology

- Embryonal:
  - Most common type.
  - Superonasal quadrant of the orbit.
  - Loose fascicles of undifferentiated spindle cells with rare cross striations.
- Alveolar:
  - Most malignant form.
  - Inferior orbit.
  - Fibrovascular strands form alveolar-like compartments, which are lined with rhabdomyoblasts.
- Pleomorphic:
  - Rarest form.
  - Occurs in adults.
  - Well differentiated with easily located cross striations.
- Botyroid embryonal:
  - Variant of embryonal that occurs in grapelike clusters with invasion from the paranasal sinuses or conjunctiva.

Disease Course

- Rapid progression of tumor with bony invasion and metastasis to lymph nodes, lung, bone marrow, and brain.
- Prognosis is based on staging of disease and histopathologic features with range from best to worse prognosis: adult pleomorphic > embryonal (including botyroid) > alveolar.

Treatment and Management

- When rhabdomyosarcoma is suspected, an immediate biopsy should be performed (complete or near-complete excisional biopsy), with an appropriate metastatic workup to stage the disease.
- Radiation therapy and chemotherapy are the mainstays of treatment, resulting in a 95% 5-year survival rate.

Differential Diagnosis

Orbital cellulitis.
Idiopathic orbital inflammation.
Neuroblastoma.
Lymphangioma with hemorrhage.
Capillary hemangioma.
Ruptured dermoid cyst.

References

Shields JA, Shields CL. Rhabdomyosarcoma: review for the ophthalmologist. *Surv Ophthalmol* 2003;48:39–57.

Wharam M, Beltangady M, Hays D, et al. Localized orbital rhabdomyosarcoma: an interim report of the intergroup rhabdomyosarcoma study committee. *Ophthalmology* 1987;94:251–254.

Fibrous Histiocytoma

Clinical Features

Most common adult mesenchymal tumor of the orbit.
Middle-aged adults.
Proptosis, decreased vision.
Range of benign to malignant based on clinical behavior.
Local recurrence, rare metastasis.
CT: well-circumscribed homogeneous mass (similar to cavernous hemangioma or schwannoma).

Pathology

Fibroblasts and histiocytes in cartwheel or storiform pattern; diagnosis of exclusion after immunohistochemistry rules out other spindle cell tumors such as solitary fibrous tumor (CD34), melanoma (S100, HMB-45), and leiomyoma (smooth muscle antigen, desmin).

Treatment

Complete surgical resection or irradiation (malignant fibrous histiocytoma).

Reference

Shields JA, Shields CL. Orbital fibrous histiocytoma. In: Shields JA, ed. *Eyelid, conjunctival, and orbital tumors*, 2nd ed. Philadelphia, PA: Lippincott Williams & Wilkins, 2008:626–631.

Solitary Fibrous Tumor

Clinical Features

- Can involve any part of the orbit, following an indolent course.
- Middle-aged adults.
- Local recurrence with incomplete excision.

Pathology

- Spindled-shaped cells uniformly reactive to CD34, unlike other benign orbital tumors.

Treatment

- Complete surgical excision.

Reference

Bernardini FP, Concilis C, Schneider S, et al. Solitary fibrous tumor of the orbit. *Ophthalmology* 2003;110:1442–1448.

Fibro-Osseous Tumors of the Orbit

See Table 7.11.

Reference

Selva D, White VA, O'Connell JX, et al. Primary bone tumors of the orbit. *Surv Ophthalmol* 2004;49:328–342.

Histiocytic Tumors

Langerhans Cell Histiocytosis (Histiocytosis X)

Clinical Features

- Tender palpable superotemporal mass, rhinorrhea.
- First decade of life.
- Results from abnormal accumulations of Langerhans cells—histiocytes normally found in the epidermis.
- Eosinophilic granuloma: solitary lytic bone lesion with soft tissue involvement.
- Hand-Schüller-Christian syndrome: triad of diabetes insipidus, exophthalmos, and multifocal bony lesions.
- Letterer-Siwe: fulminant fatal systemic disease with visceral involvement.

Pathology

- Granulomatous-histiocytic infiltrate.
- Electron microscopy: tennis-racket–shaped Birbeck granules.

Treatment

Surgical curettage, systemic or local corticosteroids, local irradiation, cytotoxic agents.

Reference

Margo CE, Goldman DR. Langerhans Cell Histiocytosis. *Surv Ophthalmol* 2008;53:332–358.

Ocular Adnexal Lymphoid Tumors

Summary

Lymphoproliferative lesions occur as a continuum from benign lymphoid hyperplasia (polyclonal) to malignant lymphoma (monoclonal) and should be regarded as a potentially systemic process. Orbital lymphoma is the most common malignant orbital tumor affecting older adults.

Signs and Symptoms

- Progressive, painless gradual proptosis.
- Motility disturbances.
- Firm nodular anterior orbital mass.
- Subconjunctival salmon patch.
- Bilateral disease in 25% of cases.
- Lacrimal gland involvement.

Demographics

Sixth and seventh decades of life.
Rare in children.

Systemic Findings

Risk of developing systemic non-Hodgkin lymphoma based on anatomic site of origin (lowest to highest): conjunctival (10%), orbital (50%), and eyelid (66%).

Table 7.11

Fibro-osseous tumors

Lesion	Clinical characteristics	Pathology
Fibrous dysplasia	Onset in late childhood Monostotic (single) or polyostotic (multiple) bony lesions Frontal bone most common monostotic site, then sphenoid, ethmoid Vision loss with sphenoid involvement Albright syndrome (polyostotic, precocious puberty, cutaneous pigmentation) CT: lucency and sclerosis of bone ("ground glass"), poorly defined	Immature woven bone and osteoid in a cellular fibrous matrix without osteoblastic rimming
Ossifying fibroma	Second and third decades, women Monostotic (frontal followed by ethmoid and maxillary bones), slowly progressive lesion with displacement of orbital structures CT: well-circumscribed homogeneous lesion with distinct margin	Lamellar bone with vascular stroma and rim of osteoblasts
Osteoma	Fourth to fifth decades, men Arises within sinuses, frontoethmoidal most common Proptosis, globe displacement, sinusitis Gardner syndrome—bone tumors, CHRPE, intestinal polyps CT: dense oval mass occluding sinus	Lamellar bone with cellular stroma
Osteogenic sarcoma	Most common primary malignancy of bone Occurs in familial retinoblastoma, especially after radiation Painful globe displacement, diplopia, decreased vision CT: lytic and sclerotic changes with soft tissue infiltration	Foci of osteoid production within anaplastic sarcomatous stroma

CT, computed tomography; CHRPE, congenital retinal pigment epithelial hypertrophy.

Special Tests

CT/MRI: usually homogeneous lesions that mold to orbital tissues without displacing them, no bony involvement.

Systemic workup: physical examination; CBC, CXR, bone marrow biopsy, bone scan; CT scan of abdomen, pelvis, chest; serum immunoprotein electrophoresis.

Fresh specimen for touch preparation, immunohistochemistry, flow cytometry, genetic studies.

Pathology

- Benign reactive lymphoid hyperplasia: lymphoid follicles with mitotic activity, polymorphous infiltration (lymphocytes, plasma cells, histiocytes), polyclonal population of lymphocytes, predomination of T cells, endothelial cell proliferation.
- Atypical lymphoid hyperplasia: lymphoid follicles, polymorphous response, but lacks mitotic activity and endothelial cell proliferation. May still be associated with systemic disease.
- Lymphoma: Follicles, if present, lack mitotic activity and endothelial cell proliferation, monoclonal population of atypical lymphocytes, usually B cell.
- Mucosa-associated lymphoid tissue (MALT) lymphoma: often presents as a conjunctival "salmon patch" that responds very well to irradiation.

Disease Course

- All forms of lymphoproliferative lesions should be examined for systemic involvement.
- Lymphoma may occur years after presentation of the orbital lymphoid lesion.

Treatment and Management

- Biopsy of the lesion should be performed with fresh tissue sent for immunohistochemical and gene rearrangement studies.
- Benign reactive or atypical lymphoid hyperplasia: irradiation of 1,000 to 2,500 rads
- Lymphoma: irradiation of 2,000 to 4,000 rads.
- Disseminated disease: chemotherapy.

Differential Diagnosis

Metastasized orbital lesions: cavernous hemangioma, schwannoma, hemangiopericytoma, fibrous histiocytoma.

Table 7.12

Lacrimal gland tumors

Inflammatory, Infectious	Idiopathic orbital inflammation (dacryoadenitis), Sjögren syndrome, sarcoid, *Mycobacterium tuberculosis*, *M. leprae*, mumps, staphylococcal species
Lymphoid	Benign reactive lymphoid hyperplasia, atypical lymphoid hyperplasia, lymphoma
Epithelial	50% benign, 50% malignant • Benign: pleomorphic adenoma Malignant (in order of frequency): adenoid cystic carcinoma, malignant mixed tumor, primary adenocarcinoma, mucoepidermoid carcinoma.

Lacrimal gland tumor, inflammation: Sjögren syndrome.

Plasma cell tumors: circumscribed orbital tumor of plasmacytoma or fulminant orbital involvement of multiple myeloma.

References

Ferry JA, Fung CY, Zukerberg L. Lymphoma of the ocular adnexa: a study of 353 cases. *Am J Surg Pathol* 2007;31:170–184.

Jakobiec FA. Ocular adnexal lymphoid tumors: progress in need of clarification. *Am J Ophthalmol* 2008;145:941–950.

Jakobiec FA, Neri A, Knowles DM. Genotypic monoclonality in immunophenotypically polyclonal orbital lymphoid tumors: a model of tumor progression in the lymphoid system. *Ophthalmology* 1987;94:980–994.

Lacrimal Gland Tumors

See Tables 7.12 and 7.13.

Table 7.13

Epithelial lacrimal gland tumors

Tumor	Clinical findings	CT appearance	Pathologic findings	Treatment
Pleomorphic adenoma (benign mixed tumor)	Fourth to fifth decade, firm mass in lacrimal fossa, slowly developing (>1 y), globe displaced down and medially, no pain	Well-circumscribed mass with pressure remodeling of lacrimal fossa	Proliferation of epithelial cells with cartilagenous, mucinous, or bony degeneration of stroma	Complete excision with pseudocapsule without a preliminary biopsy; may recur with tumor spill; malignant transformation may occur
Malignant mixed tumor	Older men, painful, rapidly progressive tumor; history of incomplete excision of benign mixed tumor	Lacrimal mass with deep extension within orbit, bony destruction	Arises *de novo* or within a benign mixed tumor, frequent mitoses, sparse stroma	Biopsy, followed by wide en bloc surgical resection, 25% survival
Adenoid cystic carcinoma	Second and fourth decade, more rapidly progressive painful lesion (<1 y), lacrimal mass, proptosis, paresthesias, motility disturbance	Lacrimal fossa mass with possible extension toward orbital apex, bony erosion, less well circumscribed	Cribiform Swiss cheese pattern—densely packed hyperchromatic cells with intervening cystic spaces; perineural invasion	Biopsy and examination of permanent sections, followed by radical orbital exenteration with removal of bone and other involved structures, possible adjuvant radiotherapy, possible intra-arterial chemotherapy in conjunction with above therapies; radical surgery may not prolong life; poor prognosis

CT, computed tomography.

Table 7.14

Metastatic orbital tumors

Age	Source	Features
Pediatric	Neuroblastoma	Primary tumor in abdomen, mediastinum, or neck Metastasis to inferior orbit, often with ecchymotic proptosis; most common orbital metastasis in children CT: bony destruction Congenital neuroblastoma of superior cervical ganglia: ipsilateral Horner syndrome with iris heterochromia
Pediatric	Leukemia	Acute lymphoblastic leukemia most likely to metastasize to orbit Granulocytic sarcoma (chloroma, primary orbital leukemia) may occur before blood or bone marrow signs of acute myelogenous leukemia
Adult	Breast	Most common metastasis in women Frequently has history of breast carcinoma May result in enophthalmos, motility disturbance, ptosis due to sclerosing lesion
Adult	Lung	Most common metastasis in men May not have prior history of lung carcinoma

Management

- Pertinent history includes duration of symptoms, associated pain: Rule out inflammatory or infectious causes mentioned above.
- Obtain imaging studies.
- Perform biopsy or excise lacrimal gland completely based on clinical presentation and CT scan.
- Pain and bony erosion tend to be associated with malignancy.
- Benign mixed tumor is the only tumor that must be removed completely without prior biopsy, to prevent seeding of the orbit with possible subsequent recurrence or malignant transformation.

References

Shields JA, Shields CL, Epstein J, et al. Review: primary epithelial malignancies of the lacrimal gland: the 2003 Ramon L. Font lecture. *Ophthal Plast Reconstr Surg* 2004;20:10–21.

Stewart WB, Krohel G, Wright J. Lacrimal gland and fossa lesions: an approach to diagnosis and management. *Ophthalmology* 1979;86:886–895.

Metastatic and Secondary Orbital Tumors

See Tables 7.14 and 7.15.

Reference

Shields JA, Shields CL, Brotman HK, et al. Cancer metastatic to the orbit. The 2000 Robert M. Curts Lecture. *Ophthal Plast Reconstr Surg* 2001;17:346–354.

ORBITAL TRAUMA

Midfacial Fractures

Le Fort classification:

Le Fort I: low transverse maxillary fracture, no orbital involvement.

Le Fort II: pyramidal fracture involving nasal, lacrimal, and maxillary bones, medial orbital walls involved.

Le Fort III: craniofacial dysjunction; watch for airway compromise, involves lateral wall, floor and medial wall.

Table 7.15

Secondary orbital tumors

Source	Tumor
Conjunctiva	Squamous cell carcinoma, melanoma
Globe	Retinoblastoma, choroidal melanoma
Eyelid	Sebaceous carcinoma, squamous carcinoma, basal cell carcinoma
Sinus	Mucocele: cystic lesion most commonly arising from frontoethmoid complex as a result of obstructed sinus drainage, erodes bone, treated with excision of mucocele and obliteration of sinus with fat Squamous cell carcinoma: originates from maxillary sinus or nasopharynx
Brain	Meningioma, encephalocele

Table 7.16

Orbital wall fractures

Location	Signs	Management
Medial wall	Orbital emphysema, decreased horizontal motility If involvement of orbital rim: telecanthus, lacrimal system injury CT: opacified ethmoid sinus, fracture	Surgical repair for muscle entrapment, telecanthus If otherwise asymptomatic, may observe, tell patient not to blow nose, consider antibiotics
Orbital roof	Ptosis, limitation of elevation, supraorbital hypesthesia, CSF rhinorrhea, pulsating exophthalmos CT: pneumocephalus, intracranial hemorrhage, fracture	Surgical repair in conjunction with neurosurgery for symptomatic displaced fractures Intravenous antibiotics
Zygoma "tripod fracture"	Inferior displacement of lateral canthus, trismus (difficulty opening mouth, malar flattening) CT: zygomatic arch, inferior orbital rim, and zygomaticofrontal suture fractures	Displaced and/or symptomatic fractures should be repaired
Optic canal	Decreased vision, afferent pupillary defect CT: fracture, sphenoid sinus opacification, nerve sheath hematoma	Treatment with high-dose corticosteroids and/or optic nerve decompression is very controversial

CT, computed tomography; CSF, cerebrospinal fluid.

Orbital Wall Fracture

See Table 7.16.

Orbital Floor Fracture

Summary

Traumatic fractures of the orbital floor, a blow-out fracture if the orbital rim is not involved, may result in enophthalmos and diplopia. Fracture repair is performed approximately 7 to 14 days after injury for enophthalmos, diplopia in a functional field of gaze, or a large fracture. Observation for up to a month following injury for cases with minimal symptoms does not seem to adversely affect outcome if surgery is performed late.

Etiology

- Direct force to orbital rim causes fracture of rim.
- Compressive force to rim causes buckling and subsequent fracture of floor.
- Increased orbital pressure causes thin portion of floor to fracture.

Signs and Symptoms

- Initially: lid edema, ecchymosis.
- Proptosis, or enophthalmos.
- Diplopia with restriction of vertical eye movements.
- Infraorbital nerve hypesthesia.
- "White eye," nausea, bradycardia in children with trap door blow-out fracture and vagal symptoms.

Ophthalmic Findings

Rule out ruptured globe.
Rule out traumatic optic neuropathy.

Special Tests

- Plain films (facial series): disruption of the floor of the orbit with opacification of the maxillary sinus. Not useful for evaluation of fractures.
- CT (Figure 7.9): floor fractures best visualized with coronal cuts; maxillary sinus air/fluid level.

Disease Course

- Observe for 1 week for resolution of motility disturbance resulting from edema, hemorrhage, or muscle contusion.
- Persistent motility defect attributable to entrapment or to extraocular muscle or nerve injury: may perform forced ductions to delineate.
- Unrepaired large fracture may result in late enophthalmos.

Treatment and Management

- Treat children with "white eyed" blow-out fracture, restriction of globe movement, and entrapment on scan immediately.
- Treat with ice compresses, possible antibiotics, no nose blowing for 1 week.
- Repair very large fractures within first week.
- Operate in 7 to 14 days for patients with entrapment, enophthalmos greater than 2 mm, fracture of more than 50% of floor, diplopia in useful fields of vision.

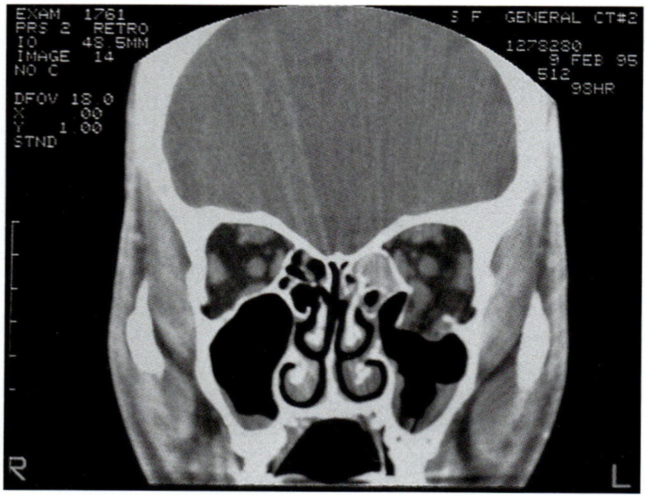

FIGURE 7.9. Coronal computed tomography scan demonstrating left-side blow-out fracture.

References

Dal Canto AJ, Linberg JV. Comparison of orbital fracture repair performed within 14 days versus 15 to 29 days after trauma. *Ophthalmic Plast Reconstr Surg* 2008;24:437–443.

Dortzbach RK. Orbital floor fractures. *Ophthalmic Plast Reconstr Surg* 1985;1:149–151.

Hawes MJ, Dortzbach RK. Surgery on orbital floor fractures: influence of time of repair and fracture size. *Ophthalmology* 1983;90:1060–1070.

Sires BS, Stanley RB Jr, Levine LM. Oculocardiac reflex caused by orbital floor trapdoor fracture: an indication for urgent repair. *Arch Ophthalmol* 1998;116:955–956.

Orbital Emphysema

Clinical Features

- May be able to palpate subcutaneous air.
- Can cause increase in orbital pressure and arterial occlusion.

Treatment

- Observe in majority of cases as long as there is no visual compromise.
- If decreased vision, arterial occlusion, can place needle into air pocket and drain into syringe filled with water.

Orbital Foreign Bodies

Clinical Features

- Localize foreign body with x-ray examination or CT.
- MRI is contraindicated for metallic foreign bodies.

Treatment

- Remove foreign body if vegetable matter or located anteriorly with sharp edges.
- Observe if posterior or an inert substance.

Orbital Hemorrhage

Clinical Features

- Upper and lower lid ecchymosis.
- Subconjunctival hemorrhage.
- Decreased ocular motility.
- Possible increased orbital tension, decreased vision, afferent pupillary defect, increased intraocular pressure, central retinal artery occlusion.

Etiology

- Retrobulbar injection.
- Traumatic injury.
- Following eyelid or orbital surgery.
- Coagulopathy.

Treatment

- If hemorrhage is postsurgical, open incisions and evacuate clot.
- If vision threatening: lateral canthotomy *and* lysis of inferior limb of lateral canthal tendon (Figures 7.10 and 7.11).
- Lower intraocular pressure: mannitol, acetazolamide, timolol, apraclonidine.
- If pressure remains elevated in orbit and globe and central retinal artery is occluded or pulsating, consider orbital decompression.

Reference

Liu D. A simplified technique of orbital decompression for severe retrobulbar hemorrhage. *Am J Ophthalmol* 1993;116:34–37.

Enucleation, Evisceration, Exenteration

See Table 7.17.

References

Afrin SI, Budenz DL, Albert DM. Does enucleation in the presence of endophthalmitis increase the risk of post-operative meningitis? *Ophthalmology* 1987;94:235–237.

Bilyk JR. Enucleation, evisceration, and sympathetic ophthalmia. *Curr Opin Ophthalmol* 2000;11(5):372–386.

Green WR, Maumenee AE, Sanders JE, et al. Sympathetic uveitis following evisceration. *Trans Am Acad Ophthalmol Otolaryngol* 1972;76:625–644.

Anophthalmic Socket: Late Complications

Clinical Features

- Implant exposure or extrusion: Porous implants may provide better motility with peg placement than nonporous implants but are associated with higher

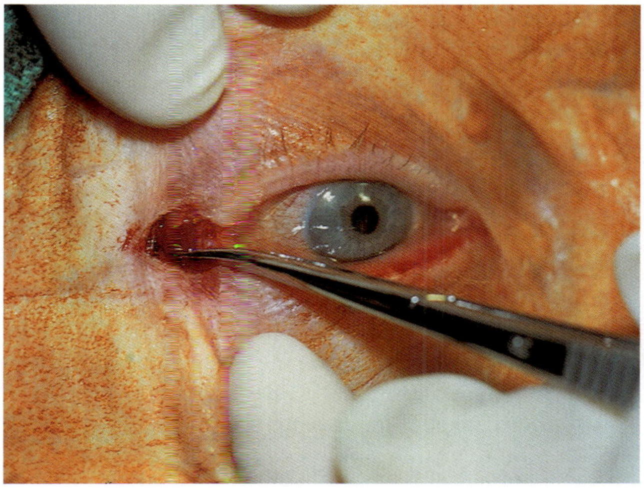

FIGURE 7.10. Lateral canthal tendon is incised.

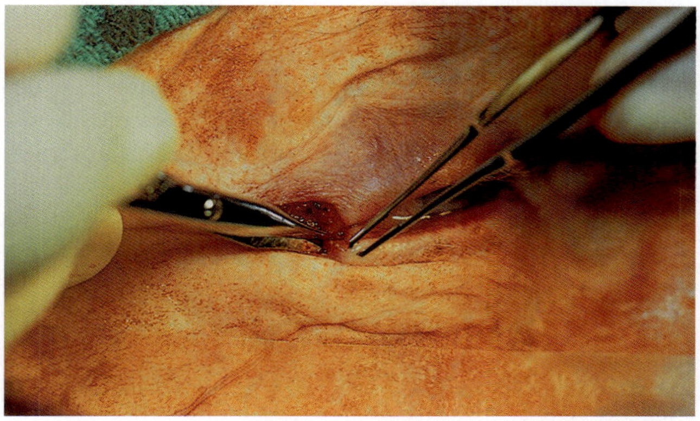

FIGURE 7.11. Lysis of inferior limb of lateral canthal tendon.

Table 7.17

Enucleation, evisceration, and exenteration

Procedure	Definition	Indications	Advantages	Disadvantages
Enucleation	Removal of globe	Intraocular tumor, blind painful eye, blind disfigured eye, prevention of posttraumatic sympathetic ophthalmia, panophthalmitis. B-scan ultrasonography pre-op with opaque media	Pathology, reduce risk of sympathetic ophthalmia, motility improving with integrated implant coupled to the prosthesis	More disruption of orbital anatomy, late socket contracture, implant exposure or extrusion
Evisceration	Removal of intraocular contents	Blind painful eye, endophthalmitis, blind disfigured eye B-scan ultasonography pre-op with opaque media to completely exclude intraocular malignancy	Usually better motility than enucleation, simple operative technique	No pathology, possibility of unsuspected tumor, possibility of sympathetic ophthalmia (very low)
Exenteration	Removal of globe and surrounding orbital soft tissues	Malignant tumors with orbital invasion, malignant lacrimal gland tumors, orbital fungal infections (e.g., *Mucor*)	Complete removal of malignancy if confined to the periorbita	Disfiguring operation, intraoperative risk of cerebrospinal fluid leak or hemorrhage, sino-orbital or naso-orbital fistulas
Retrobulbar alcohol	Injection of absolute alcohol into retrobulbar space	Blind painful eye	Eliminates pain without surgical procedure	Painful, ptosis, scarring within orbit, more difficult later enucleation, theoretical risk of intranerve sheath injection and brainstem injury

PLASTICS

exposure/extrusion rates with conjunctival and Tenon's breakdown over surface of implant.

- Deficient orbital volume: deep superior sulcus, enophthalmos, lower lid laxity or ectropion, ptosis.
- Contracted socket: failure to retain prosthesis, absent or insufficient fornices.

Treatment

Implant exposure or extrusion: conjunctival autografts, vascularized flaps, dermis fat grafts.

Deficient orbital volume: Replace spherical orbital implant with larger size, or place flat subperiosteal orbital implant on orbital floor.

Contracted socket: buccal mucus membrane grafts, hard palate grafts to reform fornix in conjunction with lateral canthoplasty, dermis fat graft.

Reference

Liu D. A comparison of implant extrusion rates and postoperative pain after evisceration with immediate or delayed implants and after enucleation with implants. *Trans Am Ophthalmol Soc* 2005;103:568–591.

EYELID

Anatomy

See Figures 7.12 and 7.13

Structures Encountered at Different Levels of the Eyelids

See Table 7.18. and Figure 7.12.

Attachments and Salient Points of Eyelid Structures

Orbicularis Muscle

- Functions as a sphincter to close the eyelids and as part of the lacrimal pump system.
- Innervated by the facial nerve (cranial nerve [CN] VII).
- Divided into pretarsal, preseptal, and orbital segments.
- Pretarsal and preseptal orbicularis involved in involuntary eyelid movements (blink), while orbital portion more involved in forced eyelid closure (winking and blepharospasm).
- Pretarsal orbicularis of upper and lower eyelids has a medial anterior attachment, which becomes part of the anterior limb of the medial canthal tendon, and a medial posterior attachment, Horner tensor tarsi muscle, which passes posterior to the canaliculi to attach to the posterior lacrimal crest; upper and lower eyelid pretarsal orbicularis muscles fuse in the lateral canthal area to become part of the lateral canthal tendon.
- Preseptal orbicularis of the upper and lower eyelids has a medial anterior attachment, which becomes part of the anterior limb of the medial canthal tendon, and a medial posterior attachment, Jones muscle, into the

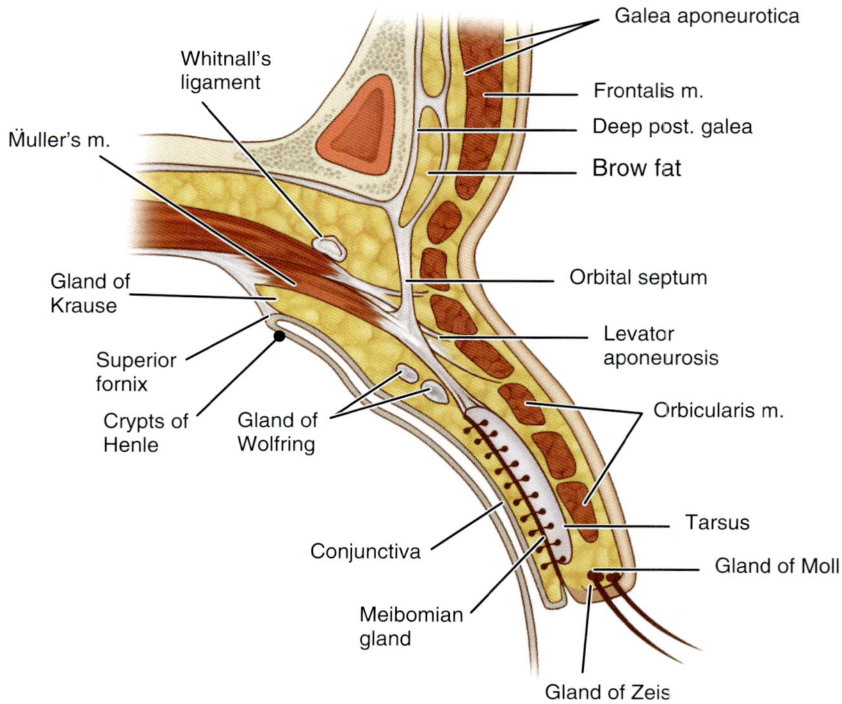

FIGURE 7.12. Sagittal section of upper eyelid.

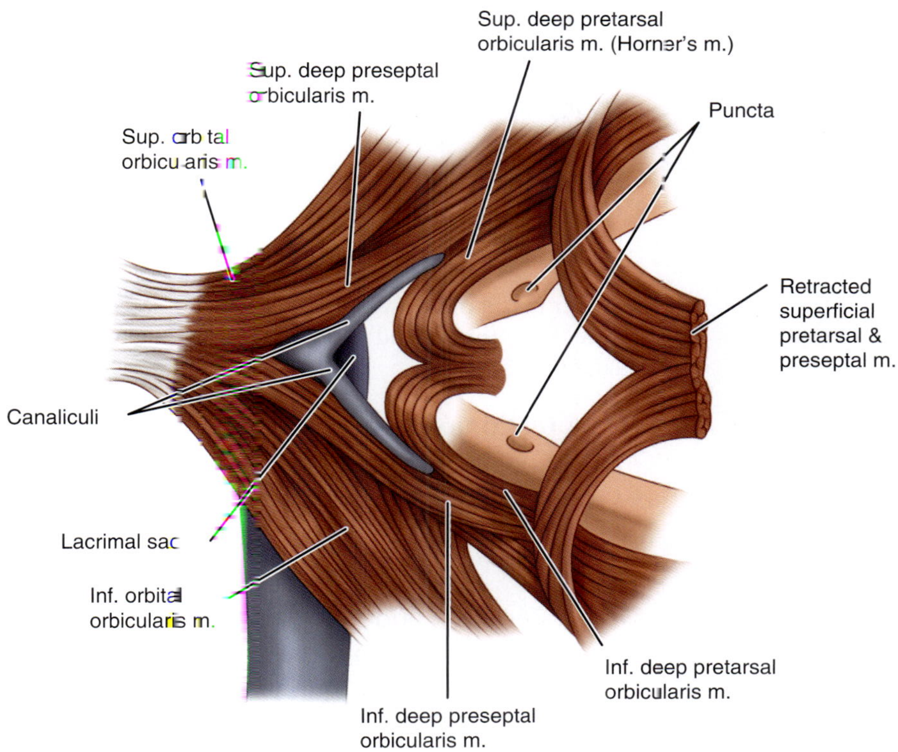

FIGURE 7.13. Medial canthal tendon attachments.

lacrimal diaphragm of the tear sac; laterally the preseptal muscles form the lateral palpebral raphe overlying the lateral orbital rim.
- The orbital orbicularis muscle arises from the anterior limb of the medial canthal tendon and periosteum and encircles the orbit.

Orbital Septum

- A barrier between the eyelid and the remainder of the orbit, limiting the spread of infection and hemorrhage, posterior to orbicularis muscle and anterior to orbital fat.
- Thin fibrous sheet arises from periosteum over the superior (arcus marginalis) and inferior orbital rims and inserts medially at the posterior lacrimal crest and laterally just anterior to the lateral orbital tubercle.
- Upper eyelid: Septum fuses with the levator aponeurosis approximately 4 mm above the superior tarsal border in Whites; closer to the eyelid margin in Asians.
- Lower eyelid: Septum fuses with the capsulopalpebral fascia approximately 4 mm below the inferior tarsal border in whites; this complex, along with the inferior tarsal smooth muscle, inserts on the tarsus.

Eyelid Fat Pads

- Located posterior to the orbital septum in the upper and lower eyelids.
- Upper lid: two preaponeurotic fat pads, medial more white, prolapsed orbital lacrimal gland can be mistaken for a lateral "fat pad."
- Lower lid: three fat pads, inferior oblique muscle courses between the medial and central fat pads.

Levator Palpebrae Superioris Muscle

- Raises the upper eyelid.
- Innervated by the superior division of the oculomotor nerve (CN III).
- Muscle originates in the apex of the orbit above the annulus of Zinn and is approximately 40 mm long.
- Whitnall ligament is a condensation of the anterior sheath of the levator muscle and acts as a fulcrum for the action of the aponeurosis in the superior orbit; medially, it attaches to connective tissue around trochlea and superior oblique tendon; laterally, it sends septa through the stroma of lacrimal gland and arches upward to attach to inner aspect of the lateral orbital wall approximately 10 mm above the lateral orbital tubercle.
- Muscle becomes aponeurosis approximately 14 to 20 mm above superior tarsal border; medial horn of the aponeurosis inserts onto the posterior lacrimal crest; lateral horn divides the orbital and palpebral lobes of the lacrimal gland and inserts onto the lateral orbital tubercle.

Table 7.18

Structures encountered at different levels of the eyelids

Level	Structures
Upper eyelid	
4 mm above the margin	Skin > pretarsal orbicularis > levator aponeurotic attachments onto anterior tarsus > tarsus > conjunctiva
13 mm above the margin	Skin > preseptal orbicularis > septum > preaponeurotic fat pads > levator aponeurosis > Müller muscle > conjunctiva
Lower eyelid	
3 mm below the margin	Skin > pretarsal orbicularis > tarsus > conjunctiva
6 mm below the margin	Skin > preseptal orbicularis > septum > fat pads > capsulopalpebral fascia > inferior tarsal muscle > conjunctiva

- Aponeurosis divides into anterior and posterior portions 3 to 4 mm above the superior border of tarsus; anterior portion sends fibers to overlying orbicularis and skin to form the upper eyelid crease; posterior portion inserts onto the anterior surface of the lower two thirds of the tarsus.

Müller Muscle

- Sympathetically innervated muscle.
- Originates from the undersurface of the levator muscle near the transition of the levator muscle to the aponeurosis.
- Inserts onto the superior border of tarsus.

Capsulopalpebral Fascia

- Arises from the inferior rectus muscle and divides to encircle the inferior oblique muscle.
- Anterior to the inferior oblique muscle, the two portions join to form Lockwood suspensory ligament (analogous to Whitnall ligament in the upper lid).
- Extends further anteriorly, sending strands to the inferior conjunctival fornix, overlying orbicularis muscle and skin.
- Inserts onto the inferior tarsus.

Inferior Tarsal Muscle

- Sympathetically innervated muscle analogous to Müller muscle.
- Originates on the posterior surface of the capsulopalpebral fascia.
- Inserts into the inferior border of tarsus, with the capsulopalpebral fascia.

Tarsus

- Composed of firm, dense connective tissue (not cartilage).
- Upper eyelid plate measures 9 to 10 mm vertically.
- Lower eyelid plate measures 4 mm or less vertically.
- One mm thick, and thins out both medially and laterally.

Palpebral Conjunctiva

- Most posterior layer of eyelids.
- Contains accessory lacrimal glands of Krause and Wolfring that are responsible for basal tear secretion and goblet cells producing mucus.

Medial Canthal Tendon

Superior and inferior limbs of tendon arise from medial aspects of tarsal plates and orbicularis muscle, split anteriorly and posteriorly to envelope the lacrimal sac, and insert on the anterior and posterior lacrimal crests.

Lateral Canthal Tendon

- Superior and inferior limbs of tendon arise from lateral aspects of tarsal plates and orbicularis muscle and insert on the inner aspect of the lateral orbital rim at the lateral orbital tubercle.
- Inserts 3 mm higher than the medial canthal tendon.

Lateral Orbital Tubercle (Whitnall's)

Attachments to this structure include the lateral canthal tendon, lateral retinaculum, and Lockwood ligament; check ligament of lateral rectus muscle and lateral horn of levator aponeurosis.

Eyelid Margin

Structures, anterior to posterior:

Eyelash follicles.

Gray line (muscle of Riolan): an isolated section of pretarsal orbicularis muscle.

Meibomian gland orifices.

Conjunctiva.

Vascular Supply of the Eyelids

- Internal carotid via the ophthalmic artery and its branches (supraorbital and lacrimal); the external carotid via the arteries of the face (angular and temporal).
- Upper eyelid: Marginal arterial arcade lies 2 mm superior to margin and anterior to tarsal plate, and a peripheral arterial arcade lies superior to tarsus and between aponeurosis and Müller muscle.

- Lower eyelid: often only one arterial arcade located at inferior tarsal border.

Venous Drainage

- Pretarsal tissues drain into angular vein medially and into the superficial temporal vein laterally.
- Posttarsal tissues drain into orbital veins and the deeper branches of the anterior facial vein and the pterygoid plexus.

Lymphatic Drainage

- Medial portion of eyelids drains into the submandibular lymph nodes.
- Lateral portion drains, first, into the superficial preauricular nodes and then into deeper cervical nodes.

Sensory Nerve Supply

- Branches of the ophthalmic division of the trigeminal nerve (V_1) innervate the forehead, upper eyelid, lateral and medial periocular areas, and tip of the nose.
- Branches of the maxillary division (V_2) innervate the lower eyelid and cheek region.

Terminology

See Table 7.19.

Congenital Eyelid Defects

See Table 7.20.

References

Kikkawa DO, Lemke BN. Orbital and eyelid anatomy. In: Dortzbach RK, ed. *Ophthalmic plastic surgery: prevention and management of complications*. New York, NY: Raven Press, 1994:1–29.

Saunders DH, Flanagan JC. Disorders of the lids. In: Nelson LB, Calhoun JH, Harley RD, eds. *Pediatric ophthalmology*, 3rd ed. Philadelphia, PA: WB Saunders, 1991:334–354.

Approach to Acquired Eyelid Disorders

Normal Eyelid Parameters

See Table 7.21.

- Upper lid examination: Evaluate for retraction and ptosis (MRD_1, LF, lid crease), inward and outward turning of eyelid margin, misdirected eyelashes, redundant upper lid skin and fat, eyelid lesions.
- Lower lid examination:
  - Evaluate for retraction (MRD_2), lid laxity (see below), inward or outward turning of the lid margin, cicatricial skin (see below), or conjunctival changes and eyelid lesions.
  - To test for lower eyelid horizontal laxity:
    - Snap test: positive if the lower eyelid, after being pulled away from the globe, does not return to its normal location without a blink.
    - Distraction test: positive if the lower eyelid can be pulled more than 8 mm away from the globe.
  - To test for cicatricial skin changes: If lower lid cannot be stretched superiorly to the superior corneal limbus without difficulty, cicatricial skin changes are present.
- Eyelid disorders are surgically repaired by attempting to restore the normal anatomy.
  - If the eyelid is lax, a horizontal shortening procedure, such as a lateral canthoplasty, should be performed.
  - If cicatricial changes in skin or conjunctiva exist, the scar tissue should be replaced with a skin graft.
  - If the levator aponeurosis is dehisced from the tarsus resulting in ptosis, it should be reattached to the tarsus.

Table 7.19

Terminology

Anterior lamella: skin, orbicularis
Middle lamella: orbital septum
Posterior lamella: structures posterior to the septum (tarsus, conjunctiva, retractor muscles)

Ectropion

Summary

An outward turning of the eyelid margin.

Signs and Symptoms

Ocular irritation and redness.
Tearing.
Loose lower lid turned away from globe.

Ophthalmic Findings

Horizontal lid laxity and/or cicatricial skin changes.
Papillary hypertrophy of the exposed palpebral conjunctiva with possible keratinization.
Pooling of tears in the lower eyelid.
Inferior exposure keratopathy.

Classification and Treatment

See Table 7.22.

Disease Course and Natural Progression

- Continued out-turning of the eyelid margin may lead to conjunctival keratinization and punctal scarring.
- Exposure keratopathy may result in corneal infection.
- Punctal ectropion and lid laxity result in epiphora.

Table 7.20

Congenital eyelid defects

Defect	Description
Ankyloblepharon	Partial or complete fusion of the eyelids by webs of skin
Blepharophimosis syndrome	Autosomal dominant Triad of telecanthus, epicanthus inversus, and ptosis Lower lid ectropion may occur
Coloboma	Cleft usually in medial upper eyelid May be associated with other facial clefts (Pierre Robin syndrome), lacrimal deformities, and Goldenhar syndrome Avoid using lid-sharing procedures (Hughes, Cutler-Beard) to repair colobomas in infants and children, which may lead to occlusion amblyopia
Cryptophthalmos	Partial or complete absence of the eyebrow, palpebral fissure, eyelashes, and conjunctiva, with fusion of the partially developed adnexal structures to underlying globe Globe is usually malformed and microphthalmic associated with dyscephaly, syndactyly, genitourinary tract abnormalities
Distichiasis	Congenital or acquired extra row of eyelashes along the openings of meibomian glands Associated with mandibulofacial dysostosis and trisomy 18 Initial treatment includes ocular lubricants and soft contact lenses Surgical treatments: cryotherapy, lid splitting with cryotherapy, or excision of the involved tarsal plate with mucosal graft
Epicanthus	Medial canthal skin fold Epicanthus tarsalis: fold most prominent in the upper eyelid Epicanthus inversus: fold most prominent in the lower eyelid Epicanthus palpebralis: fold equally distributed in the upper and lower eyelids
Epiblepharon	Excess pretarsal orbicularis muscle and skin override the eyelid margin to turn eyelashes vertically or against the globe The lid margin itself is not rotated inward, as in entropion Over time this resolves in many children Surgical repair is sometimes necessary: a strip of skin and orbicularis are excised just below or above the eyelid margin, and defect closed
Euryblepharon	Widening of palpebral fissure caused by horizontal lengthening of the temporal portion of lower eyelid and vertical skin shortening Lateral canthal tendon is often inferiorly displaced Surgical repair includes a full-thickness block resection of the involved eyelid, repositioning of the lateral canthal tendon, and full-thickness skin graft to area of vertical shortening

Reference

Anderson RL, Gordy DD. The lateral tarsal strip procedure. *Arch Ophthalmol* 1979;97:2192–2196.

Entropion

Summary

Inversion of the eyelid margin.

Signs and Symptoms

Ocular irritation and redness.

Tearing

Eyelid turned inward against globe.

Ophthalmic Findings

- Eyelid margin and lashes rotated inward against globe.
- Lid laxity.
- Entropion can be elicited in intermittent cases by having the patient forcefully squeeze the eyelids closed.
- Trichiasis with inferior bulbar conjunctival injection and chemosis, inferior keratopathy.
- Possible cicatricial conjunctival disease

Table 7.21

Normal eyelid measurements

Value	Description	Normal finding
Margin reflex distance 1 (MRD_1)	Distance from upper lid margin to pupillary light reflex	4 mm
Margin reflex distance 2 (MRD_2)	Distance from lower lid margin to pupillary light reflex	6 mm
Palpebral fissure height	Distance between upper and lower lids	10 mm
Upper lid crease height	Distance from lash line to crease	Variable, depending on sex: white men, 9–10 mm; women 8–9 mm; race: whites, 7–10 mm; Asians, 0–10 mm
Levator muscle function (LF)	Measure excursion of upper lid from downgaze to upgaze, fixating brow to prevent frontalis action	12–15 mm

Table 7.22

Classification and treatment of ectropion

Type	Etiology	Treatment
Congenital	Rare and sometimes associated with the blepharophimosis syndrome Caused by a vertical shortage of the anterior lamella	Mild: no treatment or lubrication with artificial tears or ointment Severe or symptomatic: anterior lamella must be lengthened vertically with skin graft
Involutional	Due to lower-lid laxity secondary to age- and gravity-related effects Disinsertion of lower eyelid retractors may also facilitate outward turning of the margin	Horizontal laxity addressed with a tightening procedure (i.e., lateral canthoplasty) May also attempt reinsertion of the lower eyelid retractors
Paralytic	Results from facial paralysis and loss of orbicularis tone of the lower eyelid Can also occur with local anesthetic injection	Temporary: observe Permanent: horizontal tightening procedure such as lateral and or medial canthoplasty
Cicatricial	Results from shortening of the anterior lamella from thermal or chemical burns, actinic skin damage, or scarring after trauma or lower eyelid surgery	If cicatrix is acute, treat for 6 mo with steroid massage or injections After 6 mo, surgical correction may be undertaken Scar bands, if present, are lysed with the eyelid on stretch Lateral canthoplasty with full-thickness skin graft from the upper lid or retroauricular region is used to correct the skin deficiency; midface lift may be considered to provide additional skin
Inflammatory	Results from shortening of the anterior lamella by chronic inflammation and scarring Causes include rosacea dermatitis, atopic dermatitis, eczematoid dermatitis, herpes zoster infections, and allergic reactions to chronic use of topical eye drops	Allergic reagent should be stopped if possible The inflamed eyelids should be treated with steroid ointment or injections Surgical correction is the same as for cicatricial ectropion
Mechanical	Caused by bulky eyelid tumors	Tumors should be excised If a cicatricial component is present, a full-thickness skin graft or myocutaneous advancement flap is needed

Trachoma: follicles in the upper palpebral conjunctiva, Herbert pits along the corneal limbus, Arlt line of scarring in the upper palpebral conjunctiva, superior macropannus.

Ocular cicatricial pemphigoid: older patients with symblepharon in the lower cul-de-sac, dry eye, papillary conjunctival reaction, corneal scarring.

Classification of Entropion

See Table 7.23.

Disease Course and Natural Progression

Continued rubbing of eyelashes against the corneal surface causes epithelial breakdown leading to possible scarring, thinning, perforation, or infection.

Differential Diagnosis

- Acquired misdirection of eyelashes secondary to inflammation, prior surgery, tumor
  - Lid margin is in normal position.
  - Few lashes can be treated with epilation with forceps or electrolysis.
  - Larger areas of misdirected lashes can be treated with cryotherapy using double-freeze (to –20°C) procedure; complications with cryotherapy include loss of skin pigmentation, notching of the margin, and persistent eyelid erythema and swelling.
  - Rarely, a wedge resection of the involved section of the eyelid is necessary.
- Distichiasis: see above "Congenital Eyelid Defects."
- Epiblepharon: see above "Congenital Eyelid Defects."

References

Dortzbach RK, McGetrick JJ. Involutional entropion of the lower eyelid. *Adv Ophthalmic Plast Reconstr Surg* 1983;2:257–267.

Quickert MH, Rathbun E. Suture repair of entropion. *Arch Ophth* 1971;85:304.

Blepharoptosis

Summary

Blepharoptosis, or drooping of the upper eyelid margin, is most commonly caused by age-related dehiscence of the levator aponeurosis or other involutional changes. Patients must be thoroughly examined for other neurogenic or myogenic causes.

Signs and Symptoms

Ptotic upper lid with the margin to reflex distance of the upper lid less than 3 mm.

Table 7.23

Classification of entropion

Type	Etiology	Treatment
Congenital	Associated with lower eyelid retractor dysgenesis, structural defects in the tarsal plate, and relative shortening of the posterior lamella	Mild: correct with excision of skin and muscle inferior to the lid margin Severe: may need posterior lamella lengthening procedures with spacer grafts such as hard palate
Acute spastic	Occurs with ocular irritation or inflammation after intraocular surgery Sustained squeezing or squinting of eyelids causes the eyelid margin to roll inward	Treat ocular irritation with lubrication, or intraocular inflammation with topical steroid Consider temporary Quickert-Rathbun rotation sutures
Involutional	Combination of: horizontal laxity of the lower eyelid; attenuation or disinsertion of the lower eyelid retractors; and overriding of the preseptal over the pretarsal orbicularis muscle	Temporary Quickert-Rathbun rotation sutures Horizontal tightening procedure, rotation sutures, full-thickness horizontal blepharotomy incisions, and reattachment of the lower lid retractors have all been used separately or in combination for a more permanent repair; transconjunctival retractor repair
Cicatricial	Results from shortening of the posterior lamella by cicatricial conjunctival processes: OCP, Steven-Johnson syndrome, trachoma, herpes zoster, enucleation, thermal or chemical burns, or chronic eye-drop usage	Treat underlying disease process (Cytoxan for OCP) or eliminate offending agents, such as eye drops, if possible Lengthen posterior lamella with a graft (buccal mucous membrane, hard-palate graft) in conjunction with rotation sutures and lateral canthoplasty

OCP, ocular cicatricial pemphigoid.

Obstructed superior vision.
Ocular fatigue.

Evaluation

Assessment of ptosis should include the following:
MRD_1, levator function, upper eyelid crease height.
Extraocular movements and pupil size.
Basal tear secretion test and dry eye assessment.
Brow ptosis, lower eyelid position, and laxity.
Visual field testing.
Unilateral congenital ptosis places the child at risk for amblyopia; this should be assessed early and treated promptly.

Diagnosis

- Although the most common form of ptosis seen in adults is due to levator aponeurosis dehiscence, other myogenic and neurogenic causes must be ruled out.
- Levator function is usually normal in levator aponeurosis dehiscence but poor in many myogenic and neurogenic causes
- Pupil size may help differentiate causes of neurogenic ptosis: the pupil is dilated in a third nerve palsy and miotic in Horner syndrome.
- Age of the patient is important: elderly individuals commonly develop levator dehiscence ptosis; middle-aged patients may have myasthenia, although levator dehiscence ptosis can occur with contact lens wear in this age group; children usually have congenital ptosis.
- Variability in the ptosis suggests myasthenia.

Classification of Ptosis

See Table 7.24

Differential Diagnosis

- Dermatochalasis: redundancy of upper eyelid skin, often associated with anteriorly prolapsed orbital fat; redundant skin can hang over the upper eyelid margin and give the appearance of blepharoptosis; dermatochalasis is often associated with true ptosis; surgical repair is achieved with blepharoplasty.
- Blepharochalasis: rare familial condition usually occurring in young women; episodic idiopathic inflammatory edema of the upper eyelids, which may lead to ptosis
- Pseudoptosis: contralateral eyelid retraction, enophthalmos or phthisis bulbi, hypotropia.

References

Beard C. Types of ptosis. In: Beard C, ed. *Ptosis*, 3rd ed. St. Louis, MO: Mosby, 1981:39–75.

Carter SR, Meecham WJ, Seiff SR. Silicone frontalis slings for the correction of blepharoptosis. *Ophthalmology* 1996;103:623–630.

Putterman AM, Urist MJ. Mueller's muscle—conjunctiva resection ptosis procedure. *Ophth Surg* 1978;9:27–32.

Eyelid Retraction

Summary

Upper and lower lid retraction occurs with an MRD_1 of greater than 4 mm and an MRD_2 of greater than 6 mm (Table 7.21). Frequently associated with scleral show, this leads to ocular exposure and irritation. Eyelid retraction is commonly due to thyroid ophthalmopathy.

Etiology

Thyroid eye disease: especially with lateral flare of upper lid
Congenital.
Neurologic: Parinaud syndrome, midbrain lesions, hydrocephalus, aberrant oculomotor nerve regeneration.
Contralateral ptosis: Herring phenomenon.
Postsurgical: ptosis repair, lower lid blepharoplasty. strabismus surgery, orbital fracture repair.
Posttraumatic.

Signs and Symptoms

- Ocular irritation, tearing.
- Retraction of upper lid from normal position 2 mm below superior limbus.
- Retraction of lower lid from normal position at the inferior limbus.
- Lagophthalmos.
- Conjunctival injection and keratopathy.
- Other signs of thyroid eye disease, midbrain disease.

Special Tests

- Thyroid function studies.
- MRI if pupil or motility signs of midbrain disease.

Disease Course and Natural Progression

Continued poor eyelid closure, especially with poor Bell reflex, leads to exposure keratopathy and possible corneal perforation or infection.

Treatment and Management

- Upper eyelid:
  - Mild: ocular lubrication.
  - Moderate to severe: recess the levator aponeurosis alone or in combination with an excision or recession of Müller muscle.
- Lower eyelid:
  - Mild: ocular lubrication.
  - Moderate to severe: recess the retractors with placement of graft material (e.g., hard palate graft, sclera, fascia, auricular cartilage) in combination with a lateral tarsal strip procedure and/or midface lift.

Reference

Bartley GB. The differential diagnosis and classification of eyelid retraction. *Ophthalmology* 1996;103:168–176.

Table 7.24

Classification of ptosis

Type	Etiology	Signs	Treatment
Congenital	Maldevelopment of the levator muscle Blepharophimosis syndrome Congenital ptosis with upgaze deficiency	Decreased levator function Lid lag on downgaze Lagophthalmos Weak or absent eyelid crease Chin-up position Marcus Gunn "jaw winking" (caused by abnormal connections between trigeminal and oculomotor nerves): lid opens wider with jaw movement Possible strabismus, amblyopia Epicanthus inversus, telecanthus of blepharophimosis	Good levator function (>8 mm): attempt levator resection Moderate levator function (5–7 mm): attempt maximal levator resection Poor levator function (<4 mm): attempt frontalis suspension Amount of levator resection depends on degree of ptosis and levator muscle function Frontalis suspension attaches eyelid to frontalis muscle using autogenous fascia lata or synthetic substances such as silicone rod
Myogenic (acquired)	Myasthenia gravis	Decreased levator function, weak or absent eyelid crease Variable ptosis with decreased function, increasing ptosis with fatigue, lid twitch, possible ocular motility disturbance or systemic skeletal muscle weakness Due to antibodies to acetylcholine receptors at neuromuscular junction Improvement in ptosis with edrophonium (Tensilon)	Although one may try a levator aponeurotic repair, patients with severe myogenic ptosis usually require frontalis suspension Rule out thymoma. Consider thymectomy or cholinesterase inhibitor (e.g., pyridostigmine [Mestinon]) If the ptosis is stable for more than 2 y and not controlled with medications, may attempt surgical repair In patients with severe ptosis and poor eye-protective mechanisms, perform reversible and flexible frontalis suspension with material such as silicone rod
	Chronic progressive external ophthalmoplegia (CPEO)	Gradually progressive ptosis with decreased levator function, extraocular motility weakness Kearns-Sayre syndrome: CPEO, heart block, retinal pigmentation Due to mitochondrial DNA abnormality	
	Oculopharyngeal dystrophy	Poor levator function, difficulty swallowing Occurs in French Canadians, autosomal dominant	

(Continued)

Aponeurotic	Disinsertion, dehiscence, or attenuation of levator aponeurosis from its normal position on anterior surface of tarsus usually due to aging May also be caused by eye surgery, eyelid edema (postoperative, inflammatory, blepharochalasis), eyelid tumors, contact lens wear, allergy with rubbing	Normal levator function Lid droop on downgaze (reading position) Higher than normal eyelid crease Thin eyelid	Reattachment of the levator aponeurosis to the anterior superior border of tarsus; conjunctiva-Muller muscle resection. Must assess tear function prior to repair.
Neurogenic	Horner syndrome (in congenital cases, there is iris atrophy and heterochromia)—disruption of superior cervical sympathetic chain from hypothalamus to spinal cord, spinal cord to superior cervical ganglion (SCG), SCG along internal carotid artery to Muller muscle/inferior tarsal muscle/papillary dilator muscle. Forceps delivery, trauma, neck surgery, neuroblastoma (children), apical lung tumor, carotid artery dissection	Mild ptosis, miosis, and anhidrosis Lower eyelid position may be elevated as well	Consider ordering CXR, CT of chest/head/neck (apical lung tumor in smokers), MRA (carotid dissection) Place a drop of 2.5% phenylephrine in the eye and wait 5 min; if the eyelid rises sufficiently, a Müller muscle resection is likely to be curative
	Third-nerve palsy	Other signs such as extraocular motility disorder are always present If pupil is dilated, must rule out posterior communicating artery aneurysm	For stable ptosis, may consider frontalis suspension with silicone slings Very conservative repair due to poor Bell reflex
Mechanical	Secondary to neoplasms, intraorbital foreign body, or dislodged bone fragments impinging on levator muscle or preventing eyelid from opening	Poor levator function, lid lag on downgaze, normal eyelid crease	Evaluate with CT or MRI scan or orbit Excision or removal of restrictive element
Traumatic	Secondary to blunt or sharp trauma to upper eyelid May be neurogenic, myogenic, aponeurotic, or cicatricial	Variable depending on cause Usually decreased levator function	If levator muscle has been lacerated, repair immediately Otherwise, wait at least 6 mo before performing any surgical repair, since ptosis may spontaneously improve

CPEO, chronic progressive external ophthalmoplegia; CT, computed tomography; MRI, magnetic resonance imaging.

Eyelid Tumors

See Tables 7.25 and 7.26; Figures 7.14 to 7.20.

Evaluation

Recognition of possible malignant lesions is essential.
History:

- Length of time lid lesion present.
- Change in size or appearance of the lesion.
- Recurrence of a lesion that has previously been treated.
- History of skin cancers, degree of sun exposure, previous skin radiation, diagnosis of basal cell nevus syndrome.

Treatment and Management

- Biopsy should be performed for any suspected eyelid lesions, including the following:
    - Any pigmented lesion that has changed in size, color, thickness.
    - Pearly nodules, possibly with central ulceration.
    - Nonhealing, bleeding lesions.
    - Lesions associated with lash loss, especially in patients without blepharitis.
- Chronic blepharoconjunctivitis that is not responsive to therapy may be sebaceous carcinoma; biopsy of the conjunctiva or any palpable lid nodules should be performed.
- Because malignant and benign lesions may appear similar, biopsy of the lesion should be performed if there is any doubt, especially in elderly patients.
- Long-term follow-up is necessary for all patients with an eyelid malignancy.

References

Boulos PR, Rubin PA. Cutaneous melanomas of the eyelid. *Semin Ophthalmol* 2006;21:195–206.

Donaldson MJ, Sullivan TJ, Whitehead KJ, et al. Squamous cell carcinoma of the eyelids. *Br J Ophthalmol* 2002;86:1161–1165.

Rao NA, Hidayat AA, McLean IW, et al. Sebaceous carcinomas of the ocular adnexa: a clinicopathologic study of 104 cases with five-year follow-up data. *Hum Pathol* 1982;13:113–122.

Shields JA, Demirci H, Marr BP, et al. Sebaceous carcinoma of the eyelids: personal experience with 60 cases. *Ophthalmology* 2004;111:2151–2157.

Surgical Repair of Eyelid Defects

See Table 7.27.

Reference

McCord CD Jr. System of repair of full-thickness eyelid defects. In: McCord CD Jr, Tanenbaum M, eds. *Oculoplastic surgery*, 2nd ed. New York, NY: Raven Press, 1987:117–127.

Benign Essential Blepharospasm

Summary

Bilateral condition characterized by involuntary spasms of the orbicularis oculi muscle, which is best treated with botulinum toxin injections.

Etiology

Lesions of basal ganglia, thalamus, mesencephalon, brainstem.

Signs and Symptoms

- Bilateral lid spasms preventing patient from seeing.
- Spasms are absent during sleep.
- Associated dry eyes, levator dehiscence ptosis, brow spasm, apraxia of eyelid opening.

Demographics

Women 3:1; mean age 56.

Ophthalmic Findings

Normal muscle strength.
Decreased basal tear secretion.

Disease Course

Starts as mild twitches and may progress to forceful contractures causing limitation of useful vision.

Treatment and Management

- The majority of patients are managed with botulinum toxin injections to the involved muscles; however, in patients who do not respond well to the injections, surgical myectomy is indicated. Neurectomy is much less frequently performed because of its inherent risks.
- Botulinum toxin
    - Exotoxin produced by *Clostridium botulinum* paralyzes the orbicularis muscle.
    - Duration of action: 3 to 6 months. Onset of action: 2 to 5 days.
    - Complications include ptosis and double vision from diffusion of the toxin to either the levator or inferior oblique muscle.
- Surgical myectomy of orbicularis muscle: Complications include lagophthalmos and tissue necrosis.
- Neurectomy of facial nerve branches
  Recurrence rates may be high as 30%.
  Complete facial paralysis may occur.

Medications

Patients often have dry eyes and need ocular lubrication with artificial tears.

Table 7.25

Benign eyelid lesions

Lesion	Clinical findings and treatment	Histopathology
Chalazion (hordeolum is an acute infection of a meibomian gland, gland of Zeis or Moll)	Raised nodule caused by obstruction of meibomian gland Treat with warm compresses, lid scrubs, intralesional steroid injection (risk of hypopigmentation of skin), incision, and drainage	Chronic lipogranulomatous reaction
Papilloma	Irregular, frondlike projection of skin with a central vascular pedicle	Epidermis thrown into folds over cores of proliferating fibrovascular connective tissue, and with prominent hyperkeratosis
Verruca vulgaris	Papilloma caused by epidermal infection of papovavirus (HPV 6, 11); true viral verrucae rare on eyelid	Virus induces acanthosis, hyperkeratosis, and parakeratosis, and leads to vacuolated cells in the upper squamous layer
Seborrheic keratosis	Commonly seen in the elderly Pigmented, oily or greasy, hyperkeratotic, crustlike lesions that appear to be stuck on to the epidermis	Acanthosis, hyperkeratosis, papillomatosis, and pseudohorn cysts
Actinic keratosis	Flat, white scaly surface occurring in sun-exposed areas; premalignant condition Excisional biopsy should be performed	Ranges from dysplasia to carcinoma *in situ* with dyskeratosis, hyperkeratosis, solar elastosis, and inflammation at base of lesion
Keratoacanthoma (pseudoepitheliomatous hyperplasia is a descriptive histologic term)	Rapidly growing (weeks to a few months) lesion with a central crater filled with keratin and surrounded by hyperkeratotic margins; may regress spontaneously	Rapid proliferation of epidermoid or squamous cells may look similar to squamous cell carcinoma histologically Some pathologists believe that this is a variant of SCC, and complete excision is suggested
Molluscum contagiosum	Waxy nodule with central necrotic umbilication; may produce a follicular conjunctivitis; multiple in HIV patients; treat with excision, cryotherapy, or curettage	Hyperplasia of infected epidermis with intracytoplasmic inclusion bodies
Nevus (Figure 7.14)	Well-demarcated flat or elevated, pigmented or nonpigmented congenital lesion; may become more pigmented or cystic during adolescence or young adulthood	Collection of benign-appearing dermal melanocytes often in nests

(Continued)

Table 7.25

Benign eyelid lesions (*Continued*)

Lesion	Clinical findings and treatment	Histopathology
		Intradermal nevi occur entirely in the dermis (elevated) Junctional nevi occur at the junction between epidermis and dermis (flat) and have malignant potential Compound nevi have both junctional and intradermal components (slightly elevated) Blue nevi/nevus of Ota are associated with oculodermal melanocytosis and have an increased density of melanocytes within the dermis
Xanthelasma	Soft yellowish plaques usually in the medial canthal area; treat with excision or CO_2 laser	Aggregates of lipid-laden macrophages ("foam cells") in the superficial dermis
Juvenile xanthogranuloma	Orange to yellow nodules on the head and neck of infants and young children Spontaneous regression occurs over several years. Spontaneous hyphema indicates presence of iris lesion	Collection of histiocytes with Touton giant cells: a ring of nuclei with eosinophilic cytoplasm both within and outside of the ring
Syringoma	Multiple soft papules on lower lids of young women	Benign proliferations of eccrine sweat gland structures
Trichoepithelioma	Small yellowish nodules occurring on the eyelids or the forehead	Squamous cell cysts with immature hair follicle structures
Hydrocystoma	Translucent cyst near lid margin	Cyst wall lining may be apocrine or a low-lying cuboidal eccrine epithelium
Epithelial inclusion cyst	Raised with whitish material within the walls of the cyst	Cyst lined by keratinizing stratified squamous epithelium and filled with keratin
Amyloid	Waxy elevation with purpura Cutaneous involvement suggests a systemic disease	Deposits around blood vessels Seen with Congo red stain (dichroism) and polarized light (birefringence)

Table 7.26

Malignant eyelid tumors

Tumor	Clinical appearance	Histopathology	Treatment
BCC (Figures 7.15 and 7.16)	Most common eyelid malignancy (90%) Often located in the lower eyelid and medial canthus Firm, raised pearly nodule with telangiectasia and central ulceration May be pigmented Morpheaform tumors appear plaquelike and behave aggressively	Nests of basal cells originating from the basal cell layer with peripheral palisading and retraction artifact Various types: nodular, morpheaform, and fibrosing	Mohs micrographic surgery or excision with frozen section control, followed by reconstruction Radiation or cryotreatment have greater recurrence rates than surgical resection with margin control and should never be used for medial canthal or morpheaform lesions
SCC (Figures 7.17 and 7.18)	Erythematous, raised, scaly, and centrally ulcerated lesion may arise *de novo* or from areas of actinic keratosis Regional lymph node metastasis and perineural extension may occur	Features large pink, pale cells with abundant cytoplasm, cellular atypica, dyskeratoses, and loss of normal dermal cell polarity	CT or MRI if intraorbital or other disease may be present Mohs micrographic surgery or excision with frozen section control, followed by reconstruction Cryo and radiation not used unless patient is poor surgical candidate Systemic chemotherapy for metastatic, widespread disease
Sebaceous cell carcinoma (Figures 7.19 and 7.20)	Occurs in elderly and may mimic a chalazion or chronic blepharitis; however, lash loss may be present It invades locally and spreads to regional lymph nodes Tumor <1 cm diameter, 18% mortality; >2 cm diameter, 60% mortality Distant metastasis to lung, liver, brain	Large anaplastic cells with foamy cytoplasm Pagetoid intraepithelial spread may be present with skip areas: differentiate from SCC *in situ* Oil red O fat stain must be performed on fresh tissue	CT or MRI if intraorbital or other disease may be present Wide surgical excision with conjunctival map biopsies, frozen-section control or Mohs surgery. Exenterate large or recurrent tumors Neck dissection for lymph node metastasis
Melanoma	Rare eyelid tumor—look for variation in pigmentation, irregular border, elevated nodule Classified as lentigo maligna (10%), superficial spreading (80%), and nodular (10%) Evert the eyelid to look for palpebral conjunctival involvement Systemic evaluation for regional or distant metastasis—liver, lung, brain	Atypical melanocytes with varying degree of differentiation and invasion	Possible sentinel lymph node mapping and biopsy Wide surgical excision with 1-cm margins Frozen sections unreliable: evaluate permanent sections of margins May require lymph node dissection

BCC, basal cell carcinoma; SCC, squamous cell carcinoma.

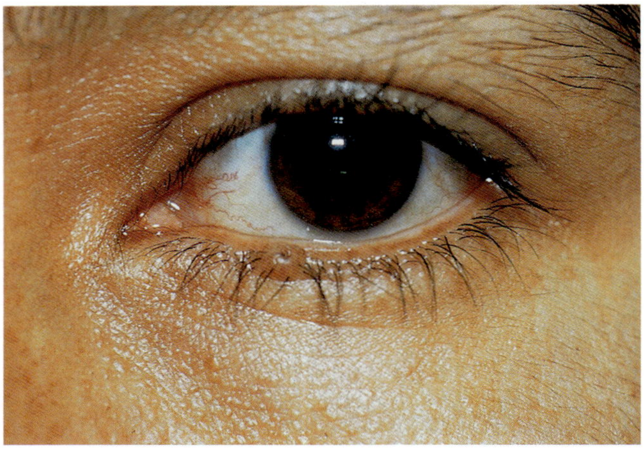

FIGURE 7.14. Lightly pigmented left lower lid nevus.

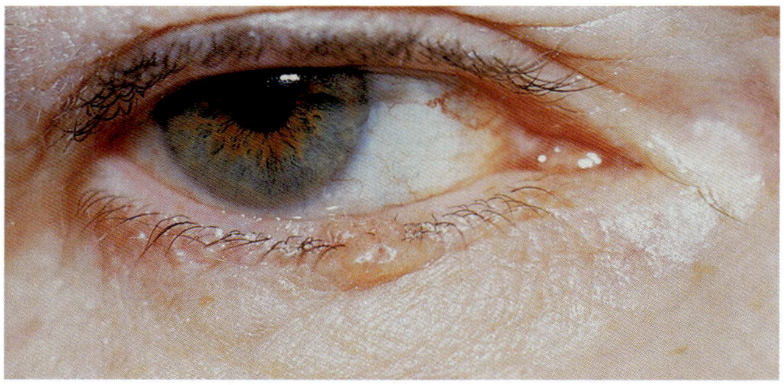

FIGURE 7.15. Right lower lid basal cell carcinoma with associated lash loss.

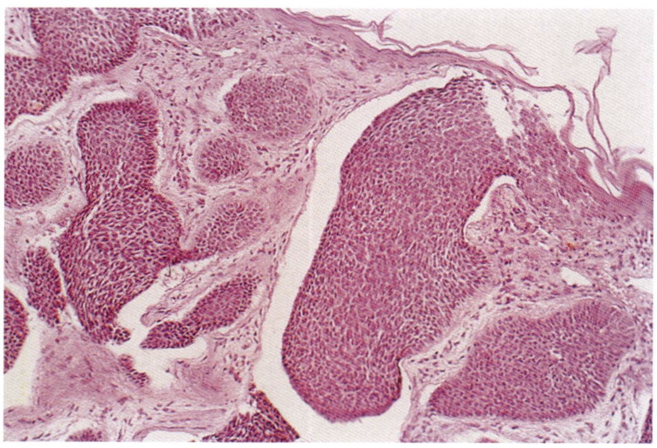

FIGURE 7.16. Basal cell carcinoma with peripheral palisading and artifactitious cleavage (H&E stain).

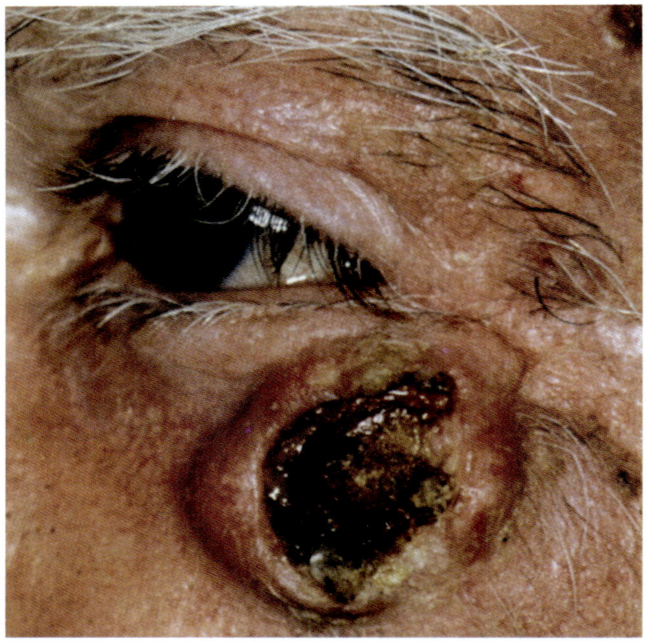

FIGURE 7.17. Squamous cell carcinoma. Large, elevated, ulcerated, and hyperkeratotic lesion.

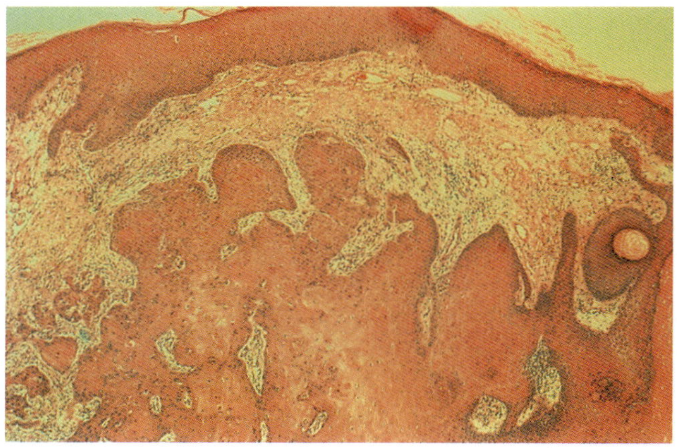

FIGURE 7.18. Squamous cell carcinoma with dermal invasion (H&E stain).

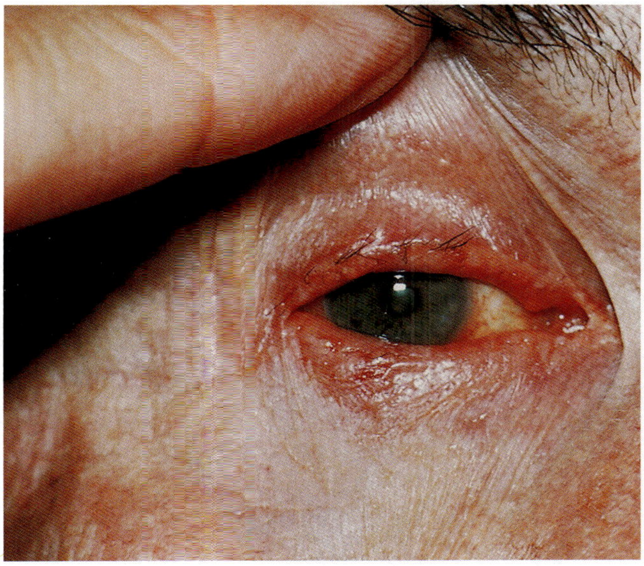

FIGURE 7.19. Sebaceous carcinoma mimicking chronic blepharitis.

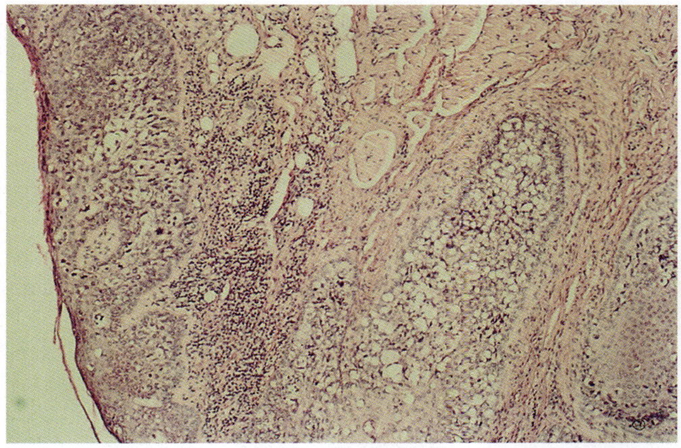

FIGURE 7.20. Anaplastic cells of sebaceous carcinoma with foamy cytoplasm.

Table 7.27

Surgical repair of eyelid defects

Defect	Repair technique
Upper eyelid	
Small (25% or less of lid margin involved)	Direct closure, may need to release the superior crus of the lateral canthal tendon
Moderate (25%–50%)	Advance lateral segment of the lid with release of the superior crus of the lateral canthal tendon alone or in combination with a semicircular skin flap (Tenzel)
Large (>50%)	Cutler-Beard: full-thickness lower eyelid advancement flap is brought superiorly
Lower eyelid	
Small	Direct closure May need to release the inferior crus of the lateral canthal tendon
Moderate	Mobilize lateral eyelid tissue with release of the inferior crus of the lateral canthal tendon alone or in combination with a semicircular skin flap (Tenzel)
Large	Hughes tarsoconjunctival flap from the central upper eyelid or Hewes tarsoconjunctival flap from the lateral upper eyelid with a full-thickness overlying skin graft or skin advancement flap Mustarde rotation cheek flap
Lateral canthus	Periosteal flap rotated to serve as lateral canthus
Medial canthus	Primary healing Full-thickness skin graft Forehead or glabellar flaps can be rotated to fill in the defect Lacrimal system must be evaluated, with possible silicone nasolacrimal intubation

PLASTICS

Differential Diagnosis

- Bilateral:
  - Meige syndrome: bilateral generalized cervicofacial spasms. Patients with benign essential blepharospasm may progress to Meige syndrome.
  - Reflex spasm: secondary to dry eyes, keratitis, entropion.
  - Neurodegenerative: Parkinson and Huntington diseases; generalized neurologic diseases not localized to the eyelids.
  - Drug induced: tardive dyskinesia–like spasms secondary to antipsychotic drugs.
- Unilateral hemifacial spasm
  - Intermittent contractures of the entire side of the face.
  - Underlying muscle weakness.
  - Present during sleep.
  - Tumor etiology (such as pontine glioma) in 0.5% to 1% of cases, MRI scan required for unilateral spasms.
  - Most common etiologic factor is vascular compression of cranial nerve VII at the brainstem by dolichoectatic basilar artery.
  - Botulinum toxin injections are effective; neurosurgical decompression of the facial nerve may be considered.
- Distal facial nerve irritative lesion: parotid tumor.
- Post–facial palsy syndrome of aberrant regeneration and synkinesis.
- Facial myokymia: rapid fine fasciculations attributable to stress, caffeine, fatigue; if condition lasts months and becomes generalized to face, consider multiple sclerosis or brainstem tumor.

References

Ben Simon GJ, McCann JD. Benign essential blepharospasm. *Int Ophthalmol Clin* 2005;45:49–75.

Bradley EA, Hodge DO, Bartley GB. Benign essential blepharospasm among residents of Olmsted County, Minnesota, 1976 to 1995: an epidemiologic study. *Ophthal Plast Reconstr Surg* 2003;19:177–181.

Dutton JJ. Botulinum-A toxin in the treatment of craniocervical muscle spasms: short- and long-term, local and systemic effects. *Surv Ophthalmol* 1996;41:51–65.

Facial Palsy

Summary

Facial palsy may result in lagophthalmos and corneal exposure, which should be treated aggressively to prevent further corneal complications.

Etiology

Tumor (cerebellopontine angle mass with associated hearing loss, vestibular dysfunction, dry eye), trauma, infection (Lyme disease, herpes zoster), surgery (for acoustic neuroma or parotid tumor), ischemia, and idiopathic (Bell palsy).

Signs and Symptoms

- Inability to close eyelids.
- Ocular irritation, pain, and tearing.
- Facial asymmetry, drooling, difficulty with speech.

Ophthalmic Findings

- Upper eyelid retraction.
- Paralytic lower eyelid ectropion.
- Lagophthalmos with exposure keratopathy.
- Pooling of tears in the lower cul-de-sac as a result of failure of the lacrimal pump.
- Forehead and eyebrow ptosis with secondary dermatochalasis.
- Check for adequacy of Bell phenomenon.
- Check for corneal sensation, as absent sensation will predispose to worse keratopathy.

Systemic Findings

- Look for other cranial nerve involvement (Bell palsy is a diagnosis of exclusion).
- Recommend examination by otolaryngologist, neurologist as necessary.

Special Tests

- May obtain MRI to look for facial nerve compression, especially when associated with an acquired hearing loss.
- Lyme disease antispirochetal antibody test.

Disease Course

- If the facial nerve function returns, observe for aberrant regeneration and hypertonicity of the muscles of facial expression.
- If the facial nerve function does not return, patients may have corneal compromise.

Treatment and Management

- Temporizing measures when the function of the facial nerve is expected to return (e.g., Bell palsy)
  - Ocular lubrication.
  - Moisture chambers and lid taping during sleep.
  - External-load weights taped to the upper eyelid.
  - Temporary tarsorrhaphy.
- Permanent facial palsy
  - Surgical placement of a gold load weight or a palpebral spring in the upper lid to treat the lagophthalmos.
  - Lateral canthoplasty for repair of the paralytic ectropion.
  - Upper lid blepharoplasty or brow lift for repair of secondary dermatochalasis.

Follow-Up

Patients with newly diagnosed facial palsy need to be followed up extremely closely; corneal drying and perforation may occur even with frequent ocular lubrication.

Reference

Seiff SR, Chang JS Jr. The staged management of ophthalmic complications of facial nerve palsy. *Ophthalmic Plast Reconstr Surg* 1993;9:241–249.

Eyelid Trauma

Evaluation

- History including blunt or sharp trauma, mode of injury, and any loss of consciousness.
- Visual acuity in both eyes.
- Examine globe to rule out rupture.
- Assess eyelids and orbit after globe integrity is ensured.
- Look for involvement of lacrimal system with laceration in medial to lacrimal puncta.

Special Tests

- Probing and irrigation of lacrimal system to assess for patency.
- Axial and coronal CT scan to rule out fractures or foreign bodies if appropriate.

Repair of Eyelid Lacerations

- The wound is irrigated with sterile saline and searched for foreign bodies.
- If orbital fat has prolapsed through the laceration, the orbital septum has been violated.
- Levator function should be assessed, and the levator repaired if lacerated.

Repair of Lid Margin Lacerations

- Good approximation and eversion of the cut edges are crucial for a good cosmetic and functional result.
- A 6-0 silk suture is placed through the gray line of the lacerated edges of the lid margin without tying it: this helps realign the lid during placement of the tarsal sutures (Figure 7.21A).
- The tarsus is reanastamosed with two (lower lid) or three (upper lid) partial-thickness 5-0 absorbable interrupted sutures.
- The grayline silk suture is tied, leaving the ends long.
- A 6-0 silk suture is placed through the lash line, leaving the ends long (Figure 7.21B).
- The skin laceration is repaired, incorporating the ends of the lid margin sutures into one of the skin sutures closest to the margin (Figure 7.21C).

Repair of Medial Canthal Lacerations

- The lacrimal system is evaluated with probing, especially if the laceration occurs medial to the punctum.
- If only one canaliculus is damaged, a monocanalicular or bicanalicular stent can be placed.
- If both canaliculi are involved, bicanalicular intubation with silicone tubing should be performed; the stents should be left in place for 3 to 6 months.
- Interrupted 8-0 absorbable sutures can be used to approximate the cut edges of the canaliculus.
- Surrounding orbicularis muscle is reapproximated with larger absorbable sutures, and the skin edges are closed.
- Avulsion of the superficial and deep heads of the medial canthal tendon results in telecanthus.
- Telecanthus is repaired either with transnasal wiring or with fixation screws drilled into the posterior lacrimal crest.

Loss of Tissue

- Because of the vascularity of the eyelid, lost tissue can be successfully implanted even after a significant amount of time.
- Eyelid tissue should not be excised at the time of primary repair.

Secondary Repair

Cicatricial changes should be addressed only after 6 months and may be treated in the interim with steroid cream massage or intralesional steroid injection.

Burns

- Ocular and eyelid lubrication with ointments and moisture chambers should be used in the short-term setting.
- Late cicatricial changes resulting from the burns can be treated with skin grafts and various types of flaps.

References

Pashby RC, Rathbun JE. Silicone tube intubation of the lacrimal drainage system. *Arch Ophthalmol* 1979;97:1318–1322.

Reifler DM: Diagnostic and surgical techniques. Management of canalicular laceration. *SurvOphthalmol* 1991;36:113–132.

PLASTICS

LACRIMAL SYSTEM

Anatomy

See Table 7.28 and Figure 7.22.

Physiology

Lacrimal pump:

Tears move from punctum to lacrimal sac, eyelids close; superficial and deep heads of pretarsal orbicularis contract, compressing the ampulla, moving the punctum medially, and horizontally shortening the

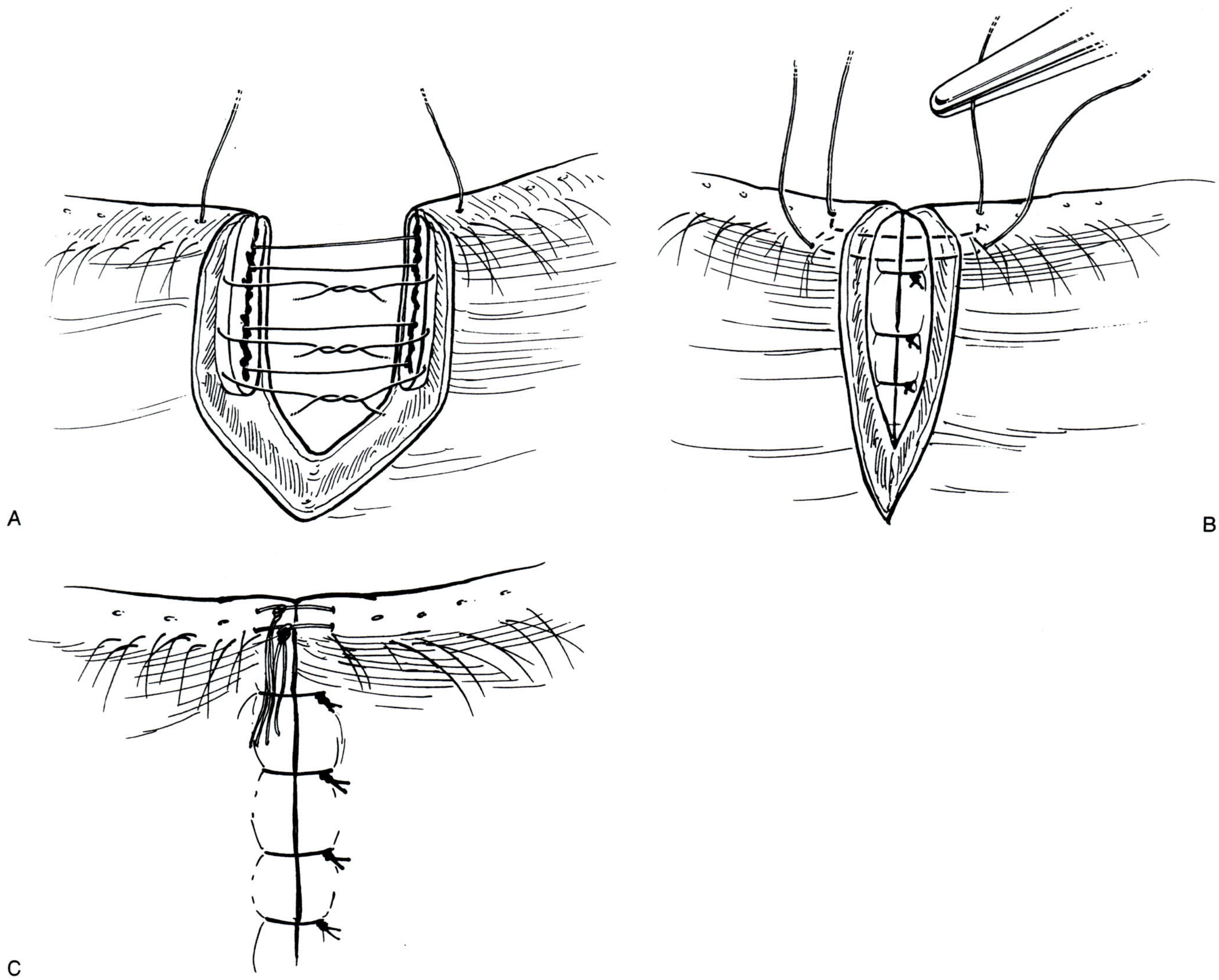

FIGURE 7.21. Repair of lid margin laceration. **A:** Place 6-0 silk suture along gray line of lid margin. Interrupted vicryl sutures realign the tarsus. **B:** A second silk suture aligns the lash line. **C:** Skin closure securing the long ends of the silk sutures away from the globe.

Table 7.28

Anatomy (Figure 7.22)

Feature	Description
Canaliculi	2 mm vertical, 8 mm horizontal, 90% of upper and lower canaliculi join to form a common canaliculus
Valve of Rosenmuller	Between common canaliculus and lacrimal sac; prevents reflux of tears from the sac to the canaliculus
Lacrimal sac	10 mm long; lies between the anterior and posterior crus of the medial canthal tendon; posterior head of the preseptal orbicularis muscle inserts onto the sac
Nasolacrimal duct	12 mm long; travels in an inferoposterolateral direction; ends beneath the inferior turbinate 30 mm from the external nares in adults, 20 mm in children
Valve of Hasner	Mucosal fold at the distal end of the nasolacrimal duct; responsible for congenital nasolacrimal duct obstruction

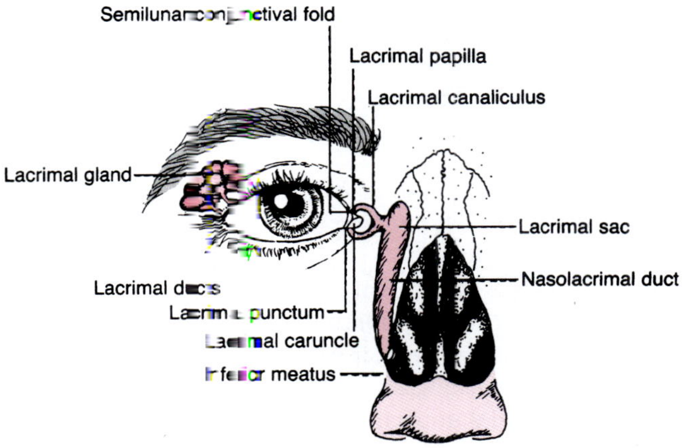

FIGURE 7.22. Anatomy of the lacrimal system.

canaliculus; superficial and deep heads of the preseptal orbicularis contract, pulling on the lacrimal sac, which expands to create negative pressure, drawing tears from canaliculi into sac.

Tears move from sac to nose, eyelids open; lacrimal sac collapses and forces tears into nose, puncta move laterally, and tears enter canaliculi.

Evaluation of Tearing Patient

See Table 7.29.

Workup

- Evaluate for hypersecretion attributable to reflex tearing associated with basal tear deficiency, corneal disease,

Table 7.29

Ancillary tests to study lacrimal system

Test	Purpose	Description
Probing and irrigation	Detects anatomic blockage	Pull lid laterally and dilate punctum; insert probe to determine patency of canaliculus Irrigate fluid to determine patency of nasolacrimal duct If fluid does not pass into the nasopharynx, the system is blocked
Dye disappearance test	Detect relative obstruction to tear outflow	Asymmetry in the amount of fluorescein 2% dye in the tear film in both eyes is observed 5 min after instillation of the fluorescein This test does not indicate origin of the problem
Jones 1 primary dye test	Detects anatomic or functional blockage	Fluorescein 2% dye is instilled in the eye and recovered from the inferior meatus after 5 min with a cotton-tipped probe Positive test result: dye is recovered; system is patent Negative test result: dye is not recovered; anatomic or functional blockage possible
Jones 2 secondary dye test	Detects functional blockage or defect in lacrimal pump	After Jones 1 test, irrigate fluorescein out of fornices Irrigate lacrimal system with saline and have patient lean forward to catch fluid from nose in basin Positive test result: dye is recovered; functional or partial blockage of nasolacrimal system Negative test result: dye is not recovered; defect in lacrimal pump because fluorescein never reached lacrimal sac
CT scan	Detect tumors, sinus disease	Obtain in cases with firm palpable medial canthal mass, bloody tears
Tear break-up time	Detects poor tear function	Tear break-up time of <10 s without blink indicates poor tear function
Basal tear secretion test	Detects basal tear secretion deficiency	With anesthesia, 10 mm or more of wetting of strips is normal at 5 min
Schirmer 1 test	Detects basal and reflex tear	Without anesthesia, wetting of 10–30 mm is normal at 5 min deficiency
Schirmer 2 test	Detects reflex tear deficiency	With anesthesia, irritate middle turbinate and watch for tearing
Dacryocystogram, dacryoscintigraphy	Detects anatomic or functional blockage	Radiopaque dye placed in tear lake or irrigated through lacrimal system and radiographs taken

CT, computed tomography.

Table 7.30

Congenital lacrimal outflow disorders

Anomaly	Description	Treatment
Punctal or canalicular dysgenesis	Absent puncta, canaliculi or extra accessory openings	Cut down over formed ampulla with absent opening may reveal patent canaliculus
Congenital dacryocystocele	Amniotic fluid and mucus-filled lacrimal sac, combined with nasolacrimal obstruction	Rule out medial encephalocele; treat with topical antibiotics and massage; if no response or infection develops, probing is necessary
Congenital NLD (Figures 7.23–7.25) NLD obstruction (Figures 7.23–7.25)	2%–4% full-term newborn infants have NLD obstruction with epiphora, one third of cases bilateral; most spontaneously resolve by 6 wk, 90% by 1 y; secondary to membranous block of the valve of Hasner	Initial: topical antibiotics, massage; probing with possible infracture of the inferior turbinate (after 6 mo, before 13 mo: success rate of probing decreases after this time) If no improvement with repeat probing, silicone tube placement or balloon dacryoplasty may help.

NLD, nasolacrimal duct.

lacrimal gland inflammation or neoplasm, central nervous system disease; slit-lamp examination, fluorescein and rose bengal staining, tear tests.

- Evaluate lower lid position, laxity, seventh-nerve function.
- Look for punctal disorders: stenosis, occlusion, ectropion.
- Probe canaliculus to rule out canalicular occlusion.
- Irrigate nasolacrimal system to evaluate for complete obstruction.
- If fluid irrigates through, Jones tests must be performed to evaluate for a partial or functional blockage on a subsequent day.
- CT scan should be obtained when tumor is suspected.

Lacrimal Outflow Disorders

See Tables 7.30 and 7.31; Figures 7.23 to 7.26.

Table 7.31

Acquired lacrimal outflow disorders

Disorder	Description	Treatment
Punctal disorders		
Punctal stenosis or occlusion	Due to inflammation, cicatrizing processes, irradiation	One-snip punctoplasty; possible silicone tube sent placement
Punctal ectropion	Poor apposition of punctum to globe, associated with lower lid laxity and ectropion	Medial conjunctival diamond-wedge resection to rotate punctum inwards; ectropion repair
Canalicular disorders		
Canaliculitis	Erythematous pouting punctum; due most commonly to *Actinomyces israelii*, a filamentous Gram-negative rod	Warm compresses, dilation and curettage, irrigate with penicillin, place on regimen of topical penicillin drops; may need canaliculotomy with curettage

(Continued)

Table 7.31

Acquired lacrimal outflow disorders (*Continued*)

Disorder	Description	Treatment
Canalicular scarring and obstruction	Due to cicatrizing conjunctivitis (herpes zoster), Stevens-Johnson syndrome, ocular cicatricial pemphigoid, medications (phospholine iodide, systemic 5-fluorouracil, docetaxel), irradiation, trauma, canaliculitis, intracanalicular plugs	Partial blockage: silicone tube stent placement; Complete blockage: conjunctivodacryocystorhinosotomy with Jones pyrex tube placement to bypass canaliculi
Lacrimal sac disorders		
Dacryocystitis (Figure 7.25)	Acute erythema, swelling, distention, and tenderness of lacrimal sac below medial canthal tendon; chronic tearing, mucopurulent discharge; secondary to *Pneumococcus*, *Streptococcus*, *Haemophilus*, or *Pseudomonas*; can be cause of orbital cellulitis; inflammatory causes include sarcoid, Wegener granulomatosis; diagnose by pressing on region of lacrimal sac and observing for reflux of pus from puncta	Acute: avoid irrigation and probing; treat with warm compresses, topical antibiotics, oral antibiotics (first-generation cephalosporin), i.v. antibiotics for severe infection; if pyocele is pointing, incise and drain, sending material for culture and sensitivity testing; dacryocystorhinostomy (DCR) should be performed when infection no longer active; DCR creates a new drainage path for tears via an anastamosis between the lacrimal sac and the nasal mucosa through a bony ostium Chronic: DCR
Dacryolith	Caused by foreign bodies such as cilia, chronic infection; may cause intermittent lacrimal obstruction	DCR
Tumors	Clinical: bloody discharge, lacrimal sac mass, intermittent epiphora; epithelial tumors most common: ratio of malignant: benign is 3:1; inverted papilloma, squamous cell carcinoma, adenocarcinoma; nonepithelial tumors: lymphoma, fibrous histiocytoma, melanoma	CT scan to evaluate firm medial canthal or lacrimal sac masses, bloody tears, suspect lesions; wide surgical resection; irradiation for lymphoid malignancies
NLD disorders		
Primary acquired NLD obstruction	Elderly women; involutional stenosis of the NLD: Inflammation and edema progress to fibrosis and cicatrization	DCR—this may be performed transcutaneously via an incision in the medial canthal region or transnasally with an endoscopic approach
Secondary acquired NLD obstruction	Midface fractures, sinus surgery, infiltrative disorders: sarcoid, Wegener granulomatosis, midline lethal granuloma; tumors: lymphoma, squamous cell carcinoma, inverting papilloma, sinonasal tumors; intranasal disease: allergic rhinitis, nasal polyps, deviated septum, tumors, previous surgery	DCR; address underlying etiology

DCR, dacryocystorhinostomy; NLD, nasolacrimal duct.

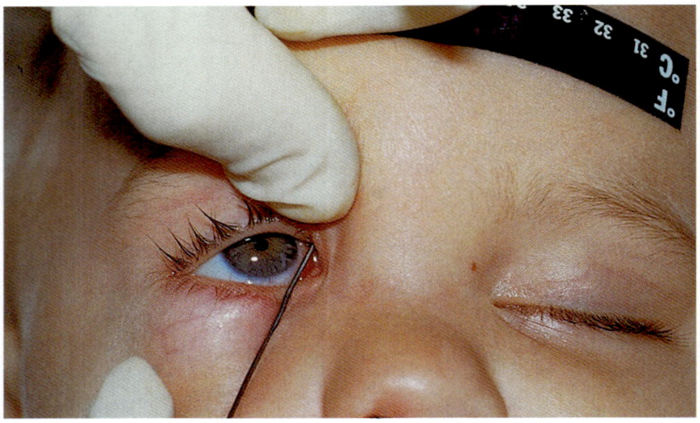

FIGURE 7.23. The probe is placed perpendicular to the eyelid margin into the superior canaliculus.

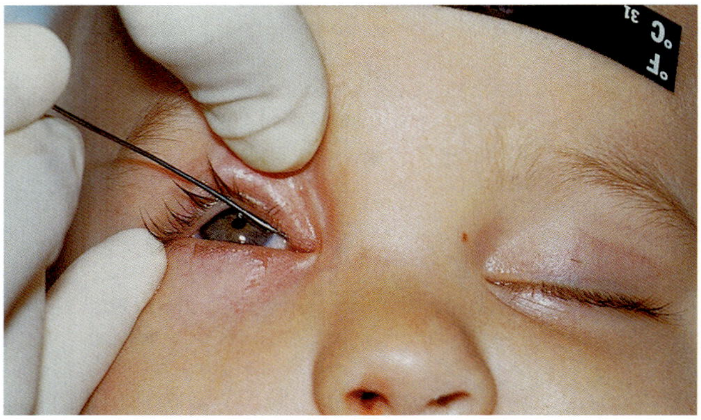

FIGURE 7.24. With the upper lid on lateral stretch, the probe is passed through the canaliculus into the lacrimal sac.

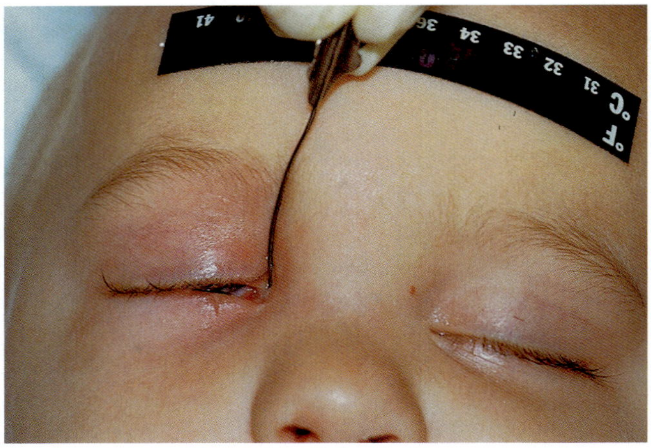

FIGURE 7.25. The probe is directed inferiorly, laterally, and posteriorly through the nasolacrimal duct.

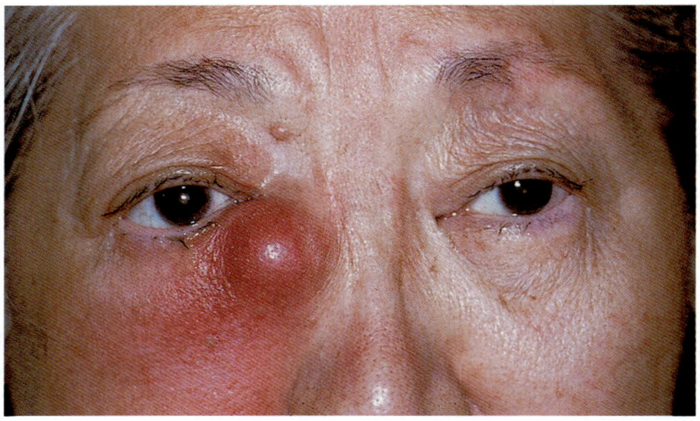

FIGURE 7.26. Acute dacryocystitis with erythema and swelling in the region of the right lacrimal sac.

References

Bartley GB. Acquired lacrimal drainage obstruction: an etiologic classification system, case reports, and a review of the literature. Part 1. *Ophthalmic Plast Reconstr Surg* 1992;8:237–242.

Bartley GB. Acquired lacrimal drainage obstruction: an etiologic classification system, case reports, and a review of the literature. Part 2. *Ophthalmic Plast Reconstr Surg* 1992;8:243–249.

Esmaeli B, Valero V, Ahmadi MA, et al. Canalicular stenosis secondary to docetaxel (taxotere): a newly recognized side effect. *Ophthalmology* 2001;08:994–995.

Katowitz JA, Welsh MG. Timing of initial probing and irrigation in congenital nasolacrimal duct obstruction. *Ophthalmology* 1987;94:698–705.

CHAPTER

8

Pediatric Ophthalmology and Strabismus

Mark J. Greenwald

EYELID DISORDERS

Epicanthus

Summary

Epicanthus is a skin fold that extends from upper to lower eyelid, overlying the medial canthus.

Demographics

- Typical in infants of Asian ethnicity.
- Common in others; diminishes over time with maturation of the face.

Symptoms and Signs

- *Pseudoesotropia* results from partial concealment of nasal sclera.
- Most evident in partial lateral gaze, which makes abducting eye appear centered in the palpebral fissure while adducting eye appears to be "in the corner" (Figure 8.1).

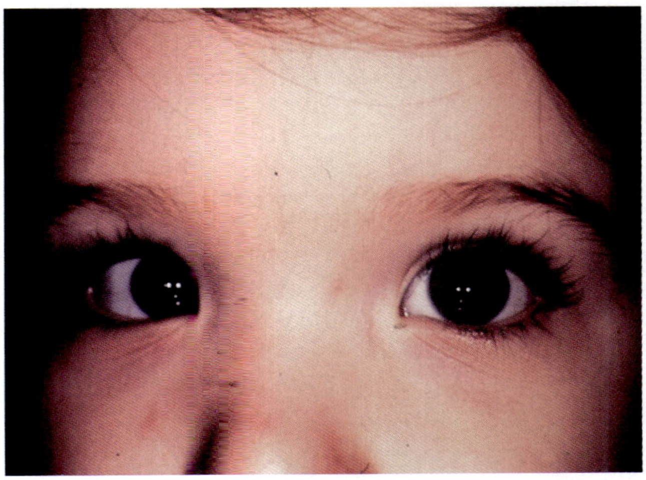

FIGURE 8.1. Pseudoesotropia caused by epicanthal folds. Slight right face turn exaggerates impression that right eye is turned inward, while left eye appears centered in the palpebral fissure.

Systemic Findings

- Many conditions involving craniofacial dysmorphism have epicanthus as a typical feature, frequently associated with additional eyelid anomaly (such as abnormal palpebral fissure slant). Foremost among these is *Down syndrome* (trisomy 21, the most common chromosomal disorder), in which epicanthus and "mongoloid" (nasal lower than temporal) fissure slant are consistently seen, and which can affect the eyes in many other ways.

  Common ocular manifestations include blepharitis, congenital nasolacrimal duct obstruction, ectropion, Brushfield spots of the iris (multiple dotlike whitish condensations of iris stroma near the pupil margin), optic disc anomalies (most commonly increased number of blood vessels), myopia, astigmatism, strabismus, and congenital nystagmus.

  There is increased incidence of cataract, glaucoma, and keratoconus in childhood. Mental impairment ranges from mild to profound. Important systemic findings include cardiac malformations and upper cervical spine instability.

  Although it occurs with much increased frequency in children born to older women, overall a majority of children with Down syndrome have younger mothers.

- *Fetal alcohol syndrome*, caused by excessive maternal alcohol consumption during pregnancy, is characterized by epicanthus, telecanthus (see below), and often ptosis, typically associated with a thin vermilion border of the upper lip and flattened philtrum. Common fundus abnormalities include mild to moderate hypoplasia or dysplasia of the optic discs, and tortuous retinal vessels. Strabismus, nystagmus, and both high hyperopia and high myopia occur with increased frequency, as do various forms of anterior segment dysgenesis (p. 440). Retardation of both physical growth and mental development to some degree is typical, and there is increased incidence of cardiac, skeletal, and other organ abnormalities.

Differential Diagnosis

- In infancy, *intermittent esotropia* may be infrequently manifest and not detectable on examination, leading to an erroneous diagnosis of pseudoesotropia. Care must be taken to differentiate these conditions and to avoid inappropriately dismissing parental concerns about strabismus merely because pseudoesotropia is present.

  Family photos believed to show esodeviation, especially when eyes are captured in partial lateral gaze (often evident from head posture that partially conceals one ear), may be used to confirm suspicion of pseudoesotropia and clarify the distinction for parents.

  Parental description of unilateral convergence movement (one eye "pulls in" momentarily at times) is strongly suggestive of true intermittent esotropia, especially when seen mainly in association with fatigue or sleepiness.

  Pseudoesotropia never gets worse. Family should be strongly cautioned to bring the child back for reevaluation if there is increasing perception of strabismus.

- *Telecanthus* is increased distance between the medial canthi, with normal interpupillary distance. (Much less common is true *hypertelorism*, or increased interpupillary distance.) Epicanthal folds, often associated, must be retracted by the examiner to make this determination. Normal intermedial canthal distance is approximately equal to the horizontal width of the palpebral fissure.

Telecanthus is a typical finding in *Waardenburg syndrome*, also characterized by laterally displaced lacrimal puncta, white forelock, decreased iris stromal pigmentation (often unilateral, causing heterochromia), and congenital sensorineural deafness (in about 20% of cases).

Cornelia de Lange syndrome also usually includes telecanthus, though synophrys ("unibrow") is the most typical facial feature (seen as well in some cases of Waardenburg). Other ocular findings include early-onset myopia, lacrimal drainage obstruction, blepharitis, ptosis, strabismus, and nystagmus. Gastroesophageal reflux and small or absent digits are characteristic, as is the presence of moderate-severe cognitive and behavioral problems and variable hearing impairment.

Abnormal Lid Apposition

Table 8.1 summarizes a number of conditions in which there is congenital or acquired disturbance of the relationship between the eyelids and/or lashes and the ocular surface. Young corneas usually are quite tolerant to moderate degrees of exposure (Figure 8.2) and contact with (relatively soft) lashes; these disorders often cause no symptoms or only mild ones, and seldom lead to scarring unless there is significant comorbidity, such as tear insufficiency.

Table 8.1

Causes of faulty eyelid apposition in childhood

Condition	Description	Other findings	Comment
Entropion	Inward rotation of entire lower lid tarsus	Microphthalmos in some cases Often significant corneal surface damage	May resolve after temporary lid taping
Epiblepharon	Horizontal skin fold spanning nasal portion of lower lid	Very common with Asian or native American ethnicity	Rarely symptomatic, or requiring treatment
Distichiasis	Extra row of lashes originating from meibomian orifices	Lower extremity lymphedema Mild if any corneal changes	May show autosomal dominant transmission
Trichiasis	Acquired misdirection of lashes toward cornea	Symblepharon after SJS (p. 435)	Treat with epilation or surgical removal of lashes
Ectropion	Outward rotation of lower lid margin	Down syndrome (p. 425) Treacher Collins syndrome (p. 427)	Lid rotation surgery if significant symptoms
Eversion	Outward rotation of upper lid with conjunctival exposure	Floppy eyelids Severe ichthyosis (Figure 8.2)	Often intermittent or transient; manage conservatively
Euryblepharon	Enlarged lower lid stands off from bulbar surface	Down syndrome	Surgical lid tightening if significant symptoms
Tarsal kink	Congenital crease in tarsal plate	Ectropion or entropion, depending on direction	Usually requires surgical correction

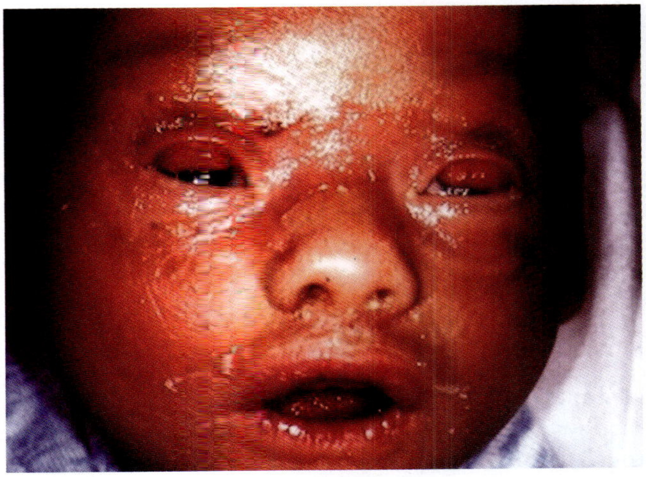

FIGURE 8.2. Eversion of upper eyelids in a newborn with lamellar ichthyosis ("collodion baby"). Skin condition improved and lids returned to normal position over several months.

Eyelid Coloboma

Summary

Eyelid coloboma is congenital absence of a portion of the lid, including margin.

Ophthalmic Findings

- Varies from small notch to absence of entire lid, usually upper.
- Absent tarsus, lashes, and meibomian glands.
- If the defect is large, exposure keratitis may quickly become a serious problem.

Systemic Findings

- *Goldenhar syndrome* (hemifacial microsomia; oculoauriculovertebral dysplasia) includes upper lid coloboma in 20% of cases. Epibulbar dermoid involving limbus or conjunctiva is the most common ocular abnormality (p. 474). Duane syndrome is also a frequent eye finding (p. 508). Other craniofacial anomalies include external (tags, microtia) and internal ear malformation (often with hearing loss), maxillary and mandibular hypoplasia, and macrostomia. Vertebral and cardiac abnormalities may be present. Findings are usually unilateral; sporadic (nonfamilial) occurrence.
- *Treacher Collins syndrome* (mandibulofacial dysostosis) typically includes temporal lower lid coloboma, with "antimongoloid" (nasal higher than temporal) slant of palpebral fissures. Malar and mandibular hypoplasia, ear malformations (often with deafness), and macrostomia are also characteristic findings. Usually bilateral; autosomal dominant inheritance, but most cases represent new mutations.
- *Amniotic band syndrome* may cause eyelid coloboma. Other findings include facial clefts, limb malformation or amputation; patterns variable and not consistent with interruption of normal developmental sequence. Typically sporadic.

Treatment and Management

- Topical lubricants if mild corneal exposure.
- Surgical closure, direct or with mobilization of adjacent tissue. Large defects may require eyelid reconstruction in early infancy to prevent severe corneal damage.

Differential Diagnosis

- Not likely to be mistaken for lid coloboma, but sometimes having similar implications, is *exorbitism*, the exophthalmic condition of eyes with very shallow bony orbits due to maldevelopment. Seen mainly in association with *craniosynostosis* (premature closure of cranial sutures) involving midfacial hypoplasia and oxycephaly (tower skull).
  - Principal forms are Crouzon syndrome, Apert syndrome (Crouzon plus syndactyly), and Pfeiffer syndrome (Crouzon plus broad thumbs)
  - Caused by allelic mutations of the gene FGFR2, chromosome locus 10q26, with autosomal dominant transmission.
  - In severe cases with markedly inadequate eyelid protection, serious corneal damage may occur in a short time, occasionally necessitating surgical reconstruction in the newborn period.
  - Other concerns include increased intracranial pressure leading to papilledema and optic atrophy (p. 472), characteristic V-pattern strabismus (p. 501), lacrimal drainage obstruction in some cases (p. 429), and varying degrees of developmental delay.

Congenital Ptosis

Summary

Ptosis (bepharoptosis) is unilateral or bilateral drooping of the upper eyelid. Congenital "dystrophic" ptosis, resulting from isolated maldevelopment of the levator palpebrae muscle (muscle tissue replaced by fibrous connective tissue), is by far the most common cause of significant lid droop in childhood.

Demographics

- Usually unilateral but bilateral (symmetric or asymmetric) not uncommon.
- Usually sporadic, but familial occurrence of both unilateral and bilateral congenital ptosis is sometimes seen.

Symptoms and Signs

- Ptosis in primary gaze position from birth; palpebral fissure height typically decreased 3 to 4 mm; may improve somewhat during early infancy.

PEDIATRIC

Table 8.2

Less common causes of childhood ptosis

Condition	Ocular findings	Other findings	Comment
Blepharophimosis syndrome	Ptosis Blepharophimosis (horizontally shortened lid fissure) Telecanthus, epicanthus inversus (mainly lower lid)	Strabismus common Autosomal dominant inheritance	Bilateral, usually symmetrical Reconstruction typically requires multiple surgical procedures
Ankyloblepharon	Partial fusion of upper and lower lid margins	May be autosomal dominant Various systemic associations	"Ankyloblepharon filiform adnatum" is a narrow bridge of tissue joining the lids
Jaw winking (Marcus Gunn eyelid phenomenon)	Ptosis (varies greatly moment to moment with jaw movement or sucking) Lid retraction at times	Nearly always sporadic and unilateral Synkinesis of levator and pterygoid muscle (CN V)	Nearly always congenital Nonintervention may be preferable to radical surgical procedures
Congenital oculomotor nerve palsy (p. 509)	Ptosis (variable severity) Exotropia (usually large angle) Variable vertical strabismus Limited adduction, elevation, depression Variable pupil findings	Variable associated neurologic defects	Some patients show little or no ptosis or mydriasis; lid and pupil movement may be disproportionately reduced
Horner syndrome (Figure 8.3)	Ptosis (mild) Lower lid elevation (mild) Miosis Heterochromia (if congenital, and intermediate iris color)	Pharmacologic testing seldom helpful in childhood Neuroblastoma originating in upper chest or neck must be considered as possible cause	Congenital or acquired Anisocoria consistently much more evident in dim light Fasanella-Servat or Mueller resection effective surgery
Rhabdomyosarcoma (p. 476)	Ptosis may be earlisest sign	Sometimes palpable mass behind orbital rim	Orbital imaging indicated in suspicious cases
Myasthenia gravis (p. 512)	Ptosis often varies moment to moment; may disappear at times, especially with transition from down to upward gaze Strabismus common; tends to be less variable than ptosis	Variable weakness of nonocular muscles; often confined to ocular muscles Pharmacologic and immunologic testing often negative when only EOMs involved	Usually acquired Surgical treatment should be considered when findings stable, consistent
Chronic progressive external ophthalmoplegia (Kearns-Sayre syndrome)	Ptosis acquired in childhood, may be asymmetrical Progressive loss of eye rotation, with or without strabismus	Pigmentary retinopathy (p. 464) Cardiac conduction defects Various other neuromuscular abnormalities; ataxia	Mitochondrial abnormality Characteristic "ragged red fibers" on muscle biopsy Usually sporadic, or in siblings with same mother

- Reduced levator palpebrae function and lid excursion, resulting in relative upper lid elevation in downgaze, sometimes to a level higher than that of the opposite normal eye in unilateral cases. This motivates a large majority of children with significant congenital ptosis to adopt a compensatory chin-elevated head posture, which usually permits maintenance of normal visual function.
- Use of frontalis contraction to raise lid level.
- Anisometropia, typically astigmatic, may develop.
- Amblyopia seldom occurs in the absence of constant strabismus or severe anisometropia. When a child with significant congenital ptosis fails to use chin-up posture, concern about vision is much increased, and there may be need for early surgical intervention.

Treatment and Management

- When vision is not threatened (i.e., is protected by use of chin-up head posture), surgical repair is usually best delayed until age 3 to 5 years.
- With fair to good levator function, and in most unilateral cases, levator resection is appropriate, usually in large amount (15 to 20 mm) via anterior (skin) incision.
- When levator function is poor, and in most bilateral cases, frontalis suspension is the preferred surgical treatment, preferably done with autogenous fascia.

Differential Diagnosis

Many dysmorphic syndromes may include ptosis. Some conditions in which ptosis is acquired and/or associated with other significant ocular or systemic findings are summarized in Table 8.2 (Figure 8.3).

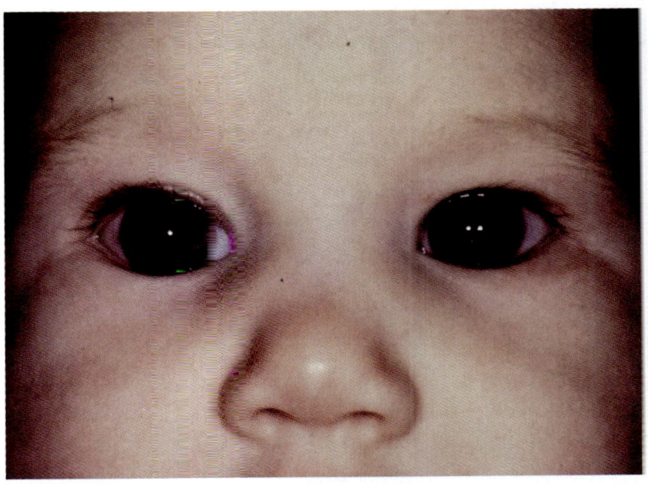

FIGURE 8.3. Congenital Horner syndrome. Note smaller size of left palpebral fissure due to displacement of both upper and lower lid margins, and relative miosis of left pupil. Heterochromia is not evident in this blue-eyed baby.

Eyelid Tic

Summary

Tic is a purposeless repetitive movement that can be (temporarily) voluntarily suppressed. Eyelid blinking is the most common form of tic.

Demographics

- More than 10% of children are affected at some point, mostly boys.
- Typical onset 6 to 10 years old, sometimes earlier.

Symptoms and Signs

- Frequent forceful eyelid closure, usually bilateral but sometimes unilateral winking.
- Eye rotation tics, typically forceful oblique conjugate gaze movements, may be seen in addition or alternatively.
- Ocular surface pathology should be ruled out, especially foreign body of the cornea or tarsal conjunctiva, but normal examination is the rule.

Treatment and Management

- Resolves spontaneously within a few months in the great majority of cases. A small minority of affected children may develop chronic tic disorder (lasting more than 12 months) or Tourette syndrome (multiple chronic motor and vocal tics).
- May be aggravated by stress but not caused by or typically associated with psychopathology. Psychiatric referral is rarely indicated.

LACRIMAL SYSTEM DISORDERS

Deficient Tear Production in Childhood

Dry eye in the pediatric population is far from the ubiquitous problem seen in adults. When it does occur, there is often little or no need for treatment, fortunately for the parents of affected infants and young children who may be more bothered by the instillation of tear supplement drops than by the condition itself. Corneal damage is most likely when there is associated lack of sensation, or when the quality as well as quantity of tear production is affected. A number of disorders in this category are summarized in Table 8.3.

Nasolacrimal Duct Obstruction

Summary

Complete congenital obstruction of the nasolacrimal duct (NLD) commonly results from membranous occlusion, most often at the lower end of the structure where it enters

Table 8.3

Causes of dry eye in infants and children

Condition	Ocular surface findings	Other findings	Comment
Absent lachrymation	Lack of emotive tearing Normal basal secretion	None	Normal variant
Congenital alacrima	Decreased tear volume	Often absent lacrimal gland Achalasia, adrenocortical insufficiency ("Triple A")	Triple A syndrome autosomal dominant
Familial dysautonomia (Riley-Day syndrome)	Decreased tear volume Corneal hypesthesia and ulceration	Exotropia Emotional lability	Autosomal recessive Ashkenazic Jewish families
Keratoconjunctivitis sicca (Sjogren syndrome)	Decreased tear volume Usually mild superficial punctate keratitis	Decreased salivary secretion Adult rheumatoid arthritis Other collagen vascular disease	Rare in childhood May be seen with graft versus host disease after BMT
Ectodermal dysplasia	Decreased tear aqueous and lipid secretion Blepharitis	*EEC syndrome:* Ectrodactyly ("claw hand") Cleft palate	Autosomal dominant, incomplete penetrance
Stevens-Johnson syndrome (p. 435)	Decreased tear aqueous and mucin secretion Symblepharon, corneal scarring	Skin and nonocular mucous membrane scarring usually mild	Cicatricial aftermath of acute disease Blindness in severe cases
Trachoma	Recurrent chlamydial infection leads to scarring Decreased tear aqueous and mucin secretion	None	Worldwide eradication may be in sight
Vitamin A deficiency (xerophthalmia)	Decreased tear aqueous and mucin secretion Bitot spots, keratomalacia	Night blindness (Table 8.15)	Dietary deficiency worldwide Malabsorption, liver disease in developed countries

the nose beneath the inferior turbinate (valve of Hasner). *Partial* obstruction or stenosis may be caused by narrowing of the lacrimal drainage passage at any point below the sac.

Demographics

- Complete obstruction occurs in up to 10% of all newborns.
- Initially bilateral in one third of cases.

Symptoms and Signs

- Complete obstruction: constant epiphora and mucus accumulation; severity may be quite variable from patient to patient and from time to time in an individual. Lashes typically bind together in "fascicles."
- Partial obstruction: intermittent epiphora, mainly at times of increased tear production; and intermittent mucus accumulation, typically associated with upper respiratory infection or congestion (which presumably results in temporary complete blockage of the stenotic passage by swollen mucous membranes.)
- Mucopurulent reflux on massage of lacrimal sac *sometimes* present with complete obstruction, not with partial.
- Mild redness and maceration of lower eyelid skin may result from chronic wetness and rubbing, but conjunctival injection is seldom seen.
- Acute dacryocystitis and periorbital cellulitis, with marked redness and swelling of eyelid skin (localized and generalized, respectively), are uncommon complications (Figure 8.4; see also discussion of lacrimal sac mucocele below.)

Special Tests

- Culture of discharge is not routinely indicated. Gram-positive isolates are obtainable from most specimens,

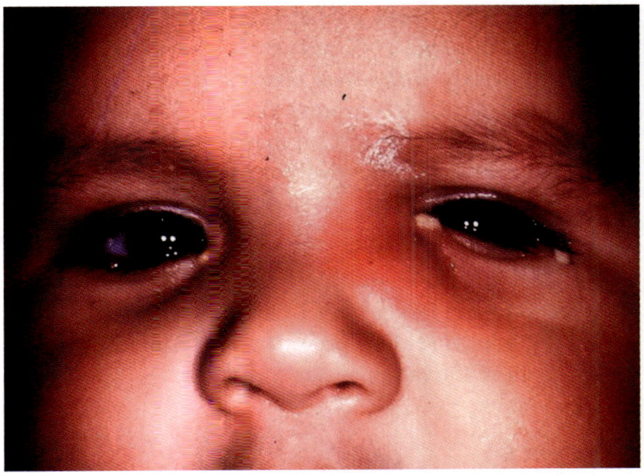

FIGURE 8.4. Acute dacryocystitis in an older infant with congenital NLD obstruction. More typically, this situation develops in a newborn with lacrimal sac mucocele.

but Gram-negatives and multiple flora are also common; treatment is seldom influenced by test results.

- Dye disappearance test: Observe eye with blue light following instillation of 1% fluorescein solution. Persistence of dye after 5 minutes is abnormal. Fluorescein may or may not become visible in the nose when passage is patent.

Disease Course

- Ninety percent resolve spontaneously by age 12 months, usually with abrupt improvement in symptoms as membranous obstruction disintegrates.
- Symptoms of partial obstruction may persist after resolution of complete obstruction; resolve gradually (months to years) as facial growth increases NLD size and capacity.

Treatment and Management

- Lacrimal sac massage: Apply firm pressure with fingertip initially over medial canthus, and then slide downward while maintaining pressure. Several times per day; with each diaper change is a convenient routine.
- Topical antibiotic: Drops preferred (unlike ointment, enter sac, and do not blur vision); polymixin-trimethoprim (Polytrim) a good choice. Use chronically as necessary (one to four times per day) to minimize mucopurulent discharge.
- Use of topical corticosteroid is suggested by some authorities, but in this author's opinion is never necessary or justified, in view of multiple risks to the infant from chronic steroid exposure including infection (highly septic ocular environment with NLD obstruction, despite concurrent antibiotic administration), intraocular pressure (IOP) elevation (steroid responders more frequent at younger ages and IOP difficult to monitor), and adrenocortical suppression (low body mass compared to dosage).
- Probing in operating room with general anesthesia if symptoms of complete obstruction persist beyond age 12 months. Earlier probing (usually after age 3 months, in outpatient setting with infant awake and securely wrapped, topical anesthesia) when symptoms are particularly bothersome, or preference to avoid general anesthesia. If initial probing is unsuccessful, repeat under general anesthesia.
- Simple probing is generally not effective for partial obstruction. If symptoms remain seriously bothersome after age 1 to 2 years, consider balloon catheter dilatation or silicone intubation under general anesthesia. A similar surgical approach is appropriate for persistent symptoms after repeated probing for complete obstruction. Dacryocystorhinostomy is rarely required for congenital NLD obstruction.

Differential Diagnosis

- In *punctal atresia*, impatency of the upper lacrimal drainage system may result from occlusion of the punctual opening by a thin membrane, absence of punctum and papilla, or partial or complete failure of canalicular differentiation. The lower system (sac and NLD) is generally intact.

  Epiphora is present, but no sticky mucoid discharge; symptoms are generally much less bothersome than with NLD obstruction, because there is no contribution from sac-secreted mucus or proliferation of bacteria in protein-rich sac fluid.

  If location of punctum can be identified visually, it is often possible to cure the condition simply by penetrating the membrane with a pointed dilator, needle, or narrow blade.

  Absent punctual differentiation, it is sometimes still possible to surgically establish access to the canaliculus; maintaining patency requires silicone tube stenting for an extended time (months). In severe cases with bothersome symptoms, there may be indication for conjunctivodacryocystorhinostomy (Jones tube), though generally not until later childhood.

- Lacrimal drainage insufficiency from congenital maldevelopment or acquired scarring is seen in association with a variety of disorders, including Down syndrome (p. 425), Cornelia de Lange syndrome (p. 426), Crouzon syndrome and related craniosynostoses (p. 427), ectodermal dysplasia (Table 8.3), Stevens-Johnson syndrome (p. 435), and Rubinstein-Taybi syndrome (p. 444). In some such cases, tearing may be aggravated by accompanying ocular surface or lid margin problems (e.g., blepharitis in Down and de Lange syndromes, ectodermal dysplasia; trichiasis or keratitis in Stevens-Johnson), while in others, it may be diminished due to decreased tear production (Table 8.3).

- Epiphora may be a symptom of congenital glaucoma. Unlike NLD obstruction, tearing is associated with clear nasal discharge, as well as corneal enlargement and photophobia in most cases.

References

Katowitz IA, Welsh MG. Timing of initial probing and irrigation in congenital nasolacrimal duct obstruction. *Ophthalmology* 1987;94:698–705.

Lueder GT. Balloon catheter dilation for treatment of older children with nasolacrimal duct obstruction. *Arch Ophthalmol* 2002;120:1685–1688.

Lacrimal Sac Mucocele

Summary

Dacryocystocele (dacryocele, amniotocele, mucocele) occurs when there is obstruction of lacrimal drainage both above and below the sac, leading to distention and frequently development of secondary infection.

Etiology

Lower obstruction is typically membranous; upper may be anatomic or physiologic (i.e., blockage of retrograde passage by unusually competent valve of Rosenmuller). Mucus secretion by goblet cells lining the sac leads to increased volume and pressure.

Symptoms and Signs

- Bluish mass in the medial canthal region, inferior to the canthal tendon, typically about 1 cm diameter and present at or soon after birth.
- Infection (*dacryocystitis*) usually develops during the first month of life if the condition persists, with onset of redness and swelling of overlying skin.
- Pressure against lower membranous obstruction may create a cystlike outpouching into the nose that can cause respiratory distress.

Treatment and Management

- Digital pressure over the distended sac (may need to be fairly vigorous) can sometimes twist open the valve of Rosenmuller and allow decompression via puncta; occasionally, this maneuver may rupture lower membrane and establish drainage into the nose.
- Topical antibiotic drop may help prevent development of infection.
- Dacryocystitis requires treatment with systemic as well as topical antibiotic; hospital admission and intravenous administration are generally indicated for a newborn. Appropriate drug is broad spectrum with good coverage for Gram-positive respiratory flora, such as a cephalosporin.
- Probing to establish full patency of drainage system should be done if possible. This is challenging in the newborn due to small size and distorted anatomy; general anesthesia and ENT assistance may be required to deal definitively with lower obstruction. Probing of the upper system to decompress the sac, in combination with appropriate nonsurgical management, is sufficient treatment for the acute situation in most cases.

Differential Diagnosis

- With encephalocele, swelling is generally above the canthal tendon and larger than 1 cm.
- Hemangioma is seldom present at birth, or confined to the region of the lacrimal sac.

Reference

Paysse EA, Coats DK, Bernstein JM, et al. Management and complications of congenital dacryocele with concurrent intranasal mucocele. *J AAPOS* 2000;4:46–53.

INFECTIOUS AND IMMUNOLOGIC DISORDERS OF OCULAR SURFACE AND ADNEXA

Neonatal Conjunctivitis (Ophthalmia Neonatorum)

Summary

Ophthalmia neonatorum is purulent conjunctivitis occurring in the first month of life. It is important to diagnose and treat this condition promptly.

Etiology

Conjunctival infection is acquired during passage through the birth canal or perinatally, especially if amniotic membranes rupture early. Timing of onset varies with etiologic agent (Table 8.4).

Symptoms and Signs

- Discharge moderate mucopurulent (bacterial, chlamydial) to hyperpurulent (gonococcus).
- Lid edema, mild to marked.
- Conjunctival hyperemia and swelling, occasionally membranes. Papillary but not follicular reaction (Figure 8.5A).
- Corneal involvement suggests Gram-negative bacteria (especially gonococcus or pseudomonas) or herpes simplex virus (HSV).

Systemic Findings

- Chlamydial conjunctivitis is often followed by development of severe pneumonitis during the first 6 weeks of life.
- Life-threatening systemic infection with HSV is a serious concern.

Table 8.4

Causes of neonatal conjunctivitis

Agent	Principal findings	Age of onset	Comment
Toxic	Mild redness, swelling Watery discharge	0–2 d	Usually caused by silver nitrate prophylaxis
Neisseria gonorrhoeae	Marked redness, swelling Serosanguinous to hyperpurulent discharge Membranes Corneal involvement	0–7 d	Gram-negative diplococci on smear
Other bacteria	Moderate redness, swelling Mucopurulent discharge	5–10 d	Cultures negative in 25%
Herpes simplex virus	80% have skin lesions Corneal ulceration may be present	3–15 d	Systemic treatment required
Chlamydia trachomatis	Mild to marked redness, swelling, discharge	7–15 d	Cytoplasmic inclusion bodies on Wright/Giemsa stain Mixed poly and mononuclear cell reaction

Special Tests

- All newborns with conjunctivitis should have conjunctival discharge Gram stained, and plated on blood, chocolate, and Thayer-Martin media for culture and sensitivity testing
- Conjunctival scraping (vigorous enough to contain a sufficient quantity of cells) should be inoculated into Chlamydia culture medium (may take up to 7 days to grow out); and may also be evaluated by Wright or Giemsa staining (to look for blue intracytoplasmic inclusion bodies) or immunologic testing (quicker but less reliable diagnostic methods) (Figure 8.5B).
- Serologic testing for syphilis and human immunodeficiency virus should be obtained in infants with gonococcal or Chlamydia infection.

Treatment and Management

- Because of the possibility of penicillin resistance, sight-threatening gonococcal infection is usually treated with a systemic third-generation cephalosporin (ceftriaxone

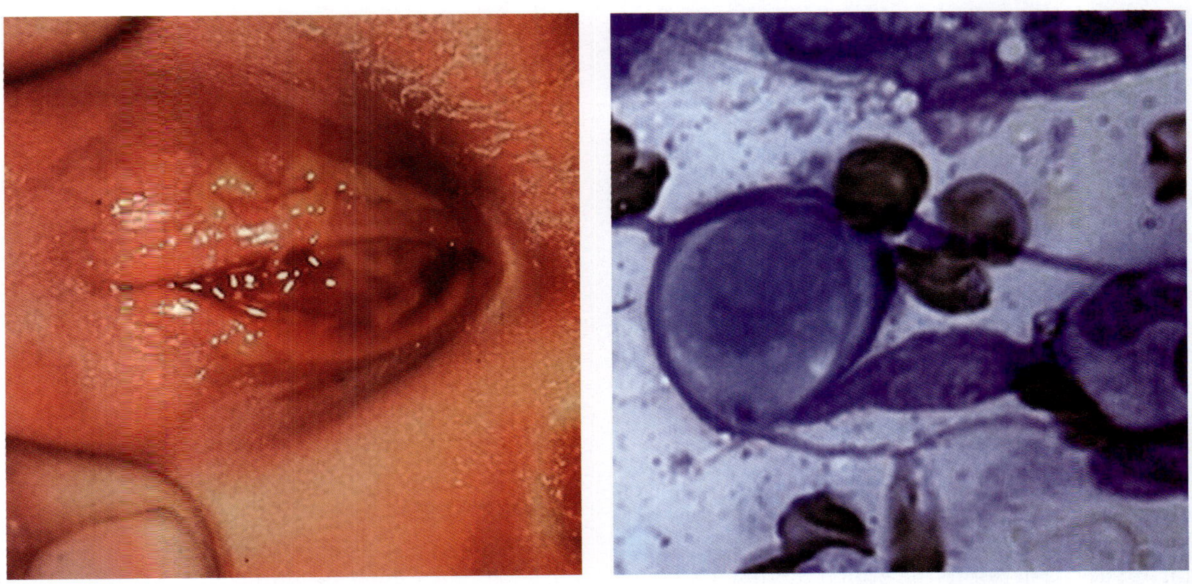

FIGURE 8.5. Chlamydia conjunctivitis in a newborn. **A:** Severe inflammation of conjunctiva and eyelids. **B:** Wright-stained scraping showing epithelial cell with blue cytoplasmic inclusion body.

or cefotaxime); topical antibiotics and frequent saline irrigation are often used in addition, but of questionable value.

- Chlamydia infection is treated with oral erythromycin 40 to 50 mg/kg per day (usually in four divided doses) for 2 to 4 weeks. Parents and sexual partners must be advised and treated for Chlamydia infection and other sexually transmitted diseases.
- Systemic treatment is also indicated for neonatal ocular HSV infection, typically intravenous acyclovir 30 mg/kg per day (usually in three divided doses) for 2 weeks. Topical trifluridine may or may not be helpful.
- Conjunctivitis without corneal involvement caused by other bacteria is treated with erythromycin ointment or bacitracin-polymixin ophthalmic ointment three times daily for 1 to 2 weeks.
- Prophylaxis for ophthalmia neonatorum is mandatory in all American states and Canadian provinces, using erythromycin ointment, tetracycline ointment, or 1% silver nitrate solution. Toxic conjunctivitis caused by silver nitrate is common and resolves spontaneously in several days. In the developing world, 2.5% povidone-iodine (Betadine) has been shown to be a highly effective, safe, and inexpensive method of prophylaxis, which may actually have advantages over methods routinely used in North America.

Differential Diagnosis

Acute conjunctivitis with onset beyond age 1 month is assumed to have been acquired postnatally, and in otherwise healthy infants and children is usually caused by Gram-positive respiratory tract flora; occasionally by adenovirus. Treatment with a topical antibiotic drop or ointment that provides good antibacterial coverage, such as polymixin-trimethoprim or erythromycin, can be initiated without need for culture in most cases, unless there is evidence suggestive of HSV infection (e.g., vesicles on the lips or eyelid skin, history of recent HSV outbreak in a close contact, corneal involvement).

References

Isenberg SJ, Apt L, Wood M. A controlled trial of povidone-iodine as prophylaxis against ophthalmia neonatorum. *N Engl J Med* 1995;332:562–566.

Weiss A, Brinser JH, Stewart VN. Acute conjunctivitis in childhood. *J Pediatr* 1993;122:10–14.

Preseptal and Orbital Cellulitis

Summary

Preseptal (periorbital) cellulitis is bacterial infection diffusely involving the eyelids. Orbital cellulitis is infection involving tissues posterior to the orbital septum.

Etiology

- Preseptal cellulitis may arise from infection of periocular skin following superficial trauma, primary skin infection (impetigo, herpes simplex), conjunctivitis with invasion of deeper tissues, or extension of upper respiratory infection from paranasal sinuses.
- By far the most common cause of orbital cellulitis is extension of infection from adjacent sinus cavities, especially the ethomoids. Infection may also arise from deep orbital trauma or bacteremia (see discussion of panophthalmitis below).
- Causative organism in all situations usually Gram-positive cocci, most often *Streptococcus* sp.
- *Haemophilus influenzae* was once a common cause of periorbital infection in childhood, presenting with rapid development of marked eyelid swelling and characteristic violaceous skin discoloration, often accompanied by signs of systemic sepsis and life-threatening meningitis. Incidence has dramatically decreased since immunization became routine in the 1980s.
- Fungal infection (especially mucormycosis) may cause severe orbital cellulitis with rapid life-threatening progression in diabetic or immunosuppressed patients.

Symptoms and Signs

- Marked diffuse edema and erythema of the upper and the lower eyelids typically develop over 24 to 48 hours in both preseptal and orbital cellulitis. Some edema fluid may track across the nose to cause mild swelling of the contralateral eyelids; this does not generally indicate spread or worsening of infection.
- Skin lesions (of similar vesicular or crusted appearance) may indicate impetigo or HSV infection.
- Conjunctival injection and discharge suggest preseptal infection; mild to severe chemosis is associated with orbital infection.
- Proptosis and limited ocular rotation present in orbital cellulitis, absent in preseptal. May be difficult to detect on examination of uncooperative sick child.
- Relative afferent papillary defect in orbital cellulitis is the most reliable and important sign of optic nerve compression, indicating serious threat to vision and urgent need for surgical intervention. Pupils should be monitored critically during early days of treatment.
- Systemic signs of sepsis, including lethargy, fever, and leukocytosis, are sometimes seen, more often with orbital cellulitis than with preseptal. Symptoms of upper respiratory infection or sinus disease (headache, nasal congestion) commonly reported.

Special Tests

- Computed tomography definitively distinguishes preseptal and orbital cellulitis. Typically shows extensive sinusitis in association with orbital cellulitis. May reveal subperiosteal abscess (typically between medial orbital wall and medial rectus muscle), sometimes with air-fluid level; occasionally, intracranial abscess is also present, especially in adolescents.

- Conjunctiva should be cultured if mucopurulent discharge present. Blood culture, lumbar puncture seldom necessary.

Treatment and Management

- Both preseptal and orbital cellulitis warrant hospitalization and initial treatment with intravenous antibiotics to cover typical respiratory flora plus other organisms as circumstances suggest. Pediatric infectious disease consultation is highly desirable for medical management.
- Clinical response may not be evident until 48 to 72 hours after optimal medical treatment is begun, but most cases of orbital cellulitis in childhood (even when medial subperiosteal abscess is present) resolve without surgery. The first sign of improvement is reduced lid swelling. Proptosis and motility may not recover fully for weeks.
- Aggressive treatment of sinusitis is indicated (with ENT consultation), possibly including endoscopic surgical drainage, which also provides the best route for draining most orbital abscesses (typically medial subperiosteal in location) that do not respond adequately to medical treatment.
- Sinus drainage via skin incision has a high frequency of complications and is now rarely if ever indicated for orbital cellulitis in childhood.

Differential Diagnosis

- Septic embolization to the orbit associated with bacteremia (often but not always from an identifiable remote focus of infection such as endocarditis or meningitis) may cause *panophthalmitis*, in which orbital cellulitis is accompanied by endophthalmitis. Loss of vision (usually to bare light perception or worse) and of media clarity (frequently with hypopyon) distinguish this condition from other forms of orbital inflammation. The prognosis is dismal, even with aggressive treatment including intraocular antibiotics; often leads to evisceration or enucleation.
- The appearance of orbital cellulitis in childhood may be mimicked by noninfectious conditions including orbital pseudotumor (see below), and a variety of cancers including rhabdomyosarcoma, advanced retinoblastoma, metastatic neuroblastoma, and orbital involvement by leukemia or lymphoma (described in sections below beginning p. 476).

References

Greenwald MJ, Wohl LG, Sell CH. Metastatic bacterial endophthalmitis: a contemporary reappraisal. *Surv Ophthalmol* 1986;31:81–101.

Weiss A, Friendly D, Eglin K, et al. Bacterial periorbital and orbital cellulitis in childhood. *Ophthalmology* 1983;90:195–203.

Inflammatory Orbital Pseudotumor

Summary

Inflammatory pseudotumor typically presents with proptosis and periocular inflammation, without evidence of sepsis or localized infection, although mild fever is sometimes present in pediatric cases.

Symptoms and Signs

- Proptosis (axial and/or downward displacement of the globe) is typical; eyelid ptosis is common.
- Pain, especially associated with eye movement.
- Bilateral involvement, often asymmetric or sequential, is not uncommon with occurrence in childhood.

Ophthalmic Findings

- Children often show evidence of anterior uveitis on slit-lamp examination.
- Fundus examination may reveal papillitis or exudative retinal detachment.
- Strabismus (often with diplopia) and limited ocular rotation when extraocular muscles involved.

Special Tests

- Orbital imaging with ultrasonography, CT, or MRI may reveal diffuse inflammatory changes, localized swelling of orbital structures including lacrimal gland or extraocular muscles (single or multiple, often involving tendon in contrast to thyroid orbitopathy), or thickening of posterior sclera and choroid.
- Biopsy is seldom necessary, but may be helpful, especially when imaging documents lacrimal gland involvement.

Treatment and Management

- Initial treatment with high-dose systemic corticosteroid (prednisone 1 mg/kg per day) typically leads to prompt resolution. Recurrence after discontinuation of medication is not unusual, but the disease typically "burns out" eventually after months to years.
- Although primary orbital lymphoma is very rare in childhood, lack of expected response to steroid treatment should prompt assessment for possible malignancy.

Stevens-Johnson Syndrome (Erythema Multiforme)

Summary

Stevens-Johnson Syndrome (SJS) is a severe acute mucocutaneous hypersensitivity disorder that typically involves conjunctiva.

Etiology

The immune response may be triggered by prior viral or other (especially mycoplasma) infection, or by drug exposure (less common in children). Usually, a specific agent cannot be identified.

Symptoms and Signs

- Initially mucopurulent discharge and papillary conjunctival reaction.
- In severe cases, extensive membranes develop, causing tenacious adherence of tarsal conjunctiva to ocular surface.

Systemic Findings

- Preceded by prodromal symptoms of malaise, fever, and upper respiratory or gastrointestinal complaints.
- Acute skin involvement is highly variable, ranging from classic discrete round "target" lesions to extensive bullous eruption, with an extreme form known as *toxic epidermal necrolysis* in which large areas of epidermis slough in response to minor mechanical stress.
- Other mucous membrane involvement besides conjunctival may include oral and genital, which are often severe but usually heal without significant scarring.

Disease Course

- Acute inflammation subsides in a few weeks.
- Chronic sequelae may range from mild to sight threatening, including tear insufficiency, punctal occlusion, keratinization of conjunctiva, symblepharon (shortening of conjunctival fornices), trichiasis, and cicatricial entropion, with potential for severe secondary corneal damage.

Treatment and Management

- There is no convincing evidence of benefit from any topical medication, including lubricants, antibiotics, or corticosteroids, and their administration is likely to cause both physical and emotional trauma to the gravely suffering child. Milder cases are best left untreated altogether.
- In severe cases, daily separation of fused eyelids is indicated. Use of Desmarres retractors after topical anesthesia is more practical and effective than the traditionally recommended glass rod. This process is excruciating for both the patient and the doctor.
- A recently developed device (ProKera) that combines a symblepharon ring with preserved amniotic membrane shows promise as a means of protecting the cornea and limiting conjunctival adhesion formation in SJS.
- Postacute phase cicatricial changes require aggressive monitoring and management by experienced clinicians to prevent or minimize corneal damage.

Reference

Prendiville JS, Hebert AA, Greenwald MJ, et al. Management of Stevens-Johnson syndrome and toxic epidermal necrolysis in children. *J Pediatr* 1989;115:881–887.

Vernal Conjunctivitis

Summary

Vernal conjunctivitis is a chronic allergic disorder characterized by seasonal exacerbations.

Demographics

- More common in boys than girls.
- Frequently a history of asthma, other seasonal allergic manifestations.

Etiology

Immune mediated by pollen- or mold-specific immunoglobulins E and G (IgE and IgG). Symptoms typically worse in spring and/or fall but may persist year round.

Symptoms and Signs

- Itching always present, proportionate to overall severity.
- Redness, tearing, and photophobia are common.
- Conjunctival injection, boggy edema; sometimes ropy mucoid discharge.
- Large "cobblestone" papillae of upper tarsal conjunctiva in palpebral form.
- Limbal vernal disease is characterized by nodular limbal swelling, usually superior sector, often accompanied by small whitish Trantas dots (Figure 8.6).
- Corneal involvement ranges from mild superficial punctate keratitis (mainly superior) to "shield" plaque or ulcer.

Treatment and Management

- Systemic allergy treatment, avoidance of allergens, cold compresses.
- In milder cases, symptomatic relief may be provided by topical tear supplement, decongestant, or antihistamine drops.

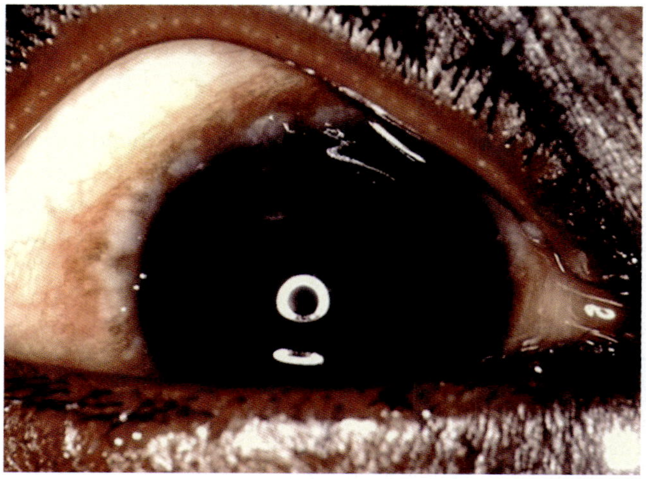

FIGURE 8.6. Limbal vernal conjunctivitis. Note limbal follicles and tiny white Trantas dots.

- Most patients require a mast-cell stabilizer such as cromolyn sodium, lodoxamide (Alomide), or olopatadine (Patanol) during active periods.
- Topical corticosteroid is often necessary, especially to achieve initial control. Use a mild formulation such as loteprednol (Lotemax) or fluorometholone (FML); monitor IOP if used for more than a few weeks.

Differential Diagnosis

Other less common causes of *chronic conjunctivitis* in childhood should be kept in mind, including molluscum contagiosum, staphylococcal lid margin disease, acne rosacea, ligneous conjunctivitis, and the various dry eye syndromes (Table 8.3).

References

Erzurum SA, Feder RS, Greenwald MJ. Acne rosacea with keratitis in childhood. *Arch Ophthalmol* 1993;111:228–230.

Friedlaender MH. Conjunctivitis of allergic origin: clinical presentation and differential diagnosis. *Surv Ophthalmol* 1993;38:105–114.

Hypersensitivity Keratoconjunctivitis (Phlyctenulosis)

Summary

Phlyctenular disease is a localized immunologic disorder of conjunctiva and cornea.

Etiology

The specific cause of hypersensitivity reaction is usually not evident in children. Staphylococcal blepharitis may be the source, but clinical signs are frequently absent. Historical association with tuberculosis and malnutrition seldom applicable in present-day cases.

Symptoms and Signs

- Localized conjunctival injection, unilateral or bilateral.
- Tearing, photophobia are common; may be severe.
- Slightly elevated, gray to pink, nodular or wedge-shaped limbal lesion, often associated with a small peripheral or paracentral corneal ulcer connected to the limbus by a narrow leash of vessels (Figure 8.7).
- Significant anterior corneal stromal scarring may result from repeated exacerbations. Rarely significant localized thinning and perforation may occur.

Treatment and Management

- Some cases respond well to treatment for blepharitis with lid hygiene and antibiotic application.
- Topical corticosteroid is usually necessary, typically bringing prompt relief of symptoms. Should be tapered as quickly as possible, though recurrence is common.

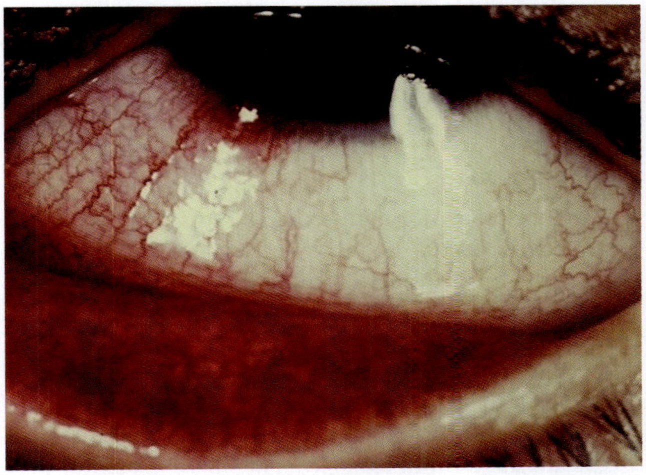

FIGURE 8.7. Phlyctenular keratoconjunctivitis, with lesion at the limbus.

Differential Diagnosis

- *Marginal ulcer* of the cornea probably represents a variant expression of the same disease process that causes phlyctenular disease. It is much less commonly seen in children than the phlyctenular variety.
- *Interstitial keratitis*, one of the characteristic late manifestations of congenital syphilis, is now rare in developed countries. Sequential onset of bilateral corneal opacities and edema with deep stromal vascularization occurs abruptly in late childhood or adolescence, usually accompanied by redness and intense photophobia, often with anterior uveitis. Associated findings may include changes in secondary dentition ("Hutchinson teeth") and progressive hearing loss; pigmentary retinopathy (p. 451).

Chalazion

Summary

Chalazia (properly pronounced with initial "k" sound) are nodular inflammatory lesions that originate from eyelid meibomian glands. The term *internal hordeolum* is now used interchangeably with chalazion by most authors.

Demographics

- By far the most common acquired adnexal lesion of childhood, representing a frequent and distressing problem in the pediatric population.
- Seen in children as young as 1 year old, both sexes, all ethnic groups.

Pathology

The material found in a chalazion (for which the name *glorp* has been suggested) has a very uniform and distinctive gross appearance, consisting of tiny yellow jellylike lobules. Microscopic examination shows granulomatous reaction (including giant cells, epithelioid macrophages, lymphocytes, and plasma cells) surrounding small fat globules.

Symptoms and Signs

- Acute or subacute, mild to moderate localized swelling with redness of overlying skin in the upper or lower eyelid may be the initial manifestation of meibomian gland inflammation. Discomfort is absent to moderate.
- Resolution of inflammatory signs occurs over a few days to a week or two, with evolution into painless nodular thickening in the lid, diameter from about 2 to 12 mm, typically a few millimeters from the margin. Nodule may develop without prior inflammatory signs; inflammation may resolve without nodule formation.
  - Initially skin intact and mobile over nodule; may remain so indefinitely, with stable, gradually increasing, or fluctuating volume.
  - In some cases after weeks to months, overlying skin becomes thin, red, and scaly, typically accompanied or followed by spontaneous partial external drainage of small amounts of serosanguinous fluid, pus, or glorp. Skin crusting and induration develop as the volume of the lesion diminishes; complete resolution typically long in coming.
  - Occasionally, a small chalazion may involve only a meibomian orifice and immediately adjacent tissue.
- Localized redness of underlying conjunctiva is typical. Fleshy polypoid excrescense of tissue from conjunctiva may appear in late stages, sometimes containing glorp but usually representing a secondary reactive phenomenon (pyogenic granuloma). These lesions may be shaved off at the (usually narrow) base followed by light cautery; care should be taken to remove also any glorp (often small in quantity) that is still present within underlying tarsus (see discussion of surgical treatment below).
- Symptomatic generalized blepharitis or meibomitis present in a minority of cases.
- Vision usually unaffected, but pressure on the cornea may produce deformation and astigmatism in some cases, which reverts to normal once the lesion is gone.

Disease Course

- Complete spontaneous resolution may occur within weeks, sometimes very quickly following the acute inflammatory phase, but chronic lesions may persist for many months or even years with stable or fluctuating symptoms and signs.
- Typically a solitary lesion, but clusters involving one or multiple lids simultaneously or sequentially (usually within a time frame of a few months to a few years) are not unusual in childhood.

Treatment and Management

- Warm compresses are the mainstay of conservative management. For maximum effectiveness should be applied for 10 to 15 minutes two to three times per day. Wrapping a moist washcloth around an object that will stay warm for sufficient time after heating (e.g., a microwaved potato or boiled egg) is recommended. Benefit should be evident within 1 to 2 weeks; often no effect on chronic lesions.
  - If present, blepharitis or meibomitis should be treated with baby shampoo lid scrubs and topical antibiotic ointment application at bedtime, which may help prevent recurrent chalazia.
  - Topical and systemic antibiotics and topical corticosteroid are generally ineffective for the chalazion itself.
- Surgery is nearly always curative (if glorp is removed completely) but does not prevent new lesions from developing.
  - Sedation (plus local anesthetic infiltration) or general anesthesia is needed for nearly all pediatric patients, including most teenagers.
  - Make 4- to 5-mm incision with No. 11 or No. 15 blade: vertical through conjunctiva and tarsus if skin intact (taking care not to extend to the lid margin), or horizontal through center of abnormal skin region.
  - Remove all glorp by scraping with a curette (force directed laterally/medially from center in plane of lid) and scrubbing with cotton-tip swabs. Excise degenerated tissue around skin incision to leave a healthy margin. It is not necessary to remove secretory membrane ("capsule" or "cyst wall") surrounding the glorp-filled cavity.
  - No sutures; rapid contraction and healing of external or internal wound by secondary intention with little or no scarring is the rule in children.

Differential Diagnosis

- An *external hordeolum* or *stye* originates from an eyelid sebaceous gland of Zeis or apocrine gland of Moll, usually closer to the lid margin and the skin surface (involving the lash line) compared with a chalazion. Inflammatory symptoms and signs are typically greater and more localized for a stye during acute phase; spontaneous resolution occurs in days to a week or two in most cases, sometimes accompanied by drainage of a small amount of pus (no glorp). Medical or surgical treatment is seldom necessary; warm compresses may be helpful.
- Eyelid abscess is the result of suppurative infection, usually caused by Gram-positive cocci, confined to a single eyelid. Usually, the entire eyelid is involved from the time of onset until spontaneous or surgical (via horizontal

Table 8.5

Congenital corneal and global abnormalities

Condition	Description	Other findings	Comment
Buphthalmos	Enlargement of cornea and globe due to high IOP	Increased axial length Variable myopia	p. 442
Megalocornea	Congenital large cornea (>13 mm) with normal IOP	Usually none Ectopia lentis (various causes)	p. 443
Keratoglobus	Central and peripheral thinning and bulging of cornea, very deep AC, blue sclera	Acute spontaneous hydrops Risk of globe rupture with minor trauma	Autosomal recessive, with deafness and lax joints (Ehlers-Danlos VIA)
Cornea plana	Abnormally flat cornea (typically 25–35 D)	Usually small diameter, often glaucoma Sometimes sclerocornea (Table 8.9)	Autosomal dominant or recessive
Microcornea	Small cornea (<10 mm diameter)	Usually associated with microphthalmos	Associated with a wide range of ocular developmental abnormalities (Table 8.6)
Microphthalmos	Small globe (short axial length)	High hyperopia if anterior segment normal	
Nanophthalmos	Small well-formed globe and cornea, shallow AC	High hyperopia, thick sclera	Risk of angle closure; uveal effusion after intraocular surgery

IOP, intraocular pressure; D, diopter; AC, anterior chamber.

skin incision) drainage. The relatively large cavity should be packed postdrainage with iodoform gauze strip, which is gradually removed over several days.

- The early acute phase of chalazion can resemble incipient cellulitis or orbital pseudotumor. Insect or spider bites can produce a very similar appearance.
- A variety of less common benign skin lesions may be mistaken for chalazion, including papilloma and pilomatrixoma. Cutaneous malignancy is extremely rare in otherwise healthy children. In questionable cases, and when no typical glob is recovered, excised tissue should be submitted for pathologic evaluation.
- Other nodular subcutaneous lesions including small hemangiomas, dermoid cysts, and rhabdomyosarcoma sometimes have a similar appearance to chalazion (see section on tumors below, beginning p. 474).

Reference

Greenwald MJ. What's in a chalazion? *Surv Ophthalmol* 1985; 30:142.

GLOBAL, ANTERIOR SEGMENT, AND LENS DISORDERS

Abnormalities of Corneal Size and Shape

Abnormally large or small size of the cornea or the entire globe, and flatter or steeper than normal corneal curvature, are important indicators of ocular maldevelopment, often but not always having serious implications for eye health and vision (Table 8.5). A wide variety of conditions may result in decreased corneal diameter. (Table 8.6 provides a partial listing.) Early-onset myopia is often found in larger than normal eyes and is also seen in association with a variety of other conditions (Table 8.7).

Keratoconus, the one significant acquired disorder affecting corneal shape, may present in late childhood as unilateral or bilateral progressive myopia with irregular astigmatism

Table 8.6

Important associations of microphthalmos and microcornea

Condition	Reference
Cornea plana	Table 8.5
Ant. segment dysgenesis	Table 8.8
Nuclear cataract	Table 8.12
Congenital infection	p. 451
PHPV	p. 452
Vitreoretinal dysplasia	p. 453
Retinopathy of prematurity	p. 457
Fundus coloboma	p. 469
Aniridia	Table 8.17

Table 8.7

Important associations of myopia in young children

Condition	Reference
Down syndrome	p. 425
Keratoglobus	Table 8.5
Glaucoma	p. 443
Ectopia lentis	p. 445
Posterior lenticonus	p. 446
Visual deprivation	p. 448
Stickler syndrome	Table 8.14
Leber congenital amaurosis	p. 461
CSNB	Table 8.15
X-linked RP	Table 8.15
Bardet-Biedl syndrome	Table 8.15
Gyrate atrophy	Table 8.15
Albinism	Table 8.17
Fundus coloboma	p. 469
Myelinated nerve fibers	p. 473

that precludes correction to normal vision with spectacles. Visualization of a "cone" by viewing the red fundus reflex remotely with direct ophthalmoscopy can help make this diagnosis, which often is missed in early stages, and may be mistaken for amblyopia (p. 491) or functional vision loss (p. 468). Keratoconus is usually sporadic, but is associated with a number of systemic disorders, including atopic dermatitis (Table 8.12), Down syndrome (p. 425), Crouzon syndrome (p. 427), and Marfan syndrome (p. 444).

References

Greenwald MJ. Refractive abnormalities in childhood. *Pediatr Clin North Am* 2003;50:197–212.

Weiss AH, Koussef BG, Ross EA, et al. Complex microphthalmos. *Arch Ophthalmol* 1989;107:1619–1624.

Anterior Segment Dysgenesis

Anterior segment dysgenesis (formerly known as *anterior chamber cleavage syndrome*) comprises a variety of ocular developmental disorders attributable to abnormal differentiation of mesenchyme-derived tissue, mainly of neural crest origin (Table 8.8). Presence of anomaly can usually be documented by careful hand-light inspection (Figure 8.8). These conditions most often occur as isolated abnormalities, sometimes are accompanied by other ocular disturbances (e.g., glaucoma), and sometimes present in the context of a complex multisystem disorder. Examples of the last category include Alagille syndrome (Table 8.8), Rubinstein-Taybi syndrome (p. 444) and fetal alcohol syndrome (p. 425). Though not generally included in discussion of this group of disorders, aniridia (Table 8.17) shares a number of features with them, including frequent origin from faulty PAX6 gene expression.

Corneal Opacity in Childhood

Localized or generalized lack of corneal transparency, present at birth or acquired during the early years of life, has numerous and disparate causes, which may involve congenital malformation, edema secondary to elevated IOP or inadequate endothelial function, or storage of

Table 8.8

Spectrum of anterior segment dysgenesis

Condition	Description	Other findings	Comment
Posterior embryotoxon	Prominent and anteriorly displaced Schwalbe line, partial or complete	Usually none *Alagille syndrome:* Pigmentary retinopathy Cholestasis, pulmonic stenosis	Alagille syndrome autosomal dominant
Axenfeld anomaly	Iris stromal extensions to posterior embryotoxon	Childhood-onset glaucoma in 50% (Axenfeld syndrome)	May be autosomal dominant, usually sporadic
Rieger anomaly	Axenfeld findings plus iris stromal hypoplasia and pupil distortion	*Rieger syndrome:* Characteristic dental anomalies Telecanthus (p. 426)	Autosomal dominant; other systemic findings variably present
Peters anomaly	Central or paracentral corneal leukoma Iris strands to edge of opacity Localized absence of endothelium and DM	Cataract with lens-cornea adherence in some cases Glaucoma common Occasional, varied systemic manifestations	Usually sporadic, unilateral Faulty PAX6 gene expression Fetal alcohol effect (p. 425)

DM, Descemet's membrane.

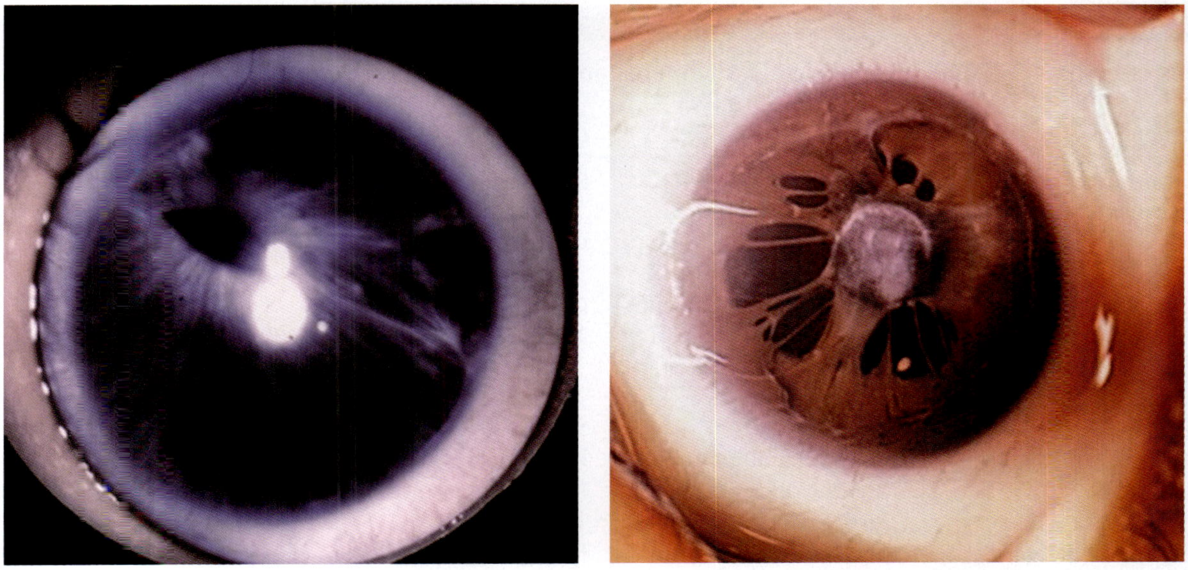

A B

FIGURE 8.3. Anterior segment dysgenesis. **A:** Rieger anomaly, viewed through a contact goniolens for magnification, with posterior embryotoxon, iridocorneal adhesions, distorted pupil, and iris stromal hypoplasia. **B:** Complex anomaly with extensive iris adherence to both posterior embryotoxon and relatively large central anterior capsular lens opacity.

abnormally accumulated metabolites (Table 8.9). Scarring from immunologic keratitis (p. 437), or secondary to inadequate tear production (Table 8.3), is covered elsewhere.

Primary Infantile Glaucoma

Summary

Childhood glaucoma most often is present at birth or develops in infancy. Abnormal development of trabecu-

Table 8.9

Causes of corneal clouding or opacification in infants and children

Condition	Description	Other findings	Comment
Infantile glaucoma	Diffuse haze and thickening, increased diameter	Haab striae Ectopia lentis (p. 444)	p. 442
Birth trauma	Vertical break in DM with overlying edema	Signs of forceps application High with-the-rule astigmatism	Risk of deprivation myopia, amblyopia
Infectious keratitis	Ulcer (HSV, bacteria; p. 432) Vascularized leukoma Diffuse keratitis (rubella)	Purulent discharge Signs of healed perforation	Rubella keratitis present at birth, clears in weeks to months
Peters anomaly, "internal ulcer"	Nonvascularized leukoma, locally absent DM	Iris, sometimes lens involvement in Peters	Table 8.8 Cornea often clears over time
Sclerocornea	Peripheral opacification and vascularization	Wide variety of reported ocular and systemic associations	Extent ranges from peripheral sector to entire cornea
Epibulbar dermoid	Discrete elevated lesion, usually at limbus	Goldenhar syndrome	p. 427, p. 474
Congenital hereditary endothelial dystrophy	Diffuse haze and thickening, normal diameter		p. 443

(*Continued*)

Table 8.9

Causes of corneal clouding or opacification in infants and children (*Continued*)

Condition	Description	Other findings	Comment
Posterior polymorphous dystrophy	Characteristic lesions of endothelium and DM Edema in most severe cases	Sometimes angle synechiae Glaucoma in small percentage of cases	Autosomal dominant, with highly variable expression
Fabry disease	Whorl-like epithelial deposits (cornea verticillata)	Cataract (Table 8.12) Tortuous conjunctival and retinal blood vessels Skin angiokeratoma	X-linked, males Similar appearance in female carriers
Cystinosis	Photophobia, often intense Crystalline deposits anterior stroma	Pigmentary retinopathy Renal tubular disease, failure	Autosomal recessive Oral and topical cysteamine treatment helpful
Mucopolysaccharidosis, types IH (Hurler), IS (Scheie), IV (Morquio), and VI (Maroteaux-Lamy)	Acquired uniform corneal haze without edema, photophobia In MPS II (Hunter) and III (Sanfilippo) clear corneas; otherwise similar to IH	Retinal and optic nerve degeneration (except IV) Characteristic facial, skeletal features ("gargoylism") Mental deficiency (mainly IH)	All autosomal recessive except Hunter (X-linked) Mucopolysaccharide in urine Specific enzyme deficiency in cells from blood or biopsy
Mucolipidosis, type IV	Uniformly cloudy cornea without edema in infancy	Retinal degeneration Progressive mental deterioration from infancy	Autosomal recessive Ashkenazic Jewish families

DM, Descemet's membrane; HSV, herpes simplex virus; MPS, mucopolysaccharidosis.

lar meshwork structures and consequent elevation of IOP lead to corneal edema and enlargement of the cornea or the entire globe (*buphthalmos*).

Demographics

- Sometimes autosomal recessive, especially in Middle Eastern countries.
- Most often sporadic, involving either sex.

Symptoms and Signs

- Corneal enlargement nearly always present, corneal clouding usually present.
- Epiphora and photophobia are typically present, but frequently absent.

Ophthalmic Findings

- Corneal diameter greater than 10 mm in newborn, or greater than 12 mm before age 1 year, is suspicious (Figure 8.9). Any detectable difference in corneal diameter between right and left eyes is potentially significant. Infant corneas larger than parent corneas are cause for concern.
- Corneal edema, typically stromal and epithelial, usually associated with horizontal or circumferential breaks in Descemet membrane (Haab striae).

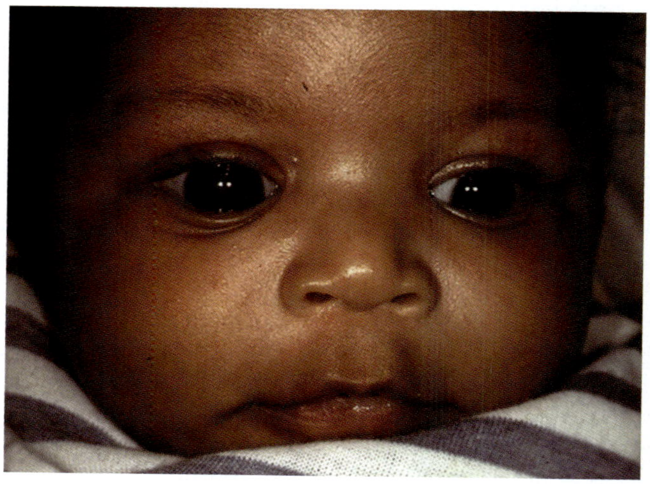

FIGURE 8.9. Infant with glaucoma, right eye. Note enlargement and clouding of cornea.

- Increased IOP, ranging from low 20s to 40s. Keep in mind that measurements in the awake infant or child, especially those made with TonoPen, may be artifactually elevated and those made under general anesthesia may be lowered.
- Gonioscopic abnormalities (Barkan membrane) classically described but difficult to document.
- Myopia ranging from mild to severe. Effect of axial elongation to some extent mitigated by associated corneal and lens flattening
- Increased optic disc cupping, in most but not all cases reversible after control of IOP.

Treatment and Management

- Estimation of corneal diameter, confirmed as necessary using a ruler (preferably marked with successively increasing multimillimeter intervals), should be a part of every infant eye examination. With practice, it is possible to estimate with accuracy to within 0.5 mm.
- Examination under anesthesia (EUA) or with monitored sedation is indicated for any infant or young child suspected of having glaucoma. Measure IOP with at least two devices (Schiotz tonometer is quite acceptable), corneal diameter, and if possible axial length using A-scan ultrasonograpy. Perform anterior segment examination with a hand-held slit lamp or operating microscope (including gonioscopy if possible), retinoscopy, and optic nerve examination (with photograph documentation if possible).
- Initial treatment is often medical, usually with a topical or a systemic carbonic anhydrase inhibitor (CAI) such as acetazolamide (10 to 15 mg/kg per day in two to four divided doses), which may be started before EUA to protect the cornea and the optic nerve from further damage and to improve visualization of angle structures and disc.
- Definitive treatment in most cases is surgical, beginning if possible with goniotomy or trabeculotomy (angle incision procedures):
  - If corneal clarity is adequate, goniotomy (incising trabecular meshwork from within the anterior chamber under direct gonioscopic visualization—ab interno) is preferred by some surgeons.
  - If the cornea is cloudy, trabeculotomy (tearing through trabecular meshwork with an instrument or suture inserted into Schlemm's canal through incision under a limbus-based scleral flap—ab externo) is the procedure of choice. Some surgeons prefer trabeculotomy, which more closely resembles other forms of anterior segment microsurgery, for cases with clear cornea as well.
  - Results from the two procedures have repeatedly been shown to be about the same.
- Inadequate pressure control after two angle incision procedures is indication for trabeculectomy. High failure rates in childhood justify initial adjunctive use of 5-fluorouracil or mitomycin-C.
- Refractory cases may require placement of a tube shunt drainage device, or ciliary body ablation with infrared diode laser or cryotherapy.
- Topical medication may play an extended role in borderline cases, especially after less than desired effect from surgery. Useful agents in addition to CAI include:
  - Beta-blockers, with attention to the possibility of adverse effects in small children with reactive airway disease.
  - Prostaglandin analog agents, increasingly used for juvenile glaucoma.
  - Alpha-adrenergic agents, specifically brimonidine (Alphagan), must be used with great caution in children. May cause severe somnolence and life-threatening systemic effects including bradycardia, hypotension, and apnea, especially in children weighing less than 20 kg.

Follow-Up

- Frequent EUAs as necessary. Developmentally normal children over 3 years old can usually be trained to cooperate for applanation tonometry at the slit lamp, after which office follow-up becomes sufficient in most cases.
- Treat amblyopia, myopia, and strabismus as necessary.

Differential Diagnosis

- *Congenital megalocornea* (symmetrical nonprogressive enlargement of clear corneas, with normal IOP and disc appearance) is often but not always familial. An X-linked variety sometimes referred to as anterior megalophthalmos is associated with corneal stromal "mosaic" dystrophy and early adult-onset cataract and glaucoma (Table 8.5). Ectopia lentis from any cause may be associated with increased corneal diameter (p. 444).
- *Congenital hereditary endothelial dystrophy* presents with bilateral corneal clouding without enlargement in infancy. May cause tearing and photophobia. Normal IOP and disc appearance. Often familial: autosomal recessive or dominant (less common, milder) (Table 8.9).
- Primary *juvenile open-angle glaucoma* is considerably rarer and more difficult to diagnose than the infantile variety. Corneal size and clarity are typically normal, and the presenting sign is most often progressive myopia, very common for other reasons in the same demographic. Visual field testing is of little value before adolescence. IOP measurements are often artifactually elevated, especially when made using TonoPen. Pressure in the upper teens is higher than average but within normal limits for children, and in the 20s may be tolerated for decades by young eyes. Cup-to-disc ratios of 0.5 or more are not exceptional for normal children, and in fact this finding is far more often physiologic than pathologic in the pediatric population. Family history of glaucoma in adult relatives is rarely

significant. Except when there is a well-documented history of glaucoma onset before age 30 in a parent, a child with suspicious discs, progressive myopia, and/or IOP in the 20s should be monitored closely for evidence of progressive optic neuropathy before treatment is initiated.

- *Rubinstein-Taybi syndrome* is a multisystem disorder with dysmorphic features (notably broad thumbs and big toes) that has a wide variety of ophthalmic associations, including glaucoma, cataract, high myopia, and anomalies of the lacrimal drainage system, anterior segment (keratoglobus, dysgenesis), and fundus (coloboma, foveal hypoplasia). Of particular importance is the frequent finding of central disc excavation that may mimic glaucomatous cupping, creating confusion with actual syndrome-related glaucoma, especially when there is associated myopia and corneal abnormality.
- Infantile glaucoma is an important concern with two of the major neurocutaneous syndromes (p. 486).

  In neurofibromatosis type 1 (NF1), glaucoma is uncommon, nearly always unilateral, and associated with either *plexiform neurofibroma* of the ipsilateral upper eyelid (which may be a subtle finding in infancy, evident as enlargement of the temporal portion of the lid causing S-shaped margin), or *ectropion uveae* (eversion of iris pigment epithelial tissue at the pupil margin; rare). Most of these eyes do poorly.

  In Sturge-Weber syndrome, glaucoma is common, nearly always associated with ipsilateral eyelid involvement by *portwine nevus* (usually unilateral, but not infrequently bilateral). Effective treatment is usually possible, but often challenging, in significant part because of the tendency of involved eyes to develop massive choroidal effusion during or after filtering surgery.
- Numerous other ocular and systemic conditions may be associated with glaucoma in childhood. (Table 8.10 provides a partial listing.) Some of these also involve microphthalmos or microcornea (Tables 8.5 and 8.6), in which case corneal diameter and axial length may remain *less* than normal in the presence of sight-threatening elevation of IOP. Greater than expected growth of a small eye in infancy should raise suspicion of glaucoma.

Table 8.10

Important associations of glaucoma in childhood

Condition	Reference
Down syndrome	p. 425
Cornea plana	Table 8.5
Nanophthalmos	Table 8.5
Ant. segment dysgenesis	Table 8.8
Post. polymorphous	Table 8.9
MPS I (Hurler, Scheie)	Table 8.9
Rubinstein-Taybi syndrome	p. 444
Ectopia lentis	p. 444
Aphakia	p. 448
Lowe syndrome	p. 449
Juvenile rheumatoid arthritis	p. 449
Congenital rubella	p. 449
PHPV	p. 452
Vitreoretinal dysplasia	Table 8.13
Retinopathy of prematurity	p. 457
Coats disease	p. 458
Aniridia	Table 8.17
Retinoblastoma	p. 484
Juvenile xanthogranuloma	p. 484
Neurofibromatosis type 1	Table 8.21
Sturge-Weber syndrome	Table 8.21

Reference

Beck AD, Freedman S, Kammer J, et al. Aqueous shunt devices compared with trabeculectomy with mitomycin-C for children in the first two years of life. *Am J Ophthalmol* 2003;136: 994–1000.

Ectopia Lentis (Lens Subluxation or Dislocation)

Summary

Lens displacement (when not attributable to trauma—Figure 8.10A) reflects abnormal laxity of zonular fibers. May occur as an isolated abnormality or in the context of a multisystem disorder.

Ophthalmic Findings

- Displacement of the lens within or perpendicular to its coronal plane. Characteristically superior/posterior in *Marfan syndrome* (MFS); inferior/anterior in *homocystinuria* (Figure 8.10B). Regardless of cause, displacement tends to increase during childhood; often undetectable in infancy.
- Spherophakia or microspherophakia (increased curvature, decreased diameter), particularly in *Weill-Marchesani syndrome*.
- Associated pupil abnormality in *ectopia lentis et pupillae* (autosomal recessive inheritance), classically displacement in opposite direction (typically downward) from the lens (typically upward), but showing much variation even between eyes and among family members. In MFS pupils often dilate poorly.
- Glaucoma may result acutely from pupillary block by anteriorly displaced lens (especially with homocystinuria or Weill-Marchesani syndrome). Ectopia lentis may be a consequence of buphthalmos or megalocornea, due to mechanical stretching of zonule. Corneal enlargement with normal IOP is also occasionally an association of ectopia lentis, regardless of origin.

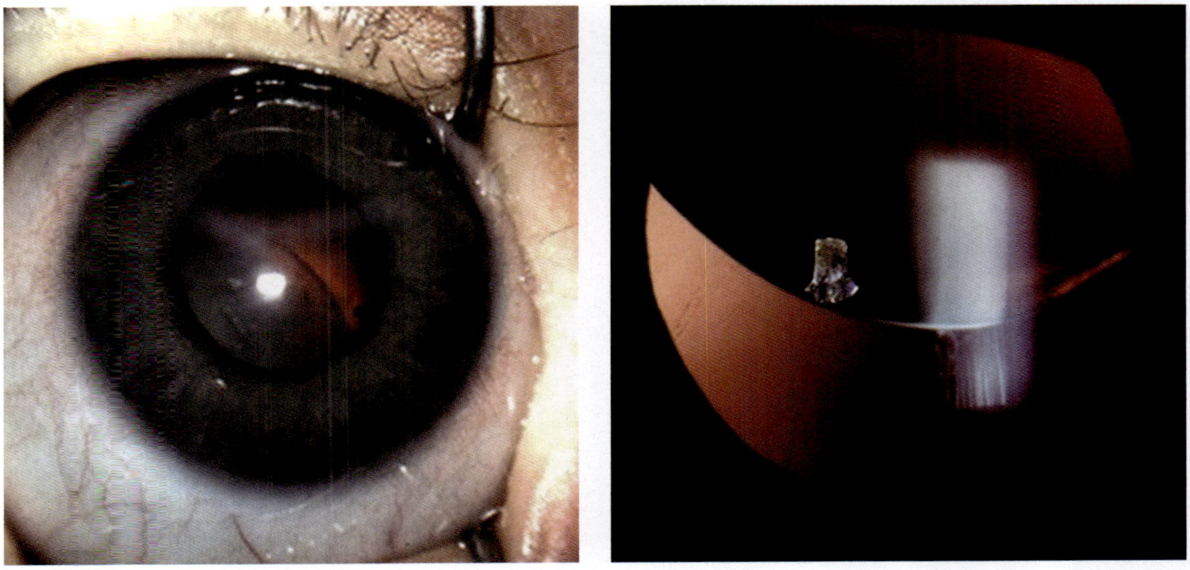

A B

FIGURE 8-10. Dislocated lenses. **A:** Traumatic dislocation with cataract in a physically abused infant; rhegmatogenous retinal detachment from a giant tear was also present in both eyes. **B:** Upward displacement in an older child with Marfan syndrome.

- Cataract develops prematurely in most dislocated lenses, and there is significant increased risk of rhegmatogenous retinal detachment possibly greater after lens extraction surgery. These complications are seldom seen in childhood.
- Refractive error (in the phakic portion of pupil) combines lenticular myopia (from steepened overall lens curvature) and astigmatism (optical power near lens edge least for axis perpendicular to edge, greatest for axis parallel to edge tangent). Many eyes with ectopia lentis (in MFS as well as other disorders) also have a significant component of axial myopia. Myopia may be the first sign of ectopia lentis, evident before displacement of the lens becomes obvious.
- With lens edge near the pupil center, retinal superimposition of phakic and aphakic images (one of which must be severely defocused) may degrade acuity to as low as 20/100 with best correction of either type, but in symmetrical cases significant amblyopia seldom occurs.

Systemic Findings

- MFS (autosomal dominant inheritance, mutation of fibrillin gene—FBN1—chromosome 15q21) is defined by characteristic cardiovascular abnormalities (aortic root dilation with valvular insufficiency, mitral valve prolapse, risk of dissecting aneurysm) and body habitus (tall stature, arachnodactyly, hyperextensible joints).
- Homocystinuria (autosomal recessive, deficiency of cystathione beta-synthase, with increased blood and urine methionine) is also associated with tall stature and other skeletal abnormalities, but tight joints. Mental deficiency and deterioration may be reduced by diet low in methionine, or in some milder cases by supplementation with pyridoxine (vitamin B_6). A major concern is high risk of thromboembolism, particularly in association with general anesthesia.
- Weill-Marchesani syndrome (autosomal recessive inheritance) is characterized by short stature, brachycephaly, and brachydactyly.
- Isolated ectopia lentis may be sporadic or show a familial pattern that is recessive or dominant (often caused by an FBN1 mutation different from those responsible for MFS).

Treatment and Management

- Refractive correction for myopia and/or astigmatism. If the lens edge is displaced to near the center of the pupil, aphakic refractive correction may be preferred.
- Lens removal is seldom necessary for visual reasons and may be associated with serious complications. Use of suture-supported lens implants remains controversial.

Congenital and Developmental Cataract

Summary

Congenital (present at birth) and developmental (onset during infancy or childhood) cataract may affect one or both eyes. Unilateral congenital cataract usually reflects localized maldevelopment of ocular structures. Bilateral cataract in childhood is often familial (Figure 8.11A), or associated with a systemic disorder, and should prompt work-up for an underlying cause. (Table 8.11 provides a partial listing; see also discussion of differential diagnosis below.)

PEDIATRIC

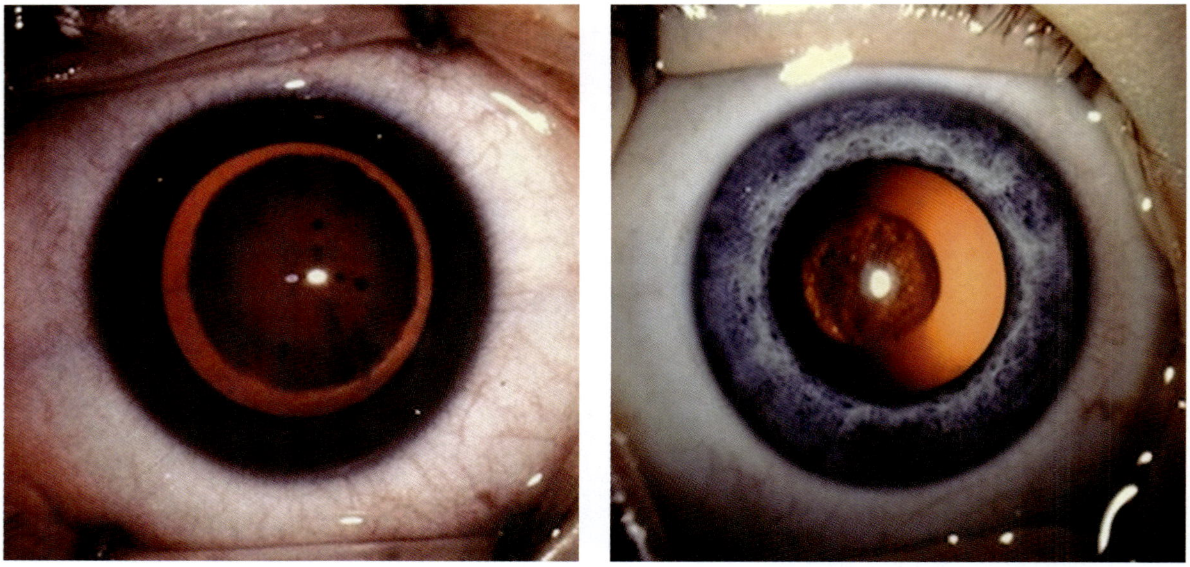

FIGURE 8.11. Developmental cataracts. **A:** Familial lamellar cataract, onset at age 3 years. Note central light transmission through clear nucleus. Amblyopia is rarely caused by this type of bilateral cataract. **B:** Posterior lenticonus with early PSC opacification.

Diagnostic Evaluation

- Critical assessment of lens and cataract morphology, with close attention to localization of opacity (Table 8.12). Of particular importance in unilateral cases is the finding of *posterior lenticonus*, thinning of the posterior capsule, usually central, that is associated with posterior bulging of cortex. Opacification, beginning at the posterior pole and often extending to the nucleus, may not develop until after infancy. Prior to cataract formation, myopia may result from steepened curvature of affected posterior capsule (Figure 8.11B).
- Comprehensive eye examination to look for associated developmental or degenerative abnormalities, including microcornea or microphthalmos (Tables 8.5 and 8.6), anterior segment dysgenesis (Table 8.8), persistent hyperplastic primary vitreous (PHPV) and other vitreoretinal disorders (p. 452), and pigmentary retinopathy (p. 451, Table 8.15). B-scan ultrasonography if fundus visualization is inadequate.
- With or without a history of maternal illness during pregnancy, serologic testing for congenital infection, including toxoplasmosis, rubella, syphilis, cytomegalovirus, and HSV (TORCH titers) is justified in infants with unexplained lens opacification (unilateral or bilateral), but only rubella (rare in North America in recent decades—see below) typically causes visually significant cataract.
- Blood chemistry testing for glucose, calcium: Both hypoglycemia and hypocalcemia may cause lens opacification. Diabetic cataract occurs rarely in childhood.
- Urine testing for reducing substance (after milk feeding, to look for galactosemia), amino acids (Lowe syndrome—test may be negative during first few months of life). (See below.)
- Comprehensive evaluation by pediatrician or genetics specialist for associated dysmorphic or systemic abnormalities (e.g., distinctive small beaklike nose in *Hallermann-Streiff syndrome*; characteristic skin and skeletal findings in *Conradi syndrome*), which may prompt additional testing (chromosome analysis, neuroimaging, etc.) Usually none found in a healthy appearing infant.

Table 8.11

Important systemic associations of cataract in childhood

Condition	Reference
Down syndrome	p. 425
Rubinstein-Taybi syndrome	p. 444
Alport syndrome	Table 8.12
Atopic dermatitis	Table 8.12
Myotonic dystrophy	Table 8.12
Wilson disease	Table 8.12
Fabry syndrome	Table 8.12
Hallerman-Streiff syndrome	p. 446
Conradi syndrome	p. 446
Lowe syndrome	p. 449
Congenital rubella	p. 449
Galactosemia	p. 449
Juvenile rheumatoid arthritis	p. 449
Stickler syndrome	Table 8.14
Zellweger syndrome	p. 461
Neurofibromatosis type 2	Table 8.21

Table 8.12

Types of pediatric cataract

Name	Description	Other findings	Comment
Anterior polar	Tiny (≤1 mm) usually central white dot on surface of anterior lens capsule	Iris strands from collarette Occasionally extends over capsule or into cortex	Present at birth Unilateral or bilateral, sporadic Seldom affects vision
Anterior lenticonus	Central bulging of anterior lens capsule and cortex, with localized opacification	*Alport sydrome:* Fleck retinopathy Renal disease, hearing loss	X-linked or recessive Late childhood or adolescence Usually not visually significant
Anterior subcapsular	Normal contour; cortex and sometimes capsule involved	*Atopic dermatitis:* Keratoconus Retinal tears, detachment	Acquired in late childhood or adolescence
Posterior polar	Involves central posterior capsule and cortex	Unilateral usually with lenticonus Bilateral usually familial	Distinguish from PSC and PHPV Often visually significant
Posterior subcapsular	Extends internally over intact posterior lens capsule	History of trauma, disease, treatment (XRT, steroid) Family hx acoustic neuroma	Usually identifiable cause in childhood Often first sign of NF2 (Table 8.21)
Persistent hyperplastic primary vitreous (p. 452)	Fibrous plaque behind lens capsule; variably evident vascular abnormality	Microphthalmos Anomalous iris vessels Variable cortical opacification	Sporadic, unilateral Cataract may conceal plaque Visual prognosis poor to good
Central pulverulent (Coppock)	Small (1–2 mm) translucent stippled disc within embryonic nucleus	None	Congenital autosomal dominant, multiple genes Minimal effect on vision
Sutural	Involves the Y-sutures of the fetal nucleus	None	Sporadic, X-linked or autosomal recessive
Fetal nuclear	Dense central opacity with surrounding clear cortex	Microphthalmos Risk of aphakic glaucoma	Usually present from birth Sporadic or dominant Amblyogenic
Lamellar zonular	Thin opaque layer between clear nucleus and cortex, typically 5–6 mm diameter	Congenital or acquired from metabolic disturbance (hypoglycemia)	Most cases symmetrical, sometimes familial Good visual prognosis
Christmas tree	Multicolored iridescent cortical flecks	*Myotonic dystrophy:* External ophthalmoplegia Pigmentary retinopathy	Dominant, late childhood Also seen with hypocalcemia, or idiopathic finding
Oil droplet	Abrupt optical discontinuity between inner/outer nucleus	Galactosemia	With continued milk feeding progresses to true cataract
Cerulean	Multiple blue-white dot-like cortical opacities	Down syndrome (p. 425) Isolated autosomal dominant	Usually not visually significant
Sunflower	Shimmering multicolored anterior subcapsular petaloid pattern	*Wilson disease:* Kaiser-Fleischer corneal ring Liver, CNS disease	Autosomal recessive Late childhood or adolescence Abnormal copper metabolism

(*Continued*)

Table 8.12

Types of pediatric cataract (*Continued*)

Name	Description	Other findings	Comment
Spoke-like	Radial linear arrays of granular opacity originating from central posterior or anterior capsule	*Fabry disease:* Corneal changes (Table 8.9) Presents with hand/foot pain Kidney, CV, skin morbidity	X-linked, late childhood onset Alpha galactosidase A defect, glycosphingolipid storage Similar cataract mannosidosis
Membranous	Small thin lens	Lowe syndrome Congenital rubella PHPV	Usually present from birth; may result from partial resorption of cortex
Total	Complete lens opacification	Unilateral traumatic or due to posterior segment disease Progression of partial cataract	Progression may be rapid Liquefication, resorption of cortex may occur

CNS, central nervous system; CV, cardiovascular; NF2, neurofibromatosis type 2; PHPV, persistent hyperplastic primary vitreous PSC, posterior subcapsular; XRT, x-ray therapy.

- Examine eyes of parents and siblings: many childhood cataracts are familial. Female relatives of boys with Lowe syndrome may show typical carrier state findings.
- Many mutations involving various genes have been identified as causes of isolated hereditary cataract, mostly with autosomal dominant transmission. Some cause highly distinctive and uniform congenital or developmental lens changes, while others show variable expression in terms of morphology, extent of opacification, and time course.

Treatment Considerations

- Dense (i.e., completely blocking light transmission) axial opacities more than 3 mm in diameter are likely to cause severe amblyopia within months of onset in infancy or early childhood, and require prompt surgical treatment whether bilateral or unilateral. Cataracts that permit light transmission centrally or that are smaller than 3 mm should be monitored closely, provided there is no development of nystagmus or nonalternating constant strabismus indicating possibly serious visual deprivation.
- Cataract extraction performed before age 6 years should include routine posterior capsulectomy and vitrectomy because of the high frequency of secondary opacification at young ages.
- Primary intraocular lens implantation is now well accepted as appropriate and even desirable in conjunction with *unilateral* cataract surgery in most children over age 2 years, and possibly as young as 6 months. To help ensure optimal visual development during the critical early years of life, IOL power selection should bring the eye as close to emmetropia as possible in the early postoperative period, recognizing the likelihood of significant myopic shift over time (see below). Close follow-up with obsessive attention to refractive and occlusion therapy needs over many years is essential to achieving best possible vision.
- Primary intraocular lens implantation is an option for *bilateral* cataract surgery in older children, but has not been shown to improve visual outcomes. Deciding whether a child is best managed with primary bilateral IOL implantation or with surgery that leaves the aphakic eyes well positioned for possible future secondary implantation requires careful consideration of options with the family.
- Currently available evidence does not support the use of primary intraocular lens implantation in infants with bilateral cataract, or less than 6 months old. Lensectomy with vitrectomy should be performed in such patients, leaving sufficient peripheral lens capsule to support possible future secondary IOL implantation. Aphakic refractive correction is provided in the form of extended wear silicone contact lenses or high plus spectacle lenses.

Disease Course

- While subnormal axial length (microphthalmos) is common with congenital cataract, when treatment is delayed excessive growth causing axial elongation and myopic refractive shift may result from visual deprivation. (Transient media opacities such as corneal clouding or vitreous hemorrhage from birth trauma may have similar effect.) After surgery in infancy, myopic shift (evident as decreased plus requirement in aphakic eyes) typically occurs as a result of normal growth of the eye, though the amount is highly variable and unpredictable.
- Open angle glaucoma is a common development following pediatric cataract surgery, requiring careful monitoring of IOP in aphakic and pseudophakic children. Risk is greatest in microphthalmic eyes with congenital nuclear or total cataract, or PHPV. Onset is usually insidious,

often more than 5 years after surgery, with more rapid than expected myopic shift in refraction as the first sign. May be challenging to treat, frequently requiring multiple surgeries, though in some cases control with topical medication is possible.

- Pupillary block with pressure elevation may occur following lensectomy/vitrectomy in early infancy, as a result of regrowth of vitreous and extension into the anterior chamber. Peripheral iridectomy should accompany L/V surgery performed before age 6 months.
- Retinal detachment, once a frequent and feared late (often decades after surgery) complication of pediatric cataract surgery, seems much less a concern with modern operative techniques. Clinically significant cystoid macular edema is rarely seen after uncomplicated cataract surgery in childhood.

Differential Diagnosis

- *Lowe syndrome* (oculocerebrorenal syndrome) is an X-linked recessive disorder that nearly always presents with bilateral congenital cataract. The lens is typically small, thin, and totally opacified. Glaucoma develops during infancy in slightly more than half of cases. Renal tubular dysfunction causes metabolic acidosis and aminoaciduria; rarely renal failure. Mental deficiency ranges from mild to severe.
- *Congenital rubella* (Gregg syndrome) is associated with cataract in up to one third of cases (75% bilateral), and glaucoma in about 10%. Pigmentary retinopathy ("salt and pepper" fundus) is seen in nearly half of cases, usually having only minor impact on vision. Important systemic findings include deafness, mental deficiency, hepatosplenomegaly, and thrombocytopenia. Live virus has been found in lens aspirates several years after birth, necessitating infection control precautions during surgery and contributing to frequently severe postoperative inflammation.
- High blood levels of galactose lead to infantile onset of cataract in patients with the autosomal recessive disorders *galactosemia* (deficiency of galactose-1-phosphate uridyl transferase—GALT) and *galactokinase* (GALK) *deficiency*, both diagnosed by assay of enzyme activity in RBCs. Prompt initiation of a soy formula diet may reverse early lens changes (beginning with the classic "oil droplet" appearance, described in Table 8.12), as well as systemic consequences (failure to thrive, signs of liver disease, mental deficiency, and often sepsis) associated with GALT galactosemia only. In North America, most cases are identified through state-mandated newborn screening programs, but both false-negative and false-positive screening results are common.

References

Francis PJ, Berry V, Bhattacharya SS, et al. The genetics of childhood cataract. *J Med Genet* 2000;37:481–488.

Greenwald MJ, Glaser SR. Visual outcomes after surgery for unilateral cataract in children over two years old: posterior chamber intraocular lens implantation versus contact lens correction of aphakia. *J AAPOS* 1998;2:168–176.

UVEITIS

Juvenile Rheumatoid Arthritis–Associated Uveitis

Summary

By far the most common and important form of pediatric uveitis is that seen with juvenile rheumatoid arthritis (JRA), typically presenting in girls under 16 years old.

Demographics

- Fifty percent or more of JRA cases are pauciarticular, and 20% of these develop uveitis.
- Female-to-male ratio is 3:1 or greater.
- Onset of arthritis before age 7 years is a risk factor for development of uveitis.

Symptoms and Signs

- Blurred vision or floaters.
- Ocular redness and discomfort typically absent to mild; occasionally more severe.
- Most patients have no ocular symptoms and are diagnosed after failing a vision test or when screened after onset of joint symptoms leads to systemic diagnosis.

Ophthalmic Findings

- Bilateral (75% of cases) or unilateral anterior nongranulomatous uveitis.
- Anterior chamber cell reaction and keratic precipitate formation are both generally of mild to moderate degree with few vitreous cells. (Perform careful slit-lamp examination using the brightest available light setting.)
- Posterior synechiae and band keratopathy are important early indicators of tissue damage.
- Cataract, glaucoma, and macular edema are late sight-threatening complications.

Systemic Findings

- Arthritis usually involves a small number of larger joints (fewer than 5, especially the knees), but uveitis occasionally occurs in polyarticular or systemic JRA.
- Uveitis may precede or follow joint involvement, or occur in its absence.

Special Tests

- ANA strongly positive in a majority of cases.
- Rheumatoid factor usually negative.
- HLA-B27 may be positive. Uveitis is more likely to be acute and symptomatic in this group, which tends also to be older and includes more males.

Treatment and Management

- Mydriatic drops and topical or periocular injected corticosteroid are used to minimize anterior chamber cell reaction and halt progression of posterior synechiae.
- Vision loss from macular edema requires periocular injection of long-acting corticosteroid (e.g., triamcinolone) or systemic steroid treatment in most cases.
- Immunosuppressive treatment (e.g., methotrexate) may be necessary in refractory cases.
- IOP may be elevated from the inflammatory process or effect of steroid treatment; must be monitored closely.
- Cataract may progress to require surgery, with significantly increased frequency of complications. Inflammation should be quiescent or maximally suppressed during the perioperative period. Intraocular lens implantation is controversial; may be appropriate in carefully selected cases.

Differential Diagnosis

- Both *childhood sarcoidosis* and *juvenile psoriatic arthritis* may present with chronic anterior uveitis and joint inflammation, sometimes before development of characteristic lesions of skin or other organs, and may be mistaken for JRA-associated uveitis. Bilateral hilar adenopathy is nearly always present in children with sarcoidosis.
- Nongranulomatous anterior uveitis (sometimes very intense but usually responding well to treatment) may accompany *tubulointerstitial nephritis* (TINU syndrome) in children (mostly girls). Abnormal laboratory findings include proteinuria, elevated serum creatinine, and high ESR.
- *Kawasaki disease* is an acute vasculitic disorder in infancy or childhood, one of whose principal manifestations is conjunctival hyperemia (without discharge), typically in a context of febrile illness and skin rash. Uveitis (nearly always mild) and joint pain/swelling may raise concern about JRA. Other findings include erythema and peeling/splitting of palms/soles/lips. Prevention of life-threatening coronary artery aneurysm, the most serious complication, requires aggressive pediatric medical management including IV immunoglobulin and high-dose aspirin.

References

Kanski JJ, Petty RE. Chronic childhood arthritis and uveitis. *Ocular Infect Immunol* 1996:40:485–493.

Lam LA, Lowder CY, Baervelt G, et al. Surgical management of cataract in children with juvenile rheumatoid arthritis. *Am J Ophthalmol* 2003;125:772–778.

Intermediate Uveitis (Pars Planitis)

Summary

The term *intermediate uveitis* is preferred for designation of chronic intraocular inflammation concentrated in the anterior vitreous.

Demographics

- Twenty-five percent of pediatric uveitis cases, second in frequency after JRA.
- Bilateral in 75% of cases.

Symptoms and Signs

- Decreased vision, floaters.
- Redness and discomfort rarely present; often diagnosed after failure on routine vision testing.

Ophthalmic Findings

- Mild anterior chamber cells and flare, usually no keratic precipitates
- Posterior synechiae and band keratopathy much less common than with JRA.
- Anterior vitreous cells always present, usually far in excess of aqueous cells.
- Posterior subcapsular (PSC) cataract common; often remains mild but may progress to require surgical treatment.
- Peripheral fundus examination (with scleral indentation if possible; employing sedation or general anesthesia if necessary) is essential to identify characteristic pars plana "snow banking," retinal vasculitis in a minority of cases, and occasionally a localized chorioretinal lesion that may indicate an infectious process (e.g., toxoplasmosis).
- Macular edema is the most frequent cause of vision loss.
- Less common complications include retinal neovascularization, retinal detachment, and glaucoma.

Special Tests

- Fluorescein angiography to look for macular edema and vasculitis.
- Chest x-ray to look for evidence of tuberculosis and sarcoidosis.
- *Lyme disease* titers if the patient has a history of possible tick bite or exposure. Intermediate uveitis is the most common intraocular manifestation of this condition. Other findings may include cranial nerve palsies (especially facial), optic neuritis, keratitis, and conjunctivitis (associated with characteristic skin rash in the acute phase).

Treatment and Management

- Topical and periocular corticosteroids; mydriatic drops if forming synechiae.
- Monitor closely for vision loss from macular edema.
- Systemic immunosuppression may be necessary in refractory cases.
- Pars plana cryotherapy and vitrectomy are sometimes performed in patients with severe disease.

Toxocariasis

Summary

Ocular toxocariasis occurs almost exclusively in children and may present either with intense posterior segment inflammation or as a cicatricial lesion involving retina and vitreous.

Demographics

- Average age of presentation is 7 years.
- Mostly boys.

Etiology

Children ingest eggs of the roundworm *Toxocara canis* with soil contaminated by dog feces; larvae develop in the intestines and disseminate via hematogenous spread throughout the body, including the posterior segment of the eye. Inflammation may increase after death of the organism.

Symptoms and Signs

- Decreased vision, floaters; nearly always unilateral.
- Mild redness and discomfort in some acute cases.
- May present with leukocoria that resembles retinoblastoma (p. 481).

Ophthalmic Findings

- In chronic cases, the usual lesion is peripheral fundus or posterior pole granuloma, an elevated whitish mass, often associated with localized tractional retinal detachment, and sometimes mild overlying vitreous cell reaction. May resemble PHPV (p. 452).
- Vitreitis in acute cases may be so severe it prevents visualization of the fundus. Anterior chamber reaction usually mild if present but occasionally there is hypopyon.
- Rarely presents with neuroretinitis or optic neuropathy.
- Macular edema, cataract, and glaucoma are occasional complications.

Systemic Findings

- Usually absent in children with ocular disease.
- The syndrome of *visceral larvae migrans*, with fever, respiratory and neurologic symptoms, and peripheral blood eosinophilia, is typically seen in children under age 3 years, without ocular involvement.

Special Tests

- Enzyme-linked immunosorbent assay (ELISA) for *T. canis* is usually diagnostic.
- CBC may show elevated eosinophil count.

Treatment and Management

- In consultation with an infectious disease specialist, consider systemic antihelminthic treatment.
- Periocular or systemic corticosteroid treatment for ocular inflammation, which may increase after antihelminthic therapy.
- Vitrectomy may be indicated for retinal detachment or vitreoretinal traction, or to remove immunogenic debris from the vitreous.

Differential Diagnosis

- Intrauterine infection with the protozoan *Toxoplasma gondii* is the most common cause of posterior uveitis in infants and children, but intraocular inflammatory activity in the great majority of cases has subsided completely by the time of postnatal diagnosis of *toxoplasmosis chorioretinitis*.
  - Disease results from maternal ingestion of raw meat or cat feces during pregnancy.
  - The usual ocular presentation is with one or more flat, sharply demarcated chorioretinal scars (characteristically showing both hyperpigmented and hypopigmented areas), typically involving the macula, often bilateral. A small minority of cases show more severe and extensive ocular damage, rarely leading to phthisis.
  - Reactivation of dormant organisms in retina, usually adjacent to a scar, may cause further loss of vision, so affected eyes need to be monitored carefully, and treated if active inflammation is found.
  - Central nervous system (CNS) involvement may cause seizures, hydrocephalus, and CT findings including loss of tissue and calcification, as well as hearing loss and mental deficiency.
  - Toxoplasmosis diagnosed in infancy or early childhood should generally receive aggressive systemic therapy with multiple drugs, primarily to minimize CNS damage, which may be progressive.
- *Lymphocytic choriomeningitis virus* infection is acquired from contact with rodent feces and may have severe effects on the fetus during pregnancy, including CNS damage and uveitis with chorioretinal scarring that may be indistinguishable from that of toxoplasmosis.
- Other congenital infection ("ORCH" agents) involving the posterior segment is diagnosed much less often than toxoplasmosis. These conditions present with similar findings, though somewhat different typical patterns of fundus pigment disturbance (e.g., "salt and pepper" appearance in congenital rubella—p. 449) and brain calcification (e.g., periventricular deposits with congenital CMV infection). Active inflammatory chorioretinal lesions are rarely seen. Except in the case of HSV with cutaneous or ocular surface disease (p. 432), treatment is seldom indicated.
- *Subacute sclerosing panencephalitis*, a pediatric neurodegenerative disease caused by chronic measles virus infection, may present with evidence of chorioretinitis in the macular region.
- Posterior uveitis from noninfectious causes is very seldom seen in children.

References

Gillespie SH, Dinning WJ, Voller A, et al. The spectrum of ocular toxocariasis. *Eye* 1993;7:415–418.

McLeod R, Boyer K, Karrison T, et al. Outcome of treatment for congenital toxoplasmosis, 1981–2004: the National Collaborative Chicago-Based Congenital Toxoplasmosis Study. *Clin Infect Dis* 2006;42:1383–1394.

VITREOUS AND RETINA

Persistent Hyperplastic Primary Vitreous

Summary

PHPV, also known as *persistent fetal vasculature*, has a broad spectrum of severity with anterior and/or posterior segment involvement. There is usually a fibrous plaque on the posterior lens capsule associated with remnants of hyaloid (embryonic vitreous) structure extending from the optic nerve. Abnormal vascular elements are frequently but not always a part of the condition, which is sporadic, unilateral in nearly all cases, and without significant systemic associations.

Symptoms and Signs

- Decreased vision, often with secondary strabismus.
- Leukocoria variably evident (Figure 8.12A).
- Smaller than normal eye.

Ophthalmic Findings

- Microphthalmos to some degree always present, unless cornea has enlarged secondary to increased IOP in infancy.
- Sometimes characteristic iris vascular abnormality, with vessels extending to pupil margin.
- Variable lens opacification from none to total; often progressive over time. Opacified cortex may resorb leaving a membranous cataract.
- Ciliary processes often dragged centrally into fibrovascular membrane adherent to posterior lens capsule. Anterior chamber may be shallow as a result of forward displacement of the lens and iris.
- IOP may be normal, increased (due to anterior displacement of lens and iris), or decreased (due to traction on ciliary body).
- Fibrovascular stalk extending from the optic disc to the posterior lens (usually central, sometimes peripheral) is common and very characteristic. May range from a slender thread to involvement of most of the vitreous.
- Significant posterior involvement, present in a minority of cases, typically takes the form of glial tissue covering a portion of the disc and adjacent retina, often with tractional distortion or elevation (Figure 8.12B), sometimes including a prominent fold.

Special Tests

Ultrasound, CT, or MRI may reveal persistent posterior segment hyaloid structures obscured by anterior membrane or cataract.

Disease Course

Milder degrees often remain stable indefinitely. With greater severity, secondary developments including progressive

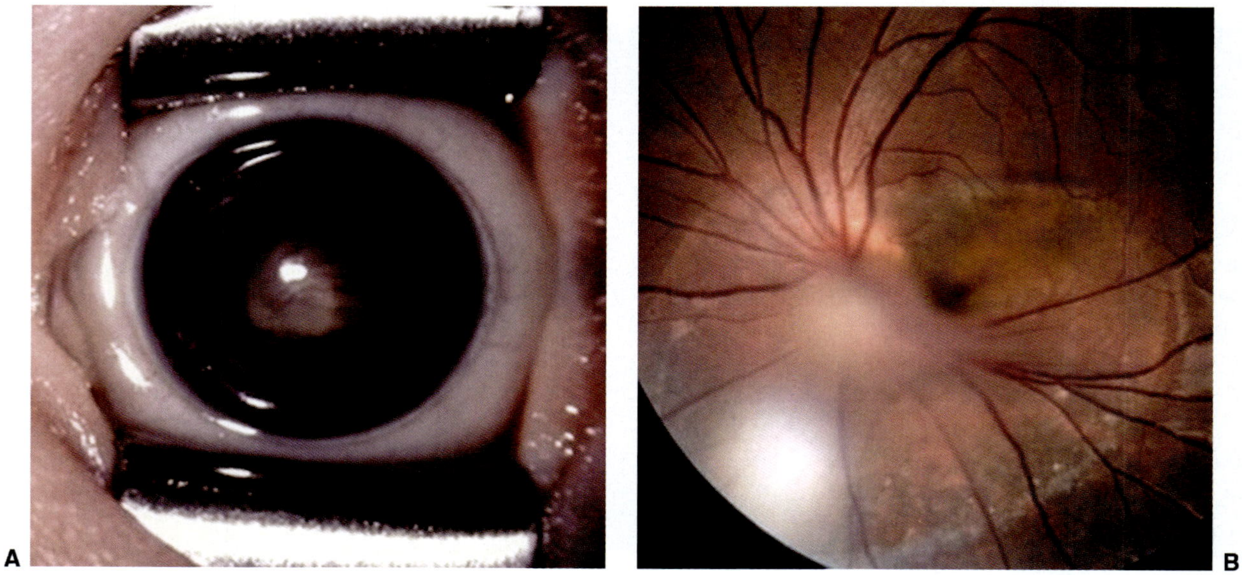

FIGURE 8.12. Persistent hyperplastic primary vitreous. **A:** Most of the posterior segment in this small eye is filled with abnormal fibrovascular tissue, causing shallowing of the anterior chamber, but lens remains clear. **B:** Posterior involvement in this eye (with 20/100 visual acuity) includes localized tractional elevation and distortion of peripapillary retina. The disc is partially obscured by fibrovascular tissue (out of focus in the image) extending toward the back of the lens, which remains clear.

lens opacification, displacement of lens and ciliary body, or vitreoretinal traction frequently lead to deterioration of vision, glaucoma or hypotony, retinal detachment, and ultimately phthisis. Posterior segment bleeding is an uncommon occurrence.

Treatment and Management

- Mild cases may require no treatment, or simply part-time occlusion of the normal eye to reverse or prevent amblyopia.
- Dense central retrolental plaque, alone or with secondary cataract, may be source of significant visual deprivation leading to severe amblyopia in infancy. Vitrectomy with lensectomy to restore media clarity, followed by contact lens correction of aphakia and occlusion for amblyopia may result in salvage of good or at least useful vision. IOL implantation is rarely an option because of age and microphthalmos.
- Surgery should be done via limbal incision; risk of retinal detachment is high after pars plana approach. Complete removal of the stalk is not necessary. Bleeding from abnormal vessels seldom a serious problem.
- When posterior segment involvement is severe, visual prognosis is poor but lensectomy may still be indicated to help stabilize IOP.

Reference

Goldberg MF. Persistent fetal vasculature (PFV): an integrated interpretation of signs and symptoms associated with persistent hyperplastic primary vitreous (PHPV). *Am J Ophthalmol* 1997;124:587–626.

Vitreoretinal Dysplasia

Summary

Vitreoretinal dysplasia (VRD) describes severe maldevelopment of the posterior segment of the globe that results in replacement of most or all of the retina and vitreous by a mass of disorganized tissue, showing limited preservation of retinal differentiation. This condition is often part of a systemic syndrome (Table 8.13).

Symptoms and Signs

- Usually bilateral; unilateral cases may be difficult to distinguish from PHPV.
- Severe vision loss in affected eyes.
- Microphthalmos.
- Leukocoria.

Special Tests

- Chromosome analysis.
- Genetic probes have been developed for several forms of retinal dysplasia, particularly Norrie disease in males.

Differential Diagnosis

- End-stage retinopathy of prematurity (ROP) may closely resemble VRD, and in many cases of incontinentia

Table 8.13

Causes of vitreoretinal dysplasia

Condition	Other ocular findings	Systemic findings	Comment
Trisomy 13 (Patau syndrome)	Anterior segment dysgenesis Fundus coloboma Intraocular cartilage	Severe CNS maldevelopment Bilateral cleft lip and palate Polydactyly Severe cardiac malformation	Usually death in infancy
Walker-Warburg syndrome	Anterior segment dysgenesis Fundus coloboma	Severe CNS maldevelopment Hydrocephalus	Autosomal recessive Severe mental deficiency
Norrie disease	Vitreous hemorrhage, ROP-like retinal folds (p. 458)	Acquired deafness, mental deterioration	X-linked recessive Genetic testing useful
Incontinentia pigmenti	Avascular peripheral retina ROP-like neovascularization (p. 458)	Characteristic skin lesions "Peg" teeth Variable mental deficiency	X-linked dominant, usually lethal in males
Vitreoretinal dysplasia	Isolated ocular disease	None	May be autosomal recessive Most cases sporadic

CNS, central nervous system; ROP, retinopathy of prematurity.

PEDIATRIC

pigmenti and Norrie disease the typical picture of VRD evolves during infancy through a vasculopathic process very similar to ROP (p. 457).

- Fundus coloboma (p. 469) may be seen as a milder expression of retinal maldevelopment in trisomy 13 and Walker-Warburg syndrome.

Vitreoretinal Degeneration

Liquefied or optically empty vitreous, sometimes with veils or hemorrhage, is associated with a variety of degenerative changes in the retina, and frequently early-onset cataract, in a number of hereditary disorders that typically manifest in childhood (Table 8.14). These conditions, particularly Stickler syndrome, are responsible for a large percentage of nontraumatic rhegmatogenous retinal detachments in the pediatric age range.

Retinopathy of Prematurity

Summary

ROP, formerly known as *retrolental fibroplasia*, is a disorder of retinal blood vessel development that occurs in infants born prematurely, prior to completion of retinal vascularization. It is characterized by neovascular proliferation in the transition zone between posterior vascularized retina and anterior avascular retina, which may cause permanent retinal damage by way of exudation or traction, and vision loss ranging from mild impairment to complete blindness.

Etiology

ROP is a complex multifactorial disorder, but considerable evidence supports the view that it originates with peripheral retinal hypoxia resulting from retinal tissue maturation in the face of arrested vascular development (at least to some degree a consequence of systemic hyperoxemia). This leads to release of vascular endothelial growth factor (VEGF), which stimulates proliferation of abnormal retinal vessels.

Risk Factors

- The incidence and severity of ROP are strongly inversely related to *birth weight* and *gestational age*. In the developed world, vision loss from ROP virtually never occurs following birth after 32 weeks' gestation and at a weight greater than 2,000 g. A substantial majority of infants born before 28 weeks and weighing less than 1,000 g at birth will show at least mild transient ROP, and many will develop sight-threatening disease regardless of other circumstances or management.
- Administration of *supplemental oxygen in excess of clinical need* has been well documented to increase the frequency and severity of ROP in vulnerable eyes. Even with carefully controlled oxygen administration, however, ROP is common in very low birth weight infants, and risk of severe vision loss cannot be eliminated by any strategy of oxygen curtailment that is compatible with optimal survival and neurologic health. There is no convincing evidence that excessive oxygen administra-

Table 8.14

Causes of vitreoretinal degeneration

Condition	Fundus findings	Other findings	Comment
Juvenile retinoschisis	Vitreous veils, hemorrhage Foveal (Table 8.16), peripheral retinoschisis Risk of rhegmatogenous RD	Loss of ERG B-wave Vascular sheathing	X-linked, males only Vision loss may progress
Stickler syndrome	Optically empty vitreous Lattice-like degeneration High-risk of rhegmatogenous RD	Early-onset high myopia Early cataract, glaucoma Flat face, Pierre-Robin chin	Autosomal dominant Cleft palate, joint problems, hearing loss common
Wagner syndrome	Optically empty vitreous Pigmentary retinopathy Low risk of RD in childhood	Moderate myopia, cataract Night blindness ERG decreased or extinguished	Autosomal dominant Progressive vision loss and fundus pigmentation
Goldman-Favre disease	Liquefied vitreous Foveal, peripheral retinoschisis Pigmentary retinopathy	Cataract Night blindness ERG decreased or extinguished	Autosomal recessive

ERG, electroretinogram; RD, retinal detachment.

tion is harmful to the retina after 32 weeks' gestational age, even when significant ROP is present.

- Risk factors of lesser importance include bronchopulmonary dysplasia, intraventricular hemorrhage, necrotizing enterocolitis, and sepsis.

Symptoms and Signs

- During the acute phase of ROP (roughly 1 to 6 months of age), when sight-saving clinical intervention is possible, ROP has no externally visible signs.
- Older infants and children with eyes that have been severely and irreversibly damaged by ROP may show leukocoria and microphthalmos. Strabismus and nystagmus may result from poor vision. End-stage ROP is characterized in some cases by inflammation and pain resulting from glaucoma in blind eyes.

International Classification of ROP

(1984, updated 2005)

ROP is characterized by *location, extent*, and *stage* of disease.

Location

- The retina is divided into three *zones*.
- **Zone 1:** A *circle* centered on the disk, the radius of which is twice the distance from the disk to the center of the macula.
- **Zone 2:** An *annulus* that extends from the edge of zone 1 to the ora serrata in the nasal meridian, and for the same distance (approximately to the fundus equator) on the temporal side.
- **Zone 3:** A *crescent* including all retina temporally, superiorly, and inferiorly that is anterior to zone 2.

Extent

- Circumferential extent is quantified by number of *clock-hours* of retina involved.

Stage of Disease

- **Stage 1:** *Demarcation line*. A narrow flat grayish structure that divides vascular from avascular retina. It consists pathologically of immature vascular channels.
- **Stage 2:** *Ridge*. A line that has developed substantial width and thickness. Arteriovenous shunting in a ridge may be associated with increased caliber and tortuosity of vessels entering and leaving the structure, and also more posteriorly (see below). The distinction between "line" and "ridge" has no well-defined clinical basis or implication.
- **Stage 3:** Ridge with *extraretinal fibrovascular proliferation* (EFP or ERP). This distinct form of neovascularization originates from the posterior edge of the ridge or further back in the retina. Fibrovascular tissue breaks through the internal limiting membrane, resulting in changes ranging from low-lying growth extending along the ridge (or behind and parallel to it, in isolated tufts or a linear configuration), to lofty veils or thick membranes rising into the vitreous and ultimately extending to the posterior lens capsule in very severe cases (Figures 8.13A and 8.14C). These structures are the cause of most retinal damage in ROP.
- **Stage 4:** *Subtotal retinal detachment*. May be *tractional, exudative*, or a combination. Typically begins with elevation of retina from which ERP originates; may evolve into a *falciform fold* extending from the disc to the far periphery (Figure 8.14A, B).
  - **4A:** Extrafoveal retina only.
  - **4B:** Including fovea.
- **Stage 5:** *Total retinal detachment*. Ultimately, extraretinal membranes extending to the back of the lens may contract and pull the entire peripheral retina into proximity with the lens, gathering the central retina into a funnel configuration (Figure 8.14D).

Plus Disease

- Defined as *dilation and tortuosity* of posterior retinal vessels equal to or exceeding that shown in a standard photograph, involving at least two quadrants (Figure 8.13B). The consequence of increased blood flow from arteriovenous shunting in peripheral neovascular structures.
- *Preplus* disease is dilation and tortuosity less than that shown in the standard photograph.

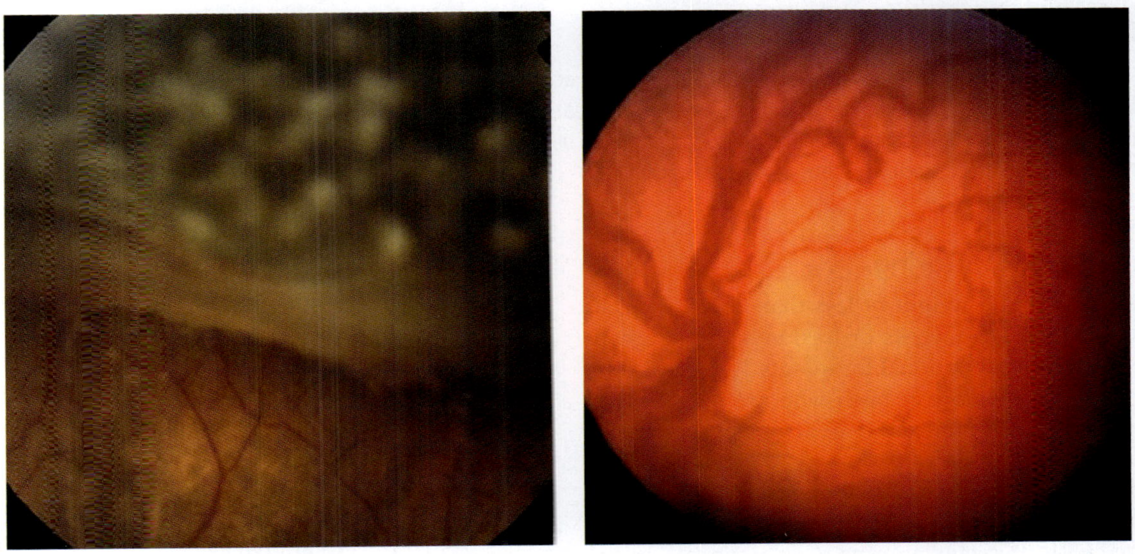

A B

FIGURE 8.13. Acute-phase ROP. **A:** Stage 3 vasoproliferation, with extraretinal fibrovascular membrane arising from the posterior edge of a terminal ridge; peripheral avascular retina shows effect of recent laser treatment. **B:** Plus disease, with marked dilation of posterior venules and tortuosity of arterioles.

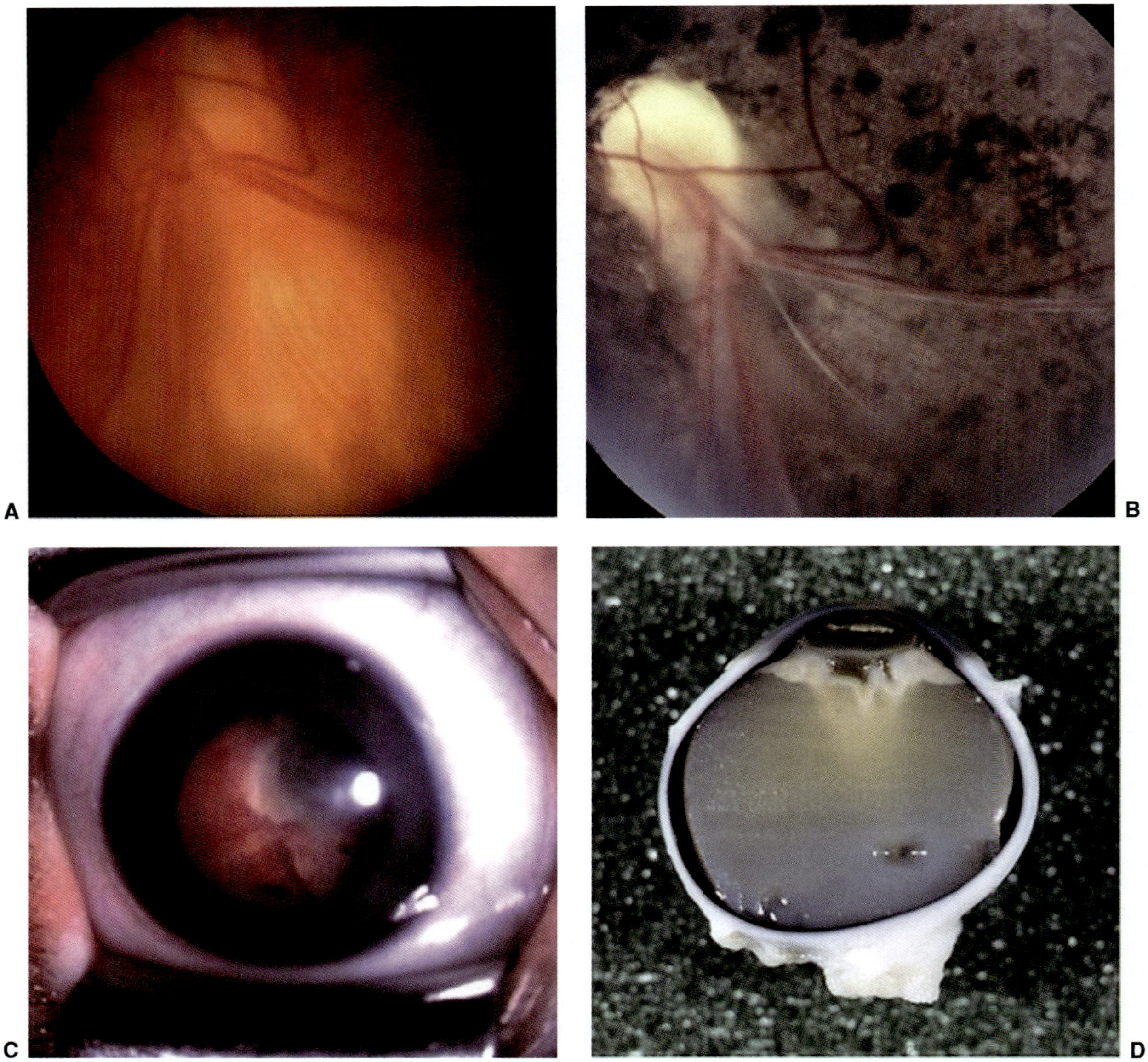

FIGURE 8.14. ROP with retinal detachment. **A:** Stage 4B with acute tractional and exudative detachment involving the macula. **B:** Same eye 13 years later, with persistent tractional detachment, and extensive pigment mottling after reabsorption of subretinal fluid. **C:** Florid fibrovascular proliferation extending to the back of the lens, leading to stage 5 funnel-shaped total detachment. **D:** Postmortem specimen showing funnel detachment.

Screening and Monitoring

- All infants born at a weight of less than 1,500 g, or at a gestational age of 30 weeks or less, must be screened for ROP. Screening is optional for infants 1,500 to 2,000 g and 31 weeks or more at birth who are judged by a responsible pediatric clinician to be at greater than usual risk.
- Screening is done following dilation of the pupils with a mild mydriatic solution (usually 0.2% cyclopentolate combined with 1% phenylephrine [Cyclomydril]), by an experienced examiner using indirect ophthalmoscopy with the aid of a lid speculum and scleral indentation. A nurse or other skilled assistant should participate to monitor the infant's vital signs, mitigate stress, and assist with positioning.
- Initial screening is done at age 4 weeks or when gestational age has reached 31 weeks, whichever comes later. In the absence of positive findings, screening should be repeated at 1- to 3-week intervals (depending on risk level) at least until zone 2 is fully vascularized (i.e., vessels have reached the nasal ora serrata) and the infant has passed the gestational age of 35 weeks.
- Once ROP is present, its course should be monitored at intervals ranging from a few days to a few weeks

(depending on severity and risk level) until complete disappearance of fundus abnormalities has occurred, or the infant has reached a developmental age of 45 to 50 weeks and shown no evidence of progression for at least 1 month.

Disease Course

- ROP is never present at birth. Onset usually occurs between ages 4 and 8 weeks, typically later for infants born at earlier gestational ages.
- Many eyes do not progress beyond stages 1 to 2. In most of these, the demarcation line or ridge gradually fades while migrating anteriorly toward the ora serrata.
- The initial development of extraretinal proliferation (stage 3 disease) or posterior vessel changes (preplus disease), both indicators of increased risk for vision loss, typically occurs 2 to 4 weeks after initial detection of a line or ridge but may not happen until as late as 42 weeks' gestational age. From this point, the criterion for treatment is often reached within 1 to 2 weeks.
- ROP that begins in zone 1 or posterior zone 2 may progress rapidly and reach severity indicating a need for treatment within 1 to 2 weeks of initial detection. This is known as *aggressive posterior ROP*, formerly called *rush* disease.
- By the end of infancy, the lesions of acute phase ROP always regress or evolve into a state of scarring or cicatrization. Findings in cicatricial ROP may include the following:

  Persistent disturbances of retinal vasculature (usually minor, intraretinal) and pigmentation. Atrophic ERP membranes may separate from retinal surface and float in the vitreous.

  Displacement of the macula ("dragging"), most often in the temporal direction, with decreased macular differentiation and loss of function to varying degree.

  Persistent tractional retinal detachment (TRD) ranging from a narrow fold, often involving the macula, to total detachment showing a "closed funnel" configuration and a retrolental fibrovascular membrane.

  Mild to moderate microphthalmos.

  Myopia, often of high degree, with significant lenticular as well as axial components.

  Glaucoma, resulting from anterior displacement of the iris and lens by retrolental cicatrix, in a minority of cases.

Treatment and Management

- Most eyes with ROP regress spontaneously, and no treatment is completely effective in preventing vision loss, or free of potentially serious complications. It is therefore standard practice to treat eyes only after ROP has reached a carefully defined level of severity.
- The multicenter CRYO-ROP study (1988) first confirmed that treatment of ROP significantly improves anatomic and functional outcomes. In this controlled randomized multicenter trial, cryotherapy was used to ablate the entire peripheral avascular retina when stage 3+ disease occupied at least 5 contiguous or 8 total clock hours of the fundus ("treatment threshold").
- Subsequent studies substituting laser ablation for cryotherapy have yielded similar or better results, making laser standard treatment in cases with sufficiently clear media. Inadequate response after initial treatment may improve following retreatment with laser (or cryo) to avascular retina that shows less than complete ablation. Close observation (1- to 2-week intervals or less) must be continued for at least 2 months after treatment.
- The ET-ROP multicenter study of earlier treatment for ROP (2003) showed greater benefit from laser treatment applied as soon as the presence of plus disease was documented, or when stage 3 was found present in zone 1. This is now the consensus criterion for treatment of ROP.
- The BEAT-ROP multicenter study (2011) recently confirmed that primary treatment with a single intravitreal injection of the VEGF inhibitor bevacizumab (Avastin) may be superior to laser for stage 3 ROP with plus disease in zone 1 or posterior zone 2. There appear to be significant advantages to anti-VEGF therapy for this group of patients, including reduced morbidity from treatment and preservation of peripheral retinal function. Close observation for months after injection is critically important, as late recurrence is more likely than after laser, though seldom requiring treatment beyond a second injection.
- Bevacizumab injection may also be beneficial for progressive ERP, after laser or in zone 3, that threatens to cause tractional detachment. Occasional development of TRD following injection in such cases makes some authorities wary of using this approach except in conjunction with surgery to relieve traction.
- In the hands of a vitreoretinal surgeon experienced with infant eyes, lens-sparing vitrectomy with or without scleral buckling can prevent progressive deterioration and partially restore vision lost to retinal detachment in stage 4 ROP. The prognosis for eyes with stage 5 ROP remains grim despite recent surgical advances. Eyes that emerge from the acute phase of ROP with significant scarring are at risk for rhegmatogenous retinal detachment from childhood through adulthood.
- Older infants and children with regressed ROP should be followed and treated as necessary for myopia and strabismus, which usually become evident by age 1 to 2 years. Asymmetric cicatricial fundus changes and refractive error increase the risk of amblyopia. Central fixation and binocular fusion may not be achievable in patients with significant macular ectopia from dragging. Children with vision loss from cicatricial changes may need blind services at an early age or low vision care at school age. Lensectomy may improve comfort in eyes with total retinal detachment and glaucoma.

Differential Diagnosis

- *Familial exudative vitreoretinopathy* (FEVR) may present at any age including early infancy, often bearing close resemblance to ROP. The condition is autosomal dominant with a wide range of expressions, frequently mild enough to be asymptomatic in parents, but also frequently of sporadic occurrence. Most cases of what appears to be ROP in infants over 2,000 g at birth are probably FEVR.
- *Norrie disease* (males only, X-linked recessive) causes a variety of posterior segment changes including vitreous hemorrhage, retinal fold or detachment, and retrolental mass (vitreoretinal dysplasia), which may be present at birth or develop during infancy. Early stages sometimes resemble ROP. Hearing loss and mental deterioration (psychosis or dementia) become evident later in life. Genetic diagnosis is now possible. Abnormality of the Norrie gene (chromosome locus Xp11.3) may play a role in cases of isolated ROP-like retinopathy that develop in larger infants.
- *Incontinentia pigmenti* (Bloch-Sulzberger syndrome) occurs almost exclusively in females, resulting from an X-linked dominant gene usually lethal in males. Retinal vascular development is incomplete at full-term birth. Neovascular lesions in the retinal periphery may closely mimic acute-phase ROP but can develop or progress after infancy. A complex sequence of characteristic skin changes in infancy (culminating in a distinctive pattern of hyperpigmented macules that gradually fade by adulthood) may be overlooked or misinterpreted. Skeletal, dental, and CNS abnormalities are found in some patients (Table 8.13). An affected mother with mild disease may be diagnosed after detection in her child.

References

Flynn JT, Bancalari E, Bachynski BN, et al. Retinopathy of prematurity: diagnosis, severity, and natural history. *Ophthalmology* 1987;94:620–629.

Reynolds JD, Dobson V, Quinn GE, et al. Evidence-based screening criteria for retinopathy of prematurity: natural history data from the CRYO-ROP and LIGHT-ROP studies. *Arch Ophthalmol* 2002;120:1470–1476.

Coats Disease

Summary

Coats disease is a form of congenital retinal telangectasia associated with exudative retinal detachment.

Demographics

- Sporadic, more common in boys; unilateral in 90% of cases.
- Usually detected between ages 3 and 10 years, often on routine vision screening.
- Cases with presentation in infancy tend to be more severe and more often involve girls.
- No significant systemic associations.

Symptoms and Signs

- Severely decreased vision.
- May present as leukocoria, or strabismus secondary to decreased vision.

Ophthalmic Findings

- Telangeictatic retinal vessels with localized aneurysmal dilation, often showing characteristic "light bulb" appearance, usually in the peripheral retina (Figure 8.15A and B). Posterior vessels are often dilated and tortuous.
- Accumulation of yellowish subretinal exudate containing cholesterol crystals may be confined to the macular region (as in Figure 8.15A), or involve the entire retina.
- Neovascular glaucoma and phthisis bulbi are seen as late complications following total retinal detachment in some cases.

A

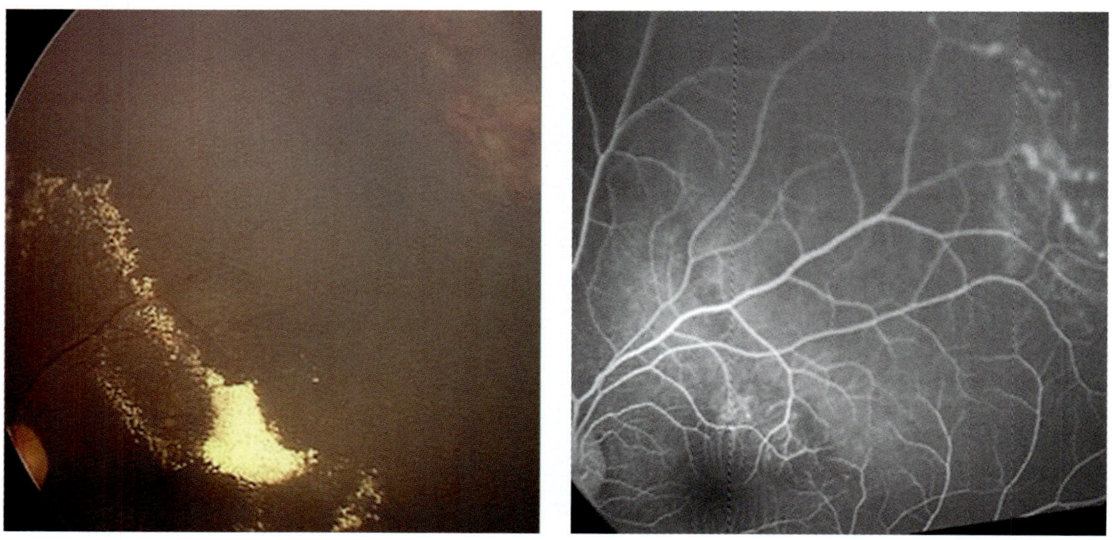

B

FIGURE 8.15. Coats disease. **A:** Wide-angle fundus image showing accumulation of hard exudate in the posterior pole as a result of leakage from abnormal vessels seen in retinal periphery. **B:** Fluorescein angiographic image of same region.

Treatment and Management

Cryotherapy or photocoagulation of abnormal blood vessels may reverse exudation or prevent progression of disease. Vision usually remains poor.

Differential Diagnosis

Coats disease with total retinal detachment in some cases so closely resembles retinoblastoma (p. 484) that enucleation and pathologic assessment is required to finally establish the nature of the problem. Absence of calcification and lower CT density in the subretinal space support the diagnosis of Coats. The poor prognosis of eyes with advanced Coats disease justifies surgical removal if there is any doubt.

Reference

Shields JA, Shields CL, Honavar SG, et al. Classification and management of Coats disease. *Am J Ophthalmol* 2001;131:572–583.

Shaken Baby Syndrome

Summary

The hallmarks of shaken baby syndrome are findings of extensive retinal hemorrhage associated with intracranial hemorrhage or other evidence of brain injury in a previously healthy infant without a history of major trauma. Usually, injuries are inflicted by a stressed isolated caregiver who loses control with an inconsolable crying infant.

Etiology

Both ocular and intracranial injury are believed due to repetitive acceleration/deceleration that occurs when the infant is held by the trunk or extremities and vigorously shaken, generating vitreoretinal traction, and rotational or shearing forces within the brain and between the brain and the meninges. Many but not all victims also sustain impact injury to the head.

Demographics

- Victim typically under age 1 year, but occasionally as old as 3 years.
- Almost always alone with a single adult caregiver at time of acute deterioration. Disproportionately often, caregiver is a nonpaternal male involved with mother.

Symptoms and Signs

- Frequently a history of minor trauma or choking; shaking is usually not mentioned.
- Presenting symptoms range from irritability, vomiting, or seizures to complete loss of consciousness, deep coma. Respiratory arrest, CPR often described.

Ophthalmic Findings

- Retinal hemorrhages in the great majority (Figure 8.16A).
  Sometimes just a few, often hundreds. Usually but not always fairly symmetrical. White centers common.
  Multiple layers including preretinal, nerve fiber, deep retinal, subretinal.
  Typically concentrated near posterior pole but extending anterior to equator, sometimes with secondary concentration in far periphery (both concentrations corresponding to areas of vitreoretinal adherence).
  Most resolve in days to weeks, without change in color but often showing thin patchy appearance during waning days.
- Internal limiting membrane separation ("traumatic retinoschisis") is commonly seen in or near macula, forming one or more cavities typically 2 to 8 mm in diameter, partially (10% to 50%) occupied by blood that usually remains bright red and fluid, and persists for weeks (Figure 8.16B–D). Cavity sometimes demarcated by a circumferential retinal fold, with or without an adjacent arc of hypopigmentation. Folds soon flatten but ILM separation may persist indefinitely; often with only minor long-term vision loss.
- Occasionally, deeper-level splitting results in cavity with inner wall containing retinal vessels, extensive retinal edema, and negative electroretinogram (ERG) from loss of B-wave amplitude. Blood in cavity often migrates into vitreous after a few days. Poor visual prognosis with this presentation.
- Optic nerve injury may result from traction or nerve sheath hemorrhage, often contributing significantly to vision loss, with acute disc edema and/or late pallor.
- Findings of hyphema, dislocated lens, or giant retinal tear with rhegmatogenous detachment suggest direct contusion of the globe rather than shaking trauma.

Systemic Findings

- Intracranial hemorrhage usually subdural, typically bilateral or interhemispheric; sometimes subarachnoid or intraparenchymal.
- Brain parenchymal injury may be direct result of rotational forces, or aggravated by hypoxia.
- Bruises (often inconspicuous) and fractures may indicate trauma to trunk or extremities from perpetrator's grasp, head impact, or other associated battering. Often such findings are completely absent.
- Mortality up to 30%; majority of survivors suffer cognitive or focal deficits.

Differential Diagnosis

- Retinal hemorrhage, sometimes extensive, is common in newborns secondary to birth process forces (occasionally even following caesarian delivery), but nearly always resolves by age 1 month.

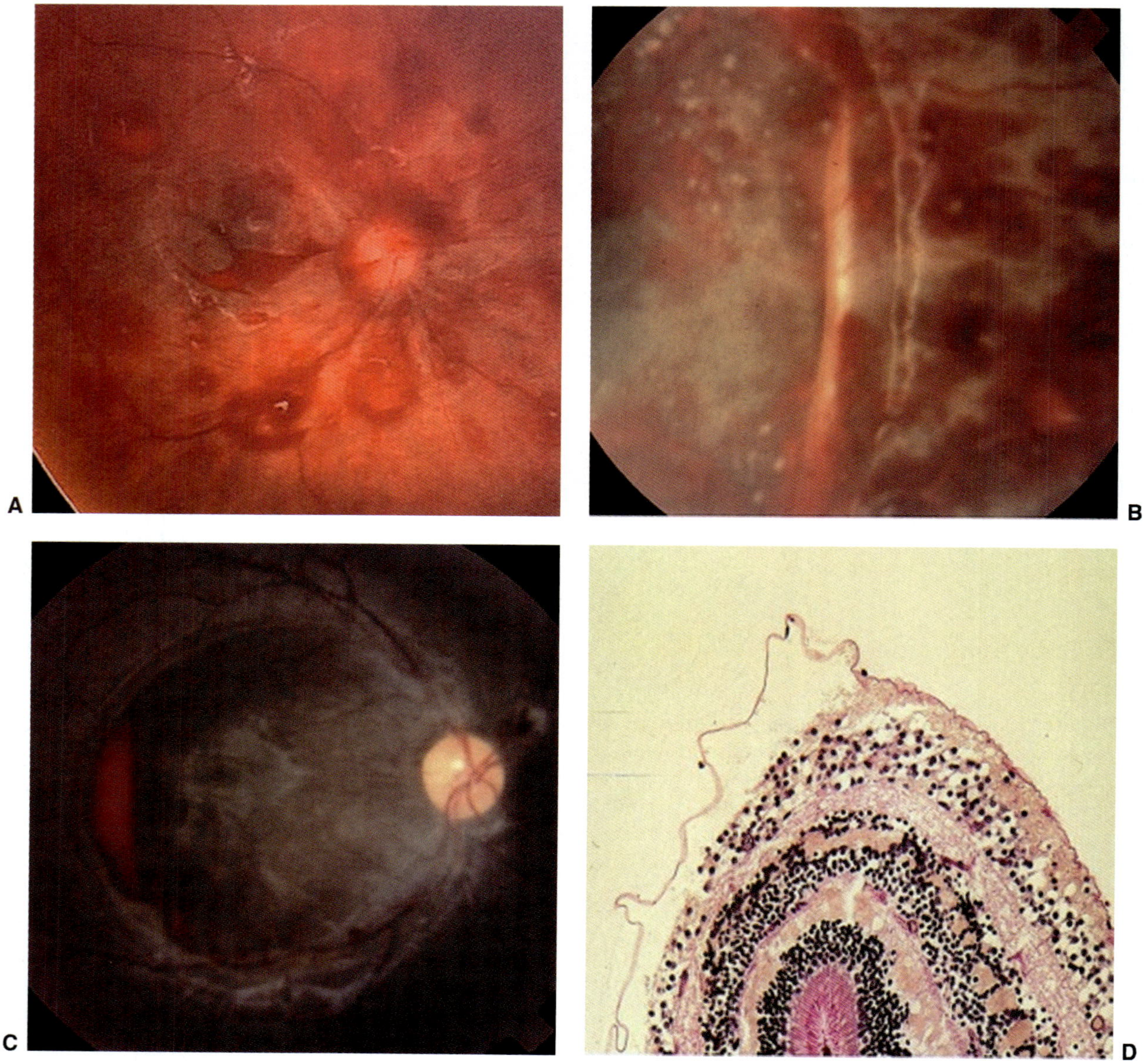

FIGURE 8.16. Retinal hemorrhage and traumatic retinoschisis secondary to presumed shaking injury. **A:** Right eye fundus showing extensive retinal hemorrhage, some in preretinal cavities with layering of blood inferiorly. **B:** Full-thickness retinal fold at the temporal edge of a schisis cavity occupying the macula, left eye. **C:** Schisis lesion weeks after injury. Other retinal hemorrhage has resolved, but a small amount of fluid blood remains in the cavity (layered temporally because patient is lying on his side for photography). **D:** Photomicrograph from a postmortem eye showing separation of internal limiting membrane, taking off from the apex of fold to span a cavity.

- Accidental injury rarely if ever causes significant retinal hemorrhage unless very severe (motor vehicle accident, fall from second story, near fatal crush).
- Expertly performed CPR may result in at most a few retinal hemorrhages. Potential for harm from resuscitative effort by untrained caregivers remains uncertain.
- Intraocular hemorrhage from abrupt rise in intracranial pressure (Terson syndrome) does not cause retinoschisis.
- Vascular and hematologic disorders need to be ruled out; usually straightforward.

References

Greenwald MJ, Weiss A, Oesterle CS, et al. Traumatic retinoschisis in battered babies. *Ophthalmology* 1986;93:618–624.

Morad Y, Wygnansky-Jaffe T, Levin AV. Retinal haemorrhage in abusive head trauma. *Clin Exp Ophthalmol* 2010;38:514–520.

Infantile Retinal Dystrophy (Leber Congenital Amaurosis)

Summary

Leber congenital amaurosis (LCA) is retinal dystrophy involving both rod and cone photoreceptors that is manifest at birth, causing severe vision loss in infancy. Inheritance is autosomal recessive, with multiple genetic loci. No effective treatment exists, though gene therapy holds promise for the future.

Symptoms and Signs

- Failure to fixate; roving eye movements present early in infancy.
- Some vision may be present at birth, but usually deteriorates during first few years of life.
- Eye pressing (oculodigital sign) is a common behavior in affected children.

Ophthalmic Findings

- Pupils react poorly to light. May show "paradoxical" response (p. 487).
- Large-amplitude pendular nystagmus.
- Fundus examination usually unremarkable at birth. Vessel attenuation, optic disc pallor, and retinal pigment changes commonly develop during infancy or early childhood.
- Often high hyperopic refractive error; occasionally myopic. Keratoconus may develop in childhood.

Special Tests

The ERG is extinguished or severely reduced. It must be recognized that mature normal responses may not yet have developed during infancy; in equivocal cases retesting at a later age may be necessary.

Systemic Findings

- Renal disease and failure are associated with infantile retinal dystrophy in Senior-Loken syndrome.
- Sensorineural hearing loss occurs in 5% of patients with LCA.
- Cognitive ability and developmental progress are usually within normal limits (see below).

Differential Diagnosis

- In *Joubert syndrome* (autosomal recessive), Leber-like retinal dystrophy is associated in infancy with rapid and/or irregular breathing, eye movement abnormalities resembling congenital oculomotor apraxia (see below), the highly characteristic finding of cerebellar vermis hypoplasia, and mental retardation. May also present later in childhood with night blindness, extinguished ERG, and progressive vision loss.
- When significant developmental delays, neurologic deficits or seizures present in association with congenital retinal dystrophy and severely reduced ERG, consider early-onset forms of peroxisomal disease (*Zellweger hepatocerebrorenal syndrome*, neonatal adrenoleukodystrophy, infantile Refsum disease) and neuronal ceroid lipofuscinosis (Batten disease). These autosomal recessive disorders are also frequently associated with cataract. Autosomal dominant *olivopontocerebellar atrophy* may have similar presentation in infancy; a parent often shows milder disease with slowly progressive ataxia, progressive external ophthalmoplegia (Table 8.2), and macular degeneration from cone-rod dystrophy (Table 8.16).
- Poor vision in infancy with nystagmus is often the presenting sign of retinal degeneration associated with disorders in which defective lysosomal enzymes cause abnormal accumulation of complex lipid breakdown products in CNS neurons, including ganglion cells. The classic early fundus finding is *cherry-red spot*, resulting from loss of transparency in perifoveal ganglion cells; this appearance may fade as affected cells atrophy and disc pallor develops (Figure 8.17). The ERG is *not* affected. Included in this category are gangliosidoses (*Tay-Sachs disease*, Sandhoff disease), leukodystrophies (metachromatic, Krabbe), Nieman-Pick disease, and rarely Gaucher disease. Hepatosplenomegaly is frequently present. Progressive CNS degeneration often leads to early death. These disorders are autosomal recessive; several of them are seen mainly in Ashkenazic Jewish families. Diagnosis is confirmed variously by finding elevated levels of metabolites in blood, characteristic deposits in biopsy tissue (bone marrow or liver), specific enzyme deficiency in cells (cultured skin fibroblasts), or gene analysis. Prenatal and carrier testing is available for most.

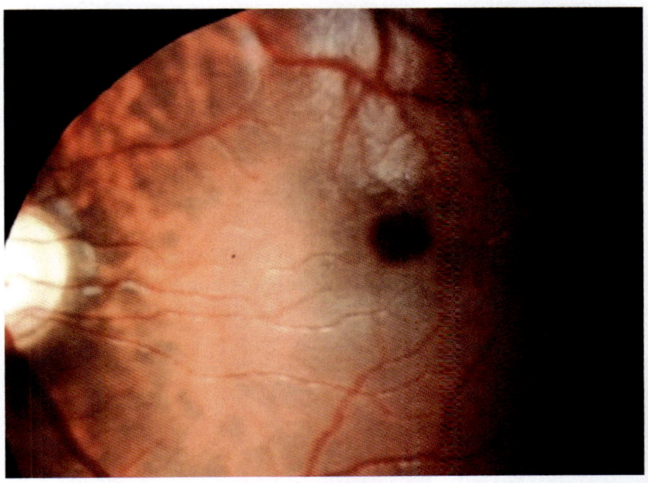

FIGURE 8.17. Cherry-red spot (with pale disc) in an infant with Tay-Sachs disease.

- In a number of not infrequently encountered situations, there is uncertainty about whether a baby can see, with possibility of LCA among the clinician's concerns.
  - Any condition causing nystagmus (Table 8.18) may delay to some degree the development of good fixation and visual attentiveness, and in early infancy nystagmoid movements from any cause tend to be coarser and less regular, as with LCA. If by age 6 to 9 months, it is still not clear that the baby can see, ERG testing should be done.
  - Any condition that severely delays overall motor development (especially if there are also cognitive deficits) may delay the development of visual fixation. If the baby is not yet rolling over, patience is indicated. Once that milestone has been passed, or if it has not been reached by age 6 months and concern about vision persists, consideration may be given to *visual evoked potential* testing, the one means of assessing visual sensory function that does not rely in any way on motor system function.
  - Loss of vision secondary to brain damage (*cortical visual impairment*, or CVI, most often caused by perinatal hypoxia) is *not* associated with nystagmus, and pupils react normally. In general, the diagnosis of CVI should be supported by neuroimaging that shows consistent anatomic findings.
  - The infant who specifically lacks capacity for normal eye movements due to gaze palsy (e.g., in Moebius syndrome, p. 498) or inability to generate refixation saccades (*congenital oculomotor apraxia*, or COMA) may appear to be blind until she has sufficient head control to compensate for the deficiency (e.g., with characteristic head-thrusting movements in COMA). The nature of the problem usually becomes evident by age 4 to 6 months.
  - Isolated *delayed visual maturation* describes visual inattentiveness in an otherwise normal infant more than 2 to 3 months old. Sometimes, responses can be elicited using a visually simple stimulus, such as OKN drum or Teller card gratings (p. 492). Normal fixation behavior is usually seen by age 6 months, with ultimately normal measured acuity.

Reference

Lambert SR, Kriss A, Taylor D, et al. Follow-up and diagnostic reappraisal of 75 patients with Leber's congenital amaurosis. *Am J Ophthalmol* 1989;107:624–631.

Night Blindness in Childhood

Summary

Night blindness (nyctalopia) is the earliest symptom in a number of hereditary retinal disorders that affect primarily the rod photoreceptors. Some are stationary while others, of which the prototype is *retinitis pigmentosa* (RP), lead to progressive loss of vision (Table 8.15).

Symptoms and Signs

- Night blindness causes children to be insecure and cling to parents in low-light situations.
- Visual acuity is normal in childhood with most progressive disorders, and nystagmus is seldom seen. Nystagmus (characteristically rapid and small amplitude) is often a feature of X-linked congenital stationary night blindness (CSNB), usually associated with mild to moderate acuity reduction.
- Early-onset high myopia (Table 8.7) may be the first indication of CSNB; also seen with some progressive disorders (especially X-linked RP, Bardet-Biedl, and gyrate atrophy).

Ophthalmic Findings

- Fundus appearance is usually normal in infants and young children with both stationary and progressive forms of night blindness.
- Distinctive fundus abnormalities, described in Table 8.15, are associated with stationary night blindness in fundus albipunctatus and Oguchi disease.
- Retinal blood vessel attenuation (narrowing), initially subtle, is often the first ophthalmoscopic manifestation of RP and related progressive disorders in older children. Vessels remain normal with stationary causes of night blindness.
- A variety of fundus pigmentary disturbances become apparent over time with progressive disorders.
  - The earliest change in RP is often generalized reduction in pigmentation in a midperipheral annulus centered on the fovea, with normal appearance in the center and far periphery, especially nasal. Look for this beginning just nasal to the disc.
  - Typical "bone-spicule" pigment clumps are usually absent or few in number during childhood.
  - Whitish "flecks" are sometimes seen; may resemble those associated with fundus albipunctatus and some forms of primarily macular or cone system degeneration (Table 8.16).
- PSC cataract and "waxy" optic disc pallor are common but usually late manifestations of progressive pigmentary retinopathies, seldom seen before adulthood.

Special Tests

- Electroretinography is critical to the diagnosis of children with night blindness.
  - In stationary forms, scotopic (dark-adapted, rod-dominated) responses are markedly reduced, but photopic (light-adapted, cone-dominated) responses remain normal or nearly so.

Table 8.15

Causes of early-onset night blindness

Condition	Other ocular findings	Systemic findings	Heredity/comment
Congenital stationary night blindness (Nonprogressive)	Moderately decreased acuity Moderate to high myopia Nystagmus frequent	None	Usually X-linked, males Dominant (Nougaret) form has normal acuity, refraction
Oguchi disease (Nonprogressive)	Green-yellow fundus becomes normal when dark adapted (Mizuo phenomenon)	None	Autosomal recessive
Fundus albipunctatus (Nonprogressive)	Whitish dots (flecks), mainly in peripheral retina	None	Autosomal recessive ERG normal after prolonged dark adaptation
Retinitis pigmentosa (Progressive)	Bone-spicule pigmentation Whitish flecks in retinitis punctata albescens	Variable depending on specific disorder (see below)	X-linked, autosomal recessive, and dominant (mildest) forms
Usher syndrome (Progressive)	Normal fundus in childhood	Congenital sensorineural hearing loss	Autosomal recessive 5% of congenital hearing loss Severe in Type I, milder in 2
Refsum disease (Progressive)	RP-like fundus changes Anterior corneal degeneration Nystagmus (motor)	Ichthyosis, anosmia, ataxia, hearing loss, neuropathies, cardiac disease	Autosomal recessive Phytanic acid accumulation; diet may limit progression
Bassen-Kornzweig disease (abetalipoproteinemia) (Progressive)	Whitish flecks Exotropia, horizontal gaze palsy	Fat, vitamin malabsorption FTT, low plasma lipid levels Anemia, acanthocytosis Spinocerebellar degeneration	Autosomal recessive Vitamins A & E may prevent retinal degeneration
Bardet-Biedl syndrome (Progressive)	In some cases, macula affected before periphery Atypical pigment clumping	Polydactyly (postaxial) Obesity, endocrine disorders Renal abnormalities	Autosomal recessive In *Laurence-Moon*, spastic diplegia, no polydactyly
Cockayne syndrome (Progressive)	Poor pupil dilation High hyperopia Corneal changes, cataract	Progeria (premature aging) Deafness, CNS degeneration Photodermatopathy	Autosomal recessive Avoiding sun exposure protects skin
Choroideremia (Progressive)	Progressive atrophy of peripheral choroid and RPE	None	X-linked, males Fundus changes with normal vision in female carriers
Gyrate atrophy (Progressive)	Sharply demarcated atrophy of peripheral choroid and RPE High myopia	None	Autosomal recessive High plasma ornithine Low arginine diet may help
Vitamin A deficiency (Progressive)	Whitish flecks in some cases	Xerophthalmia (Table 8.3) Immune system deficiency	Commonest cause worldwide

ERG, electroretinography; RP, retinitis pigmentosa; FTT, failure to thrive; RPE, retinal pigment epithelium.

In progressive forms, response amplitudes range from near normal to markedly reduced in childhood. Prolonged response latency from the cone system may be an important early predictor of future deterioration. Eventually, both photopic and scotopic responses become extinguished.

- Formal dark adaptometry is difficult to perform in children, and not often indicated. Some forms of stationary night blindness show improved function after very prolonged dark adaptation (also reflected in ERG responses).

Disease Course

- Children with stationary night blindness remain free of serious visual disability throughout their lives.
- Those with RP and other progressive forms gradually lose vision and usually are functionally blind at ages ranging from young adulthood to middle age.

Systemic Findings

- Children with Usher syndrome have congenital hearing impairment but usually do not lose vision or develop typical fundus findings until late childhood or adolescence. Many authorities recommend ERG screening of all congenitally deaf children.
- Other systemic associations are summarized in Table 8.15.

Treatment and Management

- No effective treatment is available for most conditions that cause night blindness.
- Dietary management may prevent, reduce, or delay vision deterioration in Refsum disease, abetalipoproteinemia, and of course vitamin A deficiency.
- Gene therapy remains a hope for the future; specific genetic loci have been established for many of these disorders.
- Educational and career counseling is important for both patients and families, as is genetic counseling.
- Considerable emotional support is required, both when the diagnosis is made, and when serious and progressive disability develops years later.

Differential Diagnosis

- Wagner and Goldmann-Favre forms of vitreoretinal degeneration (Table 8.14) are associated with RP-like retinal changes and vision loss.
- Progressive pigmentary retinopathy is a feature of myotonic dystrophy (Table 8.12) and of Kearns-Sayre syndrome (Table 8.2), two genetically very distinct disorders that have many overlapping features including potentially fatal cardiac conduction defects, endocrine (particularly gonadal) dysfunction, and progressive external ophthalmoplegia (especially ptosis). Night blindness and abnormal ERG are inconsistent and usually late onset in these conditions, sometimes with progression to serious visual disability.
- Patients with a number of other rare hereditary multisystem disorders develop pigmentary or fleck retinal degeneration in childhood or as they mature, but show ocular findings such as anterior segment dysgenesis (Table 8.8), corneal clouding (Table 8.9), or cataract (Table 8.12) that are more consistent, characteristic or conspicuous at early ages, and night blindness is generally not a significant concern. Progressive loss of retinal function may or may not occur.
- Abnormal fundus pigmentation associated with nonhereditary, nonprogressive conditions (e.g., congenital infection—see p. 451) may resemble that seen with RP and related disorders. Differential diagnosis is usually not a problem; ERG is likely to resolve any uncertainty.

Reference

Krill AE. *Hereditary retinal and choroidal diseases.* Hagerstown, MD: Harper & Row, 1977.

Juvenile Macular Degeneration (Stargardt Disease)

Summary

The term *juvenile macular degeneration* is often considered a synonym for Stargardt disease (STGD), but in fact, numerous disorders may present in childhood or adolescence with loss of central vision and other findings indicative of macular disease (Table 8.16). Most of these involve dysfunction of peripheral as well as central retinal elements from the beginning but have less impact on peripheral vision and the fundus periphery, especially in early stages. All cause progressive vision loss, to a greater or lesser degree. Some have significant neurologic or systemic associations.

Symptoms and Signs

- Decreased central vision, usually beginning well past infancy (typically age 5 to 15 years), and not associated with nystagmus. Initial acuity is relatively good in Best disease which (may present with complaints of metamorphopsia); for other conditions, usually between 20/60 and 20/200 when diagnosed.
- Color discrimination difficulty ranging from mild to severe (in cone-rod dystrophy).
- Light aversion and photophobia are seen especially with progressive cone-rod dystrophy; not characteristic of STGD or Best disease.

Ophthalmic Findings

- Fundus appearance often remains normal through childhood despite significant loss of vision; may lead to misdiagnosis as a functional problem or malingering (see below).

Table 8.16

Causes of macular degeneration in childhood

Condition	Fundus findings	Other findings	Comment
Stargardt disease	Normal to total atrophy of macula	"Dark choroid" on fluorescein angiography	Autosomal recessive
Fundus flavimaculatus	"Pisciform" flecks, especially in posterior pole	ERG is usually normal	Considered a variant gene expression of Stargardt
Best disease	Characteristic vitelliform "egg yolk" lesion in childhood May evolve to atrophic lesion	EOG always highly abnormal ERG is usually normal	Autosomal dominant Mild vision loss in childhood, progresses in adulthood
Juvenile retinoschisis	Stellate "cystic" foveal lesion, may resemble CME	Vitreous and peripheral retinal changes (Table 8.14) No fluorescein leakage on FA	X-linked; most common maculopathy in boys
Cone-rod dystrophy	"Bull's eye" macular lesion; later RP-like changes	Photoaversion, marked color vision deficiency Photopic (cone) ERG loss precedes scotopic (rod) loss	Autosomal dominant, recessive, or X-linked Progresses to near blindness
Alstrom syndrome	Similar to cone-rod dystrophy	Obesity, diabetes mellitus Cardiomyopathy, renal failure ERG like cone-rod dystrophy	Autosomal recessive Progresses to near blindness
Batten disease (neuronal ceroid lipofuscinosis)	"Bull's eye" lesion or decreased foveal reflex	Ataxia, neurodegeneration ERG markedly reduced	Autosomal recessive Skin biopsy confirms diagnosis
Neurofibromatosis type 2 (Table 3.21)	Epiretinal membrane or combined hamartoma	PSC cataract (Table 8.12) Cranial nerve palsies	Usually unilateral Less often seen with NF1
Pseudoxanthoma elasticum	Macular pigment mottling ("peau d'orange") Angioid streaks appear later, SRNV in some cases	Characterstic skin lesions in adults Vascular degeneration with GI bleeding (childhood), CAD	Recessive or dominant Skin biopsy confirms diagnosis Sickle cell disease, thalassemia also associated with AS
Pathologic myopia	Peripapillary atrophy, posterior staphyloma, pigmentary abnormality in macula	High myopia Lacquer cracks, Fuchs spots, SRNV in young adults	Only small minority of highly myopic children progress to degenerative changes

EOG, electrooculography; ERG, electroretinography; FA, fluorescein angiography; AS, angioid streaks; RP, retinitis pigmentosa; SRNV, subretinal neovascularization; CAD, coronary artery disease; GI, gastrointestinal; PSC, posterior subcapsular cataract.

- A wide variety of macular changes may be observed ophthalmoscopically.

  Decreased or absent foveal light reflex may be the only finding initially; if early onset may be mistaken for foveal hypoplasia (p. 468).

  "Bulls eye" pigmentary lesion (perifoveal ring of hypopigmentation) may be an early finding in STGD as well as other disorders, particularly Batten disease and cone-rod dystrophy, as indicated in Table 8.16.

PEDIATRIC

More specific findings include "beaten bronze" appearance in STGD, "peau d'orange" mottling in pseudoxanthoma elasticum (PXE—see comments in Table 8.16 and under systemic findings below), cystoid-like changes in juvenile retinoschisis (often occurring in the absence of obvious vitreous and peripheral retinal abnormality), and "egg yolk" lesion in Best disease.

Yellow-white *flecks* (described as "pisciform" or fish-shaped), concentrated in but not limited to the posterior pole, are characteristic of fundus flavimaculatus, a variant of STGD. Similar lesions are also seen in more severe retinopathies that may present in childhood with loss of central vision (e.g., Alport syndrome, Table 8.12), or with night blindness (Table 8.15). The most common flecked retina disorder, familial retinal drusen, is seldom detectable and never a cause of vision loss prior to adulthood.

Macular *epiretinal membranes* rarely develop in children, but may be an early manifestation of *combined hamartoma of the retina and retinal pigment epithelium*, possibly indicating the presence of neurofibromatosis type 2 (or type 1) (Figure 8.18).

Subretinal neovascularization (SRNV) and other typical findings of "wet" age-related macular degeneration are highly unusual before maturity but occasionally develop in adolescents with PXE or pathologic myopia who have breaks in Bruch membrane (angioid streaks; lacquer cracks).

A central area of chorioretinal atrophy is the typical end-stage appearance of STGD and Best disease, usually not observed until late adolescence or adulthood. May resemble a macular coloboma (p. 470) or postinflammatory lesion (p. 451); history is likely to resolve any confusion.

- Cone-rod dystrophy and similar disorders, as noted in Table 8.16, develop a typical RP-like fundus appearance over time, but this seldom becomes evident before maturity.

Special Tests

- Color vision testing typically shows mild defects in STGD and Best disease, severe in cone-rod and similar disorders; usually without a specific diagnostic pattern (p. 487).
- Fluorescein angiography in about half of cases of STGD shows generalized choroidal hypofluorescence (except in the immediate region of an atrophic macular lesion) that has been termed "dark choroid."
- ERG and EOG are often helpful.

  Both are normal to mildly reduced in STGD, and show no significant progression.

  Initially, photopic ERG responses are severely reduced, scotopic less so in Batten disease, cone-rod dystrophy, and related disorders; progression to extinguished responses occurs in late stages.

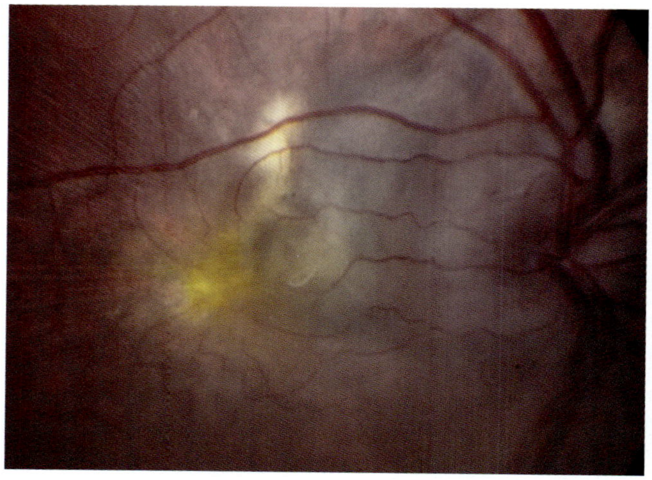

FIGURE 8.18. Combined hamartoma of retina and retinal pigment epithelium. This unilateral right macular lesion was recently acquired in a 5-year-old girl with NF1, associated with decline in vision to 20/200. Note folds radiating from the center, caused by epiretinal membrane formation. The child also had pseudotumor cerebri, causing chronic papilledema.

  EOG is consistently and diagnostically very abnormal in Best disease.

- Optical coherence tomography (OCT) may be useful, particularly for assessment of suspected juvenile retinoschisis.

Disease Course

- Best disease has the best prognosis, with relatively mild disability through middle age in most cases. Most patients with juvenile retinoschisis also progress slowly.
- Visual acuity declines steadily and then stabilizes near 20/200 within a few years after first awareness of vision loss in STGD.
- Among patients with PXE or high myopia, only the unfortunate minority who develop SRNV at young age may become legally blind by the time they reach adulthood.
- Batten disease, cone-rod dystrophy, and other disorders with severe ERG changes progress to near total blindness in adulthood, similar to RP.

Treatment and Management

- SRNV may benefit from treatment with VEGF blocking agents. No effective treatment is available for other forms of macular degeneration in childhood.
- Children and adolescents can be expected to adapt more quickly and completely to visual disability than adults with age-related macular degeneration. Those with conditions that affect central vision only are likely to do well with low vision aids. Those with conditions that progress to near total blindness need supportive care similar to that required by patients with RP (p. 464).

Table 8.17

Disorders with foveal hypoplasia

Condition	Other ocular findings	Systemic findings	Comment
Oculocutaneous albinism (OCA)	Iris transillumination Fundus hypopigmentation, grayish disk Poor stereopsis, strabismus	Skin hypopigmentation Hermansky-Pudlak: bruising *Chediak-Higashi syndrome:* immune deficiency	Autosomal recessive Defective tyrosinase or other tyrosine metabolism gene
Partial albinism	Similar to OCA but milder	Mild skin hypopigmentation	Multiple genes Usually autosomal recessive, occasionally dominant
Ocular albinism	Similar to OCA	Normal skin pigmentation	X-linked Tesselated fundus in carrier females
Aniridia	Absent central iris Microcornea, sclerocornea (Table 8.9) Polar cataract, ectopia lentis Glaucoma	Wilms tumor, seen only in sporadic cases *WAGR syndrome:* also genital abnormality, retardation	Autosomal dominant (PAX6 mutation) Often sporadic, often with 11p13 deletion
Isolated foveal hypoplasia	None	None	Usually sporadic, may be autosomal dominant Faulty PAX6 gene expression
Achromatopsia (rod monochromatism)	Total absence of color vision High hyperopia common Absent or reduced photopic ERG response	None	Autosomal recessive

Systemic Findings

- Neurodegenerative symptoms including ataxia, seizures, and dementia (often with subtle initial manifestations) may develop before, concurrent with, or months to years after macular changes in juvenile Batten disease. History should be carefully reviewed, with neurologic consultation and imaging if indicated.
- Other systemic associations are summarized in Table 8.16. Of particular importance is the potential in PXE for gastrointestinal bleeding, which may be life threatening in childhood.

Differential Diagnosis

- Disorders that typically present with night blindness (Table 8.15) may occasionally first cause decreased central vision and macular changes, particularly Bardet-Biedl syndrome.
- Subnormal acuity in a child without detectable fundus abnormality may be the initial presentation of STGD, as well as other serious conditions including hereditary optic atrophy (p. 473) and intracranial tumors (especially cran-

Table 8.18

Important associations of nystagmus in infancy*

Condition	Reference
Down syndrome	p. 425
Juvenile retinoschisis	Table 8.14
Leber congenital amaurosis	p. 461
CSNB	Table 8.15
Partial albinism	Table 8.17
Foveal hypoplasia	Table 8.17
Achromatopsia	Table 8.17
Optic nerve hypoplasia	p. 471
Optic pathway tumor	p. 488
Congenital motor nystagmus	p. 486
Manifest latent nystagmus	p. 488
Spasmus nutans	p. 488

*Any condition that causes poor vision in infancy may result in nystagmus. The disorders listed in this table are significant particularly because the eye examination is often nearly normal except for presence of nystagmus.

iopharyngioma, p. 479). Careful assessment of the pupillary light response and color vision (p. 487) should always be done, and fluorescein angiography and neuroimaging should be considered in such cases. (Also consider the possibility of early keratoconus—p. 440—in unilateral as well as bilateral situations.) The diagnosis of *functional vision loss* must be regarded as tentative (unless it can be demonstrated, with crafty acuity testing, that vision is in fact intact), especially in the absence of clear evidence of psychopathology, recent severe emotional trauma (e.g., sexual abuse), or obvious secondary gain; and reconsidered if symptoms worsen or persist over months.

Reference

Fishman GA, Farber M, Patel BS, et al. Visual acuity loss in patients with Stargardt's macular dystrophy. *Ophthalmology* 1987;94:809–814.

Foveal Hypoplasia

Summary

Foveal hypoplasia describes lack of normal differentiation of the fovea and macula. It may be seen as an isolated congenital abnormality, or in the context of albinism, aniridia, or achromatopsia (congenital absence of cone function) (Table 8.17, Figure 8.19).

Symptoms and Signs

- Decreased acuity, ranging from about 20/40 to 20/200. Typically lower end for achromatopsia; correlates with macular appearance in others. Development of fixation may be delayed, but usually good by late infancy (p. 462).
- These disorders are all among the causes of infantile-onset nystagmus (Table 8.18). Typically, oscillations are smaller than seen in Leber congenital amaurosis; usually but not always pendular in primary gaze.
- Light sensitivity (photoaversion) is severe in achromatopsia, but also present to some degree in albinism and aniridia.
- Color vision is severely impaired in achromatopsia; little or no abnormality with other causes. In *blue-cone monochromatism*, a milder variant form with X-linked inheritance, there is some preservation of color discrimination (but progressive vision loss may occur in adulthood).
- Pupillary light reaction may be normal, absent (aniridia), or paradoxical (achromatopsia, albinism) (p. 487).

Ophthalmic Findings

- Lack of normal foveal development is highly variable in degree, ranging from decreased foveolar and ring light reflexes (which may be a normal variant) to complete absence of macular pigment and foveal vascular differentiation. Mildest (or normal) in achromatopsia, most severe in complete forms of albinism.
- Iris transillumination from defective pigment epithelial layers in albinism may be complete and obvious, or patchy and subtle, sometimes detectable only on retroillumination with slit lamp. In infants, viewing iris with a direct ophthalmoscope at a high plus setting may be helpful. Iris grossly appears pinkish in the most severe cases, but "eye color" is often within normal limits, sometimes even brown.
- Residual iris tissue is present to varying degree in aniridia, sometimes sufficient to create a pupil (usually somewhat irregular) of normal diameter but completely

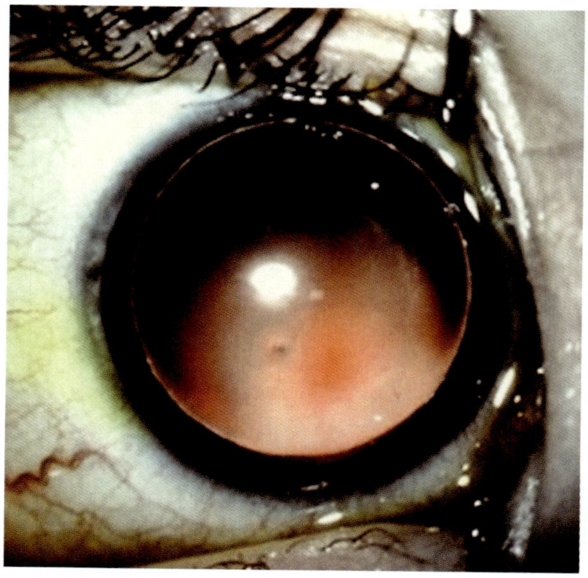

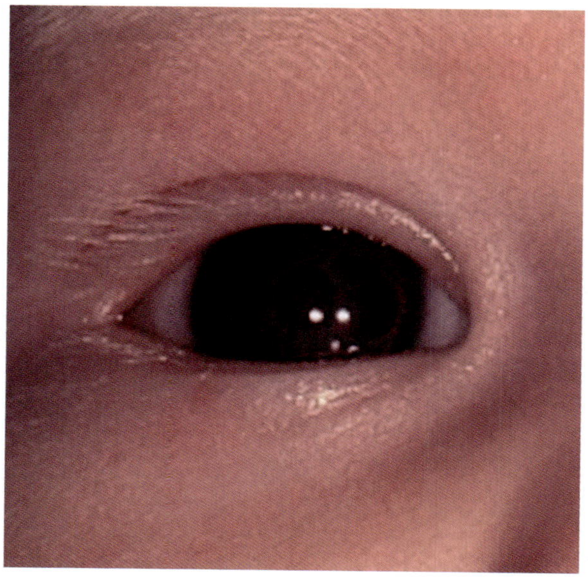

FIGURE 8.19. Associations of foveal hypoplasia. **A:** Aniridia. Note narrow remnant of blue iris tissue, visibility of entire lens equator. **B:** Complete OCA, showing extensive iris transillumination.

immobile, or resembling typical inferior iris coloboma (p. 469), may suggest Rieger anomaly (Table 8.8).

- Strabismus and high degrees of ametropia are common, especially with albinism. Optical correction may provide significant benefit. Muscle surgery is often indicated, though sensory benefit may be limited in albinism by abnormal "wiring" of the visual pathways, specifically faulty (excessive) decussation in the chiasm.

Systemic Findings

- In *Hermansky-Pudlak disease* (almost exclusively affecting persons of Puerto Rican descent), oculocutaneous albinism (OCA) is associated with abnormality of blood platelets that causes bruising but usually not more severe hemorrhage; restrictive lung disease, inflammatory bowel disease, and heart and kidney disease may develop in adulthood.
- Wilms tumor risk is a serious concern in children with sporadic aniridia, especially when 11p13 deletion is documented.

Special Tests

- ERG shows loss of photopic response with normal scotopic response in achromatopsia. Early onset of progressive cone-rod dystrophy may simulate congenital achromatopsia (e.g., in Alstrom syndrome, Table 8.16); can be differentiated by ERG. Amplitudes may be supernormal in albinism.
- Renal ultrasound screening is important in aniridia with risk of Wilms tumor, at frequent intervals from age 6 months to at least 4 years.

Disease Course

- Retinal function does not deteriorate in these conditions, and in fact with increasing age there may be some apparent improvement in vision and nystagmus often diminishes. Children can be educated as sighted persons, with accommodation for disability as necessary.
- Glaucoma becomes a serious and difficult management problem in many patients with aniridia, often requiring multiple surgeries but usually not in childhood.

References

Kinnear PE, Jay B, Witkop CJ. Albinism. *Surv Ophthalmol* 1985;30:75–101.

Oliver MD, Dotan SA, Chemke J, et al. Isolated foveal hypoplasia. *Br J Ophthalmol* 1987;71:926–930.

OPTIC NERVE DISORDERS

Fundus Coloboma

Summary

Fundus coloboma is a congenital defect variably involving optic disc, retina, and choroid, which results from incomplete closure of the embryonic fissure and subsequent partial failure of adjacent neuroectodermal and mesenchymal differentiation.

Demographics

Usually, a sporadic condition without known cause or risk factors, but familial (autosomal dominant) cases occur, often with great variation in severity among affected relatives. Mostly bilateral and approximately symmetrical, but marked asymmetry is not uncommon and some cases are unilateral.

Symptoms and Signs

- Visual acuity may be near normal (if the macula is not involved), reduced in the 20/40–20/200 range (if partial macular preservation), or very poor (if no macular differentiation and very small globe).
- Nystagmus (and often strabismus in unilateral or asymmetric cases) results from decreased vision. As with other conditions that cause nystagmus in infancy (Table 8.18), development of robust visual fixation may be significantly delayed, increasing early concern about possible blindness (p. 462).
- Microphthalmos, ranging from mild to very severe, is seen in most cases.

Ophthalmic Findings

- Optic nerve head is often highly distorted, sometimes recognizable only from location of entering/exiting retinal vessels, but milder cases may show a central or an inferior defect in variably enlarged disc, or normal disc superior to a choroidoretinal defect (Figure 8.20A). Colobomatous eyes with severely malformed discs often have surprisingly good vision when macular differentiation can be appreciated.
- Involvement of choroid and retina usually takes the form of a sharply delimited round or oval region lacking all or most pigmented tissue, extending inferiorly from the upper pole of the disc or a point below the disc, ranging in diameter from less than 1 mm to nearly that of the globe. The mildest expression may be a short linear streak of decreased pigmentation extending inferiorly from the disk.
- Underlying sclera, in or below the region of the disc, is usually thinned and ectatic to some degree, resulting in posterior bulging of the globe, or in most severe cases a cystlike structure in the inferior or the posterior orbit that may exceed the size of the adjacent small eyeball (*microphthalmos with cyst*).
- Iris, ciliary body, and lens zonule may show inferior colobomatous defects of varying degree. Iris coloboma also occurs as an isolated abnormality, possibly unrelated to embryonic fissure closure.
- Refraction is often myopic, but care should be taken in retinoscopy to base measurement only on streak reflexes from fundus area not involved in the coloboma.

Systemic Findings

- Choanal atresia is found together with coloboma in the *CHARGE association* of multiple congenital anomalies (Coloboma, Heart defects, Atresia of choana, Retarded growth/development, Genital abnormality, Ear/hearing defects).
- Goldenhar syndrome is often associated with eyelid coloboma (p. 427), rarely with fundus coloboma. Lid and globe coloboma are otherwise unrelated disorders.
- *Aicardi syndrome* (usually sporadic, always in females) often involves typical fundus coloboma, but its most characteristic lesions are "lacunae"—multiple round defects of choroid and retinal pigment epithelium typically seen near but separate from the disc. Also present are CNS malformation (especially agenesis of the corpus callosum) and seizures (typically infantile spasms).
- Basal encephalocele and other midline developmental defects occasionally accompany fundus coloboma.
- A number of rare syndromes may involve fundus coloboma, including focal dermal hypoplasia (Goltz-Gorlin syndrome), linear sebaceous nevus syndrome (Jadahsson), and Walker-Warburg syndrome (Table 8.13).

Treatment and Management

- Occlusion for amblyopic vision loss may be appropriate in unilateral or asymmetric cases, especially if there is macular function in both eyes.
- Observation for development of retinal detachment (may be either serous or rhegmatogenous); rarely occurs in childhood.

Differential Diagnosis

- *Optic pit* is a small depression near the disc margin that may accompany or resemble disc coloboma. Rarely identified in childhood; usually diagnosed in adults with characteristic associated abnormalities of adjacent retina and serous macular detachment.
- *Morning glory disc* is a congenital anomaly that may be a variant of optic disc coloboma, though very seldom bilateral or familial, and not typically associated with microphthalmos. Classic appearance is large disc with funnel-shaped central avascular region (usually occupied by glial tissue), surrounded by a neural rim from which numerous blood vessels emerge and extend radially, often with extensive peripapillary abnormality, variably including pigment disturbance, scleral ectasia, and localized subretinal fluid accumulation (Figure 8.20B).
- Sharply demarcated hypopigmented lesions of the macula are sometimes described as *atypical colobomas*. These are usually not developmental anomalies, but consequent to intrauterine infection (especially toxoplasmosis, p. 451) or macular degeneration (Table 8.16).
- The appearance of iris coloboma may be mimicked by aniridia (Table 8.17). Pupillary light reaction is absent in the latter condition, present in the former.

References

Brodsky MC. Congenital optic disc anomalies. *Surv Ophthalmol* 1994;39:89–112.

A

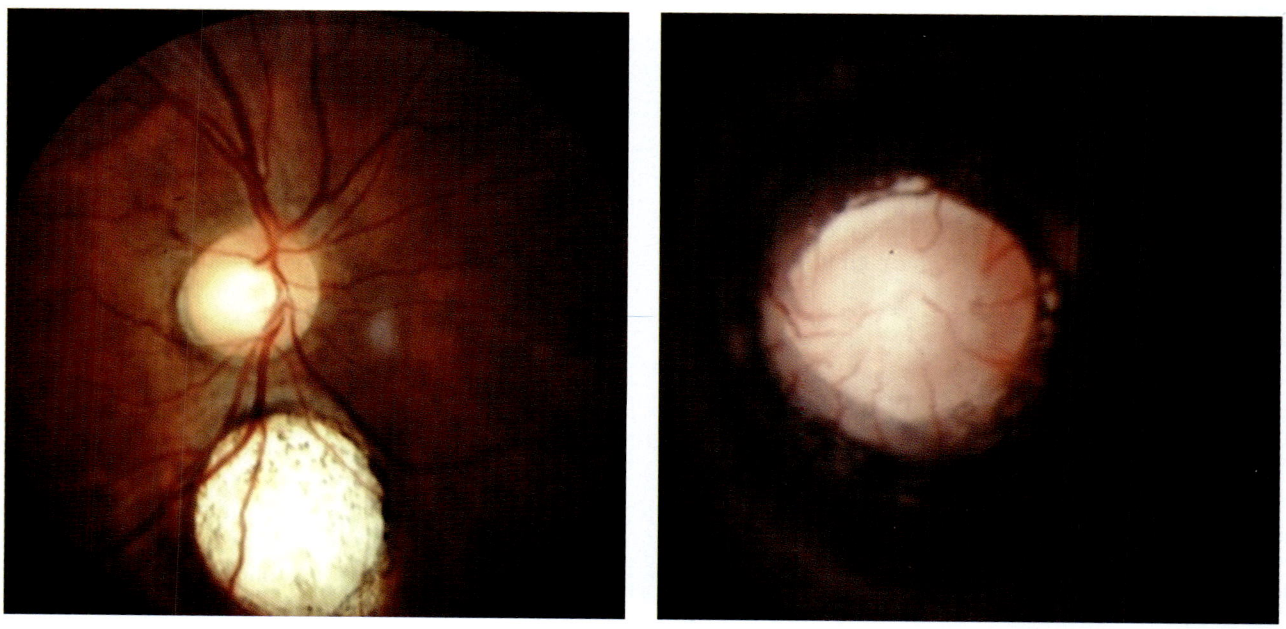

B

FIGURE 8.20. Colobomatous malformations. **A:** Small typical chorioretinal coloboma inferior to disc. Extensive disc cupping may represent mild involvement of optic nerve by coloboma. Foveal differentiation and visual acuity were normal in this eye. **B:** Morning glory disc anomaly.

Weiss A, Martinez C, Greenwald M. Microphthalmos with cyst: clinical presentations and computed tomographic findings. *J Pediatr Ophthalmol Strabismus* 1985;22:6–12.

Optic Nerve Hypoplasia

Summary

Small optic disc is the hallmark of optic nerve hypoplasia (ONH), an important cause of congenital visual impairment that is frequently associated with neuroendocrine abnormalities.

Etiology

- The cause of ONH in general is not known. It is almost always sporadic, and may be either bilateral or unilateral with no sex predilection.
- Associated with in utero exposure to teratogenic agents including alcohol (see p. 425), cocaine, lysergic acid diethylamide, phencyclidine, and phenytoin (Dilantin).
- A syndrome of bilateral superior segmental ONH associated with maternal diabetes has been described.

Symptoms and Signs

- Acuity ranges from 20/20 to no light perception, correlating poorly with disc size except in extreme cases.
- Lack of pupillary light response in most severe cases only. Relative afferent papillary defect may or may not be seen in unilateral or asymmetric cases. Paradoxical response (p. 487) is sometimes present.
- Nystagmus in more severe bilateral cases; strabismus especially when asymmetric. As with coloboma, delayed development of visual fixation may give an early impression of more severe visual disability than in fact is present (p. 462). If pupillary light reaction is well preserved, it should be anticipated that an infant with ONH will eventually be able to fixate and will not have mobility problems.

Ophthalmic Findings

- Optic nerve head is small (usually about 0.5 to 1.0 mm diameter) and often also shows significant pallor.
- Often but not always, the disc is surrounded by a whitish scleral ring (reflecting absent peripapillary choroid and retinal pigment epithelium) with sharp border that approximates normal disc size, sometimes creating the mistaken impression of a normal or an atrophied nerve (double ring sign) (Figure 8.21A).
- Tortuous retinal vessels are frequently seen.

Systemic Findings

- ONH is commonly associated with CNS abnormalities. In the syndrome of *septo-optic dysplasia* (de Morsier), neuroimaging shows absence of the septum pellucidum (diagnostic but of no clinical significance) (Figure 8.21B) and often other brain defects (particularly agenesis of the corpus callosum) that may be associated with functional impairment.
- MRI demonstrates neurohypophyseal abnormality in approximately 15% of cases of ONH, including some that are apparently unilateral.
- Associated endocrine disturbances may include frequently or variably deficient production of growth hormone, thyroid hormone, or cortisol, as well as diabetes

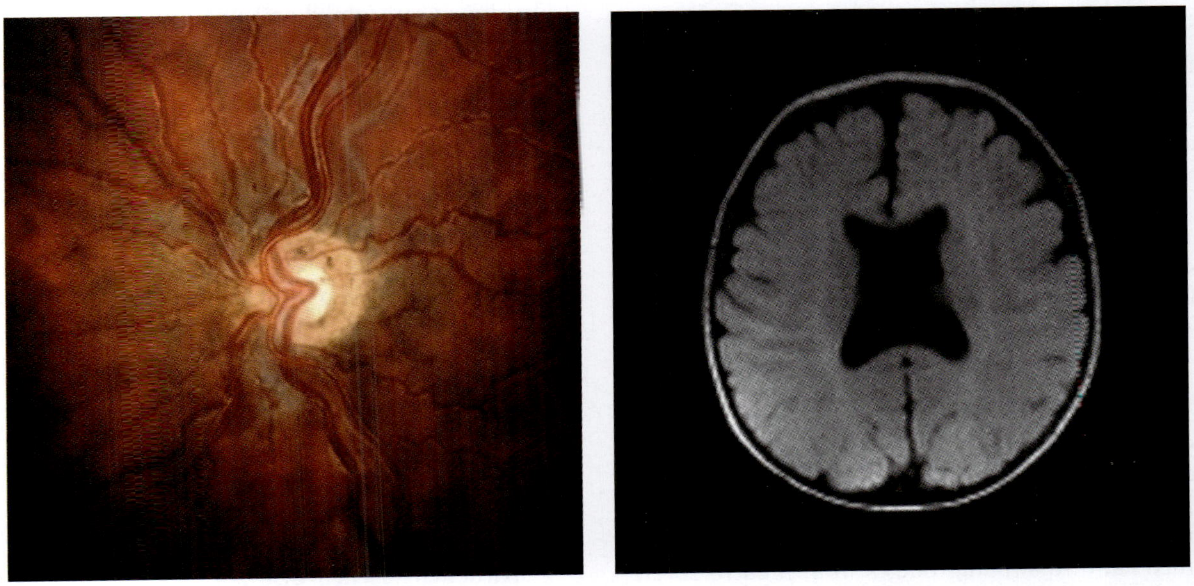

A B

FIGURE 8.21 Optic nerve hypoplasia. **A:** Small pale central region is the entire nerve head, surrounded by a ring of hypopigmentation. **B:** Magnetic resonance image showing absent septum pellucidum in de Morsier syndrome. This infant had failure to thrive secondary to hypopituitarism.

insipidus. These problems may not become evident clinically until the child is several years old.

- Of particular concern is cortisol insufficiency, secondary to low production of corticotropin (ACTH) by the pituitary. Early clinical manifestations may include recurrent infections, high fevers, seizures, and developmental delay. Sudden death during seemingly minor febrile illness has been reported in children with de Morsier syndrome, presumed to be a consequence of inadequate adrenocortical stress response.

Special Tests

Magnetic resonance imaging, with attention to the posterior pituitary, should be done on any infant or child under school age who is found to have ONH, and in older children with short stature or other evidence of endocrinopathy. Evaluation by a pediatric endocrinologist is indicated for cases with abnormal MRI or suggestive symptoms.

Differential Diagnosis

Ophthalmoscopic abnormality in ONH may be subtle enough to be overlooked on initial routine fundus examination, sometimes leading to mistaken identification of amblyopia as primary cause of unilateral decreased vision in a child with strabismus secondary to ONH, particularly exotropia. Lack of response to conscientiously applied occlusion therapy is reason for careful re-evaluation of the disc.

Reference

Lambert SR, Hoyt CS, Narahara MH. Optic nerve hypoplasia. *Surv Ophthalmol* 1987;32:1–9.

Optic Disc Swelling (Papilledema)

Summary

Symmetrical bilateral optic disc swelling in a child should prompt immediate evaluation for a posterior fossa mass lesion, especially considering that such tumors are among the more common pediatric malignancies. Other possibilities are more likely, however, in the absence of focal neurologic signs or symptoms, and when the finding is unilateral or highly asymmetrical.

Differential Diagnosis

- ***Pseudotumor cerebri*** (benign or idiopathic intracranial hypertension) in childhood may have absent or mild symptoms (typically including nonspecific headache; sometimes fluctuating vision and esodeviation). Usually symmetrical disc swelling ranges from mild to severe, without hemorrhage or cotton-wool spots; may be an incidental finding on routine fundus examination (see Figure 8.18).
  - Specific cause or precipitant can be identified in a minority of cases, and there are no important risk factors (in contrast to the predilection for obese females in adulthood).
  - Spontaneous resolution and episodic recurrence are common.
  - Most children retain normal vision, but occasionally there is severe and rapidly progressive visual loss.
  - After normal neuroimaging (computed tomography or magnetic resonance), refer to a pediatric neurologist for consideration of lumbar puncture (sedation often required) and treatment (usually initiated with oral acetazolamide).
- *Papillitis* in childhood presents with obvious disc swelling, virtually always associated with acute or subacute vision loss that is severe (sometimes to no light perception) and with marked afferent pupillary defect. Usually bilateral but frequently sequential onset, the second eye following the first by days to weeks. Typically occurs after a viral illness. Spontaneous recovery, often to near normal, is the rule, but most cases get treatment with high-dose corticosteroid. Subsequent development of multiple sclerosis is uncommon.
- *Leber hereditary optic neuropathy* initially shows characteristic disc swelling and peripapillary telangiectasia, which evolves to generalized pallor. Usually seen in young adult males but may have childhood onset. Caused by a defect in mitochondrial DNA transmitted from mother; several distinct mutations have been identified. Acuity rapidly declines to about 20/200 in one eye, followed by involvement of the other days to months later. In a minority of cases, partial recovery occurs after months to years.
- *Optic nerve head drusen* (hyaline bodies) typically develop in early childhood and may cause disc elevation and blurred margins that impressively mimic the appearance of papilledema (pseudopapilledema). Unilateral or obviously asymmetric presentation is common.
  - Usually an isolated abnormality; occasionally associated ocular or systemic findings, as in Alagille syndrome (Table 8.8).
  - In children, hyaline bodies are relatively soft and deeply buried in nerve head tissue, so that differentiation based on critical ophthalmoscopy, B-scan ultrasonography, fluorescein angiography, CT imaging, and even OCT poses a far greater challenge than in adults.
  - Detection of characteristic findings in a parent may help secure the diagnosis of this frequently familial condition.
  - Serial observation (with or without neuroimaging) is appropriate management in asymptomatic patients, particularly when disc abnormality is found on a routine examination, as is often the case. If there is progressive vision loss, onset of disc pallor, *or return to normal disc appearance* over time, other

diagnoses, particularly pseudotumor cerebri, must be reconsidered.

- *Myelinated nerve fibers* in the fundus have a distinctive appearance, but can be confused with disc edema because they typically obscure a portion of the disc margin and vessels. Occurs as a benign anomaly with no implication for vision in 1% of population, bilateral in 20% of cases; occasionally familial (autosomal dominant). Extensive unilateral myelination (sometimes involving most or all of the peripapillary and perifoveal retina) may be part of a constellation of findings that also includes ipsilateral myopia (usually but not always severe), exotropia of variable degree, and amblyopia that tends to respond poorly to treatment.
- Other conditions that can resemble papilledema include posterior PHPV and epipapillary glial membranes. Some normal variant discs with less distinct margins, usually smaller than average, may be similarly misinterpreted. Despite the often-cited association of hyperopia and pseudopapilledema, the vast majority of hyperopes have normal disc appearance, and hyperopia should never be uncritically accepted as an explanation for truly suspicious disc appearance.
- Infiltration of the disc by leukemia or other disseminated malignancy may cause swelling associated with loss of normal ophthalmoscopic features and decreased vision.
- Papilledema is seldom seen in infants with raised intracranial pressure from *hydrocephalus*, presumably because of protective effect from open cranial fontanelles and sutures, though optic atrophy may still develop. Disc swelling does occur with ICP elevation from craniosynostosis (p. 427) and may portend significant vision loss.
- Even mildly atrophic discs often fail to show evidence of swelling in response to rising intracranial pressure. This fact accounts for the absence of papilledema in most hydrocephalic children with ICP elevation due to ventriculoperitoneal shunt malfunction, and for the Foster Kennedy syndrome (unilateral disc swelling due to elevated ICP from a tumor arising near and directly compressing the contralateral optic nerve.)

Reference

Ellis GS Jr, Frey T, Gouterman RZ. Myelinated nerve fibers, axial myopia, and refractory amblyopia: an organic disease. *J Pediatr Ophthalmol Strabismus* 1987;24:111–119.

Optic Nerve Atrophy

Summary

Optic atrophy is characterized by pallor of the optic disc, resulting from any pathologic process that causes loss of retinal ganglion cell axons. This finding may be a consequence of numerous disorders in childhood and can be simulated by other conditions (Table 8.19).

Symptoms and Signs

- Decreased visual acuity. Correlates poorly with disc appearance. Nystagmus if onset in infancy.
- Relative afferent pupillary defect in asymmetric or unilateral cases.
- Optic disc pallor may be generalized, limited to the temporal portion, or (particularly when secondary to cerebral cortical damage) sectoral.
- The appearance of optic atrophy may take 6 weeks or longer to become manifest following injury to afferent visual pathways.

Special Tests

- Because primary optic atrophy from nerve compression may be the presenting sign in infancy of an intracranial mass, or of narrowing optic canals caused by *osteopetrosis* or other bone disease, CT or MRI is indicated in any case of disc pallor without an obvious explanation, or associated with progressive decline in vision.
- Color vision testing (p. 487) often shows abnormality; may provide useful diagnostic information in older children (see below).

Differential Diagnosis

- *Dominant optic atrophy* (Kjer) typically presents in childhood with mild to moderate symmetric reduction of visual acuity and temporal disc pallor (sometimes associated with temporal excavation). Family history and detection of characteristic blue-yellow color vision defect (sometimes with red-green deficiency as well) are essential to establishing the diagnosis. Visual acuity may continue to deteriorate slowly through adulthood, but usually does not reach the level of legal blindness.

Table 8.19

Important associations of optic disc pallor in infancy

Condition	Reference
Craniosynostosis	p. 427
Glaucoma	p. 443
Congenital infection	p. 451
Retinopathy of prematurity	p. 457
Leber congenital amaurosis	p. 461
Neurodegenerative disease	p. 461
Optic nerve hypoplasia	p. 471
Hydrocephalus	p. 473
Osteopetrosis	p. 473
Hereditary optic atrophy	p. 473
Perinatal brain injury	p. 474
Optic pathway tumor	p. 478
Craniopharyngioma	p. 479

- Mild to moderate disc pallor is common in children of very low birth weight, especially if periventricular leukomalacia is present or there is a history of severe intraventricular hemorrhage or hypoxia in the perinatal period.
- Congenital anomalies in which white sclera is visible within the area normally circumscribed by the disc margin may be mistaken for optic atrophy. Among these are ONH with double ring sign, small optic disc colobomas, and severely tilted, malrotated or nasalized disc variants.
- Normal disc color varies greatly. Many healthy discs are less pink temporally than nasally. Mild optic atrophy overlaps normal disc appearance to a considerable degree. Fundus imaging is generally inadequate for documenting subtle changes. Carefully described serial observations by a single examiner over time may be necessary to establish the presence or progression of optic atrophy.

Reference

Repka MX, Miller NR. Optic atrophy in children. *Am J Ophthalmol* 1988;106:191–193.

ADNEXAL AND OCULAR TUMORS

Dermoid Cyst

Summary

Dermoid cysts are choristomas (benign growths of ectopic tissue type or types) arising from surface ectodermal derivatives sequestered beneath skin during facial development.

Symptoms and Signs

- Painless periorbital subcutaneous lump or swelling, typically under 2 cm diameter.
- May slowly enlarge during early childhood or remain stable in size.

Ophthalmic Findings

- Cystic mass, most often external to superotemporal orbital rim; second most common location just internal to superonasal orbital rim.
- Fixed to underlying periosteum, but often permitting a considerable degree of movement in relation to bone; overlying skin normal and freely movable over external surface.
- Deep orbital involvement is uncommon in children but should be considered when palpable mass is fixed firmly to bone.

Special Tests

CT or MRI of orbit, including head is indicated, except in cases of small mobile extraorbital lesions. Characteristic cystic appearance with uniform low intensity interior; often remodeling but not invasion of adjacent bone.

Pathology

Cyst lined by keratinizing squamous epithelium, filled with keratin and cholesterol. Dermal appendages including hair follicles and sebaceous glands are commonly seen.

Disease Course

- Does not typically enlarge beyond early childhood.
- Cyst rupture, spontaneous or secondary to accidental or surgical trauma, may lead to moderate-severe chronic inflammation.

Treatment and Management

Excision (via lid crease, sub-brow, or conjunctival incision) usually indicated, taking care to remove the lesion completely without rupturing the capsule at the time of excision.

Differential Diagnosis

- Usually, the diagnosis is obvious. May occasionally be mistaken for orbital encephalocele, hemangioma, or lacrimal sac mucocele.
- *Orbital teratoma* presents at birth as a large cystic mass causing extreme proptosis and compromise of the globe. Tissue derived from all three embryonic layers is present. May grow rapidly, or uncommonly undergo malignant transformation. Complete excision in the newborn period is indicated, with preservation of the globe if possible, though vision likely to remain poor.
- Dermoid cyst must be distinguished from *epibulbar dermoid*, also a choristoma but with entirely different origin and implications.
  - Characterized by abnormal skinlike differentiation of a portion of the surface ectoderm-derived ocular surface (Table 8.9).
  - Presents as dome-shaped opaque cream-colored lesion involving cornea, usually straddling the limbus (typically 2 to 6 mm diameter, inferotemporal sector), or yellowish-pink growth occupying the temporal conjunctival fornix (often termed *lipodermoid* or *dermolipoma* because of predominance of deep lipoid tissue) (Figure 8.22).
  - Dermal appendages (fine hairs) are usually found on, and fat beneath, the relatively dull rough surface in both types.
  - Both are characteristic of and often a manifestation of Goldenhar syndrome (p. 427).
  - Irritation or appearance concerns justify surgical excision (complete for limbal lesions, which are discrete and readily separated from underlying thinner than normal but structurally sound mesenchyme-derived tissue in the great majority of cases; partial for

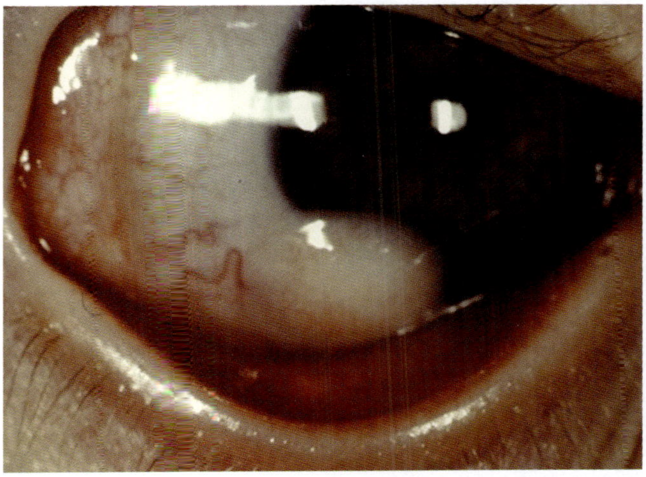

FIGURE 8.22. Limbal dermoid and conjunctival dermoid (temporal fornix) in a child with Goldenhar syndrome.

conjunctival lesions, which often extend widely and deeply, blending into orbital fat).

References

Shields JA, Shields CL. Orbital cysts of childhood: classification, clinical features, and management. *Surv Ophthalmol* 2004;49:281–299.

Weiss AH, Greenwald MJ, Margo CE, et al. Primary and secondary orbital teratomas. *J Pediatr Ophthalmol Strabismus* 1989;26:44–49.

Capillary Hemangioma

Summary

Capillary hemangioma is a benign proliferation of vascular tissue in eyelid or orbit, which may reach a size that compromises vision.

Demographics

- Most common orbital tumor in childhood.
- Female-to-male ratio is 3:2.

Symptoms and Signs

- When skin is involved, typical bright red strawberry nevus with sharp border and irregular surface.
- Subcutaneous lesions cause bluish discoloration of overlying skin.
- May be only a few millimeters in diameter or very extensive, involving entire lid and periorbita, with variable extension into orbit.
- Risk of amblyopia from occlusion of visual axis by enlarged or ptotic eyelid, or from induced astigmatism secondary to corneal deformation. Axis of plus cylinder typically runs through the center of the lesion.

Special Tests

CT or MRI of orbit necessary only if diagnosis uncertain, very large lesion, or prior to steroid injection. Shows characteristic enhancement with contrast.

Pathology

Excision or biopsy seldom indicated for diagnostic purposes. Histopathologically composed of multiply layered plump endothelial cells surrounding capillary lumens that contain few erythrocytes.

Disease Course

Typically present at birth in the form of an inconspicuous flat reddish skin lesion. Growth during the first 6 months of life often very rapid, after which stabilization followed by slow regression occurs. Color change from deep red to grayish is the first sign of involution. Complete disappearance by age 5 to 10 years is the rule, but remnants may persist indefinitely.

Treatment and Management

- Patients with periocular hemangiomas must be followed closely for development of amblyopia, and treated as necessary with refractive correction and occlusion therapy.
- Surgical excision of smaller lesions is an option.
- Medical treatment is indicated for lesions that appear to be amblyogenic or are seriously disfiguring.
- Corticosteroid given orally (prednisone 1 to 2 mg/kg per day) or as intralesional injection (0.5 to 2 mL containing up to 40 mg triamcinolone) has long been the mainstay of treatment. Responses range from rapid dramatic nearly complete regression to no change.
- Intralesional injections have been associated with local complications including focal necrosis and skin depigmentation, and intravascular injection with embolization into the ophthalmic artery leading to central retinal artery occlusion. Lesion size may rebound when systemic drug is tapered. Both methods of steroid delivery cause adrenal suppression and may affect growth or have other systemic consequences.
- Recently, there has been much interest in treatment with propranolol (0.5 mg/kg q.i.d.), which may be as effective as corticosteroid with far fewer side effects. Should be used (like steroid treatment) with involvement of a pediatric medical specialist.

Systemic Findings

- Similar lesions often present elsewhere in head and neck region, or other parts of the body.
- Very large capillary hemangiomas may cause thrombocytopenia by sequestration of platelets (Kasabach-Merritt syndrome), or high-output cardiac failure.

- Diffuse capillary hemangiomatosis can be associated with pulmonary involvement and may cause obstruction of the airways.

Differential Diagnosis

- With typical skin changes, diagnostic confusion is rare.
- Subcutaneous lesion may resemble lymphangioma, dermoid cyst, or rhabdomyosarcoma.
- Nonneoplastic vascular malformations may closely resemble hemangioma. These lesions are present at birth, show at most slow and limited growth during infancy/childhood, and do not spontaneously involute.

References

Haider KM, Plager DA, Neely DE, et al. Outpatient treatment of periocular infantile hemangiomas with oral propranolol. *J AAPOS* 2010;14:251–256.

Kushner BJ. Intralesional corticosteroid injections for infantile adnexal hemangioma. *Am J Ophthalmol* 1982;93:496–506.

Lymphangioma

Summary

Lymphangioma is a benign proliferation of vascular tissue involving conjunctiva, eyelids, or orbit, characterized by marked fluctuation in size.

Symptoms and Signs

- May present as inconspicuous swelling of conjunctiva or eyelid, or mild proptosis.
- Rapid and dramatic enlargement occurs in conjunction with upper respiratory infection, minor trauma, or without obvious cause (Figure 8.23).
- Externally visible as fleshy conjunctival mass ranging from translucent to deep red-purple color.

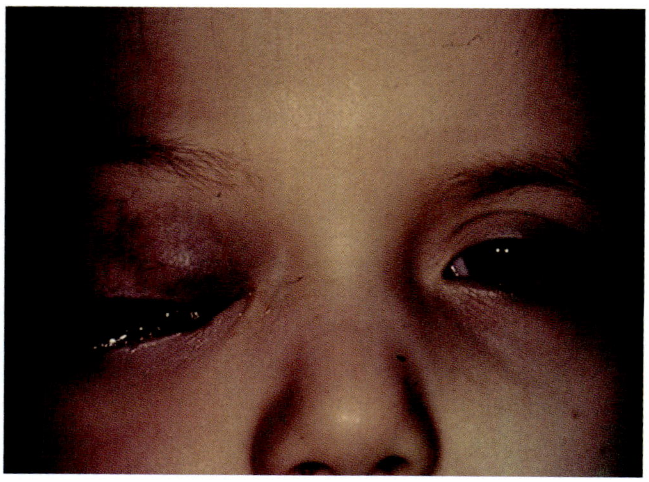

FIGURE 8.23. Orbital lymphangioma, during one of this child's numerous exacerbations.

- Strabismus or vision loss may result from expansion in orbit with compromise of extraocular muscle or optic nerve function.

Special Tests

MRI or CT of the orbit reveals characteristic cystic spaces within the tumor, often blood filled.

Pathology

Thin-walled vascular channels lined by flattened endothelial cells. Lymphoid tissue may be scattered throughout the interstitium. Diffusely infiltrative, without well-defined margins.

Disease Course

Slow growth during infancy and childhood, punctuated by sometimes repeated sudden exacerbations that gradually resolve.

Treatment and Management

- Aspiration of blood from hemorrhagic cystic spaces or orbital decompression by canthotomy/cantholysis may be indicated during hemorrhagic crises.
- Complete excision generally not possible. Surgical debulking of the lesion may be necessary but is fraught with complications.

Differential Diagnosis

- Hemangioma, rhabdomyosarcoma, or neuroblastoma may have similar presentation; in most cases easily distinguished by clinical course and findings on imaging.

Reference

Iliff WJ, Green WR. Orbital lymphangiomas. *Ophthalmology* 1979;86:914–929.

Rhabdomyosarcoma

Summary

Rhabdomyosarcoma is the most common primary orbital malignancy of childhood. It often presents with rapidly progressive proptosis.

Demographics

- More common in males.
- Most often diagnosed age 7 to 10 years but may have onset throughout childhood.

Symptoms and Signs

- Proptosis, typically progressive over days to weeks.
- Eyelid swelling, sometimes with redness, is a common feature.

- Ptosis, typically mild at onset, may be the first sign.
- Occasionally presents with thickening and redness of conjunctiva.
- Firm mass, fixed to adjacent tissues, often palpable through eyelid (Figure 8.24).

Special Tests

- CT or MRI typically shows a well-defined mass of uniform density, with or without evidence of bone destruction.
- Biopsy should be performed expeditiously, and pathologic specimen sent for electron microscopy and use of immunohistochemical stains to aid in determining the type of rhabdomyosarcoma.
- Evaluation for metastatic disease by pediatric oncologist.

Pathology

Rhabdomyosarcoma is classified into four types:

1. *Embryonal*: most common, representing majority of childhood orbital rhabdomyosarcoma. Tumor arises from undifferentiated mesenchymal tissue in the orbit, most often in the superonasal quadrant.
2. *Alveolar:* worst prognosis; commonly involves the inferior orbit or nasopharynx.
3. *Pleomorphic*: most well-differentiated, best prognosis, least common; usually older patients. Typically contains cells with cross-striations (also present in 50% of embryonal and 30% of alveolar cases).
4. *Botryoid:* distinctive gross appearance resembling a grape bunch; occurs in the orbit only by extension from paranasal sinuses or conjunctiva.

Treatment and Management

- Complete excision of smaller lesions, which are frequently encapsulated, is usually possible.

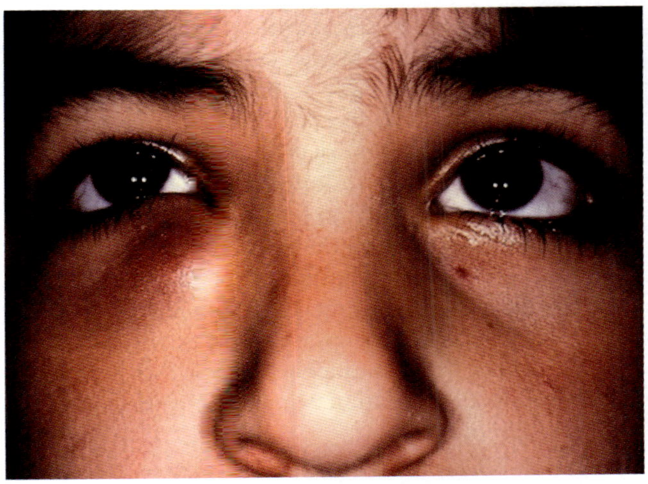

FIGURE 8.24. Orbital rhabdomyosarcoma. This lesion was initially misdiagnosed as a hemangioma.

- Chemotherapy is now the mainstay of treatment, often in conjunction with radiation.
- Greater than 90% long-term survival if tumor initially confined to the orbit.
- Ocular complications are common following radiation treatment and may be severe. Possibilities include cataract, keratoconjunctivitis sicca, retinopathy, and optic neuropathy.

Differential Diagnosis

- Initial presentation may be mistaken for or mimicked by acquired (e.g., posttraumatic) ptosis, orbital cellulitis, orbital pseudotumor, dacryoadenitis or lacrimal gland tumor, dacryocystitis, chalazion, dermoid cyst, hemangioma, lymphangioma, metastatic neuroblastoma, orbital extension of retinoblastoma, or optic nerve glioma.
- Prompt CT or MRI should be done in any case of recent-onset ptosis, proptosis, or periorbital mass of uncertain origin or significance.

Reference

Shields JA, Shields CL. Rhabdomyosarcoma: review for the ophthalmologist. *Surv Ophthalmol* 2003;48:39–57.

Neuroblastoma

Summary

The most common solid tumor of childhood, and the most frequent source of metastatic tumor to the orbit in children, is neuroblastoma, which presents as painless, progressive proptosis, often accompanied by eyelid ecchymosis.

Demographics

- Most frequent onset is around 2 years but may occur at any age from infancy through adolescence.
- No sex or racial predilection.
- Orbital disease nearly always a manifestation of metastatic tumor, most often from the abdomen.

Symptoms and Signs

- Proptosis, unilateral or bilateral (40%); may have rapid onset.
- Eyelid ecchymosis often the most striking feature; can be mistaken for trauma (accidental or inflicted).
- Horner syndrome (mild upper lid ptosis, upward displacement of lower lid, miosis of pupil) may be the presenting sign of neuroblastoma originating in, and often still confined to, the cervical sympathetic ganglia.
- Opsoclonus (dancing eyes, saccadomania; sometimes associated with myoclonus) may be the earliest indication of small occult neuroblastoma, a paraneoplastic effect presumably caused by a circulating humoral factor released from the tumor. The eye movements of opsoclonus are distinctive from oscillatory movements of nystagmus (opsoclonus chaotically variable in direction

and amplitude) or random "searching" movements seen in blind infants and children (opsoclonus ceaseless and rapid).

Special Tests

- Orbital imaging in metastatic disease shows tumor invading the bony orbit, most often superior and lateral walls.
- Any child with Horner syndrome in the absence of an evident cause should have CT or MRI of the chest and neck to look for neuroblastoma.
- Urine vanillylmandelic acid elevated. May be helpful in evaluating child with opsoclonus.

Systemic Findings

- Primary lesion in abdomen (typically originating from adrenal medulla) may be detected as a palpable mass or by means of abdominal CT or MRI. In most cases with orbital metastasis, the primary tumor has been previously identified.
- The N-myc oncogene is found in tumor cells. Multiple copies imply a poorer prognosis.

Treatment and Management

- Surgery, chemotherapy, and radiation may be employed in treating neuroblastoma.
- The prognosis for metastatic disease remains poor, but long-term survival is possible in up to 30% of cases. Prognosis for neuroblastoma presenting as Horner syndrome or opsoclonus is much better, with up to 90% survival.

Differential Diagnosis

May resemble orbital cellulitis, orbital pseudotumor, or traumatic orbitopathy (with suspicion of child abuse).

Reference

Maris JM, Hogarty MD, Bagatell R, et al. Neuroblastoma. *Lancet* 2007;369:2106–2120.

Optic Nerve Glioma (Optic Pathway Tumor)

Summary

Glioma is by far the most common tumor of the anterior visual pathway in childhood, often associated with NF1. May be confined to one optic nerve or the chiasm, or involve chiasm in addition to one or both nerves.

Demographics

- Usually presents between 3 and 10 years.
- Girls more often than boys.
- About one third of children with optic glioma have NF1 (including most with involvement of both nerves); approximately 15% of children with NF1 develop optic pathway tumors.

Signs and Symptoms

- Painless proptosis, nearly always unilateral at onset; may develop rapidly.
- Unilateral or bilateral vision loss, sometimes associated with strabismus.
- Most cases identified by neuroimaging in asymptomatic patients with NF1 never cause vision loss.

Ophthalmic Findings

- Decreased visual acuity, color vision; central and occasionally peripheral field defects.
- Relative afferent pupillary defect when unilateral or asymmetric.
- Optic disc may be swollen when onset is rapid; optic atrophy more typical, sometimes with optociliary shunt vessels.

Systemic Findings

- Children with NF1 (Table 8.21) consistently have multiple café au lait spots (more than 5 lesions more than 5 mm; axillary or inguinal "freckling" confirms the diagnosis). Lisch nodules (p. 485) usually are not yet present at the age of onset of optic glioma.
- Involvement of the hypothalamic-pituitary axis in patients with chiasmal lesions, particularly those with NF1, may cause endocrine abnormalities including precocious puberty, diabetes insipidus, or delayed growth and maturation.
- Hydrocephalus may be a consequence of glioma involving the chiasm, especially in patients without NF1.

Special Tests

- MRI is the preferred imaging procedure; better than CT for detecting chiasmal involvement. When proptosis is present, imaging typically shows fusiform swelling of the optic nerve. In the absence of proptosis, particularly in cases with NF1, cylindrical enlargement of the nerve is typical, often with kinking in the anterior portion, and contrasting perineural intrasheath signal intensity attributed to mucin accumulation in the subarachnoid space (Figure 8.25). Chiasmal involvement may cause subtle generalized enlargement (often seen in NF1 patients), or a discrete suprasellar mass, which must be differentiated from craniopharyngioma (see below).
- Endocrinologic evaluation is indicated with chiasmal or suprasellar involvement.

Pathology

Low-grade pilocytic astrocytoma.

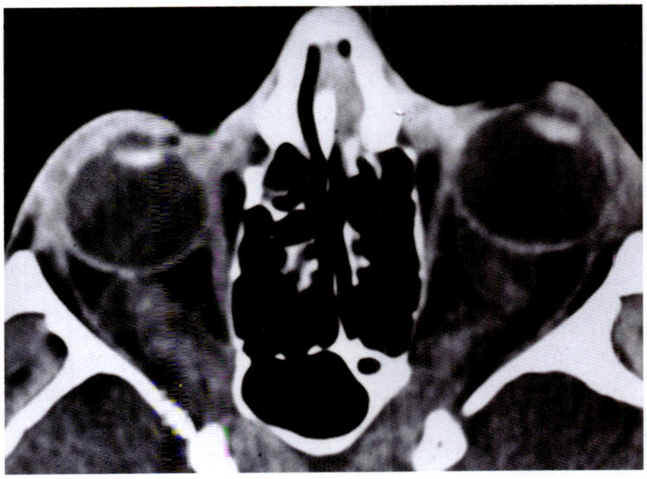

FIGURE 8.25. Axial computed tomographic image showing bilateral optic glioma extending through the optic canals toward the chiasm.

Disease Course

Progressive vision loss occurs in some but by no means all children with optic glioma. Spontaneous improvement in vision is sometimes observed.

Treatment and Management

- Patients with absent or mild findings should be observed closely.
- Surgical excision of the intraorbital nerve is seldom indicated, mainly in cases with severe unilateral proptosis and profoundly decreased vision.
- Chemotherapy is often helpful in cases with progressive loss of vision.
- Radiation may be necessary when progressive disease threatens vision or life, but complications are frequent and may be severe, especially in younger children.

Differential Diagnosis

- *Optic nerve sheath meningioma* is rare in childhood, especially in the prepubertal age range when most optic gliomas are diagnosed.
  - Sometimes associated with neurofibromatosis type 2 (Table 8.21).
  - Presents with unilateral vision loss and disc pallor; typically little if any proptosis.
  - Neuroimaging is usually diagnostic, showing tubular enlargement with perineural increased density, contrast enhancement, and sometimes calcification ("tram-track" appearance).
  - Biopsy seldom necessary and may be misleading due to the frequent association of meningeal hyperplasia with optic nerve glioma.
- *Craniopharyngioma* is a low-grade malignancy that develops as a suprasellar mass, often with cystic and calcific components. Hypothalamic signs may include diabetes isipidus and precocious puberty. Unilateral or bilateral visual loss in late infancy or childhood is the most common presentation. Often, fundus examination shows no abnormality despite very poor vision, creating a risk of confusion with functional blindness.
- Rapid onset of proptosis from optic nerve glioma may resemble that seen with orbital pseudotumor, lymphagioma, rhabdomyosarcoma, or neuroblastoma.

References

Imes RK, Hoyt WF. Childhood chiasmal gliomas: update on the fate of patients in the 1969 San Francisco Study. *Br J Ophthalmol* 1986;70:179–182.

Listernick R, Darling C, Greenwald M, et al. Optic pathway tumors in children: the effect of neurofibromatosis type 1 on clinical manifestations and natural history. *J Pediatr* 1995;127:718–722.

Retinoblastoma

Summary

Retinoblastoma (RB) is by far the most common malignant intraocular tumor of childhood, with a frequency of approximately 1 in 15,000 live births. In about 40% of cases, there is a germ-line mutation that affects all body cells, causing bilateral ocular tumors in most cases, autosomal dominant transmission to offspring, and risk of other malignancies later in life. In other cases, disease is confined to one eye, the result of mutational events in a single somatic cell.

Demographics

- Equal male and female incidence; seen in all ethnic groups.
- Germ-line cases typically diagnosed during infancy; somatic cases age 1 to 3 years, with numerous exceptions, including reported cases in adolescence or later.
- All bilateral cases (about one third of total) and about 15% of unilateral cases have germ-line mutation. A substantial majority of bilateral cases are sporadic (i.e., there is no prior family history of RB).
- A small percentage of individuals with germ-line mutation develop no ocular tumors (but may have affected offspring), and a small percentage of tumors apparently lack malignant potential, at some point ceasing to grow or involuting spontaneously. Such a lesion, termed *retinoma* or *retinocytoma*, may occasionally be found in the asymptomatic parent of a child with typical RB.

Etiology

- In the hereditary form of RB, mutation of a gene (RB1) in the q14 region of one chromosome 13 results in partial loss or dysfunction of a normally present tumor suppressing agent in all cells of the body. It is believed that a tumor results when a second mutational event then occurs in the other RB1 gene of a developing retinal cell (2-hit hypothesis of Knudson). Typically, such second mutations result in three to five tumors or more distributed between the two eyes.

- In nonhereditary RB, two mutational events occur after conception in a single developing retinal cell, leading to development of one tumor.

Symptoms and Signs

- Classic presentation is "white pupil" or *leukocoria*, usually first noted by the family; variously described as a "glow" or "gleam," often seen only intermittently or in photographs (Figure 8.26). Absent evidence of discomfort or decreased vision in the great majority of cases, delay in seeking medical attention is common. Nonophthalmologic physicians generally lack the ability to screen effectively for RB, frequently resulting in inappropriate reassurance to a family witness of leukocoria that further delays diagnosis. Finally, failure to recognize the urgency of a leukocoria history by the ophthalmologist's appointment scheduling staff may result in additional time passage before the child is seen and the condition diagnosed.
- Strabismus (esotropia or exotropia) secondary to unilaterally decreased vision is the second most common initial concern. Mistaking this for benign strabismus also often leads to delay in diagnosis.

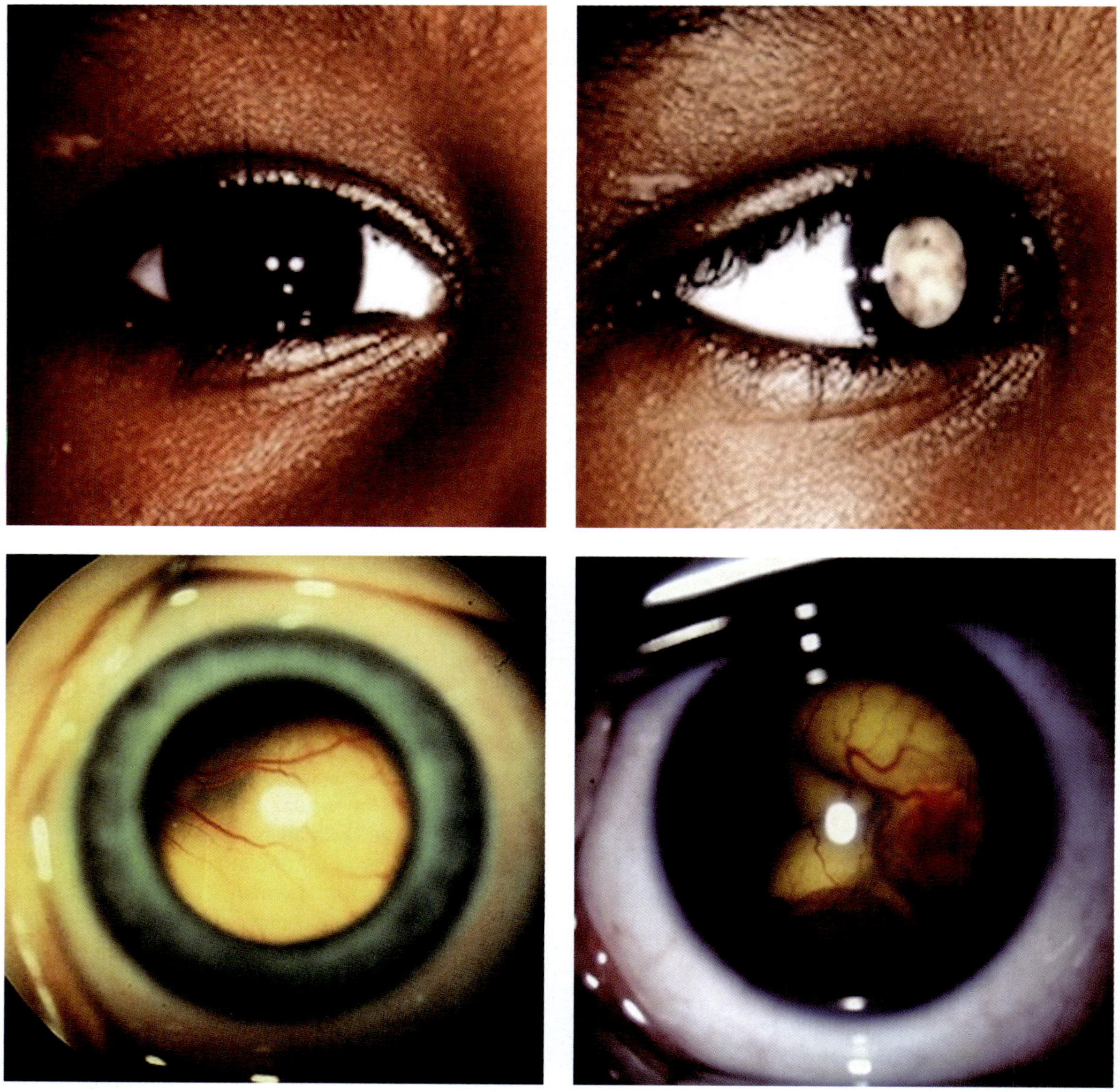

A B C D

FIGURE 8.26. Leukocoria. **A, B:** White pupil in this eye with a large endophytic RB involving the nasal retina was only visible when viewed from the side. **C:** Appearance of an eye with total exudative retinal detachment from a large exophytic RB. **D:** Very similar appearance of an eye with total exudative retinal detachment from Coats disease.

- Much less often, but important for the clinician to keep in mind (see below), advanced disease may present with redness, swelling, or pain.

Ophthalmic Findings

- In a large majority of cases (aside from those with positive family history detected by early ophthalmologic screening examinations), at least one eye contains a fairly large tumor at the time of diagnosis.
- Larger tumors that extend mainly in the subretinal space (*exophytic growth*) are usually associated with retinal detachment, typically bullous, often total; subretinal fluid is thick and proteinaceous. Overlying retina often shows dilated, tortuous blood vessels.
- Tumor that breaks through internal limiting membrane and extends into vitreous (*endophytic* growth) appears as a creamy whitish mass, with smooth or irregular surface that large or small vessels may dip into and emerge from. Tumor "seeds" in the vitreous may be present, occasionally to a degree that limits visualization of the underlying mass.
- Small tumors, still confined between the internal and the external limiting membranes, are typically grayish to pinkish white, disciform or dome-shaped, found anywhere in the fundus but with predilection for the macular region and near the ora serrata. Rarely (especially in older children) tumor may spread extensively within the retina (*diffuse*, *infiltrating* growth), creating an atypical and easily misdiagnosed clinical picture.
- Spontaneous hyphema or vitreous hemorrhage is occasionally present, and may prevent ophthalmoscopic visualization of fundus lesions.
- Tumors that occupy most of the retina or fill the posterior segment may infiltrate or seed into the anterior chamber (sometimes producing "pseudohypopyon"), cause glaucoma by compressing the angle or inducing iris neovascularization, or lead to lid edema and proptosis as a result of orbital invasion by tumor, or tumor necrosis and secondary inflammation (resembling panophthalmitis).

Systemic Findings

- A small percentage of children with germ-line RB develop primary intracranial malignancy, typically originating in the pineal body (pinealoblastoma) or parasellar region (primitive neuroectodermal tumor). The term *trilateral retinoblastoma* has been applied to such cases. Intracranial tumor may be detected at the time of RB diagnosis, or develop years later; rarely precedes the finding of intraocular disease. Extraocular disease is usually fatal in these patients.
- Survivors of germ-line RB have a high risk (20% to 40%) of developing additional primary malignancy in later life, typically from late childhood through young adulthood, which is often fatal. Osteosarcoma is the most common second tumor, followed by soft tissue sarcomas. Lesions may occur anywhere but most often are in the craniofacial region. Treatment of RB with external-beam radiation considerably increases the risk of such occurrence.
- A small minority of RB patients have a karyotype showing deletion in the 13q14 region, which in most cases also causes varying degrees of developmental delay and dysmorphic features.

Special Tests

- CT imaging and ophthalmic ultrasonography reveal characteristic dense calcification within most larger RB lesions. One or both of these tests should be performed in any case where RB is among other diagnostic possibilities (particularly unilaterally involved eyes with unexplained retinal detachment, or containing blood or cellular suspension that obscures the fundus). Absence of calcification does not rule out RB, especially in older children (who are also more likely to present with disorders that may closely mimic RB).
- Magnetic resonance imaging is helpful for determining if there is extraocular disease (optic nerve invasion, intracranial lesion) prior to initiating chemotherapy, and to monitor for disease recurrence after treatment.
- In most but not all cases, detailed genetic analysis performed on white blood cells by a qualified laboratory can distinguish germ-line from somatic RB, and refine risk estimates for family members. In sporadic cases, tumor tissue appropriately harvested and processed immediately after enucleation is usually required for informative testing.
- Karyotype analysis and tests for metastatic spread (bone marrow biopsy, lumbar puncture) are not useful or indicated in patients who appear otherwise healthy. Aspiration of intraocular fluids for cytology or biochemical analysis carries significant risk and is no longer considered appropriate in suspected RB.

Pathology

Tumors are composed mainly of poorly differentiated neuroblastic cells. More differentiated areas often contain *Flexner-Wintersteiner rosettes* or *fleurettes*. Areas of necrosis and dystrophic calcification are common.

Classification and Prognosis

- Optimal treatment of RB typically involves multiple modalities and complex decision making, but the prognosis for survival is excellent in the developed world, with mortality well under 5%.
- The outlook for saving an eye with RB depends on the extent and distribution of tumor. For many years, salvage potential was predicted using the classification system of Reese and Ellsworth. Eyes with very large tumors or extensive vitreous seeding (Reese-Ellsworth Group V) still usually require enucleation. A newer classification

Table 8.20

International classification of retinoblastoma

Group	Description	Management	Prognosis
A (small)	≤3 mm height, ≥2 DD from fovea, ≥1 DD from disc	Local treatment with laser, cryotherapy, or plaque	Excellent prognosis for salvage and vision
B (medium)	>3 mm height, clear SRF ≤3 mm from tumor margin	Chemoreduction followed by local treatment	Very good; vision depends on location of tumor(s)
C (confined)	Localized subretinal or vitreous seeding ≤3 mm from tumor	High-intensity chemotherapy (3 drugs, 6 cycles) followed by local treatment as necessary	Good; vision depends on location of tumor(s), extent of local treatment
D (diffuse)	SRF or seeding >3 mm from tumor margin	Same as C, or enucleation	Fair; high probability of intraocular recurrence
E (enucleation)	Anterior segment or orbital involvement; otherwise nonsalvageable eye	Enucleation, with or without prophylactic chemotherapy	Prognosis for survival depends on pathologic findings

Prognosis refers to likelihood of avoiding enucleation for A–D; survival prognosis excellent, visual prognosis as per comment.
DD, disc diameter (about 1.5 mm); SRF, subretinal fluid.
Adapted from Lin P, O'Brien JM. Frontiers in the management of retinoblastoma. *Am J Ophthalmol* 2009;148:192–198.

scheme is now preferred for eyes with lower levels of involvement, most of which can be preserved with appropriate treatment (Table 8.20).

- Visual outcome depends heavily on the degree of macular involvement, difficult to predict based on findings prior to treatment. Vision may be surprisingly good after regression of tumors that initially overhang or extend into the macula, sometimes despite persistent significant abnormality of macular appearance.

Treatment and Management

- Enucleation remains the initial treatment of choice for most eyes with large tumors and poor visual potential, especially in unilateral cases and when extensive vitreous seeding is present unilaterally. Removing the globe with a long segment (up to 20 mm or more) of optic nerve attached is believed to improve survival prognosis.
- Systemic chemotherapy (up to 6 monthly cycles of intravenous carboplatin, accompanied by etoposide, vincristine, or both) is now the preferred initial treatment for most bilateral RB, and for unilateral disease with good prognosis for ocular salvage (Figure 8.27). Residual tumor, often greatly decreased in volume after one to two chemo cycles, is usually treated with laser (mainly for posterior lesions) or cryotherapy (for anterior lesions). A few eyes (nearly always in familial or bilateral cases) contain only tumors small enough (<3 to 4 mm) to be treated primarily with laser or cryotherapy alone.
- External-beam radiation therapy (EBRT) was until recently widely employed in the primary management of RB. Most tumors are highly radiosensitive, but serious side effects (including cataract, severe keratopathy, retinal vasculopathy, orbital atrophy, and increased second tumor risk) are common. In the current era of effective chemotherapy-based treatment protocols, the use of EBRT for RB is limited to treatment of extraocular or recurrent disease that endangers life or sight.
- Treatment with radioisotope-bearing plaques (brachytherapy) is very useful in a subset of patients with medium-sized tumors that do not involve the disc or the macula.
- Locally administered chemotherapy (delivered by periocular injection or canulation of the ophthalmic artery) is currently under investigation as an adjunct or alternative to systemic chemotherapy.
- Given the rarity of the disease, the presence of serious threat to life and sight, and the complexity of medical decision making involved, prompt referral to a center with a high degree of relevant experience and expertise (ideally one that is a affiliated with the Children's Oncology Group) is generally in the best interest of *all* patients believed to have RB *prior to administration of any treatment*.

Disease Course

- Untreated RB is nearly always fatal after spreading to the brain (generally via invasion of the optic nerve) and/or distant sites, especially bone or bone marrow (by way of uveal tract or orbital blood vessels).
- Recurrence following enucleation, usually detected within 1 year and beginning in the orbit, is seen most often in cases where tumor was found pathologically extending beyond the lamina cribrosa into optic nerve, even though the cut end of the nerve and the meninges

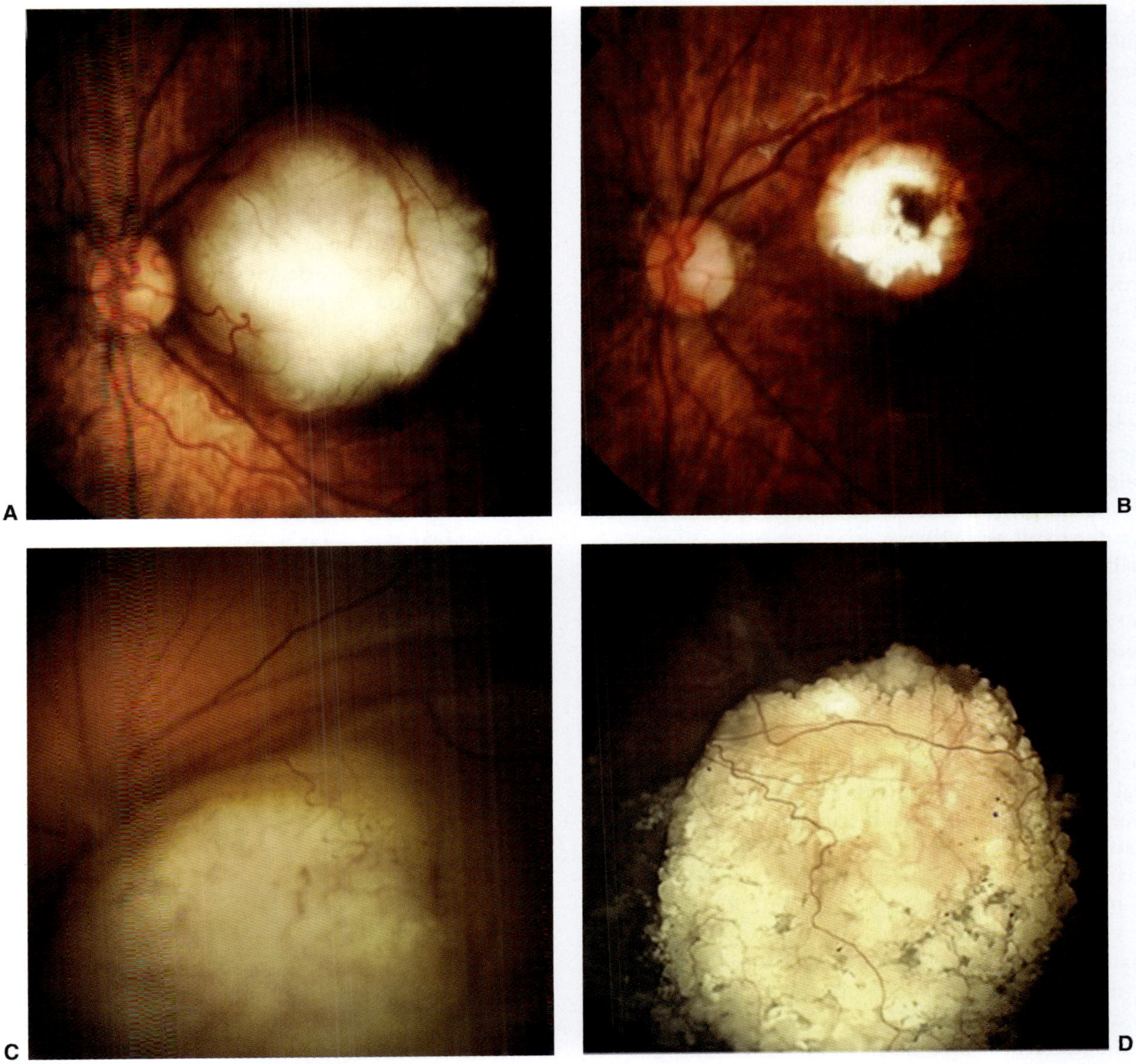

FIGURE 8.23. RB before and after successful treatment. **A, B:** Medium-sized tumor involving the macula (group B), before and after treatment with chemoreduction and laser hyperthermia. Final visual acuity was 20/30. **C, D:** Large but confined (group C) tumor, showing both endophytic and exophytic growth, with extensive subretinal fluid accumulation but without widespread tumor seeding. Regressed completely and did not recur after treatment with intensive chemotherapy alone.

may have appeared free of disease. Prophylactic postenucleation chemotherapy is of uncertain value for such patients, most of whom remain healthy without further treatment. A minority of patients with orbital recurrence, and a few with disseminated disease, can be cured with intensive chemotherapy and radiation treatment.

- Regardless of initial therapeutic approach, there is a risk of recurrent intraocular disease (reactivation of regressed lesions, retinal implantation growth from viable cells in the vitreous, and occasionally development of entirely new tumors) in retained treated eyes. Concern is greater for individual tumors with residual translucent grayish tissue ("fish-flesh" appearance), but even lesions showing complete regression to calcified remnant ("cottage-cheese" appearance) or flat pigmented scar may come back to life. Close observation with frequent examination under general anesthesia (including photographic documentation) is required for years after treatment is concluded.

Follow-Up

- Responsibility for long-term posttreatment monitoring and for screening other family members including new siblings, may be shared by the treating center with an appropriately qualified ophthalmologist in the patient's community.

- As concern about recurrent ocular disease wanes in late childhood, attention to the possibilities of second primary malignancy and transmission to offspring should become a focus of ongoing care.

Differential Diagnosis

- Listing the many causes of leukocoria is a time-honored tradition, but in fact most of the conditions that are usually found in such catalogs (including cataract and disorders like coloboma that create a flat or concave patch of high light reflectivity in the central fundus) would never be mistaken for RB by even a first-year ophthalmology resident—though a pediatrician viewing the red fundus reflex might be justifiably concerned. With usual pediatric direct ophthalmoscopic screening technique, the most common causes of asymmetrically bright red reflex are anisometropic refractive error, and detection of brighter reflection from the normal optic disc of one eye due to off-axis viewing.
- PHPV (p. 452) and conditions causing vitreoretinal dysplasia (Table 8.13) more closely resemble RB (as shown in Figure 8.12) but usually can be easily distinguished by findings on B-scan or CT imaging and by the consistent presence of microphthamos, which is rare with RB. Similar considerations, plus history in most cases, generally prevent confusion between end-stage ROP and RB.
- Just two nonneoplastic disorders have potential to create real diagnostic uncertainty for an experienced clinician. (See referenced pages for discussion of distinguishing features.)

  Toxocara uveitis (p. 451) with intense vitreous reaction may effectively simulate endophytic RB with heavy vitreous seeding.

  Coats disease (p. 458) with total or near total retinal detachment may mimic exophytic RB to a remarkable degree (Figure 8.26D).
- It should be kept in mind that advanced intraocular RB may present as glaucoma (with corneal clouding and enlargement in infancy), or with a picture of acute inflammation resembling orbital cellulitis or panophthalmitis; treatment in any such case should be initiated only after fundus examination, or appropriate imaging if the fundus cannot be visualized adequately.
- *Astrocytic hamartoma*, usually but not always associated with tuberous sclerosis (Table 8.21), may bear very close resemblance to small intraretinal or partially regressed endophytic RB lesions. An important differential diagnostic feature is that these lesions (typically a few millimeters in size, often multiple in an eye) often obscure the course of retinal blood vessels, whereas intraretinal RB does not. Larger astrocytic hamartomas, often showing a bumpy "mulberry" or "tapioca" surface and occasionally partially calcified, may arise over the disc margin. Vision is seldom affected. Skin should be carefully inspected using an ultraviolet lamp to spot ash-leaf hypopigmented macules, usually present in infants with TS.
- *Medulloepithelioma* (also known as *diktyoma*), believed to arise from ciliary body epithelium, is a very rare nonhereditary intraocular tumor without systemic associations, that usually presents in childhood (median age: 5 years). Initial signs (always unilateral) are highly variable, frequently including glaucoma and a fleshy, sometimes cystic, occasionally pigmented mass that appears to originate from iris, ciliary body, or retina; intraocular bleeding (hyphema or vitreous hemorrhage) may be seen. Many cases are diagnosed only after enucleation of a painful blind eye. Orbital extension followed by metastatic spread is exceptional, and survival is the rule.
- *Choroidal melanoma* occurs before age 20 in approximately 1% of cases, very rarely before age 10. Unless detected early as an incidental finding, most of these tumors are not diagnosed until large enough to require enucleation.

References

Greenwald MJ, Strauss LC. Treatment of intraocular retinoblastoma with carboplatin and etoposide chemotherapy. *Ophthalmology* 1996;103:1989–1997.

Lin P, O'Brien JM. Frontiers in the management of retinoblastoma. *Am J Ophthalmol* 2009:148:192–198.

Juvenile Xanthogranuloma

Summary

Juvenile xanthogranuloma (JXG) is a nonneoplastic histiocytic proliferation that typically develops in infancy with skin involvement, occasionally associated with ocular lesions.

Symptoms and Signs

- Surface lesions are typically about 1-cm-diameter papules, yellow-orange to tan color, often periocular involving eyelid skin; less commonly conjunctiva, cornea or sclera.
- Iris involvement is usually asymptomatic, or noted because of heterochromia.
- Episodes of acute redness, pain and photophobia secondary to spontaneous intraocular bleeding.

Ophthalmic Findings

- Yellow-brown nodular or diffusely infiltrating iris lesion, occasionally bilateral.
- Recurrent spontaneous hyphema may lead to inflammation, elevated IOP, secondary corneal changes and significant loss of vision.
- Rarely orbital or fundus involvement, which may be extensive.

Systemic Findings

- Skin lesions may be widely scattered over the upper portion of the body, or may be absent. Visceral involvement is rare.
- Association with NF1 and leukemia has been reported.

Pathology

Lesions consist mainly of lymphocytes and histiocytes, including Touton giant cells. Distinct from disorders of the histiocytosis X group. Biopsy of a skin lesion, or finding of histiocytes in aspirated aqueous, confirms the diagnosis.

Treatment and Management

- Spontaneous resolution of both surface and deep lesions, typically over several years.
- Excision of iris lesions should be avoided because of high risk of hemorrhage.
- Use of topical, subconjunctival, or systemic corticosteroids may accelerate regression.
- Low-dose radiation therapy has been used in cases refractory to medical treatment.

Differential Diagnosis

- The most common iris growths in childhood are *Lisch nodules*, benign proliferations of melanocytes seen in most individuals with neurofibormatosis type 1 (Table 8.21) by the time of puberty. Lesions are usually multiple, 0.5 to 2 mm in size, tan in color, with a smooth or rough surface. They have no impact on ocular health or vision, but represent a major diagnostic criterion for NF1 (two or more must be present), second in frequency only to café au lait spots of the skin.

Table 8.21

Neurocutaneous syndromes with ocular involvement

Condition	Ocular findings	Other findings	Comment
Neurofibromatosis type 1 (von Recklinghausen disease)	Lisch nodules (p. 485) Plexiform neurofibroma Glaucoma (p. 444) Optic pathway tumor (p. 478) PSC cataract (Table 8.12)	Café au lait spots (p. 478) Sphenoid wing hypoplasia (causes orbital pulsation) Learning disability	Autosomal dominant, highly variable expressivity Chromosome 17
Neurofibromatosis type 2	Combined hamartoma (p. 466) Optic nerve sheath meningioma	Acoustic neuroma Cranial nerve schwannomas Intracranial meningioma	Autosomal dominant, nearly complete penetrance Chromosome 22
Tuberous sclerosis complex (Bourneville disease)	Retinal astrocytic hamartoma (p. 484)	Hypopigmented skin macules ("ashleaf spots") Adenoma sebaceum (face) and periungual fibromas	Autosomal dominant, highly variable expressivity Chromosome 9 or 16
von Hippel–Lindau disease (angiomatosis retinae)	*Retinal hemangioblastoma,* enlarged twin feeder vessels Exudative retinal detachment	Cerebellar hemangioblastoma Renal cell carcinoma Pheochromocytoma	Autosomal dominant, variable penetrance Chromosome 3
Sturge-Weber syndrome (encephalofacial angiomatosis)	Glaucoma (p. 444) Hypervascular conjunctiva and episclera Choroidal hemangioma	Facial portwine nevus Facial hypertrophy Seizures, mental deficiency	Not hereditary Glaucoma usually a problem in childhood; choroidal abnormality usually not
Klippel-Trenaunay syndrome	Similar to Sturge-Weber in some cases	Portwine nevus, hypertrophy, hyperpigmentation, mainly trunk and extremities	Not hereditary
Wyburn-Mason syndrome (racemose angioma)	Markedly dilated and tortuous retinal vessels with arterio-venous communication	Portwine skin lesion in some Intracranial AVM (midbrain) Cranial nerve palsies	Not hereditary Seizures, hydrocephalus Risk of intracranial bleeding
Louis-Bar syndrome (ataxia telangiectasia)	Conjunctival hypervascularity, skin telangiectasia Oculomotor apraxia (p. 462)	Ataxia, neurodegeneration Immune deficiency causing infection, malignancy	Autosomal recessive Chromosome 11

AVM, arteriovenous malformation; PSC, posterior subcapsular.

- Anomalous concentrations or deficits of iris stromal pigment, sometimes strikingly evident, are common in children, but rarely a serious concern. Iris melanoma is very rare. Monitoring of appearance and IOP is appropriate management.
- The most common early acquired ocular surface neoplasm is *conjunctival nevus*, typically a 3 to 6 mm diameter slightly elevated fleshy lesion near the limbus, noted in late childhood with evidence of growth or color change. Color varies from pink to brown. Recurrence after excision is rare. Histopathology shows compound or junctional melanocyte proliferation.
- Spontaneous hyphema may also result from retinoblastoma (p. 481). Given that history is often unreliable or misleading in childhood injuries, JXG and RB should be considered in the differential diagnosis of apparently *traumatic hyphema*. With any hyphema, the possibilities of inflicted (abusive) injury and of acute sight-threatening pressure elevation should be kept in mind. IOP should be measured, even if this requires sedation. If pressure is high (or unknown), screening for *sickle trait* (the most frequent culprit) should be done, even in patients without known African ancestry.

Reference

Zimmerman LE. Ocular lesions of juvenile xanthogranuloma: nevoxanthogranuloma. *Trans Am Acad Ophthalmol Otolaryngol* 1965;69:412–442.

Neurocutaneous Syndromes (Phakomatoses)

The neurocutaneous syndromes are a group of disorders with manifestations involving skin and elements of the peripheral and/or CNS, frequently including benign neoplasms (hamartomas or phakomas) of the eye. These conditions are summarized in Table 8.21, and some of their major ocular findings are described more fully elsewhere in this chapter (page references in table). Most show familial occurrence with variable expression; recognition in a parent after diagnosis in a more severely affected child may have important implications for the older relative.

Reference

Greenwald MJ, Paller AS. Ocular and dermatologic manifestations of neurocutaneous syndromes. *Dermatolog Clin* 1992;10:623–639.

NYSTAGMUS

Congenital Nystagmus

Summary

Nystagmus that appears in early infancy (usually referred to as congenital nystagmus or CN) may represent an isolated developmental disturbance of the oculomotor control system (congenital motor or idiopathic nystagmus), or be associated with one of numerous other conditions, some previously listed in Table 8.18.

Etiology

- Primary motor defect may have a genetic basis (most often autosomal dominant), be part of a multisystem disorder (e.g., Down syndrome—p. 425), or present in association with infantile-onset strabismus.
- Decreased central vision in both eyes (and occasionally monocular visual deprivation) from any cause in infancy, if sufficiently severe, is likely to lead to development of nystagmus with similar properties.

Symptoms and Signs

- Onset of abnormal eye movements is usually between birth and 6 months; may not be noticed until later.
- Movements are always bilateral and conjugate; typically moderate frequency, amplitude, intensity.
- Nearly always horizontal oscillations; sometimes vertical and/or torsional component as well. Axis of movement does not vary with gaze direction.
- Usually, there is an identifiable null/neutral gaze position/region characterized by pendular movement, minimum intensity, optimal vision; usually along the horizontal gaze axis but occasionally a vertical gaze component as well. Head posture often maintained to facilitate use of preferred gaze direction.
- Typically jerk-type movement seen to both left and right of null zone, fast component in direction of gaze, intensity increasing with distance from null.
- Intensity may increase with visual concentration, or occlusion of one eye; may decrease with convergence, or during sleep.
- No oscillopsia or sensation of movement.
- Development of visual interest and fixation may be somewhat delayed when CN is present, regardless of the underlying disorder, and whether there is a primary sensory abnormality or not. This often leads to concern about blindness in the young infant (p. 462). If there is a good pupillary response to light, good visual fixation by late infancy can be anticipated.
- Associated "shaking" or "nodding" head movements often become conspicuous in later infancy.

Ophthalmic Findings

- Characteristics of eye movements do not distinguish primary motor from sensory defect nystagmus.
- Ophthalmologic evaluation in any case of infantile-onset nystagmus must include careful attention to multiple elements:

  Visual fixation quality (see p. 462), and acuity if measurable. Test with isolated letters—linear presentation may artifactually lower score. Also, test vision at near point (as close as the child wants to hold print); record print size type read, and distance from preferred eye. This is valuable in determining adequacy of vision for educational needs.)

Color vision, if cooperation adequate. The *HRR test* (Richmond Products) and *Color Vision Testing Made Easy* (T. L. Waggoner) are far superior to standard Ishihara plates for this purpose: less confusing for children and designed to screen with just a few plates. The HRR test is also valuable for detecting blue-yellow (*tritan*) defects; for distinguishing *deutan* (red-green confusion alone) from less common *protan* (red-green confusion plus decreased sensitivity for red) anomalies in males with normal acuity and X-linked congenital "color blindness"; and for quantifying the degree of abnormality (*dichromacy* vs. milder *anomalous trichromacy*).

Pupillary light reaction, absolute and relative. Look for "paradoxical light response" by observing pupils in bright, then dim illumination: positive response is constriction rather than expected dilation. This finding confirms the presence of congenitally abnormal anterior visual pathway function, but is nonspecific; seen in both rod- and cone-system disorders (p. 461), as well as hypoplasia of the fovea (p. 468) or optic nerve (p. 471).

Ocular alignment: If strabismus is present and examination otherwise normal, usually no need to search for other causes of nystagmus.

Corneal diameter and clarity: Microphthalmos alone rarely causes nystagmus; associated disorders often do (Tables 8.5 and 8.11).

Iris transillumination: May be subtle in milder forms of albinism (p. 463).

Lens clarity: Usually, no nystagmus from congenital cataract unless complete blockage of light transmission in central 3 mm, both eyes (p. 448).

Optic disc size and configuration: Hypoplasia and dysplasia may be challenging to detect or distinguish from other anomalies (p. 471).

Quality of macular/foveal differentiation: Subtle abnormalities may be difficult to distinguish from normal variation, especially in young infants.

Distribution and caliber of retinal blood vessels: Vessel narrowing may be the only ophthalmoscopic evidence of LCA or other early-onset rod-cone dystrophy (p. 461).

Amount and distribution of fundus pigmentation, both macular and peripheral (p. 461, Table 8.17).

- High degree of ametropia may be clue to presence of retinal dystrophy (e.g., hyperopia with LCA; myopia with CSNB). Nystagmus is rarely if ever caused by purely refractive visual impairment.

Special Tests

- Neuroimaging (usually MRI) is indicated in infancy if evidence for ocular sensory origin of nystagmus is lacking, and if there is cause for concern about intracranial abnormality, such as optic atrophy, deteriorating vision, developmental delay or regression, seizures, or focal deficits such as ataxia. Infantile-onset nystagmus with movement characteristics different from typical CN (e.g., primarily vertical oscillation) should prompt neuroimaging.
- Electroretinography is indicated in infancy if there is any abnormality of retinal vessels, pigmentation, or macular differentiation that suggests retinal dystrophy (p. 461); if there is high ametropia; or if the baby does not consistently fixate by age 6 months in the absence of a neurodevelopemental explanation.
- ERG should be considered for the older child with nystagmus of infantile onset and uncertain origin if there is evidence of night blindness, deficient color vision, progressive visual impairment, or visual acuity measuring less than 20/50 to 20/100. At any age, ERG is indicated if family planning considerations require diagnostic precision.
- If available, eye movement recording may be helpful by demonstrating the characteristic waveform of CN (accelerating slow-phase movement).

Disease Course

- Regardless of origin, CN in early infancy tends to be less regular, with relatively slow and large amplitude movements, and without well-defined jerk direction.
- With increasing age, nystagmus intensity tends to diminish gradually, accompanied by improved visual acuity measurements, especially in nonsensory cases.
- Most children with primary motor nystagmus and many with sensory causes require little if any special assistance in the classroom. A minority may qualify for motor vehicle operator licensing as adults.

Treatment and Management

- Various medical and surgical treatments have been advocated for reduction of nystagmus movements; none has become established as standard management.
- Eye muscle surgery is generally effective for shifting the null zone position toward primary gaze. The Kestenbaum-Anderson procedure is most often used: recess-resect for "ET" on eye that is adducted in null, for "XT" on eye that is abducted. Various formulas for surgical dosage have been proposed; simplest approach is to derive from prism diopter equivalent of face turn angle (1 degree = 2 prism diopters).
- Cataract surgery performed urgently in early infancy within a few weeks of nystagmus onset may restore steady fixation in some cases.

Differential Diagnosis

- *Periodic alternating nystagmus* may be indistinguishable from CN, except for the fact that null position migrates between left and right gaze with a period of several minutes. Diagnostic possibilities are similar to CN; especially common in albinism. Must be ruled out before undertaking surgery to shift null zone.
- Latent nystagmus that is present during binocular viewing (often termed *manifest-latent* or MLN) may easily be mistaken for CN, but has significantly different implications for diagnosis and treatment (see below). Most important differentiating feature is reversal of nystagmus jerk direction with shift of fixation between right and left eyes in LN.

References

Scott WE, Kraft SP. Surgical treatment of compensatory head position in congenital nystagmus. *J Pediatr Ophthalmol Strabismus* 1984;21:85–93.

Weiss AH, Biersdorf WR. Visual sensory disorders in congenital nystagmus. *Ophthalmology* 1989;96:517–523.

Latent Nystagmus

Summary

Latent nystagmus (LN) is generally considered to be an expression of the same poorly understood disturbance of oculomotor function that is responsible for essential or idiopathic infantile esotropia (p. 496).

Symptoms and Signs

- Always bilateral horizontal conjugate jerk movements; occasional torsional component.
- Nearly always associated with strabismus but may persist after surgical realignment; dissociated vertical deviation (DVD) commonly present.
- Characteristically increases in intensity with occlusion of one eye; may or may not be detectable during binocular viewing.
- Jerk-phase direction *always* toward the fixating eye; reverses with alternating occlusion.
- Intensity least with fixating eye in adduction, greatest in abduction; may lead to face turn that maintains fixating eye in adduction. Does not show gaze null zone like CN.
- LN may be an obstacle to reliable monocular acuity testing; effect minimized by testing in adduction or with partial occlusion of other eye (central field only, or optical blur).

Special Tests

- LN is not a sign of visual sensory loss or neurologic disease; no requirement for imaging or electrophysiologic evaluation of retinal function when findings are typical.
- Nystagmus wave-form recording shows characteristic pattern of decelerating slow-phase movement.

Treatment and Management

- Often improves following medial rectus muscle recession for esotropia.
- Kestenbaum-Anderson procedure may be helpful for face-turn, provided preferred gaze direction is consistently unilateral. May be modifiable to correct strabismus as well as nystagmus.

Reference

Dell'Osso LF, Schmidt D, Daroff RB. Latent, manifest latent, and INS. *Arch Ophthalmol* 1979;97:1877–1885.

Spasmus Nutans

Summary

Spasmus nutans is an early acquired disorder characterized by high-frequency pendular nystagmus associated with head nodding and torticollis.

Symptoms and Signs

- Rapid, pendular, small-amplitude nystagmus; "shimmering" quality.
- Right and left eye movements are dysconjugate.
- No variation with gaze direction or fixating eye.
- Usually bilateral but asymmetric; sometimes appears strictly unilateral.
- Nystagmus typically horizontal but may have vertical or torsional component.
- Head movement usually horizontal, sometimes vertical (especially with vertical nystagmus). Nystagmus may diminish with head nodding.

Disease Course

- Onset of nystagmus age 3 months to 2 years, occasionally older.
- Head nodding and torticollis may develop later than nystagmus, or not at all.
- Resolves spontaneously in most cases within 2 years, nearly always by age 5 years.

Differential Diagnosis

- Virtually identical findings may result from intracranial tumor, especially glioma involving the chiasm, or occasionally from uniocular decreased vision of any origin.
- Most authorities recommend MRI in any case of apparent spasmus nutans, especially if over age 6 months at onset.

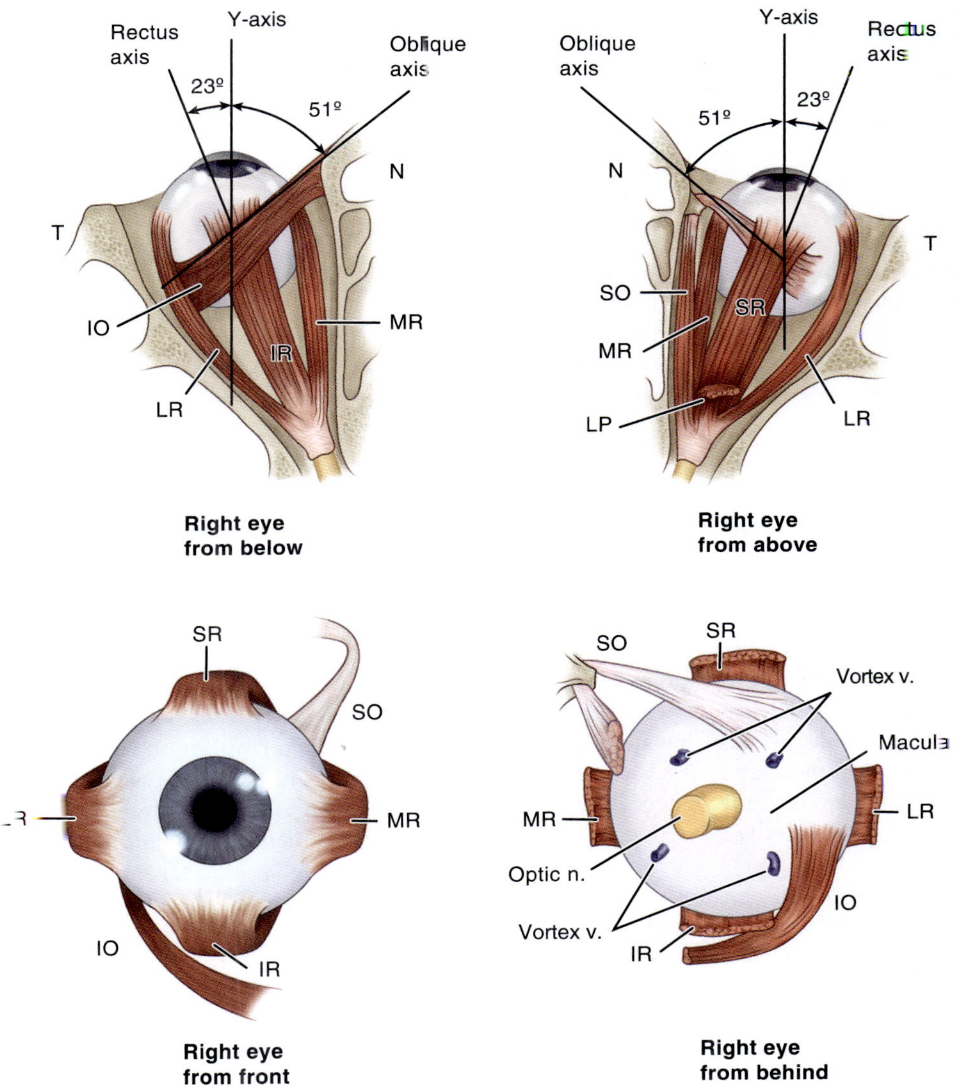

FIGURE 8.28. Anatomy of the extraocular muscles.

- Some retinal disorders (e.g., CSNB) may cause nystagmus closely resembling spasmus nutans. ERG is indicated if symptoms suggestive of retinal dystrophy are present.

Reference

Albright AL, Sclabassi RJ, Slamovits TL, et al. Spasmus nutans associated with optic gliomas in infants. *J Pediatr* 1984;105:778–780.

STRABISMUS

Motor Anatomy and Physiology

- Ocular rotation

  Fick axes: X axis, horizontal; Y axis, anteroposterior; Z axis, vertical

  Listing plane: defined by X and Z axes (equator of globe); contains all axes about which rotation to redirect gaze occurs.
- Anatomy of extraocular muscles is diagrammed in Figure 8.28 and described in Table 8.22.
- Increasing distance of rectus muscle insertions from the limbus (MR closest, SR furthest) defines the "spiral of Tillaux".
- Action of extraocular muscles from primary position, and test positions, are summarized in Table 8.23.
- *Yoke muscles* (pairs of muscles that move the eyes in a direction of gaze):

  Eyes right: right LR and left MR.

  Eyes up in right gaze: right SR and left IO.

  Eyes up in left gaze: left SR and right IO.

  Eyes left: left LR and right MR.

  Eyes down in left gaze: left IR and right SO.

Table 8.22

Structure of extraocular muscles

Muscle	Overall/tendon length (mm)	Insertion distance from limbus (mm)	Angle (degrees) with sagittal plane
Medial rectus	38/3	5	
Lateral rectus	36/7	7	
Inferior rectus	37/5	6	23
Superior rectus	37/5	8	23
Inferior oblique	37/2	17–20	57
Superior oblique	60/20	14–18	57

Eyes down in right gaze: right IR and left SO.

- *Hering's Law*: Innervation flows equally and simultaneously to synergistic (yoke) muscles during conjugate gaze. For example, in left gaze, there is equal innervation to the right medial rectus and the left lateral rectus.
  - Accounts for the increase in strabismic deviation caused by a paretic muscle when the paretic eye assumes straight-ahead viewing position (secondary deviation), compared with that seen when the normal eye occupies this position (primary deviation).
  - A high level innervation must go to the week muscle to generate force sufficient to center its eye. The same innervation going to the intact yoke of the sound eye pulls that eye far from the center.
  - Similar considerations apply in strabismus due to a single muscle with restrictive change (abnormal tightness). Centering the restrited eye requires a high level of innervation to the antagonist of the tight muscle, which also goes to the yoke of the antagonist, which pulls the other eye way out of alignment.
- *Sherrington's Law:* Increased innervation of an extraocular muscle is accompanied by decreased innervation of its antagonist. For example, in left gaze, the left lateral rectus (agonist) is stimulated and the left medial rectus (antagonist) is inhibited.

Normal and Abnormal Binocular Vision

Binocular Fusion

- *Sensory fusion:* Unification of similar visual input from the two eyes into a single visual perception.
- *Motor fusion:* Ability to align the eyes (by means of vergence movement, in which the two eyes rotate in opposite directions) so that sensory fusion can be maintained or recovered. Normal fusional convergence amplitude is 40 prism diopters or more; divergence less, vertical very small.
- *Stereopsis:* The relative ordering in depth which occurs when objects at different distances stimulate retinal elements in the two eyes of slightly differing horizontal disparity.

Table 8.23

Function of extraocular muscles

Muscle	Primary action in primary position	Secondary and tertiary actions in primary position	Test position
Medial rectus	Adduction		Adduction
Lateral rectus	Abduction		Abduction
Inferior rectus	Depression	Excyclorotation Adduction	Depression with ABduction
Superior rectus	Elevation	Incyclorotation Adduction	Elevation with ABduction
Inferior oblique	Elevation	Excyclorotation Abduction	Elevation with ADduction
Superior oblique	Depression	Incyclorotation Abduction	Depression with ADduction

Ab, away from the midline; Ad, toward the midline; Excyclo, 12:00 meridian tilts away from the midline; Incyclo, 12:00 meridian tilts toward the midline.

Normal *stereoacuity* (minimum disparity that allows depth discrimination) is 15- to 30-arc seconds.

A form of "hyperacuity": 20/20 visual acuity discriminates at a level of only 60 seconds. *Vernier acuity*—the ability to detect offset in edges—is similarly hyperacute.

- *Rivalry:* Alternating perception when highly dissimilar (and therefore not fusible) images are presented to corresponding retinal areas near the foveas.

Strabismic Binocularity

- *Confusion:* Simultaneous perception of two different images in the same visual direction, as a result of projection on corresponding retinal areas (such as the two foveas) in misaligned eyes.
- *Diplopia:* Double vision produced when images of the same object are projected on noncorresponding retinal areas in misaligned eyes.
- *Suppression:* An adaptation to ocular misalignment that eliminates diplopia by excluding input of the deviating eye from conscious perception.
  - A facultative scotoma occupies part or all of the visual field in the deviating eye that overlaps the fixating eye.
  - Input from the deviating eye may remain accessible to sensorimotor centers to guide motor fusional movements.
  - The scotoma disappears when the originally fixating eye is occluded and the originally deviating eye takes up fixation, or when fusion is reestablished.
- *Anomalous retinal correspondence (ARC):* An adaptation to ocular misalignment that eliminates diplopia *without* excluding input of the deviating eye from conscious perception.
  - During binocular viewing with ARC (but reverting to normal with monocular viewing), the two foveas have different subjective visual directions.
  - ARC is "harmonious" when the angle of anomaly (subjective sensory angle between the two foveas) equals the angle of the strabismic deviation.
  - ARC does not produce a scotoma, but "fusion" based on ARC does not support stereopsis or stabilize alignment, and provides no significant functional advantage over suppression.
- Suppression and ARC frequently occur simultaneously in different parts of the visual field. One or both mechanisms prevent diplopia in the great majority of patients with childhood-onset strabismus, and in a minority with apparent onset in visual maturity (after about age 10 years).
  - Even after years of suppression and/or ARC, patients with alternating fixation retain normal vision in each eye, and those with intermittent strabismus are still able to fuse normally when alignment is recovered.
  - It is not unusual for suppression/ARC to fail at times, resulting in diplopia awareness. This may occur after a change in strabismus angle, during a period of stress or fatigue, or for no apparent reason.

Monofixation Syndrome (Subnormal Binocular Vision)

- Definition: A defective form of binocular vision in which there is absence of central fusion with preservation of "normal" peripheral fusion.
- Clinical demonstration of absent central fusion
  - Small (3 to 5 degrees) facultative central scotoma in nonfixating eye, detected by testing with *Worth 4-dot lights* or *Bagolini lenses*. As in suppression, the scotoma disappears when fixation shifts to the originally nonfixating eye.
  - *Microtropia* (constant deviation of 10 prism diopters or less) without diplopia during binocular viewing, detected by cover test to the fixating eye.
- Clinical demonstration of preserved peripheral fusion ("looser" than fully normal *bifixational* fusion)
  - Subnormal stereoacuity (60 to 3,000 seconds of arc).
  - Latent deviation detected by alternate cover testing. Alignment returns to microtropia when binocular viewing is reestablished.
- Frequently but not always associated with mild to moderate amblyopia. When no amblyopia, scotoma may alternate from eye to eye with fixation switches.
- Monofixation syndrome is a common sensory outcome when alignment is restored after a period of constant strabismus during infancy or childhood, more desirable than complete lack of useful binocularity, but less desirable than normal binocular function.

Reference

Greenwald MJ, Coates CM. Normal and abnormal binocular vision. *Ophthalmol Clin North Am* 1990;3:303–324.

Amblyopia

Definition

Amblyopia is an acquired defect in monocular vision caused by abnormal visual experience early in life. Amblyopia is NOT a defense against diplopia: Suppression eliminates diplopia without harm to monocular vision, and individuals with profound amblyopia may still experience diplopia in certain circumstances.

Classification

- *Strabismic:* Caused by constant nonalternating deviation, most often esotropia. Characterized by relative preservation of function at low light levels, disproportionate reduction of vernier acuity, and frequently monocular fixation with an eccentric (nonfoveolar, usually nasal) retinal locus. *Haidinger brush* or *Maxwell spot entoptic phenomena*, or *visuscopy* with direct ophthalmoscope (patient directs fixation to small circle projected on the retina) may reveal subtle degrees of eccentric fixation.

- *Anisometropic:* Unequal refractive errors. Most amenable to therapy.
- *Visual deprivation:* Congenital cataract, corneal opacity, vitreous hemorrhage. Most profound and most difficult to reverse.
- *Bilateral amblyopia* may result from bilateral deprivation (often severe vision loss) or high ametropia (usually mild vision loss). Usually hyperopia of 8 diopters or more, or astigmatism of 4 diopters or more; astigmatic ("meridional") amblyopia primarily reduces discrimination along axis of maximum defocus.

Detection and Monitoring

Assumes refractive error insignificant, corrected, or equal right and left; no physical defect causing poor vision.

- *Binocular fixation pattern:* Suspect amblyopia in a patient with constant strabismus if fixation in the deviating eye is "not maintained," that is, reverts to preferred eye immediately after removal of occluder forcing shift to the deviating eye.
- *Induced tropia test* (for patient without strabismus): 10- to 20-diopter prism is placed before either eye; if a refixation saccade is consistently observed only when prism in front of right eye, or only in front of left eye, other eye may be amblyopic.
- Visual acuity difference (two lines or more is usual criterion). Use *Lea symbols* (circle, square, "apple," "house"), HOTV letters, tumbling E, or pictures (in descending order of reliability) for preliterate children. Discrimination may be poorer for, and should be tested with, linear presentation of symbols or interactive bars around isolated symbols, *if and only if mild strabismic amblyopia is suspected* ("crowding phenomenon").
- *Teller cards* permit measurement of visual acuity in infants by determining the narrowest width of black-and-white stripes ("gratings") the baby can distinguish from a gray background. Very helpful in monitoring visual rehabilitation postcataract surgery but may underestimate the degree of strabismic amblyopia.

Treatment and Management

- *Occlusion therapy*
  Adhesive patch applied to skin over the nonamblyopic eye. Skin irritation or inadequate adherence may benefit from painting skin with tincture of benzoin before application.
  Fabric patch or occlusive foil applied to spectacle lens; must be monitored closely to avoid "peeking."
- Part-time versus full-time patching
  Full-time patching puts the patient at risk for developing occlusion-induced amblyopia in the good eye, or strabismus, and requires monitoring at intervals of 1 week (in infant) to 1 month.
  Two hours per day is sufficient for most mild-moderate amblyopia; 40 hours per week nearly as effective as full time.
- *Penalization*
  Use atropine 1% in better eye to blur the image for near; withdrawal of plus spectacle correction adds blur for distance.
  One drop on 2 to 3 successive days per week is usually sufficient.
- Both atropine and patching are effective treatments for moderate amblyopia (20/40 to 20/80) in children 3 to 6 years old; sometimes effective for older children (especially with anisometropic amblyopia).
  Patching has advantage of more rapid improvement than atropine. However, results equalize after 6 months of treatment for moderate amblyopia.
  Atropine has advantage of easier administration and lower cost.
- Consider stopping treatment if no initial improvement after 2 months (with adequate compliance), or no continuing improvement after 6 months. Maintenance therapy (1 to 2 hours per day patching or 1 to 2 days per week atropine, until age 9 to 10 years) may be necessary to prevent recurrence in up to ½ of patients.
- Nearly half of adult amblyopes experience improvement in amblyopic vision (seldom to normal) following complete loss of vision in the good eye.
- Even in preschool children, some amblyopia, with acuity as good as 20/40, is highly resistant to treatment.
  If expected improvement does not occur with treatment, carefully recheck refraction, fundus examination for subtle optic nerve malformation.
  If acuity decreases during treatment for amblyopia, carefully inspect fundus for optic atrophy and consider neuroimaging.

References

Greenwald MJ, Parks MM. Amblyopia. In: Tasman W, Jaeger EA, eds. *Duane's Clinical Ophthalmology*, vol 1, ch 10, Philadelphia, PA: Lippincott Williams & Wilkins, 2002.

Pediatric Eye Disease Investigator Group. A randomized trial of atropine versus patching for treatment of moderate amblyopia in children. *Arch Ophthalmol* 2002;120:260–278.

Sensorimotor Evaluation

History

- Age ocular deviation first noted; circumstances (recent trauma, illness)?
- Does the deviation appear constant? If so, was it previously intermittent? Until when? Do eyes occasionally straighten, even momentarily?
- If intermittent, approximate time percentage eyes appear straight; trend over past months, years?
- Strictly unilateral deviation or alternating fixation? Which eye preferred?

- Usual direction (in, out, up) of deviation? Other directions observed?
- Variability, aggravating factors (gaze direction, fatigue)?
- Is there a preferred head posture?
- Does there appear to be a problem with vision?
- Is diplopia present? How much of the time, what circumstances?
- Family history of strabismus (close relatives)?
- Prior treatment with occlusion, glasses (compliance?); surgery.
- Difficulty with work, school, recreational activities? Specific tasks?

Screening for Strabismus

- *Cover test for heterotropia* (constant deviation): With visual attention directed toward a small target, an opaque occluder is used to cover one eye. The uncovered eye is observed for rapid *saccadic refixation* movement outward (*esotropia*, ET), inward (*exotropia*, XT), downward (*hypertropia* of uncovered eye, RHT or LHT), upward (*hypotropia* of uncovered eye, RHoT or LHoT). If no movement, test is repeated for the opposite eye.
- *Cover/uncover test* for *heterophoria* (latent or controlled deviation): An occluder is used to cover one eye. The cover is then removed and the uncovered eye is observed. Slow *vergence* movement of the eye to realign indicates that a latent deviation is present.
- Deviation that is *only* evident following dissociation of the two eyes in such manner is termed a *phoria* and designated, for example, as X or XP. Deviation that is sometimes but not always manifest during binocular viewing is described as *intermittent tropia* and designated, for example, as X(T). Lack of any movement on cover/uncover test (or alternate cover test—see below), in the presence of normal monocular fixation with each eye, is *orthophoria*, sometimes designated EX.

Quantification of Deviation

- Measure deviation in *primary gaze* (straight ahead viewing) for distance and near. (Near measurement is designated with a "prime" symbol—not an apostrophe—at the end of the description, e.g., ET′.) Measure with corrective lenses (and without if patient is hyperopic); with and without bifocal (or +3.00 trial lenses) for near if *esodeviation* (excessive convergence) is present; in *secondary gaze* positions (right, left, up, down) to determine if deviation is *comitant* (magnitude same in all gazes) or *incomitant* (shows consistent variation with gaze); in right and left head tilt if vertical deviation is present.
- *Hirschberg test*

  Technique: Reflection (reflex) of light from both corneas is observed while the patient views a small bright light source positioned near the bridge of the examiner's nose. The position of the reflex from the deviating eye in relation to the center of the cornea (which would normally be symmetric to the reflection from the fixating eye) estimates deviation. One millimeter of decentration equals 7 to 8 degrees or 15 prism diopters. Reflex at the pupil margin typically indicates a deviation of about 30 prism diopters.

  Advantages: Rapid estimation of deviation; does not require prolonged fixation by the patient.

  Disadvantages: Not very precise; does not account for abnormal angle kappa (difference between the eye's visual and optical axes).
- *Krimsky test*

  Technique: Corneal light reflexes are observed as in the Hirschberg test while prism is placed in front of the deviating eye (or fixating eye) to make the reflections from both eyes appear centered or symmetric.

  Advantages: More precise than Hirschberg; does not require central fixation by deviating eye.

  Disadvantages: Requires more cooperation than Hirschberg.
- *Prism alternate cover test*

  Technique: An occluder is used to alternately cover each eye, breaking down fusion, while the patient continuously views a small object. This dissociates the eyes and brings out the maximum deviation (including latent component). Prism of increasing power is placed in front of either eye until no refixation movement occurs (deviation is "neutralized").

  Advantages: Accurate and reliable; detects deviation as small as 2 prism diopters.

  Disadvantages: Requires central steady fixation in each eye, good cooperation.
- *Maddox rod test* (for vertical deviation)

  Technique: The eyes are dissociated by a vertically oriented (bars at 90 degrees) red Maddox rod disc in front of one eye. The patient views a small bright light source in a darkened room, and sees a horizontal red line and a white spot. If images are superimposed ("line touches light"), no vertical phoria or tropia is present. If images are separated, prism is added (base-down over the eye that sees the lower image) until they are superimposed.

  Advantages: Extremely sensitive; detects deviation as small as ½ prism diopter.

  Disadvantages: Requires central steady fixation in each eye, very good cooperation, no suppression or ARC. Less useful for horizontal deviation because accommodation not controlled.
- *Double Maddox rod test* (for cyclodeviation—eyes differently rotated in relation to Y-axis; not detectable with other tests): A red and a white Maddox rod disc are placed with bars oriented vertically (at 90 degrees), one in front of each eye. If necessary a low-power base-down prism is placed before one eye to separate the red and white lines viewed by the right and left eyes.

Rods are rotated until patient reports lines are parallel and level. Angle between final rod positions indicates total amount of cyclodeviation; less reliably the degree of cyclotorsion in each eye is estimated.

Estimation of Ocular Rotations

- Secondary gaze amplitudes are scored on a scale of 0 (normal) to 4-, as percentage of normal, by estimated degrees of rotation, or with the *Urist version test* (Figure 8.29).
- *Tertiary* (oblique or diagonal) *gaze* position vertical deviation is graded in terms of corresponding oblique muscle overaction or underaction, +N to –N (N = mm difference between eyes in level of top or bottom of limbus).
  Up-left: RIO (right eye higher by 4 mm = 4+)
  Down-left: RSO (right eye higher by 2 mm = 2–)
  Up-right: LIO (left eye lower by 3 mm = 3–)
  Down-right: LSO (left eye lower by 1 mm = 1+)

Binocular Sensory Testing

- Testing for a suppression scotoma with Worth lights or Bagolini lenses (p. 491), or for ARC with Bagolini lenses or *afterimage test*, is seldom clinically useful. A patient with manifest strabismus who is not experiencing diplopia can be assumed to have one of these adaptations, and it matters little which.
- *Testing for stereopsis should be part of complete evaluation of any patient who appears capable of fusion at any time*. Test in viewing circumstances (e.g., with plus or prism lenses, in preferred head position) that optimize alignment. Keep in mind that a patient with intermittent strabismus and normal stereoacuity when fusing, will demonstrate NO stereopsis when fusion is not occurring.
- *"Fly" test* (Stereo Optical Company; often erroneously called *Titmus*)
  Uses Polaroid viewing lenses, vectographic figures.
  Fly panel tests gross stereopsis, level as low as 3,000 seconds of arc. Normal observer perceives wing tips 4 to 5 cm in front of background; subnormal observer (monofixator) typically perceives at 1 to 3 cm. Tilting figure 45 degrees completely eliminates depth illusion; useful check on reliability.
  Circle and animal panels quantify stereoacuity from 800 to 40 seconds. When viewed through Polaroid lenses, monocular cues are confounding only for first and possibly second circle panels; NO monocular cues for animals. Stereodefective observer sees first circle in laterally displaced position.
- *Randot test*
  Also uses Polaroid vectographic image separation.
  Based on random dot stereogram technique developed by Julesz; more difficult for some normal observers.
  Tests to 20 seconds of arc.
- *TNO test* uses red-green anaglyphic figures with color separating lenses; some random dot stereograms.
- *Verhoeff stereopter* employs objects with actual physical depth.

Accommodative Esotropia

Summary

Accommodative esotropia is an acquired strabismic deviation that results from accommodative convergence in

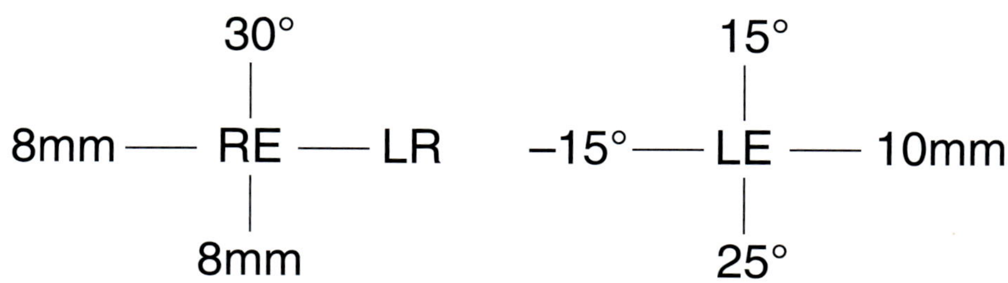

FIGURE 8.29. The Urist version reflex test quantifies rotation in secondary gaze directions with light reflex observations similar to those used in the Hirschberg assessment of strabismic deviation (p. 493). The diagram shows Urist measurements for a normal right eye (RE) and a left eye (LE) with incomplete oculomotor nerve palsy (p. 510). To perform the test, an examiner faces the patient holding a small bright light source just in front of the bridge of his own nose, directed toward the same point on the patient's face, and instructs the patient to look in each direction as far as possible with eye movement alone. In the illustrated case, normal RE abduction results in reflection of light from a point on nasal conjunctiva 8 mm posterior to the limbus; adduction, from the temporal "limbal region" (designated LR) with dual reflections from cornea and conjunctiva straddling the limbus; elevation, from cornea about 4 mm below its center (corresponding to the displacement produced by a 30 degree or 60 prism diopter vertical strabismus); depression, from conjunctiva 8 mm above the limbus. (Apparent nonequality of normal abduction and adduction measured in this manner is an artifact resulting from the light source not being directly in front of the observed eye; nonequality of elevation and depression reflects a true excess of downward rotation in the normal person.) Measurements for the paretic left eye indicate severely reduced adduction that falls short of the midline, with reflection from cornea 2 mm nasal to its center; moderately reduced elevation and depression; and slightly greater than normal abduction.

hyperopic eyes, and can be eliminated by corrective plus lenses.

Etiology

- A synkinetic relationship exists between accommodation and convergence.
- In some hyperopic children, maintaining accommodation required for sharp focus leads to excessive convergence and esotropia for both distant and near viewing.
- Some children generate more convergence than is usual, necessary or appropriate with each diopter of accommodation (*high accommodative-convergence-to-accommodation ratio*, or AC/A), which leads to esodeviation that is greater for near than for distant viewing.

Demographics

- Usual onset between 18 and 36 months but may present from 6 months to 8 years.
- Family history of strabismus is common.

Symptoms and Signs

- "Crossed" in-turning eye.
- Deviation often intermittent, especially early after time of onset.
- May be more evident when the child is ill or fatigued.
- Patient may complain of diplopia before development of suppression.

Ophthalmic Findings

- Esotropia, typically 20 to 40 prism diopters.
- Hyperopia, typically 4 to 6 diopters but sometimes less, especially with high AC/A.
- With full correction of hyperopia by plus lenses, esodeviation should be *eliminated*.
- In the absence of high AC/A (most cases), near deviation should NOT be substantially greater than distance deviation.
- Amblyopia is common when strabismus is constant, especially if there is significant anisometropia; the more hyperopic eye is nearly always the amblyopic eye.
- Normal acuity and stereopsis are typically preserved when strabismus is intermittent.
- Many children with hyperopia and esotropia show reduction of esodeviation (decreased angle or decreased frequency or both) but not complete restoration of alignment when accommodative convergence is eliminated with plus lenses. Such cases are usually referred to as partially accommodative, or having an accommodative component. Treatment often involves surgery as well as refractive correction.

Special Tests and Considerations

- Refraction with *cycloplegia* (pharmacologic suspension of accommodation) is essential for proper diagnosis. In most cases, use *1% cyclopentolate* drops, instilled one to two times, followed by 30- to 60-minute wait prior to refraction. In older children with darkly pigmented eyes, 2% cyclopentolate may provide better cycloplegia.
- Use of atropine for maximally complete cycloplegia is seldom required but should be considered when residual accommodation is detected after cyclopentolate, or when improvement with glasses is substantial but falls a bit short of restoring alignment. (Repeating refraction with cyclopentolate in the latter situation may also be helpful.) Parents instill atropine 1% at home for 3 days prior to examination, one to three times per day.
- Calculation of AC/A ratio (gradient method):
  - Measure deviation for near using accommodative target without correction, and with +3.00 lenses in trial frame; alternatively, measure deviation for distance with and without plus spectacles.
  - AC/A = (Deviation without lens – Deviation with lens)/ Power of lens.
  - Example: ET = 40 without correction, ET = 20 with +4 glasses, AC/A = 5.
  - Normal value of AC/A is 3 to 5. When AC/A equals the interpupillary distance in centimeters (typically about 5 for a child), near deviation should equal distance; AC/A > 5 implies near deviation > distance.
- In many children with esotropia who benefit from wearing plus lenses, near deviation exceeds distance despite normal AC/A as calculated above. This situation is more appropriately termed *convergence excess*, for which the physiologic basis is unknown. Bifocal lenses are sometimes but not always helpful (see below).
- Most children (and adults) with hyperopia, sometimes of impressive degree, do not show any evidence of accommodative esotropia. Many children with esotropia and hyperopia, sometimes of impressive degree, obtain little or no benefit from wearing plus lenses.

Disease Course

- Progression from intermittent to constant strabismus is common but not seen in all cases. Some patients develop A- or V-pattern with SO or IO overaction (p. 501). DVD and latent nystagmus are not associated with accommodative esotropia.
- Accommodative esotropia that initially responded well to treatment with glasses not uncommonly shows a progressively increasing nonaccommodative component that may lead to need for surgical treatment (see below).
- Hyperopia tends to decrease with age, but most children with accommodative esotropia that is well controlled with glasses alone continue to require or benefit from plus refractive correction through adolescence and adulthood. Some may be able to cultivate increased fusional ability with gradual reduction in lens power

("weaning from correction"), or learn to avoid accommodating when glasses are removed for social reasons. Others make a transition to contact lenses, but many prefer to remain in spectacle correction.

Treatment and Management

- Hyperopic glasses are the mainstay of treatment for accommodative esotropia. Prescription should be for the *full plus power determined with cycloplegia* if strabismus is *constant*. *Partial* correction of hyperopia is preferred by many clinicians for *intermittent* esotropia, which allows the patient to continue relying in part on good-quality motor fusion to maintain alignment.
- Bifocal lenses are appropriately used *to promote fusion for near viewing*, based on observation of near deviation reduced below 10 prism diopters, or significantly increased frequency of fusion for near, with additional plus power.
  AC/A-based calculations that predict near deviation less than 10 prism diopters with add also justify bifocal prescription, but *the mere presence of excess deviation for near does not.*
  Bifocal prescription should specify large flat-top or executive segments, with top of segment at pupil level, or slightly above the center of the lens.
  Most clinicians usually use an add power of +2.50 or +3.00, but lesser amounts may be sufficient, particularly when AC/A is high.
  Progressive lenses may be a good alternative for the older child with bifocal experience who effectively uses and benefits from conventional segments.
- Pharmacologic management
  Anticholinesterase drops (Phospholine Iodide [echothiophate] 0.06%) induce accommodation locally, eliminating or reducing the need for accommodative innervation, and thereby reducing the stimulus for convergence. There may also be some reduction of the AC/A ratio. Because of side effects, notably formation of iris sphincter cysts or nodules (which risk may be reduced by concurrent administration of phenylephrine drops), this approach is no longer very popular.
  Atropine drops may be used short term to block accommodation and improve acceptance of glasses. Abandonment of accommodative effort by the atropinized child sometimes allows the eyes to align even without glasses.
- Surgical management
  Surgery is indicated when there is unacceptable residual esodeviation with full plus correction. Surgery is NOT indicated for esodeviation that is adequately controlled with glasses.
  Traditionally, surgical dosage has been based on the measured nonaccommodative component (in amounts the same as for fully nonaccommodative deviation of the same magnitude; recession of one medial recuts is often sufficient), with expectation of continued spectacle wear postoperatively. Some surgeons now increase surgical dosage slightly beyond the expected requirement for the nonaccommodative component in hope of reducing both the frequency of undercorrection and dependence on glasses postoperatively. Rates of overcorrection and consecutive exodeviation appear not to be much affected by this strategy.
  Preoperative *prism adaptation* is used by some surgeons as an aid to safely maximizing surgical dosage. (See references below.)
- Amblyopia management must be done concurrently with strabismus treatment, usually with requirement for occlusion or atropinization, although some improvement may follow restoration of fusion with glasses alone. Spectacle corrected accommodative esotropia provides natural opportunity for use of spectacle-mounted occlusion devices, and for withdrawal of plus correction from the nonamblyopic eye to enhance the effect of atropine penalization.

References

Greenwald MJ, Eagle JR, Peters C, et al. Treatment of acquired esotropia: for augmented surgery. *Am Orthopt J* 1998;48:16–20.

Prism Adaptation Study Research Group. Efficacy of prism adaptation in the surgical management of acquired esotropia. *Arch Ophthalmol* 1990;108:1248–1256.

Essential (Infantile) Esotropia

Summary

Essential esotropia is convergent strabismus that is not attributable to accommodative convergence, or to any identifiable abnormality of extraocular muscles or their innervation. This term was advocated by von Noorden to replace the misleading designation *congenital esotropia*, as the condition is rarely present at birth, developing during the first year of life in most cases.

Etiology

Unknown.

Demographics

- Onset most often occurs between ages 2 and 6 months, but otherwise indistinguishable strabismus becomes evident in many children during the second year of life, or at later ages with decreasing frequency.
- Family history of strabismus is often present, but with no clear inheritance pattern. Most patients with this very common condition are the only affected member of their immediate family.

Symptoms and Signs

- Obviously inturned eye; typically alternating fixation.
- Often intermittent at onset; becomes constant in most but not all cases within weeks to months. Parents often volunteer or confirm that the eyes occasionally straighten momentarily even after years of nearly constant strabismus.

Ophthalmic Findings

- Large esodeviation is typical, usually 40 prism diopters or more, but smaller angles are not uncommon, especially in the early period after onset (Figure 8.30). Variable angle in many cases, sometimes increasing with fatigue (even when constant, i.e., never fusing).
- In most cases, either eye can be observed to maintain fixation, though often only with lateral gaze that keeps the eye in an adducted position ("cross-fixation"). When the same eye retains fixation regardless of gaze direction, and deviation is constant, amblyopia typically develops.
- Resistance to abduction may be striking, mimicking sixth nerve palsy. Can usually but not always be elicited by vestibulo-ocular reflex stimulation (VOR; "doll's head maneuver") or after a period of monocular occlusion.
- Near deviation is frequently greater than distance, but AC/A ratio calculated by gradient method (p. 495) is usually normal.
- Typically mild to moderate hyperopia.
- Asymmetric horizontal pursuit movement and optokinetic nystagmus are characteristic, with greater facility in nasalward direction for the fixating eye.
- Motor findings that frequently develop later include oblique muscle overaction (usually inferior, with V-pattern—p. 50[illegible]), DVD (p. 503), and latent nystagmus (p. 488). May first be noted years after successful treatment of esodeviation.

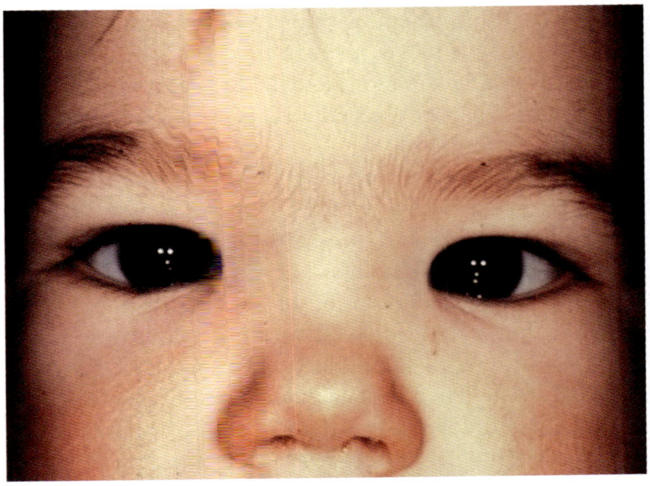

FIGURE 8.30. Infantile-onset essential esotropia, with small-moderate angle deviation of left eye. Note also the confounding presence of pseudoesotropia caused by conspicuous epicanthal folds.

Systemic Findings

Infants with neurologic deficits, notably *cerebral palsy*, and with many multisystem syndromes, often develop strabismus indistinguishable from essential esotropia, though variability of deviation tends to be greater. In particular, hydrocephalus (p. 473) is often associated with what appears to be nonparalytic esotropia, worsening when the condition is exacerbated by ventriculoperitoneal shunt malfunction. Management in such cases is generally the same as for isolated essential esotropia of similar appearance. Surgery is appropriate once consistency over time has been confirmed, though outcome is considered less predictable and less stable.

Disease Course

- Without treatment, angle of deviation tends to increase during infancy and to decrease after infancy. Rarely spontaneous resolution may occur.
- In the minority of cases that remain intermittent, binocular function often remains intact.
- Prolonged persistence of early-onset constant strabismus may result in complete loss of binocular fusion ability, though patients who recover alignment in late childhood or even adulthood sometimes show surprisingly good stereoscopic vision, presumably because intermittency was present, unrecognized, until a relatively advanced age.
- Elimination of esodeviation at any age results in expansion of the peripheral binocular field of vision, assuming the peripheral monocular field of the deviating eye is intact (true even in most cases with profound amblyopia).

Treatment and Management

- Treatment of amblyopia, if present, is the first priority, usually with part-time occlusion in infancy.
- Glasses for hyperopia are frequently helpful and indicated.
  - Consider correction of hyperopia greater than +1.00 for any *intermittent* deviation (may increase frequency of fusion considerably even if little reduction in angle).
  - For constant esotropia, prescribe glasses if anticipated effect (calculated based on assumption of AC/A = 5) might eliminate or reduce need for surgery. Example: +3.00 glasses might reduce angle from 45 to 30 prism diopters (3 D × 5 pd/D = 15 pd), changing surgical dose for most surgeons.
- Surgical treatment is usually required.
  - It is well established that restoration of ocular alignment in patients with infantile onset of constant esotropia should be accomplished by age 2 years in order to recover binocular fusion in most cases. Recent studies have confirmed the value of surgery even before age 6 months if stable constant large angle esotropia is present. With later onset of constant deviation,

PEDIATRIC

alignment should be restored within a few months if possible.

Initial surgery in most cases is bilateral medial rectus muscle recession. Dosage formula varies among surgeons. The author bases surgical amounts on near deviation with correction, recessing both MR 5 mm for ET measuring 30 to 35 prism diopters, 6 mm for 40 to 50, 7 mm for 60 or more.

Some surgeons include resection of one or both lateral rectus muscles in the initial procedure for very large angles, while others prefer to reserve lateral rectus resection for a second operation if needed. Unilateral recess-resect surgery, once the most widely used approach, is still sometimes employed for early-onset esotropia, especially when vision is irreversibly reduced in one eye.

- Outcome of surgery

  Satisfactory outcome is achieved in a large majority (80% to 90% or more) of cases with initial surgery for essential infantile esotropia.

  Early postoperative alignment after medial rectus recession surgery is often obviously divergent. By the time of final postoperative assessment 6 to 8 weeks out, persistent exotropia (at this point appropriately described as *surgical overcorrection*) is seen in only a small minority of cases. Divergent strabismus that develops more than 2 months after surgery for esotropia is termed *consecutive exotropia*; this becomes increasingly common with further passage of time.

  Intermittent strabismus with reduced angle and frequent fusion (typically with subnormal binocularity and microesotropia—p. 491) may be considered a satisfactory surgical outcome, which is likely to prevent further deterioration of binocular function. Further surgery for residual intermittent esodeviation may be delayed for years, until it becomes clear that the patient needs better alignment, or the situation deteriorates again to constant strabismus. Over time, it is also possible that alignment will spontaneously improve.

  Up to 50% of children operated on in infancy for essential esotropia will need a second surgical procedure (for residual or recurrent esotropia, consecutive exotropia, or DVD) sometime later in life, even if the outcome of initial treatment is good to excellent.

- Botulinum toxin injection into one or both medial rectus muscles may provide lasting benefit in infantile esotropia, but anticipation of transitory effect in most cases limits usefulness.

Differential Diagnosis

- Accommodative esotropia (p. 494) may present during infancy; complete response to treatment with high plus lenses differentiates.
- Monocular or binocular sensory deprivation in infancy or early childhood (e.g., from cataract, coloboma, RB) may cause strabismus motorically indistinguishable from essential esotropia. Sensory exodeviation occurs less commonly in childhood but typically develops after severe monocular vision loss in older individuals.
- Bilateral abducens palsy (p. 510) may be suspected when abduction cannot be elicited by above-described maneuvers. Recovery of normal abduction after medial rectus recession surgery confirms the diagnosis of essential esotropia. Muscle transposition should never be performed as a primary procedure in infancy.
- Bilateral Duane syndrome (p. 508) may be difficult to distinguish from essential esotropia in infancy. Typically shows marked ABduction deficits out of proportion to relatively small angle esodeviation, with subnormal ADduction.
- *Moebius syndrome* is often characterized as bilateral sixth and seventh nerve palsies, but the primary motility defect is paralysis of horizontal gaze due to failure of the pontine lateral gaze centers to develop.

  Convergence usually remains intact; may be used to help redirect the fixating eye. Typically presents as total abduction deficit with or without variable/intermittent esotropia; constant large-angle deviation suggestive of true bilateral sixth nerve palsies is seen in some cases.

  Associated partial or complete bilateral facial nerve palsy (which may lead to exposure keratopathy in later life) is often overlooked in infancy. Other associated findings include underdeveloped tongue, poor sucking ability, and extremity abnormalities including clubfoot, fused or absent digits, maldeveloped pectoralis muscle (Poland anomaly).

  Surgical treatment is often indicated. Very large recessions of both medical rectus muscles may be necessary.

- *Nystagmus blockage syndrome* refers to large-angle esotropia, often intermittent, with increasing nystagmus when the fixating eye moves away from adduction. Once considered an indication for medial rectus posterior fixation suture (p. 511); now usually treated the same as essential esotropia.
- *Arnold-Chiari type 1 malformation* of the lower brain may be associated with a variety of motility disturbances, including comitant esotropia, often intermittent, typically onset in late childhood or adolescence, sometimes as the earliest manifestation of the condition. Presence of associated vertical nystagmus, typically *downbeating*, is diagnostic. MRI should be done in suspicious circumstances (e.g., when associated occipital headaches).
- Comitant esodeviation, intermittent or constant, with or without diplopia, closely resembling early-onset essential esotropia, may develop in otherwise asymptomatic and healthy young to middle-aged adults with no prior strabismus history (sometimes family history of typical childhood strabismus). Moderate *myopia* often

present. Especially if near deviation exceeds distance, neuroimaging is probably unnecessary. Typically excellent response to bilateral medial rectus recession, with recovery of good stereopsis.

- Older adults may present with comitant small-angle esodeviation and diplopia, greater for distance than near. Neuroimaging is justified in view of the differential diagnosis of sixth nerve palsy in this age group but is normal in the great majority of cases. Recession of one medial rectus muscle usually provides relief if prism management is inadequate.

References

Greenwald MJ. Surgical management of essential esotropia. *Ophthalmol Clin North Am* 1992;5:9–23.

Miller MT, Ray V, Owens P, et al. Möbius and Möbius-like syndromes. *J Pediatr Ophthalmol Strabismus* 1989;26:176–188.

Pediatric Eye Disease Investigator Group. Spontaneous resolution of early-onset esotropia: experience of the Congenital Esotropia Observational Study. *Am J Ophthalmol* 2002;133:109–118.

Comitant Exodeviation

Summary

Any divergent misalignment of the visual axes is an exodeviation. The deviation may be kept latent by fusion (exophoria), may be intermittently manifest (intermittent exotropia) or present at all times (constant exotropia). The great majority of cases cannot be attributed to any identifiable disorder involving the orbits or CNS.

Symptoms and Signs

- Exophoria usually asymptomatic; may cause asthenopia (eyestrain) or occasional diplopia.
- Intermittent exotropia usually first evident as occasional momentary eye wandering before age 2 years, worse with fatigue (Figure 8.31).

  Symptoms of intermittent exotropia include asthenopia from effort required to maintain fusion, intermittent diplopia (typically present much less of the time than manifest strabismus, resulting from occasional failure of suppression), losing place when reading (due to unconscious fixation shift from one eye to the other), unilateral eyelid closure in bright surroundings (specific cause unknown), and clumsiness or visual discomfort resulting from stereoscopic depth perception turning on and off.

  Surprisingly, most individuals with intermittent exotropia do not notice abrupt and dramatic changes in binocular sensory status, and many claim to lack subjective awareness of eye position.

  The most common reason by far for seeking treatment is concern about appearance, which may represent a major social handicap.
- Constant exotropia can develop at any age beginning in infancy; symptoms other than concern about appearance are seldom bothersome.

Ophthalmic Findings

- Typically greater deviation with distant viewing ("divergence excess"); often deviation in both lateral gaze directions is smaller than primary gaze measurement.
- Suppression develops readily, even with infrequent intermittent deviation.
- Usually normal stereoacuity with intermittent exotropia.
- Amblyopia uncommon, generally only in association with early-onset constant tropia.

Systemic Findings

Comitant exotropia is less often associated with neurologic deficits and multisystem disorders than esotropia, but is nevertheless quite common in such situations; may be constant or intermittent. Conditions as diverse as Crouzon syndrome (p. 427), Riley-Day syndrome (Table 8.3), and Marfan syndrome (p. 444) are particularly linked to exodeviation.

Special Tests

- Prolonged occlusion: Covering one eye for 30 to 60 minutes dissociates the eyes more completely than standard

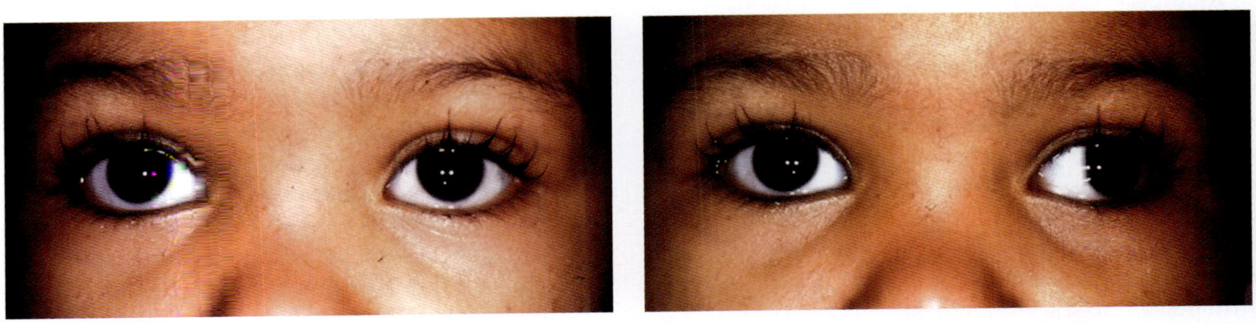

A B

FIGURE 8.31. Intermittent left exotropia. **A:** During binocular fusion, with normal stereoacuity. **B:** During manifest deviation, with absent stereopsis.

alternate cover testing; may cause near deviation to increase to match distance measurement ("simulated divergence excess").

- Suspending accommodation with +3.00 lenses for near viewing may also result in increased near measurement.
- Remote viewing: Measuring deviation while patient views a distant target (preferably out a window) helps determine maximum angle for surgical dosage.
- Office prism adaptation: Patient views through base-in prism matching initially measured distance deviation for up to 60 minutes; prism power increased to match increased deviation until stable maximum reached. Allows determination of maximum angle for surgical dosage; may reduce risk of both under- and over-correction.

Disease Course

- True exophoria (manifest deviation never visible, generally measuring <10 prism diopters) usually remains stable and asymptomatic.
- Intermittent exotropia, especially if small angle (<20 prism diopters), often shows spontaneous improvement during childhood; otherwise, typically remains stable for many years or even decades.
- Some intermittent exodeviations show progressively increasing angle and frequency, with tendency for near deviation to increase toward or beyond distance measurement.
- Deviations that approach constancy in childhood may cause damage to binocularity (monofixation syndrome) and amblyopia, but those that progress similarly in adulthood (often not until middle age) generally cause no lasting harm and permit recovery of normal stereoacuity.

Treatment and Management

- Occlusion for amblyopia when indicated in constant exotropia. Rarely necessary with intermittent exotropia, even when deviation is strictly unilateral. Part-time occlusion as an antisuppression measure is of questionable value. There is little evidence that diplopia awareness actually promotes motor fusion, which functions very effectively in most cases of intermittent exotropia despite consistent suppression during tropic periods.
- Minus lenses (up to –3.00) stimulate accommodation, leading to convergence that may improve control of intermittent exotropia, or reduce asthenopia by substituting accommodative effort for fusional effort. Base-in prism may help relieve asthenopic symptoms if surgical treatment is considered inappropriate.
- Orthoptic exercises are often helpful for convergence insufficiency (p. 502) but usually not indicated for other forms of exodeviation.
- Surgical treatment is indicated in nearly all cases of constant exotropia (after treatment of amblyopia, if needed, has been completed) and is the preferred treatment for most cases of intermittent exotropia that cause bothersome symptoms.
  - Initial surgical treatment usually involves recession of one or both lateral rectus muscles, resection of one or both medial rectus muscles, or a unilateral recession/resection combination.
  - Preferences vary widely among individual surgeons, with only a minority continuing to make choices based primarily on traditional categories defined by distance-near relationships.
- Postoperative diplopia is commonly experienced by exotropes rendered esotropic after surgery, regardless of age, because they lack the ability to suppress (or to fuse) in that condition. (Exceptions, most of whom have a history of past esodeviation, can be identified preoperatively by demonstrating lack of diplopia recognition when viewing through base-in prism power exceeding the magnitude of their deviation.)
  - Especially following bilateral LR recessions for intermittent exotropia, a period of esodeviation (up to 20 prism diopters or more) lasting days to weeks is typically experienced before alignment stabilizes appropriately, associated initially with near-constant diplopia awareness. Many surgeons view this transitional period as having a desirable antisuppression effect, but patients should be warned preoperatively. With recovery of tone in the operated muscles, alignment improves to allow fusion, first for near viewing, and last for lateral gaze. Complete recovery occasionally takes several months, and lasting overcorrection occurs in a small minority, often requiring treatment with prism lenses or additional surgery for esotropia.
  - Some overcorrected intermittent exotropes, especially younger children, develop suppression for esotropia within a short time, but these patients are at risk of losing high-grade binocularity and becoming amblyopic if allowed to remain constantly esodeviated, and should be "rescued" with prism within a few weeks, even if the angle of esotropia is small.
  - Some adults with longstanding constant exotropia, especially those whose strabismus began as esotropia in early life (including some with significant amblyopia), who totally lack fusion ability, may after surgury cease to suppress and suffer from diplopia that persists regardless of ocular alignment status. Fortunately, most such patients eventually start to suppress again, over time ranging from hours to months, typically days to weeks. A small minority continue to experience double vision indefinitely, though with time its obtrusiveness tends to diminish. There is no known effective treatment other than occluding one eye. This possibility should be discussed preoperatively with every adult patient who recognizes a

second image when viewing through prism of any power (especially if less than the magnitude of preoperative deviation), though it seldom justifies avoiding surgery altogether when motivation is appropriate.

- Recurrent exotropia of some degree develops over time (typically years) in a fairly large percentage of surgically treated patients, but further surgery is required for only a small minority (even in occasional cases where the angle of deviation ultimately returns to preoperative magnitude), owing to persistent reduced frequency of manifest deviation.
- Exotropia in adults and adolescents, especially if the angle is large or there was previous muscle surgery, is treated by many surgeons with the aid of lateral rectus muscle *adjustable suture*.

  When surgery comprises only lateral rectus recession, it is customary to adjust to small esodeviation, even though this leaves the patient diplopic, because of anticipated exo drift during early postoperative weeks.

  Alignment after LR recession combined with MR resection tends to be more stable, and therefore this procedure lends itself particularly to adjustable technique. The opportunity it provides to achieve single vision by adjustment in most cases is reassuring to patients concerned about the possibility of diplopia.

Differential Diagnosis

- Exotropia not uncommonly develops in patients with a history of esotropia, typically following an extended period (months to many years) during with the eyes appeared well aligned. Consecutive exodeviation is often initially intermittent, usually becoming constant over time. Some cases are identifiable as dissociated horizontal deviations (p. 503). Distinguishing from primary exotropia in the absence of reliable history (or evidence of previous medial rectus recession on inspection of the nasal ocular surface) may not be possible. In contrast to those with primary comitant exodeviations, such patients typically lack potential for high-grade binocular vision, and amblyopia is common, probably both consequences of constant esotropia early in life.
- Third-nerve palsy (p. 510), especially when complete and unilateral, usually can be easily distinguished from comitant exotropia by disturbance of vertical motility, incomitance of horizontal deviation, and presence of ptosis and pupil mydriasis. Incomplete congenital third-nerve palsy (often lacking obvious lid or pupil involvement) may create confusion; this possibility should be considered when exodeviation presents in early infancy.
- Duane syndrome Type 2 (p. 508) causes exodeviation in primary gaze, and especially if bilateral may mimic comitant exotropia. Should also be considered in the differential diagnosis of infantile-onset exodeviation. Distinguishing features including leash effect and globe retraction are not always evident.
- It is not rare for comitant exotropia to present with nearly constant large-angle deviation in middle-aged or older adults. In such cases, however, consideration should be given to the possibilities of myasthenia gravis (exotropia is the most frequent associated strabismus—p. 512) and WEBINO syndrome (wall-eyed bilateral internuclear ophthalmoplegia), with referral for neuro-ophthalmologic evaluation if indicated.

References

Baker JD. Twenty-year follow-up of surgery for intermittent exotropia. *J AAPOS* 2008;12:227–232.

Hiles DA, Davies GT, Costenbader FD. Long-term observation of unoperated intermittent exotropia. *Arch Ophthalmol* 1968;80:436–442.

A and V Patterns

Summary

The terms A- and V- pattern apply to strabismus in which horizontal deviation magnitude changes with upgaze and downgaze. A clinically significant A-pattern has vertical incomitance of at least 10 prism diopters with relative convergence in upgaze, and a clinically significant V-pattern has vertical incomitance of 15 prism diopters or more with relative convergence in downgaze.

Symptoms and Signs

- Strabismus may be observed or cause symptoms only in the upgaze or the downgaze position that maximizes deviation, while fusion occurs elsewhere.
- Horizontal strabismus with A- or V-pattern may result in a compensatory head posture that facilitates fusion by maintaining gaze in the position of least deviation. This is a reassuring observation that implies intermittency of strabismus, with minimal threat to vision. A child's abandonment of chin-up or chin-down posture should raise concern about deteriorating alignment and sensory status (with risk of losing stereoacuity and developing amblyopia), and lead to consideration of prompt surgical treatment.

Ophthalmic Findings

- The great majority of patients with A- or V-pattern have horizontal strabismus that may be classified as essential esotropia or "comitant" exotropia; deviation may be constant or intermittent.
- V-pattern is often but not always associated with bilateral inferior oblique overaction (hypertropia of the adducting eye in gaze up and to the side), and variable degree (usually but not always lesser) of bilateral superior oblique underaction.
- A-pattern is often but not always associated with bilateral superior oblique overaction (hypotropia of the adducting eye in gaze down and to the side), and variable

degree (usually but not always lesser) of bilateral inferior oblique underaction.
- Medial rectus overaction in esotropia may be associated with a small V-pattern in downgaze, which is usually eliminated by medial rectus recession.
- V-pattern with IO overaction is more common in children; A-pattern with SO overaction is seen more often in adults with horizontal strabismus.
- Fundus examination often shows evidence of excyclorotation with IO overaction and incyclorotation with SO overaction. In the indirect ophthalmoscopic view, appearance of the fovea above the upper (actually below the lower) pole of the disc indicates excyclo; fovea below (actually above) the center of the disc indicates incyclo.
- Mongoloid slant (p. 425) of the palpebral fissures is associated with A-pattern; antimongoloid slant (p. 427) with V-pattern.

Systemic Findings

- Neurologic conditions associated with A-pattern esotropia include hydrocephalus (p. 473), Arnold-Chiari malformation (look for downbeating nystagmus—p. 498), and posterior fossa masses.
- Craniosynostosis associated with excyclo tilting of the orbits, specifically Crouzon syndrome and its variants (p. 427), produces very striking V-pattern and IO overaction that are difficult to correct surgically. Congenital absence of one or both superior rectus muscles (leaving IO as the sole elevator) may contribute to this situation.

Treatment and Management

- Every horizontal deviation should be measured or at least observed in both upgaze (25 degrees) and downgaze (25 degrees) prior to surgical treatment. In a child with limited ability to cooperate, this can be quickly done by maintaining fixation on a near object while using a hand to tilt the head back into chin-up posture, then forward into chin-down posture, and watching for relative convergence or divergence.
- If no significant oblique muscle dysfunction is noted, A- or V-pattern may be reduced by transposing horizontal muscles vertically, usually by ½ tendon width, to shift the effect of surgery toward the direction of greater deviation.
  Whether surgery is for exotropia or esotropia, and whether recession or resection is planned, medial rectus muscles are moved toward the apex or point of the A or V, and lateral rectus muscles are moved toward the wide part. (Mnemonic: M for medial has multiple points.)
  Example: V-pattern esotropia is treated by recessing both medial rectus muscles and transposing the muscles downward, or by resecting both lateral rectus muscles and transposing the muscles upward.
  This approach typically reduces the pattern by 10 to 15 prism diopters.
- Surgery for V-pattern strabismus associated with significant inferior oblique overaction, particularly when the lateral rectus muscles are to be involved (permitting access to both muscles through a single fornix incision), usually includes bilateral inferior oblique weakening, which may reduce the pattern by 15 to 25 prism diopters. Effective IO weakening can be accomplished in a number of ways, including disinsertion, recession, myotomy, and myectomy.
- Bilateral superior oblique tenotomy for A-pattern with SO overaction may correct up to 40 prism diopters or more of vertical gaze incomitance; the effect tends to be greater when preoperative incomitance is greater. The tendon is transected nasal to the superior rectus muscle.
  SO tenotomy unfortunately sometimes results in excyclodeviation with vexing torsional diplopia, especially in patients with high-grade binocular fusion.
  Using a graded approach to lengthening the SO tendon, such as suturing a short length of silicone band material between the cut ends following tenotomy, reduces the risk of this complication.
  Safer still is posterior partial tenotomy or tenectomy, with preservation of the anterior one eighth to one quarter of the tendon to minimize torsional effect.
- Oblique weakening should never be performed unilaterally for A- or V-pattern. Vertical transposition of both horizontal rectus muscles in opposite directions may be combined with recess-resect surgery for A- or V-pattern esodeviation or exodeviation.

Reference

Jampolsky A. Oblique muscle surgery of the A-V patterns. *J Pediatr Ophthalmol* 1965;2:31–36.

Convergence Insufficiency

Summary

Convergence insufficiency (CI) is a common condition in which there is difficulty maintaining eye alignment as viewing approaches from distance to near.

Etiology

Unknown.

Symptoms and Signs

- Asthenopia and headache, especially after prolonged near viewing.
- Diplopia at near.
- Blurred vision complaints.

Ophthalmic Findings

- Remote near point of convergence (>5 to 10 cm).

- Low accommodative convergence/accommodation (AC/A) ratio
- Exophoria or intermittent exotropia only with near viewing.
- Low fusional convergence amplitude for near.

Treatment and Management

- Convergence exercises, preferably supervised by an orthoptist, are usually very effective in increasing convergence amplitude and relieving symptoms.
- Base-in prism may be helpful if motor function cannot be improved.

Differential Diagnosis

- Uncorrected hyperopia may cause asthenopic symptoms with near viewing similar to those of CI.
- Uncorrected mild myopia allows clear vision for near without accommodation (or accommodative convergence); may result in symptoms identical to CI.
- Small-angle comitant exodeviation may produce CI-like symptoms, especially if deviation increases with near viewing.
- Convergence paralysis (due to closed head trauma, lesion in the midbrain, toxic encephalopathy, or encephalitis), myasthenia gravis, and rarely partial third-nerve palsy may simulate CI.

Dissociated Vertical Deviation

Summary

DVD, also known as *dissociated vertical divergence*, *alternating sursumduction*, or *alternating hypertropia*, is a peculiar form of strabismus seen mainly in patients with history of infantile-onset essential esotropia, characterized by vertical (and sometimes horizontal) misalignment that appears to result from uniocular movement, in apparent violation of Hering's Law (p. 490).

Etiology

Unknown.

Symptoms and Signs

- Because suppression is nearly always present in patients with DVD, there is seldom diplopia.
- Main concern is appearance of one eye drifting up at times, to highly variable degree.

Ophthalmic Findings

- Nonfixating eye behind occluder, or during binocular viewing after fixation shift) drifts upward (typically 5 to 20 prism diopters), characteristically with a slow movement that may also include elements of abduction and excyclorotation. Reversal of occlusion or fixation causes similar (symmetric or asymmetric) movement of the other eye.
- Magnitude is often greater with occlusion of the deviating eye. Removal of occluder is followed by slow reversal of induced movement, while the fixating eye remains stationary. Small (5 to 10 prism diopters or less) hyperdeviation typically persists during binocular viewing. Stereopsis is sometimes preserved but nearly always reduced.
- Exo drift is sometimes dominant (may be up to 30 prism diopters) with little or no visible hyper. One eye may drift mainly up, the other out. When exodeviation is relatively large and symmetric, and vertical is consistently small with both right and left fixation, recognition of dissociated horizontal or exodeviation (sometimes referred to as DHD or DXD) may be problematic.
- Magnitude varies greatly over time. Often much worse with fatigue. Sometimes greater in one direction of lateral gaze or head tilt without clear physiologic basis.

Special Tests

Bielschowsky phenomenon refers to the tendency for the elevated eye in DVD to descend (sometimes into a hypotropic position) when illumination to the fixing eye is reduced (traditionally using progressively darker filters).

Treatment and Management

- If DVD is asymmetric, it may be helpful to encourage fixation with the eye whose fellow drifts less by using a lens to induce blur in other eye.
- Bilateral superior rectus muscle recession using "hang-back" technique (suture extending forward from the recessed muscle to anchor in sclera near the center of the original insertion) is the preferred procedure of most surgeons when there is no significant inferior oblique overaction.
  - Large amounts of surgery are necessary: 8 to 12 mm, either symmetrical or greater recession for the eye with larger deviation.
  - Nonabsorbable suture material (e.g., Mersilene) should be used, as the presence of superior oblique tendon between the recessed muscle and sclera may interfere with development of secure adherence to the globe.
- Anterior transposition of the inferior oblique muscles is also an effective approach for treatment of DVD in cases that also involve significant IO overaction.

Differential Diagnosis

- Distinguishing DVD from inferior oblique overaction may be a challenge, particularly because they often are seen in the same patient.
- Observation of slow upward drift when fusion is disrupted supports the diagnosis of DVD.
- IO overaction is generally not associated with hyperdeviation in primary gaze. Alternate cover test in lateral

gaze should confirm that the adducting eye is consistently higher in IO overaction.

Reference

Wilson ME. Dissociated deviations. In: Plager DA, ed. *Strabismus surgery: basic and advanced strategies*. Oxford, UK: Oxford University Press, 2004:69–82.

Double Elevator Palsy

Summary

Vertical strabismus that increases in upward gaze and shows similar magnitude in right and left gaze is termed *double elevator palsy* (DEP).

Etiology

The name and description imply weakness of both the superior rectus muscle and the inferior oblique muscle of one eye, but this is rarely the actual cause. Most cases represent isolated paresis of the superior rectus muscle (the more important elevator) or palsy of the superior division of the oculomotor nerve (in which case ptosis, which may be mild, is also present). Primary restrictive change in the inferior rectus may create a very similar appearance.

Symptoms and Signs

- Limited elevation of one eye.
- Typically chin-up head posture to maintain fusion.
- Often mild ptosis in the lower eye.

Ophthalmic Findings

- Hypotropia in primary position, increasing with upward gaze and much reduced or eliminated in downward gaze. Deviation with the hypotropic eye in abduction is equal to or greater than in adduction.
- Ptosis may appear to vanish when fixation is shifted to the hypotropic eye, giving rise to the term *pseudoptosis*. However, close observation shows that the contralateral lid has assumed a higher level, suggesting a true difference in levator palpebrae function.

Special Tests

- *Passive rotation* (forced duction testing) often reveals resistance to elevation caused by inferior rectus restriction. This may be secondary to the chronically downward deviated position of the hypotropic eye, or represent the primary cause of the deviation.
- *Saccadic velocity assessment*, either quantitative using electrooculographic technique, or a clinical approximation, can help distinguish between paretic and restrictive causes of DEP. With primary restriction, upward movement of the hypotropic eye has normal speed when refixation saccade is initiated from downgaze position, decelerating abruptly when restrictive effect is met in primary or upward gaze. In paretic cases, movement is slower in the hypotropic eye than in the fellow eye from the beginning of the saccade.

Treatment and Management

- Surgery is indicated if there is manifest hypotropia in primary gaze or a significant chin-up head posture is maintained. A variety of surgical approaches may be employed for this condition, depending on specific findings and the surgeon's preference.
  - Recession of the inferior rectus muscle may be necessary if there is significant restriction, but this is likely to create at least some degree of hypertropia in downgaze, which may be treated with posterior fixation of the contralateral inferior rectus, usually in a second surgery (p. 511).
  - Resection of the superior rectus muscle is seldom the best choice for improving elevation: Resection is in essence a tightening, not a strengthening procedure, and does not provide the desired greater effect in upward gaze.
  - Transposition of the medial and lateral rectus muscles to attach to sclera adjacent to the superior rectus insertion (Knapp procedure) is an effective and often-used approach for DEP. Effect is somewhat unpredictable, and a second procedure, most often on the contralateral eye, may be required.
  - In some cases, the best approach may be to weaken one or both elevators of the other eye (superior rectus, the primary elevator; inferior oblique, the yoke of the paretic muscle.) Resulting mild symmetric limitation of evevation almost never causes symptoms.
- Consideration of surgical correction for ptosis should be deferred until after acceptable vertical alignment of the eyes has been achieved.

Differential Diagnosis

- Thyroid orbital disease (p. 512), orbital floor fracture (p. 511), and Brown syndrome (p. 507) may cause restriction of elevation that resembles DEP. Differentiating features are discussed under each of these headings.
- *Monocular paralysis of elevation* is an acquired supranuclear disorder, usually a consequence of cerebrovascular disease ("small stroke"). Damage to the midbrain center (in the pretectum) that coordinates upward gaze innervation to the ipsilateral eye causes complete unilateral loss of elevation without hypotropia in primary or downgaze.
- Vertical strabismus following cataract or other intraocular surgery with local anesthetic injection (retrobulbar or peribulbar, particularly bupivicaine) is an increasingly recognized disorder that is considered to be a consequence of *anesthetic myotoxicity*. It may take the form

of apparent restriction, paresis, or overaction of the inferior rectus or (less commonly) superior rectus on the involved side, simulating DEP in some cases. Onset of vertical diplopia within days after cataract surgery usually makes the diagnosis straightforward. Response to surgical treatment is typically good.

- *Orbital adherence syndrome* (inferior oblique or fat adherence) is a situation that develops as a consequence of orbital fat prolapse through an opening in the posterior portion of Tenon's capsule created during surgery (usually inferior oblique weakening or retinal detachment repair). The resulting scar tissue formation may create restriction of elevation that is nearly impossible to remedy. Great care must always be taken to avoid damage to Tenon's when operating on the posterior aspect of the globe.
- *Congenital fibrosis of extraocular muscles* (CFEOM, or congenital fibrosis syndrome) is a disorder in which muscles develop as thin fibrotic bands, possibly secondary to congenitally defective innervation. Generalized involvement is usually familial, with presentation that includes bilateral ptosis and near immobilization of the eyes in downgaze with or without horizontal misalignment. The condition may be unilateral or limited to one inferior rectus muscle, in which case it simulates the appearance of DEP.
- Small (10 prism diopters or less) comitant vertical deviation is often seen in conjunction with larger horizontal comitant or essential horizontal strabismus. This may be treated by vertical transposition of one horizontal rectus muscle at the time of surgery for esotropia or exotropia. Occasionally, comitant vertical deviation appears to be the dominant expression of essential strabismus, in which case recession of one or two vertical rectus muscles or a vertical recess-resect procedure may be indicated.

Reference

Knapp P. The surgical treatment of double-elevator paralysis. *Trans Am Ophthalmol Soc* 1969;67:304–323.

Fourth Nerve Palsy

Summary

Isolated fourth (trochlear) cranial nerve palsy or superior oblique muscle paresis (SOP) is one of the more common forms of vertical strabismus, and by far the most frequent isolated cranial nerve palsy or EOM paralysis.

Etiology

- SOP of presumed congenital origin (no trauma history or evidence of underlying disorder) may not become symptomatic until late childhood or even adulthood.
- Closed head impact involving considerable force, often but not always producing loss of consciousness, is a frequent cause of acquired unilateral or bilateral SOP.
- Much less often, SOP may be the presenting sign of neurologic disease including stroke, brain tumor, or myasthenia gravis.

Symptoms and Signs

- Upward deviation or drifting of one eye, often showing cosiderable variability.
- Head tilt to the side of the lower (nonparetic) eye, often accompanied by face turn to the same side, and sometimes with a component of chin-up or down posture (Figure 8.32).
- Vertical and/or torsional diplopia.

Ophthalmic Findings

- Hypertropia, ranging from less than 5 to more than 25 prism diopters in primary gaze.
- Vertical deviation is consistently greater in lateral gaze to the side opposite the paretic eye, and with head tilt toward the paretic side (*Bielschowsky tilt effect*).
- Overaction of the inferior oblique muscle ipsilateral to paretic superior oblique muscle is seen in most cases, sometimes overshadowing the effect of the primary paresis. For this reason, deviation in downward gaze (including the field of action of the SO) is not always greater than that in upward gaze. Occasionally, preferred fixation with the paretic eye creates an appearance of contralateral SR underaction ("inhibitional palsy"); 3-step test (see below) reveals the true nature of the condition.
- Presumed congenital SOP is often associated with horizontal strabismus of mild to moderate degree (usually exotropia), and often shows considerable "intrinsic"

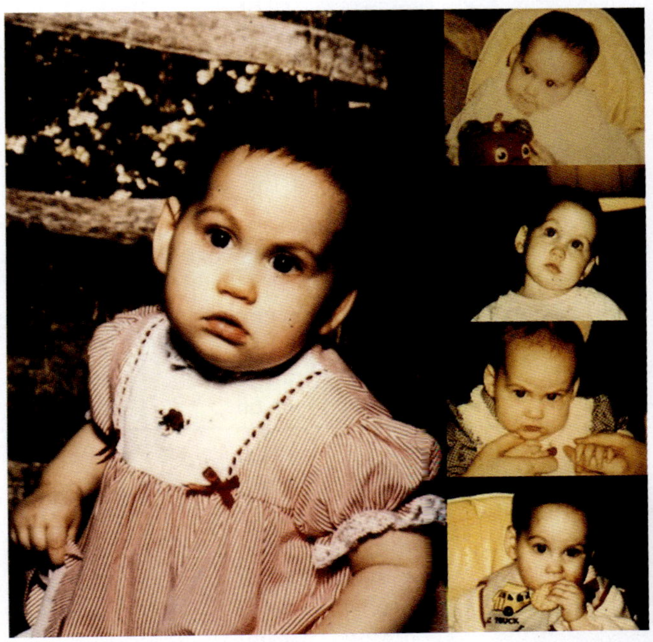

FIGURE 8.32. Family photographs document consistent left head tilt in this infant with right superior oblique paresis.

variation, that is, variability unrelated to gaze direction, completeness of binocular dissociation, or other identifiable cause.

- In nearly all cases of unilateral SOP, fusion is maintained most of the time with the aid of head posture and movement, and there is no loss of binocular capability or development of amblyopia. Especially with congenital SOP, vertical fusion amplitudes may be impressively large.
- Facial asymmetry is often seen in association with long-standing SOP (relative hypoplasia of the contralateral side of the face), believed to result from reduced blood flow through a carotid artery that is "kinked" by head tilting.
- *Bilateral superior oblique paresis*, usually posttraumatic, is characterized by
  - Absent or small hyperdeviation in primary gaze, with emergence of hypertropia of the contralateral (adducting) eye on right or left gaze, and of the ipsilateral eye on right or left tilt.
  - V-pattern with esotropia in downward gaze.
  - Excyclotropia (typically 10 degrees or more measured by double Maddox rod test) with torsional diplopia, worse in downward gaze.
  - Primarily chin down head posture is often used to maintain fusion, sometimes associated with a tilt or turn in asymmetric cases.

Special Tests

- The *3-step test*, as formulated and popularized by Parks, is a generalization of the Bielschowsky tilt test that provides a convenient and systematic way to diagnose SOP as well as isolated paralysis of any other cyclovertical muscle.
  - The number of paretic muscle possiblities is reduced from 8 to 4 by the side of hyperdeviation, from 4 to 2 by the lateral gaze direction that increases hyperdeviation (leaving a rectus of the abducting eye and an oblique of the adducting eye), and from 2 to 1 based on head tilt effect.
  - Head tilt toward the side of a paretic superior oblique stimulates the intorters of the paretic eye (SO and SR); force generated in the nonparetic SR (an elevator) is NOT balanced by the paretic SO (a depressor), so the eye goes up, increasing hyperdeviation.
  - Each muscle can be considered to have a 3-letter "signature" derived from the side of the higher eye, the lateral gaze direction with greater deviation, and the tilt direction with greater deviation (Table 8.24).
  - The SOP signatures are fortunately easy to memorize: RLR (for RSO), and LRL (for LSO). Need a mnemonic? Remember "SOusa marches"!
- Isolated paralysis of cyclovertical muscles other than SO (all of which are innervated by the third cranial nerve) is relatively uncommon.
- Use of the 3-step test for incomitant vertical strabismus that is NOT caused by an isolated muscle paresis yields a meaningless result.

Treatment and Management

- Superior oblique tendon tightening (tuck or plication, using a nonabsorbable suture such as 5-0 or 6-0 Mersilene) has unique advantages among the numerous options for surgical management of SOP.
  - Most effective procedure for cyclodeviation; may correct 20 prism diopters or more of hyperdeviation.
  - Similarly effective for hyperdeviation in upward and downward gaze.
  - Directly addresses the apparent underlying abnormality (tendon laxity or "floppiness" in many cases of congenital SOP).
  - Quantified based on operative findings (degree of tendon slack), making critical preoperative measurements unnecessary.
  - Readily reversible or modifiable with early revision of suture, or later tendon lengthening surgery.
- Postoperative IO underaction (iatrogenic Brown syndrome) is seldom a problem when SO tightening is appropriately quantified. Rarely, the tendon is found to be absent in congenital SOP, and a change in plan must be made intraoperatively.

Table 8.24

Three-step test for isolated cyclovertical muscle paresis

Higher eye	Increase in gaze	Increase on tilt	Step signature	Muscle monogram		Muscle identity	
Right	Right	Right	RRR	LIO	Left	Inferior	Oblique
		Left	RRL	RIR	Right	Inferior	Rectus
	Left	Right	RLR	RSO	Right	Superior	Oblique
		Left	RLL	LSR	Left	Superior	Rectus
Left	Right	Right	LRR	RSR	Right	Superior	Rectus
		Left	LRL	LSO	Left	Superior	Oblique
	Left	Right	LLR	LIR	Left	Inferior	Rectus
		Left	LLL	RIO	Right	Inferior	Oblique

- Ipsilateral IO weakening is appropriate for primary gaze deviation of 15 prism diopters or less associated with moderate to marked IO overaction.
- Contralateral IR recession is useful for cases with greater deviation in downward gaze, especially when incomitance is mild; may be effectively combined with IO weakening for larger and less comitant deviations.
- Ipsilateral superior rectus recession may be helpful for large-angle deviations, especially when longstanding elevation has caused tightness (contracture) to develop in this muscle.
- Bilateral SOP is generally best treated with bilateral tendon tightening: Symmetric or asymmetric plication (depending on degree of hypertropia in primary gaze), or Harada-Ito procedure (anterior transposition and advancement of the anterior portion of both tendons) for cases in which cyclodeviation is the sole indication.

Differential Diagnosis

- When the three-step test confirms a superior oblique pattern, differential diagnosis is rarely an issue.
- Isolated frontal *plagiocephaly*, a relatively common and benign form of craniosynostosis in which there is premature closure of the coronal suture on one side, may be associated with strabismus that closely mimics ipsilateral congenital SOP, attributed to posterior displacement of the trochlea.

References

Saunders RA. When and how to strengthen the superior oblique muscle. *J AAPOS* 2009;13:430–437.

Scott WE, Kraft SP. Classification and surgical treatment of superior oblique palsies. I. Unilateral superior oblique palsy. *Trans New Orleans Acad Ophthalmol* 1986;34:15–38.

Brown Syndrome

Summary

Brown syndrome is a restrictive form of strabismus in which there is limitation of elevation, particularly when the involved eye is in adduction.

Etiology

May be congenital or acquired, resulting from any abnormality of the superior oblique muscle, tendon, or trochlea that prevents extension to full length in relaxation, including contractured muscle, congenitally short tendon or tendon sheath, and presence of localized swelling in the tendon or damage to internal tendon structure or to the trochlea itself that prevents normal movement in relation to the trochlea. Orbital trauma or infection, tumor metastasis, and inflammatory disorders such as rheumatoid arthritis are among possible causes of acquired Brown syndrome.

Symptoms and Signs

- Diplopia in upward gaze.
- Chin-up head posture (sometimes with face turn) to avoid elevation or adduction of the involved eye.
- Occasionally pain in the region of the trochlea.
- A "click" or other abnormal sensation in the region of the trochlea may be felt or heard when the eye is elevated and adducted, resulting from resistance followed by yielding as abnormal tendon passes through trochlea.

Ophthalmic Findings

- Limitation of elevation, greatest in adduction, resembling IO underaction.
- Ipsilateral superior oblique shows little if any overaction.
- Hypotropia may or may not be present in primary gaze; affected eye may downshoot in adduction.
- Resistance to passive elevation in adduction (positive forced duction test) in all cases.
- V-pattern with exotropia in upgaze is a consistent finding that is very helpful in differentiating Brown syndrome from the A-pattern strabismus that is usually seen with IO paresis and inferior rectus restrictive syndromes (thyroid, floor fracture, congenital fibrosis).

Special Tests

MRI should be considered in cases of acquired Brown syndrome that lack an obvious explanation (e.g., trauma, localized infection, associated rheumatoid arthritis).

Treatment and Management

- It is not unusual to see spontaneous resolution in either congenital or acquired Brown syndrome, particularly when findings are mild. Observation is usually the best approach for cases in which there is no hypotropia in primary gaze or bothersome symptoms.
- Acquired Brown syndrome caused by inflammation (with nodular swelling in the tendon that prevents passage through the trochlea) can often be relieved by injecting a small amount of long-acting corticosteroid (e.g., triamcinolone) in the trochlear region. Repeated treatment may be necessary. Orbital imaging prior to injection is recommended.
- SO tendon lengthening is indicated for more severe cases. Insertion of a silicone-band spacer after tenotomy nasal to the superior rectus muscle is considered safer than free tenotomy by many surgeons.
- Care must be taken to ensure complete transection of the tendon, or the problem will persist. A maneuver popularized by Guyton is helpful in confirming that this has been accomplished.
  After cutting the tendon, the eye is grasped at the limbus with two forceps, then excyclorotated 45 to 90 degrees,

displaced posteriorly, and rotated into elevation and adduction, all of which contribute to maximal elongation of the SO muscle-tendon complex.

Gently rocking the globe with alternate pressure on the two forceps creates a sense of rolling over a taut cable (or a "speed bump") when there are intact tendon fibers. If the tendon has been fully severed, the sensation is of rolling on a flat surface.

- Up to 50% of eyes after successful tenotomy for Brown syndrome will develop signs of superior oblique paresis, which may need to be treated with ipsilateral inferior oblique weakening. Some surgeons prophylactically weaken the IO at the time of SO surgery.

Differential Diagnosis

- The presence of implanted orbital hardware following retinal detachment repair or glaucoma shunt surgery may limit elevation similar to Brown syndrome, but the cause is usually obvious.
- Other causes of hypotropia in upward gaze are reviewed under the heading of double elevator palsy (p. 504).

Reference

Wilson ME, Eustis HS Jr, Parks MM. Brown's syndrome. *Surv Ophthalmol* 1989;34:153–172.

Duane Syndrome

Summary

Duane syndrome is a common disorder of horizontal eye movement that results from innervational abnormality of the lateral rectus muscle.

Demographics

- Usually sporadic, but occasionally familial (autosomal dominant).
- Bilateral in 10% to 20% of cases.
- Most patients are female, and most show left eye involvement.

Etiology

Congenital aplasia of the abducens nucleus is associated with innervation of the lateral rectus muscle by an anomalous branch of the oculomotor nerve. Lateral rectus tone in primary gaze may be normal or reduced (Type 1), or increased (Type 2). Effort to abduct generates less than normal force in the lateral rectus, while adduction fails to inhibit the muscle normally, resulting in "co-contraction" of the lateral and the medial rectus (in violation of Sherrington's Law, p. 490). An uncommon variant (Type 3) is associated with abnormal innervation of both medial and lateral rectus muscles and severe limitation of both abduction and adduction.

Symptoms and Signs

- Face turn to maintain fusion and avoid diplopia; use of head movement to follow horizontally moving objects.
- Lid fissure narrowing (Figure 8.33), "upshoot" or "downshoot" of the Duane eye with gaze to the opposite side.
- In infants, the most obvious abnormality is often large-angle esodeviation with gaze toward the abnormal side, the result of normal adduction of the opposite eye while the Duane eye fails to abduct. Families usually perceive this as a problem with the normal eye.

Ophthalmic Findings

- Primary gaze esodeviation with Type 1, usually small angle (20 prism diopters or less), may be ortho; variable exotropia with Type 2.
- Both abduction and adduction are reduced to some degree in all cases.

  ABduction reduced secondary to lateral rectus underaction, striking in Type 1, mild in Type 2. Esodeviation is always present in far ipsilateral gaze, large angle in Type 1, small in Type 2. Occasionally, abduction is better in downgaze or upgaze, resulting in A- or V-pattern.

  ADduction reduced secondary to resistance from the co-contracting lateral rectus, subtle in Type 1, obvious in Type 2. Exodeviation is usually detectable in far contralateral gaze, minimal in Type 1, moderate to marked in Type 2.
- Despite the often-used designation *retraction syndrome*, posterior displacement of the globe on adduction, a consequence of co-contraction, is usually inconspicuous and often clinically undetectable, especially in infants and young children.
- The appearance of IO or SO overaction or both (generated by vertical force from the co-contracting horizontal muscles with adduction above and below the horizontal, respectively—also called *leash effect*) may be very striking or completely absent.
- Nearly all patients with unilateral Duane syndrome are orthophoric and fuse with normal stereoacuity at some point in the horizontal gaze range (and for a slight distance to either side); most actively maintain this viewing direction with head posture and movement. Strabismic deviation is therefore intermittent, and binocular capability is preserved. Diplopia may or may not occur when fusion is lost in other gaze positions (depending on whether suppression has developed.) Amblyopia is rarely seen unless other cause (e.g., anisometropia) is also present.
- Patients with *bilateral* Duane syndrome usually lack an orthophoric direction and fusion range. Constant strabismus leads to permanent complete loss of binocularity, with potential for amblyopia (if fixation does not alternate).

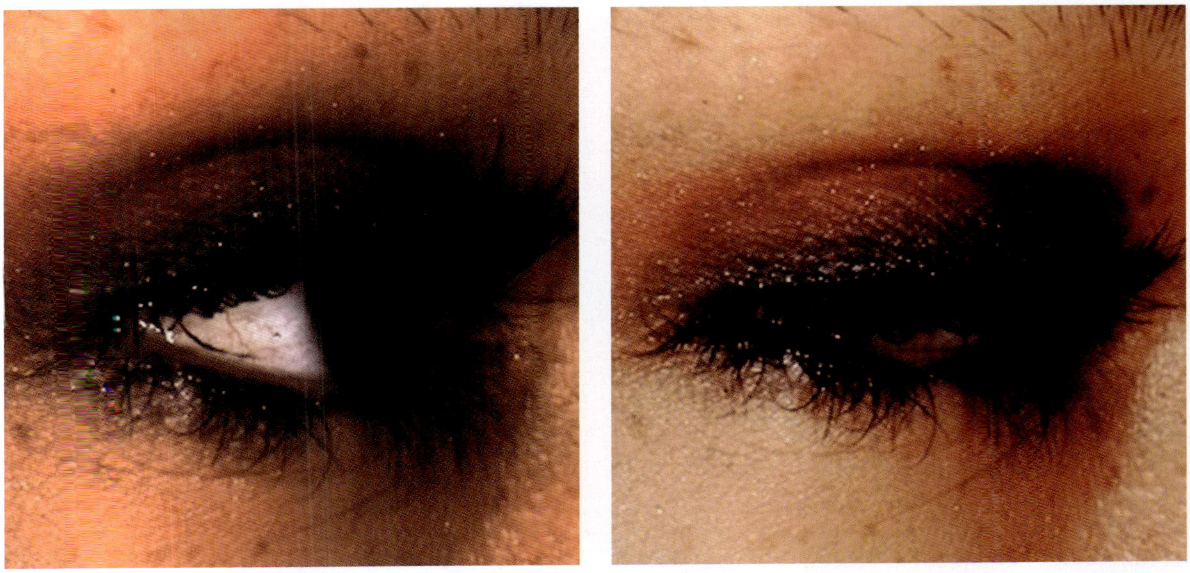

A B

FIGURE 8.33. Duane syndrome. **A:** Primary gaze. **B:** Left gaze, showing retraction of right globe and lid fissure narrowing with adduction.

Systemic Findings

- Duane syndrome is usually an isolated abnormality, but associated ocular and systemic findings are common (up to 30% to 50% of cases), most notably sensorineural hearing loss (10% to 20%).
- Goldenhar syndrome (p. 427) and Wildervanck syndrome (includes Klippel-Feil skull malformation) frequently incorporate Duane syndrome.
- Duane syndrome is an element of thalidomide embryopathy (most prominently characterized by severe developmental abnormalities of the extremities), seen in a cohort of Europeans exposed *in utero* to this potently teratogenic drug in the early 1960s.

Treatment and Management

- Normal ocular motility cannot be achieved in patients with Duane syndrome. Surgery is justified by a need to relieve one or more specific bothersome symptoms.
  For face turn, recession of the ipsilateral medial rectus (Type 1) or lateral rectus (Type 2) is effective, but may significantly reduce already subnormal rotation in the field of action of the operated muscle, and further narrow fusional range.
  For retraction and leash effect, combined recession of both the lateral and the medial rectus may be helpful. Other approaches for leash include Y-splitting or posterior fixation (p. 511) of the lateral rectus, and oblique weakening procedures.
- Surgery on the horizontal rectus muscles of the normal eye that reduces its rotation (recession, posterior fixation—p. 511) to more closely match the Duane eye may help by increasing the width of the fusional range but is seldom done.
- Resection of the lateral rectus muscle is likely to have unexpected and undesired consequences and is generally to be avoided in Duane syndrome.
- Transposition of superior and inferior rectus attachments to sclera near the lateral rectus insertion is very effective in reducing esodeviation and ipsilateral face-turn. This approach may be superior to MR recession in terms of preserving fusional range and improving abduction.

Differential Diagnosis

- Obviously reduced abduction (Type 1) and adduction (Type 2) often lead to confusion with lateral or medial rectus paresis. Mild limitation in the opposite direction distinguishes Duane syndrome, as does disproportion between primary gaze esodeviation (usually small) and abduction deficit (usually large).
- Medial orbital wall fracture with MR entrapment may closely resemble Duane syndrome.

References

Greenwald MJ. Paretic strabismus. In: Cibis GW, Tongue AC, Stass-Isern ML, eds. *Decision making in pediatric ophthalmology*. St. Louis, MO: Decker (Mosby-Year Book), 1993:230–233.

Rosenbaum AL. The efficacy of rectus muscle transposition surgery in esotropic Duane syndrome and VI nerve palsy. *J AAPOS* 2004;8:409–419.

Third Nerve Palsy

Summary

Complete third (oculomotor) cranial nerve palsy eliminates function in the medial rectus, inferior rectus, inferior oblique, superior rectus, levator palpebrae, pupilloconstrictor, and ciliary muscles. Partial third nerve palsy may have effects limited to a subset of these muscles, or cause incomplete loss of function, or both. This condition is more extensively considered in Chapter 6.

Ophthalmic Findings

- With complete palsy, the eye is nearly immobile, "down and out"—exotropic and hypotropic, but exodeviation is dominant. Incyclorotation from contraction of the superior oblique unaccompanied by inferior rectus may be noted on attempted downgaze.
- In partial palsy, exodeviation increasing in adduction is typical, with hypo- or hypertropia in primary gaze depending on distribution of residual function in vertical muscles. Limitation of both elevation and depression is usually evident, with hypotropia in upgaze, hypertropia in downgaze regardless of primary position deviation.
- Ptosis ranges from complete to absent. Especially when palsy is congenital or shows "aberrant regeneration," lid droop may be mild but excursion (levator function) reduced or paradoxical.
- Pupil may be fixed in dilation, or small but poorly reactive (not unusual with congenital palsy).

Treatment and Management

- Monocular occlusion of paretic eye in adults to prevent diplopia, nonparetic eye in children to prevent amblyopia. Hyperopic child may need full plus correction with bifocal if ciliary muscle is involved.
- For complete palsy with closed lid, no treatment may be the best option: Risk of corneal exposure damage, likelihood of intractable diplopia or unacceptably narrow fusion range, undesirable appearance with best possible motility outcome.
- If lid open and poor function in all third nerve EOMs, immobile globe in primary position is the surgical goal, often requiring more than one operation. Inactivate LR with supermaximal recession or extirpation, or by suturing muscle to lateral orbital wall. Very large medial rectus resection is helpful despite lack of contractile function. Tenotomy of SO for hypotropia, with reattachment to sclera just above MR insertion if additional correction is needed for exotropia.
- Strategies for partial third nerve palsy are complex. If rotation into the paretic fields of gaze is reasonably preserved (20 degrees or more), good results can often be obtained by weakening the yoke muscles on the other eye, usually in combination with recess/resect surgery for exotropia on the paretic eye.

Differential Diagnosis

See discussion under comitant exotropia (p. 501), double elevator palsy (p. 504), Duane syndrome (p. 509), and myasthenia gravis (p. 512).

Sixth Nerve Palsy

Summary

Palsy of the sixth (abducens) cranial nerve causes isolated paralysis or paresis of the lateral rectus muscle and esotropia. Even in childhood, the condition is usually acquired. Clinical features of sixth nerve palsy in adulthood are further considered in Chapter 6.

Ophthalmic Findings

- Unilateral sixth nerve palsy, complete or partial, produces obviously incomitant esotropia that increases steadily from near ortho in contralateral gaze to a maximum in ipsilateral gaze. Binocular fusion is usually preserved and maintained with the aid of face turn toward the paretic side.
- Bilateral sixth nerve palsy may show little or no evidence of horizontal gaze incomitance. Deviation for distance is typically greater than for near viewing, a finding seldom noted in esotropia that is nonparalytic and nonrestrictive.

Systemic Findings

- Unilateral sixth nerve palsy in childhood is most often a benign postviral occurrence with acute onset, followed by resolution over a period of weeks to months. Sometimes, strabismus evolves into a persistent comitant deviation.
- The apparently healthy child with recent onset of unilateral sixth nerve palsy should undergo careful motility evaluation for evidence of other cranial nerve dysfunction (especially mild underaction of the opposite lateral rectus), fundus examination to look for papilledema, and assessment for cerebellar signs such as ataxia. In the absence of any such findings, especially if there is a history of recent viral illness, observation at 1- to 2-week intervals without further diagnostic studies is acceptable management.
- Neuroimaging is indicated if any of the above-mentioned findings are present, or if there is progressive loss of function or lack of any improvement after 4 weeks; may be justified in other cases depending on circumstances. Imaging is not generally required after recent onset of comitant esotropia without other findings, unless deviation is greater for distance than near.

Treatment and Management

- Partial sixth nerve palsy with relatively good preservation of abduction can be treated effectively by recession of the contralateral medial rectus (yoke of the paretic muscle) and resection of the contralateral lateral rectus. These procedures combine to provide greater effect in the paretic gaze direction, where it is needed; similar surgery performed on the paretic eye has its greatest effect in the gaze direction of least deviation. The dosage of surgery with this approach must be based on the *secondary deviation* (measured with the paretic eye centered in primary gaze, prism before the sound eye).

- Complete lateral rectus paralysis requires surgery on the paretic eye. Very large recession of the antagonist medial rectus combined with very large resection of the paralyzed lateral rectus may center the eye, but leaves it with little horizontal movement. Partial transposition procedures involving the SR and IR (Jensen, Hummelsheim operations) have little if any advantage over LR resection.
- Most surgeons now treat complete sixth nerve palsy with full-tendon transposition of the superior and inferior rectus muscles.
  - Scleral reattachments adjoin the lateral rectus insertion, oriented roughly parallel to the limbus with SR slightly more posterior than IR (as are original insertions).
  - Usually augmented by anchoring a nonabsorbable suture near the temporal edge of each transposed muscle, 6 to 8 mm posterior to the insertion, and securing it to the adjacent lateral rectus, or to sclera alongside the edge of the LR (Foster modification).
  - This procedure is often supplemented by moderate weakening of the ipsilateral medial rectus.
- Surgery on three rectus muscles, particularly in older adults, may result in *anterior segment ischemia* (with postoperative iritis and corneal decompensation) due to loss of most anterior ciliary blood supply. Risk can be reduced by using vessel-sparing technique, performing MR surgery after an interval of weeks or months, substituting botulinum toxin injection for surgical recession of the MR, or using fornix conjunctival incisions.

Differential Diagnosis

See discussion under essential esotropia (p. 498), Duane syndrome (p. [illegible]).

Orbital "Blow-Out" Fracture

Summary

Orbital wall fractures often have significant effect on ocular motility, in addition to other consequences detailed in Chapter 7.

Etiology

- Compression of orbital bone and soft tissues by impact from an object of appropriate size and shape causes fracture with prolapse of orbital contents due to increased pressure gradient between the orbit and adjacent sinus cavity, probably also requiring significant deflection of bone from the primary impact. Inferior wall (orbital floor) is the most common site, followed by medial wall. In young children, orbital roof fracture is a frequent consequence of brow or forehead impact, but EOM function is seldom disturbed.
- EOM action may be affected by mechanical entrapment of muscle, direct trauma to the muscle or its nerve supply, hematoma or edema of surrounding tissues (early and transient), or scarring of orbital fat and connective tissue (late and lasting).

Ophthalmic Findings

- Primary gaze deviation after floor fracture is usually hypotropia, sometimes hypertropia or no deviation; typically, esotropia is seen with medial wall fracture.
- Paretic as well as restrictive components are often present, limiting both elevation and depression (or abduction and adduction with medial wall); forced duction and saccadic velocity testing help differentiate.

Systemic Findings

Muscle entrapment may cause bradycardia via oculocardiac reflex, particularly with small "trapdoor" floor fractures in childhood.

Treatment and Management

- Early orbital surgery is indicated if imaging (noncontrast CT with thin cuts through orbit) confirms entrapment of muscle (especially when vagal effects present) or significant prolapse of orbital contents likely to cause enophthalmos.
- Consider EOM surgery for motility defects persisting beyond 2 weeks after injury or primary repair of fracture.
- Cautious recession of restricting muscle (to avoid excessive limitation in field of action); transposition of adjacent recti for paretic muscle in appropriate cases.
- Surgery on the other eye to create matching limitation is often the most appropriate strategy when there is significant reduction of rotation in the involved eye, especially when primary gaze deviation is small. Possible approaches include recession or posterior fixation of one or both vertical recti (inferior wall) or horizontal recti (medial wall).
- *Posterior fixation* (also known as fadenoperation, retroequatorial myopexy) involves placing nonabsorbable suture(s) to create attachment between muscle and sclera posterior to the equator (10 to 15 mm behind the normal insertion). This limits rotation in the field of action of the muscle to approximate that of the underacting yoke muscle without altering primary gaze alignment. May be combined with moderate recession when there is a small primary gaze deviation associated with large deviation in the field of action.

References

Buckley EG, Meekins BB. Fadenoperation for the management of complicated incomitant vertical strabismus. *Am J Ophthalmol* 1988;150:304–312.

Greenwald MJ, Boston D, Pensler JM, et al. Orbital roof fractures in childhood. *Ophthalmology* 1989;96:491–496.

Thyroid Eye Disease

Summary

Orbital myopathy associated with Graves disease is the most common cause of acquired strabismus with diplopia in adults. This topic is considered at length in Chapter 7.

Ophthalmic Findings

- Inferior rectus muscle most often involved, followed by medial rectus, superior rectus, and then lateral rectus.
- Restrictive change is typical, with increasing deviation and diplopia in gaze direction opposite the involved muscle's field of action, and positive forced duction test. Inferior rectus restriction may cause increased IOP in primary and upward gaze.
- A-pattern is common, in consequence of adduction generated by tight inferior rectus on upward gaze; may worsen after IR recession with tendency toward abduction in downgaze (superior obliques become more important as depressors).
- The presence of exotropia, or any evidence of muscle paresis, raises concern about myasthenia gravis (see below), which is found concurrent with Graves disease in many patients. Occasionally, however, paresis is a direct consequence of Graves myopathy.

Treatment and Management

- In the acute stage of thyroid eye disease, systemic corticosteroid treatment can lead to improvement of ocular motility. Botulinum toxin injection into restricting muscles may be helpful. Prism lenses are sometimes useful. Strabismus surgery should be deferred until the patient is euthyroid, treatment for optic neuropathy (including surgical decompression) is completed, and alignment has been stable by history for 4 to 6 months, with confirmation over at least 2 months of reliable observation.
- Hypotropia is usually treated with inferior rectus muscle recession, unilateral or asymmetric bilateral depending on degree to which elevation is limited. Late overcorrections are common, leading many surgeons to use adjustable suture technique and leave the operated eye slightly hypotropic. IR recession should always include complete severance of attachments to the lower eyelid (relatively stiff fascial projections going back 15 mm or more from the insertion) to minimize postoperative downward lid displacement (likely to occur by about 1 mm even with optimal technique)
- Medial rectus recession for esotopia is usually effective; lateral rectus resection occasionally indicated as a second procedure, in the absence of severe restriction.

Myasthenia Gravis

Summary

Myasthenia gravis (MG) is a complex autoimmune neuromuscular disease with highly variable expression that may be limited to the extraocular muscles (ocular myasthenia), producing ptosis and/or strabismus. Pathophysiology, diagnostic considerations, systemic findings, and nonsurgical management are discussed fully in Chapter 6.

Ophthalmic Findings

- Highly variable, often intermittent ptosis is the hallmark of MG, but is not always present, and may be overlooked when symmetrical and of mild to moderate degree. Observation of transient lid elevation after downgaze (Cogan sign) is helpful.
- Strabismus also typically shows considerable variability, but generally less than MG ptosis, and often no more than is commonly seen with idiopathic comitant strabismus, especially exotropia, which MG may closely resemble.
- Incomitancy not always present, but may be striking. Can mimic any paretic deviation, most typically pupil-sparing third nerve or double elevator palsy with ptosis; Duane syndrome if lateral and medial recti involved. Should be suspected in any situation with apparent weakness of EOMs (and normal pupils) not comprising a neuroanatomically meaningful constellation.
- Ocular rotation may be quite limited in multiple directions (diagnostically helpful if antagonist of suspected paretic muscle is also involved), or near normal.

Special Tests

- Clinical tests (pharmacologic, cooling with ice) often show much greater response from ptosis than from strabismus.
- Laboratory tests (acetylcholine receptor antibodies, electromyography) are often negative because of the small mass and unique qualities of extraocular muscle.
- The diagnosis of MG may simply not be confirmable when confined to the EOMs.

Treatment and Management

- Cholinergic drugs such as Mestinon are frequently ineffective for strabismus and may have significant side effects, but a trial is usually indicated when there is sufficient suspicion of MG.
- Surgery is an option that should definitely be considered for strabismus when findings are stable and bothersome. Resection may be preferable to recession when there is significant limitation of rotation.

Differential Diagnosis

In addition to the various strabismus entities mentioned above, MG may resemble chronic progressive external ophthalmoplegia (CPEO), a mitochondrial myopathy often associated with pigmentary retinopathy and potentially fatal cardiac conduction defects (Table 8.2).

Reference

Ellenhorn N, Lucchese N, Greenwald M. Juvenile myasthenia gravis and amblyopia. *Am J Ophthalmol* 1986;101:214–217.

Appendix A

Ophthalmic Drugs and Medications

Table A.1

Select medications used in ophthalmology

Class	Drug	Route	Mechanism of action	Side effects
Antiglaucoma				
Beta-blockers	Betaxolol	Drop	Decreased aqueous production	Exacerbation of asthma, bradycardia, fatigue, impotence, blunting of hypoglycemia in diabetics
	Carteolol	Drop		
	Levobunolol	Drop		
	Metipranolol	Drop		
	Timolol	Drop		
Alpha-adrenergic agonists	Apraclonidine	Drop	Decreased aqueous production	Allergy
	Brimonidine	Drop		Tachyphylaxis
Carbonic anhydrase inhibitors	Acetazolamide	Oral	Decreased aqueous production	Tingling in fingers and toes dysgeusia, fatigue, GI tract upset, urination
	Methazolamide	Oral		Similar to acetazolamide, but better tolerated
	Dichlorphenamide	Oral		Similar to acetazolamide
	Brinzolamide	Drop		
	Dorzolamide	Drop		Metallic taste
Osmotics	Glycerin	Oral	Dehydration of vitreous	Exacerbation of congestive heart failure, fluid shifts
	Isosorbide	Oral		
	Mannitol	i.v.		
	Urea	i.v.		
Prostaglandin analogues	Latanoprost	Drop	Increased uveoscleral outflow	Darkening of iris color Exacerbation of uveitis
Sympathomimetics	Epinephrine	Drop	Increased aqueous outflow	Adrenochrome deposits, allergy
	Dipivefrin	Drop		Allergy
Direct-acting cholinergic agents	Carbachol	Drop	Increased trabecular outflow	Brow ache, retinal detachment, cataract formation
	Pilocarpine	Drop, gel		
Indirect-acting cholinergic agents	Demecarium	Drop	Increased trabecular outflow	Brow ache, retinal detachment, cataract formation
	Echothiophate	Drop		
	Isoflurophate	Ointment		
	Physostigmine	Ointment		

(Continued)

Table A.1

Select medications used in ophthalmology (*Continued*)

Class	Drug	Route	Mechanism of action	Side effects
Antibiotics				
Sulfonamides	Sulfacetamide	Drop, ointment	Interferes with bacterial synthesis of folic acid	Allergy
	Sulfisoxazole	Drop		
Fluoroquinolone	Ciprofloxacin	Drop	Interference with bacterial DNA gyrase	Precipitation of drug on epithelial surface
	Norfloxacin	Drop		
	Ofloxacin	Drop		
	Moxifloxacin	Drop		
	Gatifloxacin	Drop		
Aminoglycoside	Amikacin	Intravitreal	Blocks protein synthesis	Epithelial toxicity
	Gentamicin	Drop, ointment		
	Tobramycin	Drop, ointment		Epithelial toxicity
Cell wall active	Vancomycin	Drop, intravitreal	Disruption of the cell wall	
Macrolide	Erythromycin	Ointment	Blocks protein synthesis	
	Azithromycin	Oral		
Tetracyclines	Tetracycline	Ointment, oral	Inhibits protein synthesis	
	Doxycycline	Oral		
	Minocycline	Oral		
Miscellaneous	Chloramphenicol	Drop	Inhibits protein synthesis	Aplastic anemia
	Bacitracin	Ointment	Inhibits cell wall synthesis	
	Clindamycin	Intravitreal	Suppresses protein synthesis	
	Polymyxin B	Drop, ointment	Disruption of the cell wall	
Antifungals				
Polyene	Amphotericin B	Drop, intravitreal, i.v.	Disrupts fungal cell wall	Renal toxicity with i.v. dosing
Pyrimidine	Flucytosine	Oral	Inhibits RNA synthesis	
Imidazole	Ketoconazole	Oral	Inhibits synthesis of ergosterol	
	Miconazole	Oral		
	Clotrimazole	Oral		
Triazole	Fluconazole	Oral	Inhibits fungal cytochrome P450	
	Voriconazole	Oral, topical	Inhibits fungal cytochrome P450 blocking synthesis of erosterol	GI distress, visual disturbance
	Posaconazole	Oral	Blocks synthesis of erosterol	

Table A.

Select medications used in ophthalmology (*Continued*)

Class	Drug	Route	Mechanism of action	Side effects
Antivirals				
Nucleoside analogue	Trifluridine	Drop	Interferes with viral DNA synthesis	
	Idoxuridine	Drop		
	Vidarabine	Ointment		
	Acyclovir	Oral		
	Valacyclovir	Oral		
	Valgancyclovir	Oral		
	Foscarnet	Intravitreal, i.v.		
	Ganciclovir	Intravitreal, i.v.		
Anti-inflammatory				
Corticosteroids (topical)	Dexamethasone	Drop	Suppression of immune system	Cataract formation
	Fluorometholone	Drop		Steroid-induced glaucoma
	Loteprednol	Drop		
	Medrysone	Drop		
	Prednisolone acetate	Drop		
	Prednisolone phosphate	Drop		
	Rimexolone	Drop		
Corticosteroids (injectable)	Dexamethasone		Suppression of immune system	Shortest duration
	Betamethasone			
	Triamcinolone			Depost steroid
Nonsteroidal anti-inflammatory medication	Ketorolac	Drop	Interruption of prostaglandin synthesis	
	Diclofenac	Drop		
	Flurbiprofen	Drop		
	Suprofen	Drop		
Mast cell stabilizers	Cromolyn sodium	Drop	Stabilizes mast cell membranes	
	Lodoxamine	Drop		
Antihistamine	Levocabastine	Drop	H_1-Specific antagonist	
	Olopatadine	Drop		
	Emedastine	Drop		
	Epinastine	Drop		
	Bepotastine	Drop		
	Ketotifen	Drop		
	Naphazoline	Drop		
Mydratics and cycloplegics				
Alpha-adrenergic agonist	Phenylephrine	Drop		Hypertension with 10% solution
Parasympatholytics	Atropine	Drop		Anticholinergic toxicity
	Scopolamine	Drop		
	Homatropine	Drop		
	Cyclopentolate	Drop		
	Tropicamide	Drop		
Alpha-adrenergic blocker	Dapiprazole	Drop	Reverses dilation of pupil	

(*Continued*)

Table A.1

Select medications used in ophthalmology (*Continued*)

Class	Drug	Route	Mechanism of action	Side effects
Anesthetics				
	Proparacaine	Drop		Epithelial toxicity
	Tetracaine	Drop		
	Cocaine	Drop		Most epithelial toxic
Miscellaneous				
Hypertonic agents	Glucose 40%	Drop		
	Hypertonic saline 5%	Drop	Dehydrates corneal epithelium and stroma	
	Glycerin	Drop		
Mucolytic	Acetylcysteine	Drop	Dissolves mucus	

Note: There are many new drugs in the pipeline. Their use in the armamentarium of ophthalmology has not yet been established.
GI, gastrointestinal; CHF, congestive heart failure.

Appendix B

Microorganisms Infecting the Eye

Table B.1

Common microorganisms and their characteristics

Organism	Staining characteristics	Risk factors for infection	Ocular diseases
Gram-positive organisms			
Staphylococcus aureus	Gram-positive cocci in clusters		Blepharitis, keratitis, endophthalmitis, conjunctivitis, cellulitis, dacryocystitis
Staphylococcus epidermidis	Gram-positive cocci in clusters		Blepharitis, keratitis, endophthalmitis
Streptococcus viridans and nutritionally variant streptococci	Gram-positive cocci in pairs, short chains, or single cocci		Keratitis, endophthalmitis, infectious crystalline keratopathy
Streptococcus pneumoniae	Gram-positive, lancet-shaped cocci in pairs, encapsulated		Keratitis, conjunctivitis, endophthalmitis, scleritis, dacryocystitis, bleb infections
Streptococcus pyogenes (beta-hemolytic group A *Streptococcus*)	Gram-positive cocci in pairs, short chains, or single cocci		Cellulitis, dacryoadenitis, conjunctivitis, keratitis
Bacillus spp	Gram-positive rods, straight sided with rounded or square ends, single or in chains	Trauma, especially with organic matter	Endophthalmitis
Propionibacterium acnes	Gram-positive pleomorphic rods, anaerobic	Intraocular surgery	Endophthalmitis
Corynebacterium spp., excluding *C. diphtheriae*	Gram-positive pleomorphic rods, aerobic	Compromised corneas	Keratitis
Enterococcus spp.	Gram-positive cocci, single or in pairs		Endophthalmitis, keratitis
Actinomyces spp.	Gram-positive filamentous rods, anaerobic		Canaliculitis
Norcardia spp.	Gram-positive filamentous, rods, aerobic, partially acid-fast		Keratitis, scleritis

(*Continued*)

Table B.1

Common microorganisms and their characteristics (*Continued*)

Organism	Staining characteristics	Risk factors for infection	Ocular diseases
Mycobacterium fortuitum and *Myobacterium chelonei*	Acid-fast, slightly curved or straight rods	Trauma, especially with contaminated water	Keratitis
Gram-negative organisms			
Pseudomonas aeruginosa	Gram-negative slender rods	Contact lens wear	Keratitis, endophthalmitis
Enteric Gram-negative rods (*Serratia marcescens, Escherichia coli, Klebsiella pneumoniae, Proteus mirabilis, Enterobacter aerogenes, Citrobacter* spp., etc.)	Gram-negative straight rods, single and in pairs	Debilitated patients	Keratitis, endophthalmitis
Moraxella catarrhalis	Gram-negative cocci, single or in pairs		Conjunctivitis, keratitis
Moraxella lacunata and *Moraxella nonliquefaciens*	Gram-negative rod, short, plump, in pairs (diplobacilli)		Keratitis, angular blepharitis
Haemophilus influenzae	Gram-negative rod, tiny, coccobacillary Grow on chocolate agar	Thin avascular blebs, children	Keratitis, conjunctivitis, endophthalmitis, bleb infection, dacryocystitis, cellulitis
Neisseria gonorrhoeae	Gram-negative cocci, in pairs with adjacent sides flattened Grow on chocolate agar		Conjunctivitis, keratitis
Capnocytophaga spp.	Gram-negative fusiform rods		Keratitis
Fungi			
Yeasts: *Candida albicans*	Gram-positive, oval-to-round budding cells	Compromised corneas, immunosuppression	Keratitis, endophthalmitis
Molds: *Fusarium* spp., *Curvularia* spp., *Acremonium* spp., *Aspergillus* spp., *Alternaria* spp.	Filamentous hyphae seen with special fungal stains	Trauma, especially with organic matter, compromised corneas	Keratitis, endophthalmitis
Other organisms			
Acanthamoeba	Double-walled cysts seen with Giemsa and Gram stains	Contact lens wear, homemade saline, exposure to contaminated water	Keratitis, scleritis
Microsporidia	Round-to-oval intracellular spores seen with Giemsa and Gram stains	Patients with AIDS	Keratoconjunctivitis

AIDS, acquired immunodeficiency syndrome.

Index

Note: Page numbers in *italics* denote figures; those followed by a t denote tables.

R